SURGERY OF THE UPPER RESPIRATORY SYSTEM

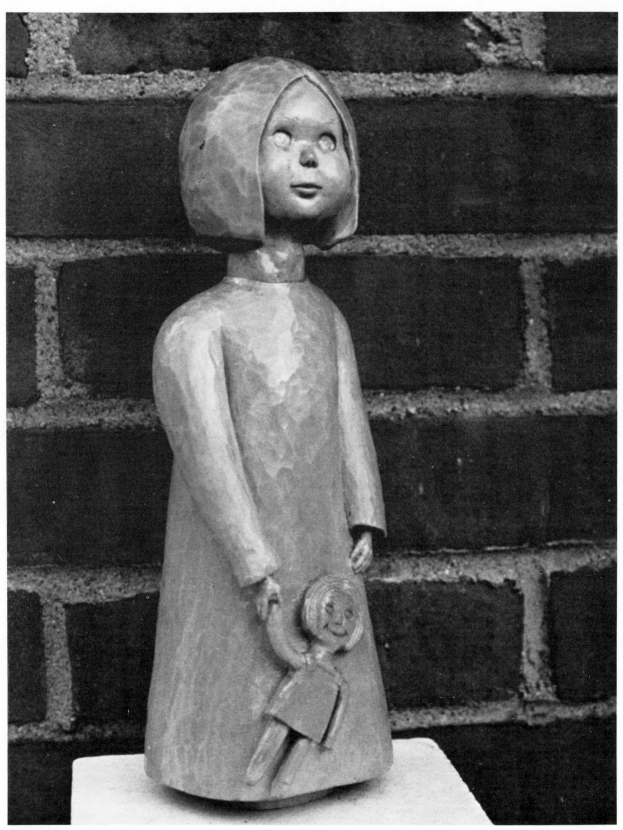

This edition, like the first, is dedicated to Natasha—the subject of my woodcarving. The original was carved from Vermont basswood and was later cast in bronze.

Surgery
of the Upper Respiratory
System

WILLIAM W. MONTGOMERY, M.D.

Professor of Otolaryngology,
Harvard Medical School, Boston, Massachusetts
(Senior) Surgeon, Massachusetts Eye and Ear Infirmary,
Boston, Massachusetts
Consultant in Otolaryngology, Children's Hospital
Medical Center, Boston, Massachusetts

Volume One · Second Edition

LEA & FEBIGER · 1979 · PHILADELPHIA

Library of Congress Cataloging in Publication Data

Montgomery, William W   1928–
    Surgery of the upper respiratory system.

    Includes index.
    1. Otolaryngology, Operative.   I. Title.
[DNLM: 1. Head—Surgery.   2. Respiratory system—
Surgery.   WV168 M788s]
RF51.M56 1978   617'.523   78-9004
ISBN 0-8121-0640-7

Published in Great Britain by Henry Kimpton, London

PRINTED IN THE UNITED STATES OF AMERICA

Print Number   3   2   1

TO NATASHA

Preface

This atlas of otolaryngologic surgery has been compiled for both the physician in training and the practicing specialist.

In this second edition, various techniques of surgery have been expanded to include recent developments.

In Chapter 3, surgery of the ethmoid and sphenoid sinuses, the discussion emphasizes the detailed technique for performing an external ethmoidectomy. Emphasis is also placed on mucocele of the ethmoid sinuses, transethmoido-sphenoidal approach to cystic lesions of the petrous apex, and decompression of the optic nerve.

Chapter 4, surgery for frontal sinus disease, pays special attention to advances in our technique for performing the osteoplastic frontal sinus obliteration. This chapter also includes a statistical analysis of more than 20 years' experience with 250 operations.

In Chapter 5, surgery of dural defects of the paranasal sinuses, cribriform region, and temporal bone is considerably expanded to reflect an additional 6 years' experience. As a result of this recent experience, our techniques for diagnosis of cerebral spinal fluid otorrhea and rhinorrhea have become more definitive.

Chapter 6 reports on changes in our surgical approach to malignant tumors of the maxillary sinus. In this discussion, particular emphasis has been placed on the partial maxillectomy with postoperative radiation therapy. Vidian nerve neurectomy for vasomotor rhinitis has been updated.

Chapter 7 includes a complete revision of the diagnosis and therapy of facial fractures.

In Chapter 11, the translabyrinthine resection for acoustic neurinoma has been rewritten in much more detail with new illustrations.

The past decades have seen otolaryngology expand to the point where many otolaryngologists have limited their surgery to one aspect of the specialty, such as otology, head and neck surgery, plastic procedures, or surgery of the paranasal sinuses. This trend, however, is only practicable in large medical centers that can be staffed by many specialists.

The modern otolaryngologist must be an accomplished surgeon, for a single operation can require the versatility and dexterity needed for handling soft tissues and bones, as well as various macro- and microsurgical procedures. The otolaryngologist must also be proficient in the diagnostic procedures associated with head and neck surgery and possess acumen in the interpretation of the results. He must have thorough knowledge of the anatomy and physiology of the upper respiratory system to enable him to deal effectively with diseases of the nose, paranasal sinuses, nasopharynx, oropharynx, laryngopharynx, cervical esophagus, and neck.

In this volume, it has been my aim to provide the student and the practicing otolaryngologist with guidelines for the diagnosis and treatment of the various conditions requiring otolaryngologic surgery. To this end, the volume contains descriptions and illustrations pertaining to examination, diagnosis, and treatment of paranasal sinus disease, cerebrospinal fistula, facial fractures, and nasal and nasopharyngeal disorders. Because otologic operations have been dealt with extensively in a number of recently published textbooks, discussions on surgery of the ear have been limited to reconstructive surgery of the auricle, operations for acoustic neurinoma, in which I am particularly interested, and carcinoma of the ear. Although I have endeavored to present the latest techniques, with the rapid advancement in the field of otolaryngologic surgery, new diagnostic procedures and methods of treatment may evolve while this book is in press. Comments by the reader concerning these new techniques as well as any criticisms will be appreciated. By such means, progress is advanced and goals are attained.

I am indebted to Dr. Alexander S. MacMillan, Jr., Dr. Edgar Holmes, Dr. James E. Gamble, Dr. Charles W. Cummings, and Dr. Charles Gruenwald, Jr., for their assistance with techniques of paranasal sinus radiography, rhinoplasty, otoplasty, nasoseptal perforations, and facial fractures.

To the surgeons of the Massachusetts Eye and Ear Infirmary and the Massachusetts General Hospital who have contributed to my learning I owe my sincere gratitude.

My thanks are due to Miss Edith Tagrin and Mr. Joshua B. Clark; the excellence of their drawings will be immediately apparent to the reader. Thanks are also extended to Mr. Norman R. Archambault and Mr. David Tilden, who contributed to the artwork in Chapter 8.

To Miss Patricia Perrier, Mrs. Judith Bond, and Mrs. Pamela A. Elbasher, who spent tedious hours in manuscript editing and preparation, I express my appreciation.

WILLIAM W. MONTGOMERY, M.D.

Boston, Massachusetts

Special Acknowledgment

The support and frequent words of advice of Howard Dearing Johnson (1897–1972) have contributed substantially to the completion of this work. The forthright character revealed in this man who has been able to so successfully define and pursue his own goals is one which a younger generation of men was brought up to respect and revere.

Mr. Johnson's interest in the needs of modern medicine, leading among other things to this present volume, is only one facet of the personality of this "Tall Man." The author wishes to express his gratitude to him.

W. W. M.

Contents

1

The Examination

NOSE

History

Patients with disease of the nose or paranasal sinuses will complain of anterior nasal discharge, posterior nasal discharge, nasal stuffiness or obstruction, localized pain over a sinus, headache, bleeding, sneezing, and/or external swelling. The following inquiries should be made and the replies carefully recorded for each patient who comes to the physician for the first time with potential nasal or sinus disease.

1. When did the trouble start?
2. What was it like at that time?
3. How has it progressed until the present time?
4. Nasal discharge:
   a. Is it anterior or posterior?
   b. Is it unilateral or bilateral?
   c. Is it persistent or intermittent?
   d. Is the amount slight, moderate, or profuse?
   e. Is it purulent, watery, mucoid, or bloody in character?
   f. Does it have an odor or taste?
   g. Does it have an unusual color?
5. Sneezing:
   a. Amount?
   b. Frequency?
   c. During what time of the day?
   d. Is it accompanied by rhinorrhea and/or epiphora?
   e. Is it seasonal?
6. Nasal obstruction:
   a. Is the obstruction partial or complete?

b. Is it unilateral or bilateral?

c. Does it have any time-of-day relationship?

d. Is it associated with environmental factors?

e. Is it associated with the ingestion of liquids or food?

7. Olfactory system:

a. Is there any distortion of smell?

b. Is there partial or complete absence of smell?

c. How long has the anosmia persisted?

d. Is the anosmia associated with other signs or symptoms?

8. Pain:

a. Does the pain consist of generalized headache, or is it localized to the distribution of the nose and paranasal sinuses? (Generalized headache is usually not a symptom of intranasal or sinus disease.)

b. Is it true pain or a sensation of pressure?

c. Is the pain associated with other symptoms, such as nasal blockage, rhinorrhea, or sneezing?

9. Has there been a history of redness or swelling in relation to the external nose and paranasal sinuses.

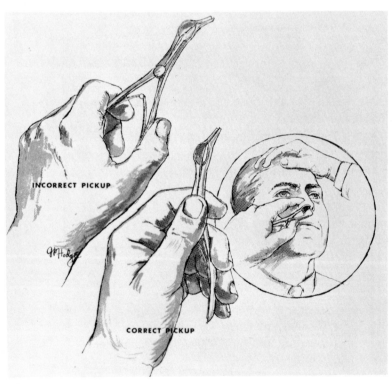

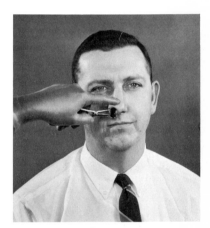

Correct

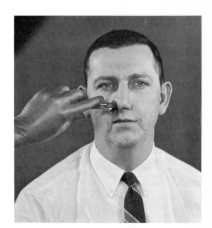

Incorrect

FIGURE 1.1. *Intranasal examination.*

Above. The nasal speculum is grasped with the left hand (by the right-handed examiner) so that it feels comfortable and well balanced between the examiner's palm and fingers.

Right. The tip of the nasal speculum is inserted in a slightly lateral direction so that discomfort will not be caused by touching the nasal septum. As the speculum is inserted, the examiner's index finger may be placed on the side of the patient's nose for support. Overdilatation of the external nasal orifice is unnecessary and produces pain. The correct and incorrect methods of insertion of the speculum are shown.

Local Examination

For examination of the nose, a head mirror, light source (100-watt bulb), and instrument tray containing a nasal speculum, finger cots, an atomizer, bayonet forceps, cotton strips, sterile swabs (for culture), nasal decongestants, and topical anesthesia are essential.

After the patient has been seated directly facing the examiner, and without any extension or flexion of his head, the external nose, as well as the remainder of the face, is first carefully examined by observation and palpation. The presence of redness, swelling, or ecchymosis, or loss of structure or support is determined. The nasal speculum is inserted into the nose and directed away from the nasal septum in order to avoid unnecessary discomfort for the patient (Fig. 1.1). Also overdilating the external nasal orifice is avoided, for this can cause the patient an undue amount of pain. The color of the nasal mucous membrane is observed and it is determined whether the turbinates are normal, hypertrophic, or atrophic. The nasal septum is observed carefully for deviations. Abnormalities in the nasal vestibule can be readily seen.

Next, the nose is sprayed with 0.25% Neo-Synephrine, 1% ephedrine solution, or 0.50% cocaine solution and, after a few minutes, is reexamined. If the posterior aspect of the nasal cavities cannot be seen, additional spray decongestant is applied to the nasal mucous membrane. With adequate decongestion of the mucous membrane, the entire nasal cavity and superior aspect of the nasopharynx can be seen. If instrumental palpating or probing is to be carried out, or if a biopsy specimen of a lesion is to be obtained, it is best to anesthetize the mucous membrane of the nasal cavity with cotton strips impregnated with 4% cocaine or 2% Pontocaine solution (Fig. 1.2). Cultures and smears are taken as soon as abnormal discharge is seen.

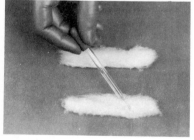

a

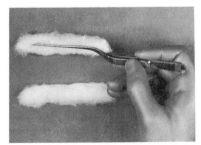

b

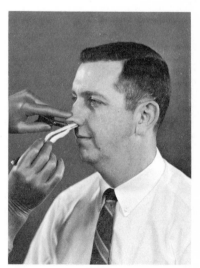

c

FIGURE 1.2

a. Cotton strips impregnated either with a vasoconstricting solution, a topical anesthetic solution, or both are most valuable in the diagnosis and treatment of intranasal disease. They are cut approximately 4 inches in length and placed on a disposable mat or on the palm of the hand. Medication is applied to these cotton strips with either a dropper or an atomizer spray.

b. The cotton strip is grasped by the bayonet forceps as is shown.

c. The cotton is inserted gently into the nasal cavity. One strip in each nostril is usually sufficient to constrict the mucous membrane for diagnosis. Two or three strips are necessary for intranasal anesthesia.

Physiology

A sound knowledge of nasal physiology is necessary in order to evaluate normal and abnormal findings properly. The three major functions of the nose are: (1) respiration, (2) olfaction, and (3) phonation. Only a brief review of these functions is included in this text.

Respiration. Approximately 500 cubic feet of air pass through the nasal cavities every 24 hours. The nose warms, filters, and moistens this air. In order to accomplish these functions, there must be a large surface area of moist mucous membrane. The mucous film covering the nasal mucosa must be in constant motion as it replenishes itself. There must be normal airways, a sufficient air supply from the cavernous spaces, and a constant pH for the nasal secretions. On inspiration, very little air passes through the middle and superior meatuses. The reverse is true with expiration. The ostia of the paranasal sinuses are thus not subjected to cold or dry air. The negative pressure caused by inspiration is important in the evacuation of the paranasal sinuses. There is gross filtration by the vibrissae in the nasal vestibule. The mucous film and ciliary action take care of fine particles. Lysozyme found in the mucous film destroys certain bacteria. A secondary line of defense against infection is situated in the stroma of the mucous membrane. It is made up of histiocytes which engulf and destroy bacteria. The nasal cilia are 7 microns in length and beat eight to twelve times a second, with a rapid effective stroke followed by a slower recovery stroke. The direction of sweep of these cilia is away from the ostia of the sinuses and in the direction of the nasopharynx. The action of these cilia in the anterior third of the nasal cavity is relatively slow, but rather rapid from the tip of the turbinates, posteriorly.

Olfaction. The olfactory epithelium is located in the superior aspect of the nasal cavity. The olfactory mucous membrane is yellow or brownish in color and extends down onto the septum and lateral nasal wall for a distance of 5 to 8 mm. The total olfactory area is approximately 500 sq. mm. The sense of smell is sometimes referred to as "taste at a distance." Taste and smell are closely connected in the central nervous system, and it is often difficult to disassociate one from the other. Constant exposure to any odor can produce fatigue. This fatigue also interferes with new or different stimuli. The mechanism of olfactory discrimination is unknown. Reflexes from the olfactory system can produce salivation and gastric secretion. Reflexes from the nasal mucous membrane can result in sneezing, lacrimation, respiratory inhibition, or vasomotor response.

Phonation. Together with the paranasal sinuses the nose gives resonance to the sounds produced by the vocal cords.

Nerve Supply

Included in the nerve supply to the nose are the following:
1. The nasociliary nerve. This nerve arises from the ophthalmic nerve and lies in the lateral wall of the cavernous sinus. It enters the orbit through the superior orbital fissure and passes obliquely across the orbital cavity to the anterior ethmoid foramen, which lies in the medial wall of the orbit. The posterior ethmoid branch leaves the orbit by way of the posterior ethmoid foramen. The other branch of the nasociliary nerve inside the orbit is the infratrochlear nerve. The anterior and posterior

ethmoid nerves leave the orbit through the ethmoid foramina and thus reenter the cranial cavity. They then pass along the cranial surface of the cribriform plate before entering the nasal cavity.

2. The anterior ethmoidal nerve. The medial or septal branch of this nerve supplies the anterior septum as far as the nares. Its lateral branch supplies the anterior portions of the middle and inferior turbinates, anterior ethmoid cells, frontal sinus, and anterior middle and inferior meatuses. Its lateral nasal nerve is a branch which passes between the nasal bone and upper lateral cartilage to supply the tip of the nose.

3. The posterior ethmoidal nerve. This nerve supplies only a small area of mucous membrane, posterior ethmoid cells, and sphenoid sinus.

4. The sphenopalatine nerve. The maxillary nerve leaves the cranial cavity by way of the foramen rotundum and enters the pterygopalatine fossa where the sphenopalatine ganglion is found. The nasal branches of the sphenopalatine ganglion enter the nasal cavity through the spheno-palatine foramen, located just behind the posterior end of the middle turbinate.

The medial posterosuperior branch of the sphenopalatine nerve supplies the posterior nasal septum and continues on as the nasopalatine nerve which passes through the anterior palatine (Scarpa's) foramen to supply the hard palate. Before reaching the foramen it anastomoses with the nasal branch of the anterosuperior alveolar nerve. Here the medial posterosuperior branch of the sphenopalatine nerve and the nasal branch of the anterosuperior alveolar nerve supply the infero-anterior surface of the inferior turbinate and the adjacent floor. After anasto-mosing they pass together through the intermaxillary suture (foramina of Scarpa) to supply the hard palate behind the upper teeth. At this location they anastomose with branches of the greater palatine nerve.

The lateral posterosuperior branch of the sphenopalatine nerve supplies the superior and middle turbinates (large portion) and has branches to the posterior ethmoids.

The lateral postero-inferior branch of the sphenopalatine nerve is where the sphenopalatine ganglion gives off the great or anterior palatine nerve which passes through the pterygopalatine canal within the lateral nasal wall. Here it gives off branches to the postero-inferior turbinate and posterior middle and inferior meatuses.

5. The infraorbital nerve. This nerve gives off a branch which supplies the lateral surfaces of the external nose, the ala nasi and also the lower end of the septum, by way of the external nares.

6. The anterosuperior alveolar (dental) nerve. This nerve gives off a branch which pierces the lateral wall of the nose to supply the anterior portion of the inferior meatus and adjacent nasal floor.

7. The nervi terminales. The ganglion cells of these nerves, which pass through the cribriform plate, lie between the crista galli and the olfactory bulb. The nerves lie in the deepest portion of the nasal septal mucosa, over the cartilaginous portion of the septum. Their function is not known. They are thought to be both sensory and autonomic.

The parasympathetic system of the nose includes the facial nerve, interme-diary nerve, greater superficial petrosal nerve, and the sphenopalatine ganglion. This system has a vasodilatory and secretory function.

The sympathetic system of the nose includes the superior cervical sympathetic ganglion, the internal carotid arteries, the deep petrosal nerve, vidian nerve, vidian canal, and sphenopalatine ganglion. Its function is vasoconstrictory.

The sensory elements of the external nose are:

1. Branches of the infraorbital nerve.
2. Branches of the infratrochlear nerve, which is a branch of the nasociliary, and thus of the ophthalmic branch of the fifth cranial nerve.
3. The lateral nasal nerve, with its branch of anterior ethmoid nerves.

The motor elements of the external nose are in the muscles supplied by the seventh nerve.

Included in the arterial supply to the nose are the following:

1. Branches of the internal carotid artery. These include the anterior ethmoid arteries with their branch of the ophthalmic arteries, and the posterior ethmoid arteries with their branch of ophthalmic arteries. The course and distribution of the ethmoid arteries are similar to those of the nerves.
2. Branches of the internal maxillary artery. The sphenopalatine arteries pass with the nerve through the sphenopalatine foramen. The lateral branches supply most of the turbinates. The nasopalatine or septal branch courses along with the nerve.

The descending palatine artery accompanies the greater palatine nerve down into the pterygopalatine canal. Like the nerve, it sends twigs to the lower posterior part of the nasal cavity. It passes through the greater palatine foramen, sends branches to the soft palate, and runs forward as the major palatine artery. Anteriorly it passes through the incisive foramen to the septum and laterally through the foramen of Stensen to anastomose with the nasopalatine branch of the sphenopalatine artery to supply the anterior floor. The infraorbital artery has the same distribution as the nerve.

The posterosuperior alveolar branch arises near the pterygopalatine fossa, courses through the alveolar foramina of the maxilla and goes on to supply the maxillary antrums.

3. The external maxillary artery. The angular branch includes the branch of the facial artery and supplies the lateral aspect of the nose, the skin of the vestibule, and the dorsum of the nose. The superior labial artery supplies the vestibular portion of the septum.

Little's (Kiesselbach's) area includes the anterior ethmoidal arteries, the nasopalatine (septal) branch of the sphenopalatine arteries, the branch of greater palatine arteries which passes from the palate through the incisive foramen, and the branch of the superior labial arteries.

Normal Findings

The nasal vestibule varies considerably in different individuals as to size and shape. It is bound medially and laterally by the crura of the greater alar cartilage. It is lined with fibro-elastic tissue and skin which are tightly adherent to the underlying cartilage. The anterior nasal septum (Fig 1.3) and anterior tips of the middle and inferior turbinates can be seen without the use of a nasal decongestant. The line of transition from squamous to respiratory epithelium can be easily identified.

After the nasal cavity has been decongested, the four walls are easily seen unless some abnormality is present. The floor is mostly made up of the hard palate. A portion of the nasal surface of the soft palate can also be seen. The nasal septum makes up the medial wall. By palpation, the anterior cartilaginous portion can be distinguished from the bony portion, which is made up of the septal process of the palate, the vomer, and the perpendicular plate of the ethmoid bone (Fig. 1.3). The mucous membrane is rather tightly adherent to the septum. Superficial blood vessels, especially those located anteriorly in Little's area, can be seen. A thickening of the mucous membrane of the septum opposite the anterior tip of the middle turbinate is known as the septal tubercle. The roof of the nasal cavity is quite difficult to view. Where the mucous membrane changes from a pinkish to a yellowish hue the olfactory epithelium begins. The most prominent structure on the lateral nasal wall is the inferior turbinate (Fig. 1.3). This is a separate bone which articulates with the lacrimal, ethmoid, and palatal bones. The mucous membrane is quite thick, for it contains numerous venous plexus in the form of cavernous erectile tissue. The inferior meatus is inferior to the inferior turbinate. For the most part it corresponds to the medial wall of the maxillary sinus. The nasolacrimal duct opens high in the anterior portion of the inferior meatus. The middle turbinate is a projection of the ethmoid bone. It obstructs a good view of the middle meatus. In some patients the middle meatus can be seen, especially when the mucous membrane of the middle turbinate is atrophic. The ethmoidal infundibulum is a crescent-shaped groove seen just anterior to an elevation known as the ethmoidal bulla. The opening into the infundibulum is known as the semi-lunar hiatus. The nasofrontal duct may be positioned in the superior aspect of the infundibulum. Just inferior to this are the openings for the anterior ethmoid cells. The ostium of the maxillary sinus is found inferiorly and posteriorly in the infundibulum. The nasofrontal duct usually enters anterosuperiorly to the infundibulum in the area known as the nasofrontal recess. In some individuals a superior turbinate can be seen; usually, however, only a thickening of the mucous membrane can be identified. The superior meatus and the ostia of the posterior ethmoid cells are found in this area. Posterior to this area is the spheno-ethmoidal recess. The ostium of the sphenoid sinus is located posteriorly.

Abnormal Findings

Disorders of Nasal Vestibule. The nasal vestibule is a common site for furuncles and fissures. Most deformities of the nasal vestibule are caused by dislocation of the septal cartilage at the columella. These deformities may also be due to the variation in size and shape of the alar cartilages. This area is not an uncommon site of benign and malignant skin tumors.

Disorders of Mucous Membrane. The color of the mucous membrane is noted. Normally it is a deep pink, but with inflammatory processes or nasal allergy, it may be reddened or pale and of a bluish-gray color. The mucous membrane should be evaluated for the presence of hypertrophy or atrophy; also the quantity and character of nasal secretions should be carefully studied. The swollen mucous membrane associated with allergy usually has a watery discharge. When vasomotor rhinitis is suspected, it is most important to determine whether or not there is an excessive amount of mucous secretion. Hypertrophy of the turbinates and mucous membrane associated with hypersecretion of mucus is probably not due

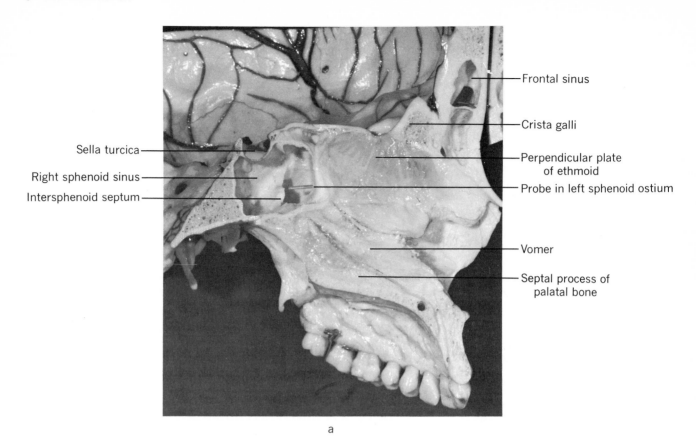

Frontal sinus

Crista galli

Sella turcica

Perpendicular plate
of ethmoid

Right sphenoid sinus

Probe in left sphenoid ostium

Intersphenoid septum

Vomer

Septal process of
palatal bone

a

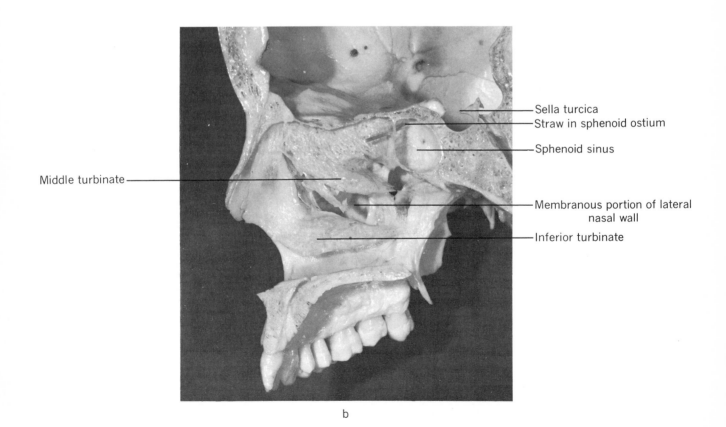

Sella turcica

Straw in sphenoid ostium

Sphenoid sinus

Middle turbinate

Membranous portion of lateral
nasal wall

Inferior turbinate

b

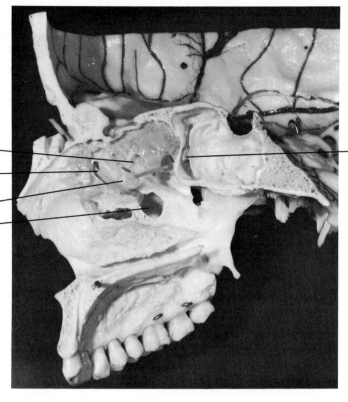

Attachment of middle turbinate

Straw from frontal sinus

Ethmoid bulla

Membranous portion of lateral nasal wall

Straw through sphenoid ostium

c

FIGURE 1.3

a. A midsagittal section gives a view of the right frontal sinus, bony nasal septum, and sphenoid sinus. A portion of the left frontal sinus is seen, indicating that the intrafrontal septum is not in the midline. The intrasphenoid septum is often displaced from the midline. In this specimen, it is in an oblique plane. The sphenoid sinus is well pneumatized, rendering the sella turcica accessible for transsphenoid surgery. The quadrangular cartilage of the nasal septum is absent, but its outline is described by the anterior borders of the perpendicular plate of the ethmoid and the vomer. The septal process of the palatal bone makes up the remaining portion of the bony nasal septum.

b. A sagittal section just to the right of the midline gives a view of the lateral nasal wall. The frontal sinus on this side is not developed and pneumatization of the sphenoid sinus is not extensive. The thickness of bone between the sella turcica and the sphenoid sinus would, on this specimen, render the pituitary inaccessible to transsphenoid surgery. The sphenoid ostium is quite high. The relationship of the middle turbinate, membranous lateral nasal wall, and inferior turbinate can be visualized.

c. In this specimen, the middle turbinate has been removed. The attachment of the middle turbinate with its upper extension makes up the medial wall of the ethmoid labyrinth. The right frontal sinus opens into the semilunar hiatus. The ostium of the right sphenoid sinus is in its usual position. A good view of the membranous portion of the lateral nasal wall is obtained. With the absence of the middle turbinate, any point of the maxillary sinus ostium can be seen.

to a true vasomotor rhinitis, and therefore a good response to either a medical or a surgical regimen directed toward therapy of this type of rhinitis cannot be expected. The hypertrophy may represent an early phase of atrophic rhinitis. Smears should be made to determine whether or not eosinophils are present. The protein and sugar content of the secretions can be easily ascertained with a lab stick. A watery rhinorrhea can represent leakage of spinal fluid. It is usually best to take samples for cultures before applying vasoconstrictors; on the other hand, purulent secretions may not be obtained prior to vasoconstriction.

Irregularities of Septum. There is almost always some degree of septal irregularity (except, possibly, in the Bantu people of South Africa). Quite commonly there is a ridge located inferiorly on one or both sides where the septal cartilage joins the septal process of the palatal and vomer bones. As a rule these minor irregularities are symptomless; too often they are taken as a cause for nasal stuffiness which is due to other factors and an unnecessary submucous resection of the nasal septum may be performed. On occasion, ridges, spurs, or deflections of the nasal septum, which do interfere with normal nasal respiration, can be seen. Septal spurs can, on occasion, initiate nasal neuralgia manifested by a severe, intermittent or constant, boring pain, usually in the lateral aspect of the nose, over the maxilla, but may be located in any area supplied by the second division of the fifth cranial nerve. In making the diagnosis, the spur and surrounding area should be anesthetized with a topical agent. If this is not effective in relieving the pain, the sphenopalatine ganglion should be anesthetized to determine if the pain is due to sphenopalatine neuralgia.

Stuffiness or Obstruction. The most common symptom of nasal disease is stuffiness or obstruction. This may be unilateral or bilateral. A deviated nasal septum is the most common cause of unilateral stuffiness or obstruction. Operation for its correction should be advised only if the symptom is distressing or the deviation causes complicating sinus disease.

Foreign bodies are not uncommonly found in the nasal cavity. They may produce a reaction which in turn leads to stuffiness or obstruction. They are encountered most commonly in children and in psychotic patients. In addition to stuffiness, they may be responsible for pain, bleeding, and a foul discharge. The diagnosis is made by palpation with a probe, after a topical anesthetic has been applied, and also by x-ray examination. Removal of intranasal foreign bodies can be quite difficult and often a general anesthetic is required.

Acute and chronic rhinitis, hay fever, and vasomotor rhinitis are the most common causes of bilateral nasal stuffiness and obstruction in adults; adenoid hypertrophy is the most common cause in children. If adenoid hypertrophy is persistent or associated with recurrent or persistent sinusitus or middle ear disease, an adenoidectomy is indicated. A deviated septum may cause bilateral nasal stuffiness, especially when the septum is deviated to one side anteriorly and to the other posteriorly. Nasal polyps, a chronic edematous inflammatory process of the nasal mucous membrane, may be responsible for bilateral obstruction. They appear as yellowish, grape-like masses and are usually associated with bilateral chronic allergic ethmoiditis. Other sinuses may also be involved.

Hematoma of the septum produces bilateral nasal obstruction. It is usually of traumatic origin, or it may follow submucous resection of the nasal septum. Abscess of the nasal septum presents as bilateral nasal obstruction with pain, redness, and swelling of the septum on both sides. Both hematoma and abscess of the nasal septum require surgical therapy (p. 349).

Benign Tumors. Papillomas appear in the region of the nasal vestibule as viable, sessile masses. Osteomas can extend into the nasal cavity. They quite often produce external deformity as well as nasal obstruction. Juvenile angiofibromas occur posteriorly. They are more common in males than in females and rarely are seen in persons beyond 20 years of age.

Malignant Tumors. The most frequently occurring intranasal malignant lesions are of epithelial origin. Often their presenting symptom is unilateral nasal obstruction; therefore, an excellent course to follow is to regard unilateral nasal obstruction as due to a malignant tumor until proven otherwise. Adenocarcinoma is the next most common malignant lesion. Lymphosarcoma, melanoma, and other malignant tumors also may occur in the nose. Malignant intranasal tumors may be manifested by bilateral as well as unilateral nasal stuffiness or obstruction, by external swelling, bleeding, discharge due to secondary infection, pain, and/or epiphora.

Perforation of Nasal Septum. The nasal septum may be perforated either anteriorly or posteriorly. Although such association is uncommon today, we still must think of an anterior perforation as indicative of tuberculosis and a posterior perforation as due to syphilis. At the present time, most perforations are anterior and are the result of trauma from chronic nose picking or are due to surgical procedures. Small anterior perforations are quite troublesome, for they produce a whistling nasal respiration. These can be repaired surgically. The nasal stuffiness or obstruction associated with septal perforation is due to crusting. Epistaxis from the margin of a perforation is common, especially if the patient has not learned how to use saline irrigations and to apply petroleum jelly to the margins of the perforation.

Unilateral Partial or Complete Choanal Atresia. Unilateral choanal atresia often remains undiagnosed, even in adults. In addition to the nasal obstruction, a mucoid or purulent nasal discharge is present. The diagnosis can be made by anterior rhinoscopy, probing, or contrast radiography. Bilateral choanal atresia becomes apparent in the neonatal period. Since the newborn cannot breathe through his mouth, if he has this congenital abnormality he will die from asphyxiation unless the attending physician is alerted to the necessity of an oral airway. Diagnosis is made by attempting to pass rubber catheters from the nose into the pharynx. To confirm the diagnosis and outline the obstruction, radiopaque substances are instilled into the nasal cavity, and lateral x-ray views are obtained with the infant in the recumbent position.

PARANASAL SINUSES

History

Much of the history of sinus disease is obtained during the interrogation for nasal signs and symptoms. The most common symptom of sinus disease is nasal discharge. It is, however, important to review carefully the history of discomfort or pain related to the various paranasal sinuses. Generalized headache is usually not a symptom of sinusitis. Pain from the frontal sinus can be present directly over the sinus or in the orbit. This pain appears each morning and progresses in severity until late afternoon, at which time it subsides spontaneously. Pain from the maxillary sinus can occur directly over the sinus, in the orbit, or at the upper teeth. Pain from the ethmoid sinus is usually in, or medial to, the orbit on the affected side. The pain resulting from sphenoid sinus disease is most difficult for the patient to describe. It is usually severe, persistent, and emanates from the "center of the head." A change of head position may either worsen or relieve the pain.

There are numerous orbital manifestations of sinus disease. These include orbital pain, exophthalmos, enophthalmos, lid swelling, mass in the orbit, epiphora, orbital cellulitis, and abscess (see Chapter 2).

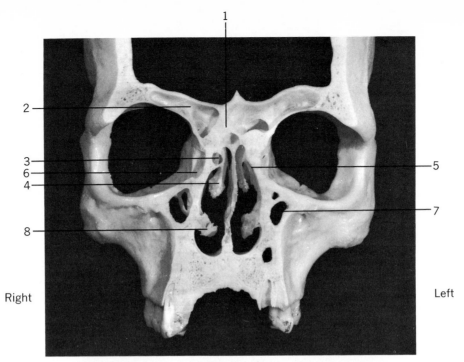

1

2

3
6
4

5

8

7

Right

Left

a. Anterior view

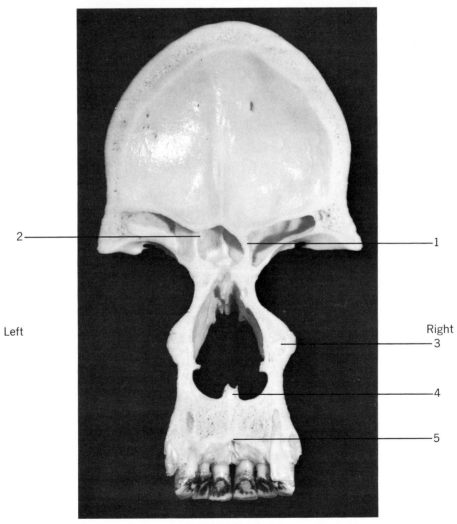

2

Left

1

Right

3

4

5

b. Posterior view

Anatomy

The anatomy of the paranasal sinuses will be discussed in detail in the following chapters along with surgical technique. A thorough knowledge of the anatomy, with its variations, is essential for the diagnosis and treatment of sinus disease. For general orientation, photographs of skull sections are included in this chapter (Figs. 1.4–1.6).

Technique of Examination

Examination of the sinuses should include palpation of the roof and floor of the orbits, of the ascending process of the maxillae, and of the canine fossae. Tenderness may be elicited in these areas, and masses or defects may be felt. Transillumination is of limited value but should not be excluded. Its use is limited to the diagnosis of frontal and maxillary sinus disease. For the frontal sinuses the light is placed under the medial aspect of the supraorbital rim for observation of the forehead; for the maxillary sinuses it is placed above the infraorbital rim for observation of the hard palate (Fig. 1.7). The test is not of true diagnostic value, for both the frontal and maxillary sinuses vary considerably in their degree of development. A sinus filled with clear liquid will transilluminate well. The presence of a mass, thickness, or reaction in the surrounding bone will interfere with transillumination. Transillumination is most useful as a tool for following the patient's progress once a clinical or radiographic diagnosis has been made.

FIGURE 1.4. *A coronal section through the anterior nasal cavity and paranasal sinuses.*

a. Looking from anterior to posterior, both frontal sinuses are well pneumatized. The inner frontal septum is to the right of the midline. The nasal frontal orifice can be seen from above on the right. An anterior ethmoid cell is apparent on the right. The middle turbinate below this remains intact. On the left side the middle turbinate is partially resected giving a view of the semilunar hiatus and middle meatus and a glimpse of the nasofrontal orifice from below. Both lacrimal fossae can be seen. The three openings in the left maxillary bone indicate the irregularity of the left maxillary sinus. A partition can be seen subdividing the right antrum. Both inferior turbinates are intact. The intranasal openings of the nasolacrimal ducts cannot be seen from this view.

    1. Interfrontal septum
    2. Right frontal sinus
    3. Anterior ethmoid cell
    4. Middle turbinate
    5. Left middle meatus and nasofrontal orifice
    6. Lacrimal fossa
    7. Left maxillary sinus
    8. Right inferior turbinate

b. Looking from posterior to anterior, the interfrontal septum is seen to the right of the midline. The left frontal sinus is larger than the right and is partially subdivided by incomplete septa. The anterior aspect of the right antrum can be identified. The anterior tip of the vomer bone is seen as it attaches to the anterior septal spine. Directly below this, on the anterior aspect of the hard palate, the incisive foramen can be visualized.

    1. Interfrontal septum
    2. Left frontal sinus
    3. Right maxillary sinus
    4. Vomer
    5. Incisive foramen

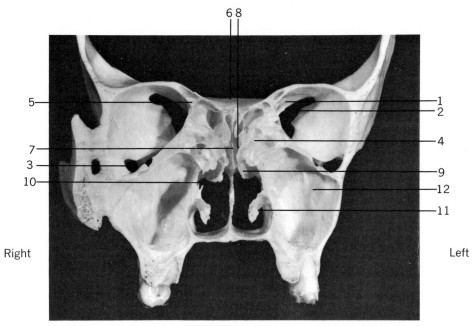

a. Anterior view

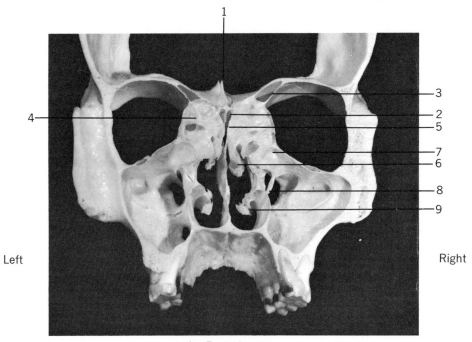

b. Posterior view

During infancy, the frontal and sphenoid sinuses are not clinical entities. The frontal sinus is an extension of an anterior ethmoid cell and is usually not fully developed until puberty. In approximately 5% of the population there is no frontal sinus development; in 15 to 20%, only unilateral pneumatization is found above the supraorbital rim. The sphenoid sinus at birth is a definite structure in the posterior nasal cavity. Pneumatization extends into the sphenoid bone when the child is approximately 3 years of age. Full pneumatization is reached during adolescence. The maxillary and ethmoid sinuses are present at birth and thus can be diseased during infancy. This is especially true of the ethmoid sinuses. Neither the maxillary nor the ethmoid sinuses, however, reach full development until adolescence.

FIGURE 1.5. *Coronal section through the midnasal cavities and paranasal sinuses.*

a. Looking from anterior to posterior aspect, the openings into the orbit include the optic foramen, the superior orbital fissure, and the inferior orbital fissure. A rather large number of ethmoid cells can be seen on each side. A supraorbital ethmoid cell is present on each side. (These cells are best viewed from below.) The posterior aspect of the cribriform plate can be seen above the perpendicular plate of the ethmoid bone. Below and behind this is the front face of the sphenoid sinuses, and just lateral to the latter on each side are the sphenoid ostia. These ostia can be seen in Figure 1.6b. The posterior half of each middle and inferior turbinate is present. The defect representing the membranous portion of the lateral wall of the nose and ostia to the maxillary sinuses can be found between the middle and inferior turbinates. The posterior half of each maxillary sinus is shown in this specimen.

1. The optic foramen
2. Superior orbital fissure
3. Inferior orbital fissure
4. Left ethmoid cells
5. Right supraorbital ethmoid
6. Right cribriform plate
7. Perpendicular plate of the ethmoid bone
8. Front face of sphenoid sinuses
9. Middle turbinate
10. Ostium of the right antrum
11. Left inferior turbinate
12. Left maxillary sinus

b. Looking from the posterior to the anterior aspect, an excellent view of the crista galli is afforded in this section. The cribriform plate is seen end-on but is not clearly demonstrated. The supra-orbital ethmoid cell on each side could easily be mistaken for the posterior aspect of a frontal sinus. Both of these ethmoid cells are completely separated from the frontal sinuses and are directly posterior to them. On the right side is a fairly good demonstration of the attachment of the middle turbinate forming the medial wall of the ethmoid labyrinth and clearly dividing the cribriform from the ethmoid bone. Both maxillary sinuses are well pneumatized, especially in the direction of the ethmoid labyrinth. A transantral ethmoidectomy in an individual in whom the anatomic structure is similar to that in this specimen would not be at all difficult.

1. Crista galli
2. Cribriform plate
3. Supraorbital ethmoid cell
4. Ethmoid labyrinth
5. Upper extension of attachment of right middle turbinate
6. Middle turbinate
7. Pneumatization of the right antrum and the close proximity of the ethmoid labyrinth
8. Partial subdivision of the right antrum
9. Inferior turbinate

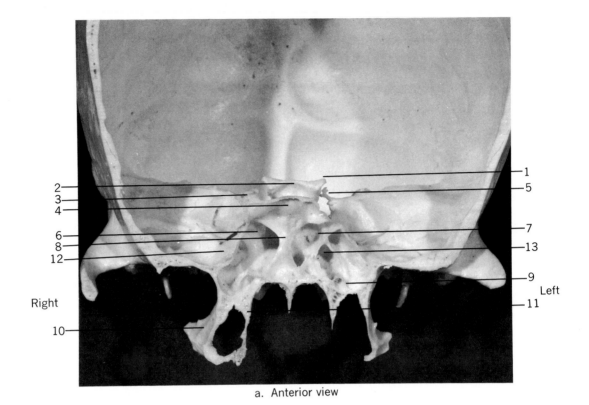

a. Anterior view

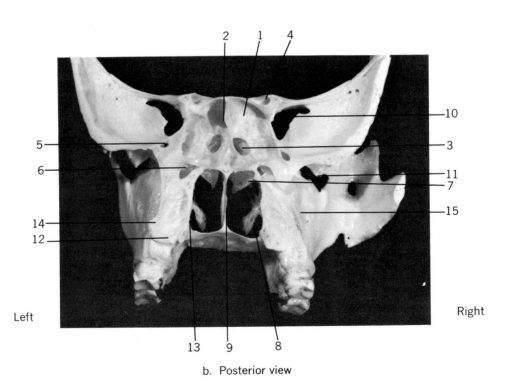

b. Posterior view

FIGURE 1.6.   *A coronal section through the posterior nasal cavities and sphenoid sinus.*

a. Looking from anterior to posterior aspect, both posterior clinoid processes, the sella turcica, and the right anterior clinoid process can be seen. The petroclinoid ligament on the left side is calcified. The left sphenoid sinus is larger and multiloculated. The intersphenoid septum, because of its oblique position, is not visible. The anterior bulge of the sella turcica is quite clear and is mostly in the right sphenoid sinus. This specimen shows the vidian canal on each side. Note its proximity to the floor of the sphenoid sinus. The medial and lateral pterygoid plates are fairly well intact on the right side.

1. Left posterior clinoid process
2. Sella turcica
3. Right anterior clinoid process
4. Anterior bulge of posterior sphenoid sinus caused by the sella turcica
5. Calcified petroclinoid ligament
6. Right sphenoid sinus
7. Left sphenoid sinus
8. Intersphenoid septum
9. Left vidian canal
10. Lateral pterygoid plate
11. Medial pterygoid plate
12. Foramen rotundum
13. Posterior ethmoid cells

b. Looking from posterior to anterior aspect. The anterior half of both sphenoid sinuses is in clear view as are the sphenoid ostia. The posterior portion of the middle turbinate can be seen in the sphenoid through the sphenoid ostia. The intrasphenoid septum appears to be near the midline anteriorly in contrast to its oblique position. The posterior portion of the sinus is seen above.

The optic canal, foramen rotundum, and dilated portion of the vidian canal can be seen on the left side. The posterior tips of the inferior and middle turbinates, as well as the nasal septum, are in view. The posterior wall of the maxillary sinus is intact on each side. The superior and inferior orbital fissures are viewed from behind. The pterygoid process and superior aspect of the medial and lateral plates are seen on the left side.

1. Right sphenoid sinus
2. Intersphenoid septum
3. Right sphenoid ostium
4. Optic foramen
5. Foramen rotundum (seen from behind)
6. Anterior enlarged portion of vidian canal
7. Right middle turbinate
8. Right inferior turbinate
9. Posterior nasal septum
10. Superior orbital fissure
11. Inferior orbital fissure
12. Pterygoid process
13. Medial pterygoid plate
14. Lateral pterygoid plate
15. Posterior wall of antrum

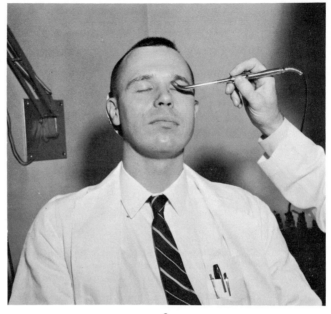

a

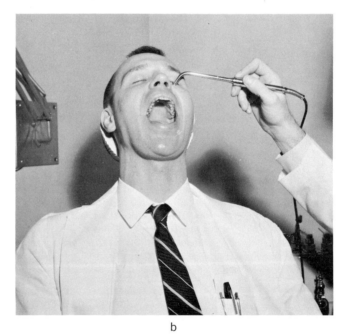

b

FIGURE 1.7.   *Transillumination of the sinuses.*

a. To transilluminate the frontal sinuses, the light is placed against the floor of the frontal sinus, posterior to the supraorbital rim. This examination, of course, must be conducted in a dark room. No illumination of the outline of the frontal sinus on the forehead is indicative of an underdeveloped sinus, a diseased frontal sinus, or a frontal sinus with a thick bony wall.

b. In order to transilluminate the maxillary sinuses the patient's head is extended and the light placed against the floor of the orbit, just behind the infraorbital rim. Illumination will occur in the hard palate. Decreased illumination is indicative of an underdeveloped maxillary sinus, diseased sinus, extremely thick bones surrounding the sinus, or sclerosis following a radical antrum operation.

Technique of Radiography*

By Alexander S. Macmillan, Jr., M.D.

Tabletop screen technics are very effective in paranasal sinus radiography. A stainless steel lead-backed mask, 6 inches in diameter, is placed over a 6½ x 8½-inch cassette for each view. An off-center mask, 4 inches in diameter, is useful for obtaining both optic foramina on one film and for stereoscopic views (Fig. 1.8). Five standard projections are used: (1) PA (Caldwell), (2) erect Waters', (3) prone Waters', (4) basal, and (5) lateral.

The following accessory projections are employed when necessary to show more clearly areas that are not well defined on the standard views: (1) optic foramina, (2) dental films, (3) AP and lateral laminograms, and (4) lateral soft-tissue films. Various film combinations can be used for special purposes: (1) upright and cross-table lateral views for fluid levels, especially in the sphenoid sinus, (2) lateral and basal views for nasopharyngeal neoplasm, and (3) PA, Waters', basal, lateral and optic foramen views plus laminography to determine the extent of injury after trauma.

Tabletop screen technic is adaptable to all ages and conditions of patients because of the optimal object-film distance and short exposure time. Infants are wrapped in a sheet, mummy style, for immobilization, and the standard or accessory projections are used.

We line up our five views in the above order much as one would study the facial bones and sinuses of an anatomical skull:

(1) On the Caldwell view (Fig. 1.9) we look the skull 'in the eye.' This is the best view of the frontal bone and sinuses, the ethmoids, and orbits and the upper aspect of the antra. The floor of the back or apex of the orbit projects above the inferior orbital rim.

---

* The section "Technique in Radiography" is reproduced from the article "Technics in Paranasal Sinus Radiography" by Alexander S. Macmillan, Jr., M.D., published in *Seminars in Roentgenology*, Vol. III, No. 2, pp. 115–122, April 1968, with permission of author and publisher.

CASSETTE

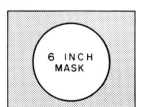

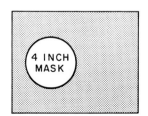

FIGURE 1.8. *Diagrammatic representation of lead-backed masks.*

Above is a cassette 6½ x 8½ inches. The 6 inch mask is used on all but the lateral sinus film. The eccentric 4 inch mask is used for views of the optic foramina.

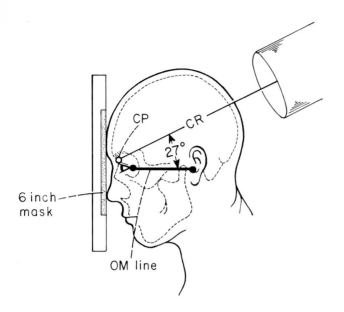

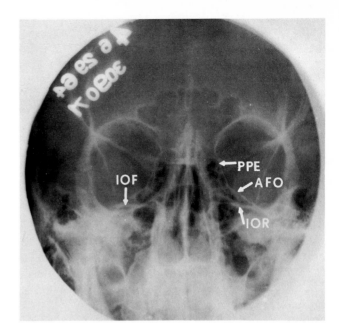

FIGURE 1.9. *PA (Caldwell) projection.*

a. The drawing is depicted with the patient erect, but the same angles are used for prone or prone-angled board views. CP = centering point-nasion; OM line = orbito-meatal line—perpendicular to cassette; CR = central ray-angled 27° caudally. The nasion is positioned at the center of the cassette.

b. An example of the Caldwell projection. The following landmarks are indicated: AFO = floor of the apex (posterior portion) of the orbit or antral roof at its highest point; IOF = infraorbital foramen; IOR = inferior orbital rim; PPE = paper plate of ethmoid. The petrous ridge projects at the level of the inferior orbital rim. The upper part of each antrum is visualized.

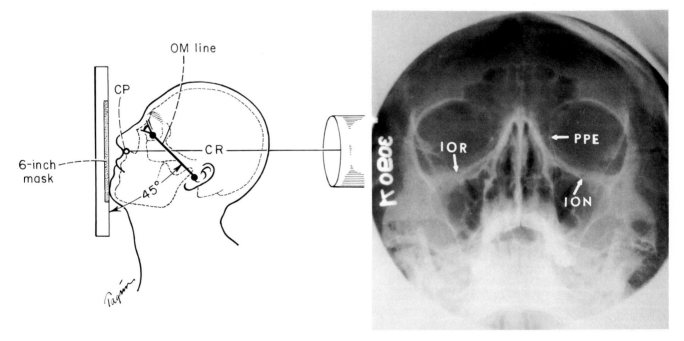

FIGURE 1.10. *Erect Waters' view.*

a. The patient's mouth is closed to avoid confusing the film with the prone Waters' view. CP = centering point—inferior nasal spine; OML = orbito-meatal line—45° angle to cassette; CR = central ray—perpendicular to center of cassette.

b. Erect Waters' view—normal appearance. Note location of PPE (paper plate of ethmoid), ION (infraorbital nerve groove), and IOR (inferior orbital rim) in relation to the maxillary sinus and the orbit.

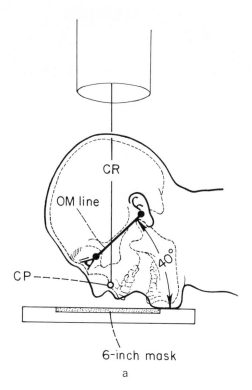

a

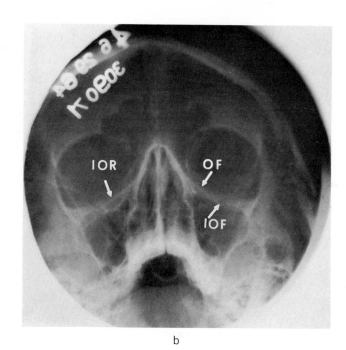

b

FIGURE 1.11. *Prone Waters' view.*

a. The mouth is open. The orbito-meatal line is angled 40° from the horizontal.

b. The petrous ridges lie just below the inferior margins of the antra. IOR = inferior orbital rim; OF = orbital floor; IOF = infra-orbital foramen. The entire floor is seen (an exception); usually only the medial two-thirds is well seen. The soft tissue line parallels the rim and is a useful area to examine for swelling and emphysema.

(2) The erect Waters' view (Fig. 1.10) is taken with the orbito-meatal line at a 45° angle to the central beam. This gives the most satisfactory view of the facial bones, especially for injuries. The orbital floor is projected below the lower rim of the orbit due to parallax.

(3) In the prone Waters' view (Fig. 1.11), the skull is tilted back a little more. The prone and upright Waters' views will often permit stereoscopy.

(4) The basal view (Fig. 1.12) is best made in the prone position with the orbito-meatal line as close to parallel to the cassette as possible and the central beam angled slightly caudally and passing through the angle of the mandible.

(5) The [erect] lateral view (Fig. 1.13) is usually made with the patient facing left.

Individual variations in facial features (size, shape, etc.) need not be considered in positioning the patient or in angling the beam. The orbito-meatal line, sagittal plane and other surface landmarks guarantee consistent reproducibility on subsequent examinations. The central ray is always aligned to the center of the film. The mask, slightly raised above the cassette, is a convenience in accurate positioning and provides sharp edges to the exposure area on the films. We omit the mask on the lateral view.

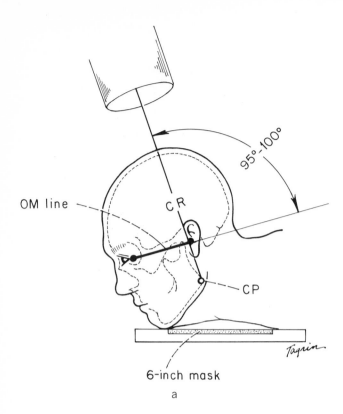

OM line

CR

95°-100°

CP

6-inch mask

a

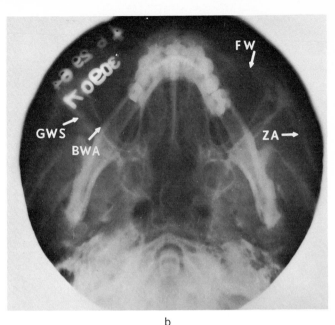

FW

GWS

BWA

ZA →

b

FIGURE 1.12. *Basal view.*

a. The prone projection is preferable to the supine with elevated shoulders and head markedly extended because of greater patient comfort and ease of attaining proper angles. CP = centering point—angle of mandible; OM line = orbito-meatal line—as close to parallel with the cassette as possible; CR = central ray—slightly more than perpendicular to the orbitomeatal line.

b. Note the relative symmetry, helpful for interpreting unilateral abnormalities of the antra, mandible, base of skull and nasopharyngeal air column. The sphenoid sinuses are usually asymmetrical. BWA = back wall of antrum (this is usually sigmoid-shaped and may overlap the greater wing of the sphenoid); FW = front wall of the antrum, depressed in zygomatic fractures (this may be the only view that convincingly indicates the need to elevate the fracture fragments); GWS = greater wing of sphenoid or outer wall of the orbit: ZA = zygomatic arch.

Some Principles of Interpretation

1. The radiologist must have the patient's history at hand when reporting the films.

2. Be specific in recording your impressions. We use the term, 'density due to . . .', thereby committing us to attempt a pathologic correlation, much as Fleischner [F. Fleischner, personal communication], in describing a blunted costophrenic angle, says, 'It is obscured by fluid, old pleurisy, tumor, etc.'

3. Displacement of air from a sinus results in increased density. An overlapping lesion outside the sinus usually has a negligible effect on the density. Feldman [M. Feldman, personal communication] demonstrated this by placing bolus material over a maxillary sinus and exposing a film. It is well recognized that only the peripheral contours of a breast shadow are seen on a chest film while an epicardial fat pad is usually as dense as the heart.

4. Mucosal thickening can be determined only when seen in true tangent, as on the antronasal wall [Alexander S. Macmillan, Sr., personal communication].

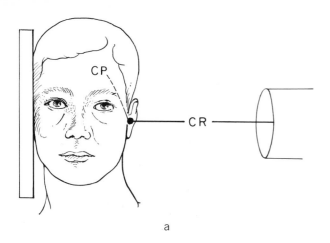

a

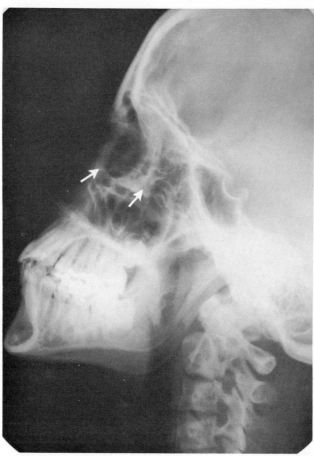

b

FIGURE 1.13. *Erect lateral view.*

This view is important in that it provides the anteroposterior dimensions of the sinuses and is the most informative projection for lesions of the nasopharynx.

a. The key to the ideal lateral view is to rotate the nose 5° toward the cassette from the true lateral position. The mask is not used. CP = centering point—midpoint of the orbito-meatal line; CR = central ray—horizontal. The orbito-meatal line is horizontal or tipped up slightly.

b. The anterior arrow points to the inferior orbital rim. The posterior arrow marks the floor of the apex of the orbit. Note how much higher it is than the inferior rim. Lateral tomograms show this especially well.

5. Blood in a maxillary sinus from an orbital floor fracture does not obscure the fragments. The fragments cannot be seen because they are displaced so that their flat side faces the central beam.

6. The orbital floor and optic foramina are bilaterally symmetrical.

7. An asymptomatic primary focus of cancer is commonly found in the nasopharynx but seldom in the sinuses.

8. Maxillary retention cysts are smooth in outline and are seen on the roof, lateral wall, or floor of the sinus. Rarely does cancer present in a sinus as an isolated mass unless it is irregular and then there usually is bone destruction.

9. Bone destruction usually means malignant disease but infection and benign lesions may on occasion erode bone.

10. Cellulitis over a maxillary sinus should alert the radiologist to study the teeth carefully for a periapical abscess in the upper jaw. It is rare for maxillary sinusitis to 'break out' of its confines whereas such extension from the frontal and ethmoid sinuses is common.

Polytomography and computer tomography (CT) body scanning of the paranasal sinuses has greatly improved our armamentarium for diagnosis of sinus disease. This added detail not only allows for more accurate diagnosis but also allows the surgeon to better plan his surgery.

For an example of the value of polytomography and CT body scanning, refer to diagnosis of the ethmoid mucocele on page 48 and osteoma of the frontal sinus on page 119.

NASOPHARYNX

Anatomy

The nasopharynx extends from the bony choanae to the inferior border of the soft palate. Looking anteriorly from the nasopharynx into the nose, the posterior border of the nasal septum dividing the two choanae is seen. The posterior tips of the middle and inferior turbinates can be identified in each choana (Fig. 1.14b). The lateral and posterior walls of the nasopharynx are formed by mucous membrane which covers the superior constrictor muscles.

Adenoid tissue, a mass of lymphoid tissue also known as the pharyngeal tonsil, is found on the posterior wall of the nasopharynx. It is connected with the palatine and lingual tonsils by a band of lymphoid tissue extending down the lateral pharyngeal wall. This entire lymphoid complex is known as Waldeyer's ring.

In the superior aspect of the lateral wall of the nasopharynx is a depression known as the pharyngeal recess (sinus of Morgagni or fossa of Rosenmüller). This is formed by a deficiency in the muscle insertion of the superior constrictor to the base of the skull. Below the pharyngeal recess is the eustachian tube cartilage. This is called the torus tubarius. A ridge extending downward from the torus tubarius to the lateral pharyngeal wall is often referred to as the salpingopharyngeal fold.

The anterior wall of the nasopharynx is formed by the hard and soft palate.

Physiology

Inspired air passes into the oropharynx from the nose by way of the nasopharynx. The mucous blanket (mentioned under the discussion of nasal physiology) passes from the nose into the oropharynx by way of the nasopharynx. The nasal mucosa, under normal conditions, produces approximately a quart of seromucinous fluid a day. When this amount is decreased by intranasal and environmental factors, the mucous blanket becomes greatly thickened. This blanket, which is normally insensible, thus becomes sensitive by virtue of being concentrated and is referred to as a postnasal drip.

The nasopharyngeal space, with the nasal cavities, is also concerned with the resonant quality of the voice.

Technique of Examination

Mirror Examination (Fig. 1.14a). A mirror, size #0 to #00, is used to examine the nasopharynx. It is warmed by a flame, hot water, or by holding it over an electric light bulb. If no heat is available, a thick soapy solution is placed on the mirror and wiped off without rinsing. The patient should be sitting directly in front of the examiner, with his head at the same level as that of the examiner. The patient is asked to sit erect, all the way back in the chair, with his head projected slightly forward.

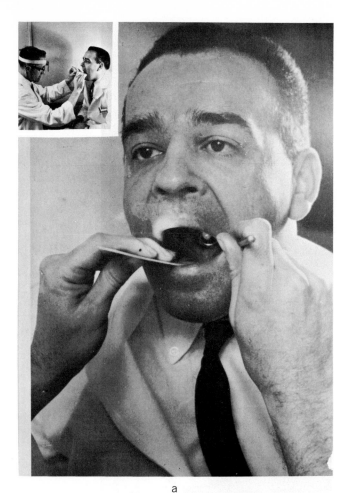

a

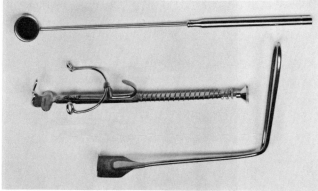

b

FIGURE 1.14

    a. The examiner should be sitting directly in front of and at the same level as the patient.

    b. The instruments used for an examination of the nasopharynx include, from top to bottom, a size # 0 or # 00 mirror, a self-retaining soft-palate retractor, and a Latrobe soft-palate retractor.

    The examiner depresses the patient's tongue onto the floor of the patient's mouth with the left hand, making sure not to extend the tip of the tongue blade beyond the patient's mid-tongue area. Light is reflected into the pharynx with the head mirror. The examiner grasps the mirror with his right hand as he would grasp a pencil and slips it behind and to one side of the patient's uvula. The patient is requested to breathe quietly and not to hold his breath. Care is taken not to touch the base of the patient's tongue. Two percent Pontocaine, or 4% cocaine, solution may be sprayed into the pharynx to control the gag reflex. The soft palate may be retracted anteriorly for a better view of the nasopharynx by placing a rubber catheter, which exits through the oropharynx, into each nostril. The catheters are stretched and clamped over a piece of rolled-up gauze placed just below the nose (Fig. 1.15).

    Anterior Rhinoscopy. The upper nasopharynx can be examined, after proper shrinkage of the nasal mucosa (with 1% ephedrine or 0.5% cocaine), by direct examination of the nose through a nasal speculum (see p. 2).

    Nasopharyngoscope. The nasopharyngoscope (Fig. 1.16b) is an instrument similar to the cystoscope. It provides an excellent view of all areas of the nasopharynx.

    Palpation. Palpation is usually reserved for examination with the patient under general anesthesia. Topical anesthesia relieves some of the discomfort of this examination.

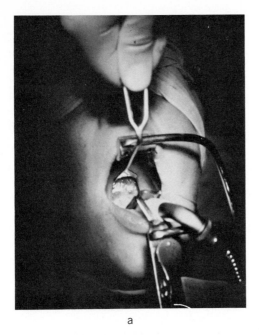

a

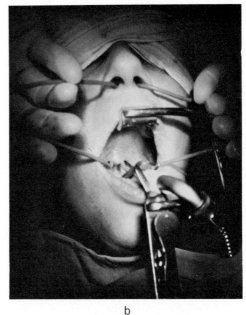

b

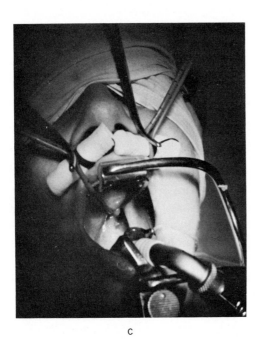

c

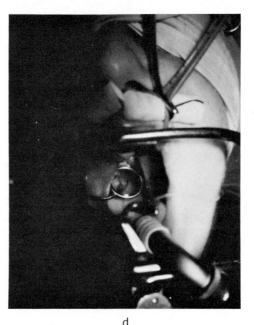

d

FIGURE 1.15

Quite frequently, an adequate examination of the nasopharynx cannot be made even after a topical anesthetic has been applied. Elevation and anterior retraction can, however, afford an excellent view of the nasopharynx.

a. The soft palate is retracted with a hand retractor. An assistant or a self-retaining soft-palate retractor is required for this maneuver.

b. Excellent retraction of the soft palate can be obtained by inserting a catheter through each nasal cavity into the pharynx and out the mouth.

c. These catheters are slightly stretched, crossed, clamped over a gauze or cotton roll, and placed on the upper lip.

d. The soft palate has been retracted anteriorly and superiorly by the catheters, and an excellent view of the nasopharynx can be obtained with a large mirror.

FIGURE 1.16

a. A sketch of the mirror view of the nasopharynx. The most obvious landmark is the posterior border of the nasal septum dividing the two choanae. The posterior tip of the middle and inferior turbinates can be seen in each choana. Adenoid tissue may be noted on the posterior wall. The posterior surface of the hard and soft palate can be seen anteriorly. There is a pocket or depression, known as the pharyngeal recess, sinus of Morgagni, or fossa of Rosenmüller, in the superior lateral wall. The torus tubarius is an elevation of a projection of the eustachian tube cartilage above and behind the orifice of the eustachian tube. The salpingopharyngeal fold is a ridge extending inferiorly from the torus tubarius.

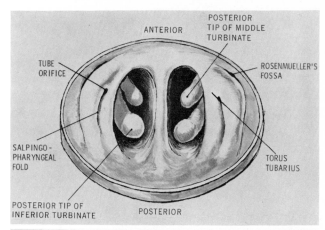

b. The nasopharyngoscope is similar in construction to the cystoscope but is 12 cm in length and 0.4 cm in diameter. Illumination is provided by an electric bulb located at the tip of the scope, just beyond the prism. A small knob on the periphery of the eyepiece indicates the direction of vision. The nasopharyngoscope is inserted along the floor of the nose into the nasopharynx, after the nasal mucous membrane has been topically anesthetized.

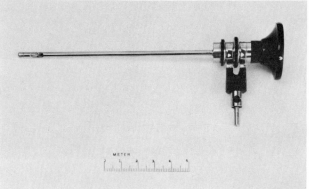

c. The Yankauer nasopharyngeal speculum is used only when the patient is under general anesthesia. The tip of the scope is inserted beneath the soft palate. The instrument is useful only for viewing the posterior and lateral nasopharyngeal walls.

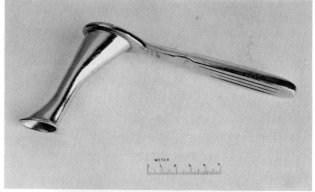

d. The nasopharynx is being examined with a Yankauer nasopharyngeal speculum. A Brown-Davis mouth gag, with a Ring attachment for placement of the endotracheal tube, is used to expose the pharynx.

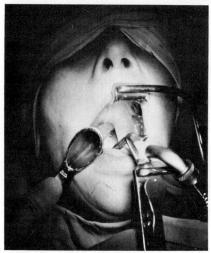

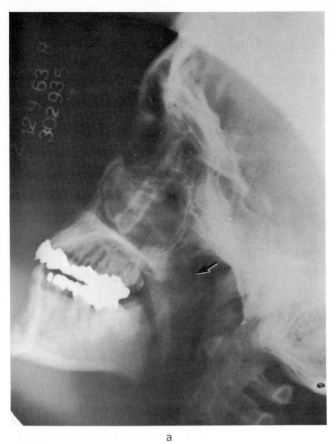

a

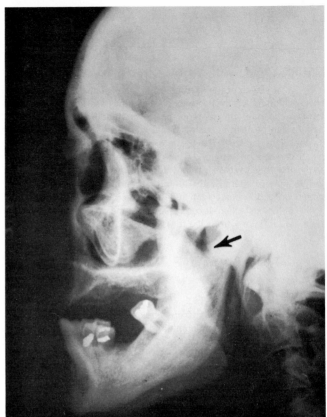

b

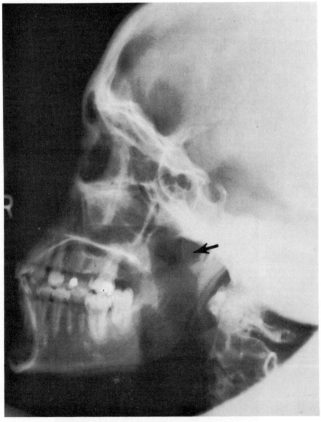

c

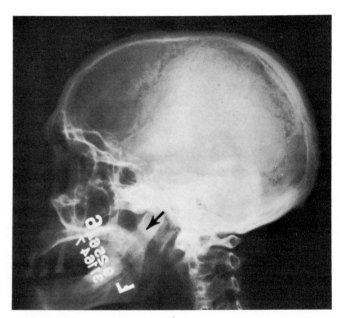

d

Direct Examination. A tubular instrument known as the Yankauer speculum (Fig. 1.15) provides direct inspection of the nasopharynx by lifting the soft palate out of the way. This instrument, however, is only suitable for examination of the lower half of the nasopharynx.

X ray. The lateral view of the nasopharynx (Fig. 1.13) is used to determine the following:

1. Size of adenoids
2. Status of eustachian tubes
3. Size of nasopharyngeal airway
4. Presence of tumors
5. Patency of choanae (using radiopaque substance)
6. Disorders of hard and soft palate
7. Ability of soft palate and transverse ridge of contracted superior constrictor (known as Passavant's ridge), at level of soft palate, to close the velopharyngeal space
8. The boundary between the nasopharynx and the oropharynx (this x ray is taken during the act of swallowing).

The base of skull view demonstrates:

1. Presence of lesions
2. Size of lesion
3. Extension of disease beyond the nasopharynx (bony destruction).

Symptoms of Nasopharyngeal Disease

Nasal Obstruction. Impaired or obstructed nasal airways are not always due to intranasal disease.

Unilateral or bilateral choanal atresia may be due to bony or membranous obstruction. Bilateral atresia occurring in the neonatal period presents an emergency situation, for mouth-breathing is an acquired habit.

Choanal Polyp. A large polyp (Fig. 1.17a) may extend from the middle meatus into the nasopharynx and cause obstruction.

Benign Tumors. Fibromas and other benign tumors (neurofibroma, hemangioma, mixed tumor, chondroma, and lipoma) may arise in the nasopharynx.

Cancer of the Nasopharynx. Cancer of the nasopharynx represents 2% of all malignant growths. It is most common in the Oriental population. A mass in the neck or serous otitis media due to blockage of the eustachian tube may be the first symptom.

Cysts. Cysts may form in the upper posterior wall of the nasopharynx at the site of evagination of embryonic structures which form the pituitary gland (Rathke's pouch) (Fig. 1.17b).

FIGURE 1.17

a. A rather large choanal polyp is seen projecting into the nasopharynx. Such a growth usually has its origin in a maxillary sinus and at times can be seen below the level of the soft palate.

b. The arrow points to a mass arising from the upper posterior wall of the nasopharynx. This entodermic pouch (Rathke's) is a remnant from the buccopharyngeal membrane of the embryo from which the anterior lobe of the pituitary gland develops.

c and d. A smooth, dome-like bulge of the lower posterior wall of the nasopharynx usually designates the presence of a Thornwaldt's cyst or bursa. The lesion is said to originate from degenerated notochord remaining in contact with the pharyngeal ectoderm.

On the lower posterior wall, a cyst may form from the sac-like depression known as the pharyngeal bursa. This area is the point of union between the anterior end of the notochord and the pharyngeal endoderm (Thornwaldt's cyst, Fig. 1.17c).

Adenoid Hypertrophy. Adenoid hypertrophy is the most common cause of nasopharyngeal obstruction.

Bleeding. Bleeding from the nasopharynx may have its origin in the nose. Benign and malignant tumors, varices, and atrophic mucous membrane may be the sites of hemorrhage.

Discharge. In addition to "postnasal drip," described under the heading "Physiology," the following may account for nasopharyngeal discharge:

1. Purulent sinusitis
2. Nasal allergy
3. Atrophic nasopharyngitis
4. Infected pharyngeal bursa
5. Acute infection of the nasopharynx.

Cranial Nerve Paralysis. Cranial nerve palsy may result from extension of disease from the nasopharynx. The sixth cranial nerve is the one most commonly paralyzed. Next in order are the third, fourth, and fifth cranial nerves.

Hearing Loss and Otalgia. Almost any disease process in the nasopharynx may obstruct the eustachian tube orifice, producing discomfort and blockage of the ear. The blockage of the eustachian tube results in a negative middle ear pressure and thus exudation of serum.

REFERENCES

Commission on Neuroradiology of the World Federation of Neurology: Radiography of the Skull and Brain. June, 1961. E. I. DuPont de Nemours and Co.

Etter, L. E.: *Roentgenography and Roentgenology of the Middle Ear and Mastoid Process.* Springfield, Ill., Charles C Thomas, 1965.

Macmillan, A. S., Jr.: Technics in Paranasal Sinus Radiography. Seminars in Roentgenology *3*:2:115–122, (April) 1968.

Macmillan, A. S., Jr.: Radiographic Technics for Facial Injuries. In W. C. Guralnick (Ed.): *Textbook of Oral Surgery.* Boston, Little, Brown and Co., 1968, Chapter 19, pp. 285–315.

Montgomery, W. W.: Ears, Nose and Throat. In R. D. Judge and G. D. Zuidema (Eds.): *Physical Diagnosis,* 2nd ed. Boston, Little, Brown and Co., 1963, Chapter 8, pp. 113–129.

2

Introduction to Sinus Surgery

INDICATIONS FOR SURGERY OF THE SINUSES

As a general rule, surgical treatment is indicated for those patients with chronic sinusitis who do not respond to medical therapy. The advent of biochemotherapy and of a better understanding of sinus and intranasal physiology has been instrumental in a reduction of the frequency with which sinus surgery must be undertaken.

Routine indications for sinus surgery are:

1. Intracranial extension of infections such as meningitis, subdural abscess, or brain abscess
2. Persistent pain and/or purulent discharge which has not responded to conservative therapy
3. Necrosis of the sinus wall as shown by fistula formation
4. Mucocele or pyocele formation
5. Orbital cellulitis or retrobulbar neuritis
6. Venous sinus thrombosis.

The objective of surgical treatment of a sinus is either to (1) provide free and easy drainage from the sinus into the nose (while at the same time not interfering with intranasal physiology); or (2) eliminate the sinus (obliteration). Before resorting to any of the radical sinus procedures it is most often preferable to perform simple intranasal operations in order to establish better drainage. Such operations as submucous resection of the nasal septum, removal of nasal polyps, resection of the anterior half of the middle turbinate, intranasal antrostomy, and intranasal ethmoidectomy are often sufficient to effect a cure.

COMPLICATIONS OF SINUS DISEASE

Orbital Manifestations of Sinus Disease

The paranasal sinuses might also be referred to as the paraorbital sinuses, for the orbit is surrounded (except laterally) by these sinuses (Fig. 2.1). The first indication of sinus disease is often manifested by orbital symptoms.

Orbital Pain. Generalized headache is not a usual manifestation of sinus disease, whereas pain in or above the orbit is a common symptom of this malady.

Pain in the eye may be the presenting complaint in a patient with acute maxillary sinusitis. Orbital pain is a less common complaint associated with chronic maxillary sinusitis. Benign and malignant tumors which extend through the roof of the antrum may cause orbital pain.

Acute frontal sinusitis frequently produces orbital pain. Pain elicited by palpation of the floor of the frontal sinus just posterior to the medial aspect of the supraorbital rim is indicative of such infection. Orbital pain is increased if the infection extends into the orbit, either directly through the floor of the frontal sinus or by phlebitis. Chronic frontal sinusitis and benign and malignant tumors may, if they extend into or in the direction of the orbit, also produce orbital pain.

Orbital pain is an early manifestation of acute ethmoiditis. This is, of course, increased with the onset of orbital cellulitis or abscess. Chronic ethmoiditis does not usually produce orbital pain unless the disease extends in the direction of the orbit. Benign and malignant tumors of the ethmoid may produce orbital pain.

Acute and chronic sphenoiditis produce pain which the patient describes as being behind the eye(s). Extension of disease beyond the confines of the sphenoid sinus, whether the disease be inflammatory or neoplastic, may produce severe retrobulbar pain.

Exophthalmos. Exophthalmos is a protrusion of the eyeball from the orbit. It is usually a manifestation of a disease other than that of sinus origin.

Acute and chronic maxillary sinusitis are rarely complicated by exophthalmos unless infection has extended by means of phlebitis into the retrobulbar space.

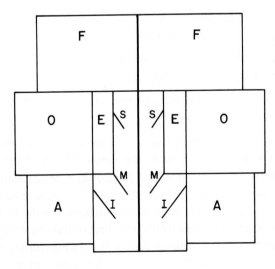

FIGURE 2.1. *Box sketch showing the relationship of the sinuses to the orbit and nasal cavity.*

A = antrum
O = orbit
F = frontal sinus
E = ethmoid cells
I = inferior turbinate
M = middle turbinate
S = superior turbinate

Cystic lesions of the maxillary sinus include mucocele, dentigerous cyst, dermoid cyst, and cystadenoma. Any of these lesions may expand so as to destroy the roof of the antrum and extend into the orbit, thus producing exophthalmos. The pressure exerted in the direction of the orbit may also cause a ptosis of the upper lid which is produced by a restriction of elevation of the upper lid. Epiphora may accompany this proptosis. Diplopia results from the upward displacement of the orbital contents. On occasion, the lesion may be palpated posterior to the infra-orbital rim. Malignant lesions of the maxillary sinus which occur high in the sinus will cause early destruction of the roof of the antrum and extend into the orbit, producing exophthalmos. Malignant lesions which have their origins elsewhere in the antrum may also extend into the orbit. In these cases the prognosis is poor because, as a rule, the disease has also spread in other directions such as through the posterior wall of the antrum into the pharyngomaxillary fossa. A fracture of the maxilla rarely produces exophthalmos, but exophthalmos does occur, however, in association with certain tripod fractures (see Fig. 7.9).

Acute and chronic ethmoiditis may produce exophthalmos as a result of extension of infection through the lamina papyracea. This will be discussed under the headings "Orbital Cellulitis and Abscess" and "Cavernous Sinus Thrombosis." Tumors of the ethmoid sinuses are not common. They extend in the direction of least resistance, which is the lamina papyracea, thus causing outward and lateral displacement of the orbital contents. The most common benign lesions of the ethmoid sinus are mucoceles, osteomas, papillomas, and fibromas. Primary carcinoma of the ethmoid is unusual. A fracture of the ethmoid labyrinth and lamina papyracea may cause a degree of proptosis following nose-blowing. The subcutaneous emphysema of the lids is indicative of fracture.

Acute or chronic frontal sinusitis may extend into the orbit by way of the floor of the frontal sinus with resultant cellulitis and orbital abscess attended with proptosis. Other diseases of a frontal sinus may penetrate through the orbital roof and cause displacement of the orbital contents in an outward and downward direction. The upper lid may be involved in an inflammatory process, or a mass may be palpated between the upper lid and the supraorbital rim. The two most common tumors of the frontal sinus causing displacement of the orbital contents are mucocele and osteoma. The progression of downward and outward displacement of the orbital contents by either of these lesions can be very slow and insidious. The displacement can also have a rapid onset if the mucocele becomes infected (pyocele) or if the osteoma becomes complicated by acute frontal sinusitis. Other benign lesions and malignant lesions of the frontal sinuses are rare, but, when present, they also may produce exophthalmos by extension through the floor of the frontal sinus.

Acute and chronic sphenoiditis, cystic (mucocele) and solid benign tumors, and primary or secondary carcinomas of the sphenoid sinus may extend into the retrobulbar area and produce exophthalmos simply by occupying space or by interfering with the venous return from the orbit. These conditions are usually also accompanied by interference with the nerves and blood vessels entering the orbit as manifested by visual defects and extraocular muscular dysfunction. There have been numerous reports of metastatic lesions of the sphenoid sinuses with orbital complications. These malignant lesions may arise in the nasal cavity, nasopharynx, other sinuses, intracranial spaces (pituitary), and distant points, such as the bowel, or kidney.

Enophthalmos. Enophthalmos is a recession of the eyeball into the orbit. It may result from contractures following orbital cellulitis, orbital and sinus operations, orbital injuries, and fractures of the orbital walls.

The blow-out fracture is a relatively common cause of enophthalmos. This is a fracture of the floor of the orbit with prolapse of the orbital contents into the antrum. There may be also a fracture and medial displacement of the lamina papyracea with prolapse of the orbital contents into the ethmoid labyrinth. Varying degrees of interference with ocular motility may accompany these fractures when the extraocular muscles (especially inferior rectus and inferior oblique) are trapped between the bony fragments. This situation requires immediate surgical intervention.

Two cases of enophthalmos resulting from mucocele of the maxillary antrum have been reported (Montgomery, 1964). The pathogenesis is not absolutely clear. It is assumed that the mucocele expands, destroying the roof of the antrum by pressure, and that the enophthalmos occurs with subsequent rupture and partial evacuation of the mucocele.

Lid Swelling. Inflammatory edema of the eyelids may occur with acute maxillary, ethmoid, or frontal sinusitis. This edema is soft with no point of tenderness or localization such as that found in acute meibomian gland infection. Ocular motility and vision are not affected. If the inflammatory process extends into the orbit from the sinuses, this inflammatory edema may become more severe as orbital cellulitis progresses. As a general rule, the upper lid is more swollen with frontal than with ethmoid or maxillary sinusitis. Both upper and lower lids are swollen with ethmoiditis, and the lower lid may be more swollen than the upper with extension of infection from the maxillary sinus.

Mass in the Orbit. A mass palpated in the orbit may be the first sign of sinus disease. A mass in the region of the infraorbital rim may represent extension of disease from the maxillary sinus. The most common diseases of the antrum producing a mass behind the infraorbital rim are carcinoma, mucocele, and osteoma of the maxillary sinus. A mass medial to the inner canthus may indicate a disease in the ethmoid sinuses, the most common being carcinoma, mucocele, and osteoma. A mass behind the supraorbital rim may indicate disease extending through the floor of the frontal sinus; the lesions most commonly responsible are mucocele, pyocele, osteoma, chronic inflammatory process, recurrent or persistent disease following the Lynch frontal sinus procedure (which entails removal of the floor of the frontal sinus), and carcinoma of the frontal sinus.

Epiphora. A prolonged inflammatory process of the nasal mucosa is said to cause epiphora, either by stenosis of the nasal lacrimal duct or by obstruction of the orifice in the inferior meatus. It is also within the realm of possibility that an inflammatory process could extend from the ethmoid sinuses to the lacrimal sac. Epiphora may also accompany exophthalmos of sinus origin.

Orbital Cellulitis and Abscess. An inflammatory process may extend from any of the paranasal sinuses into the orbit by direct extension through the bony wall or by way of the venous circulation. At first there is an inflammatory edema of the lid(s). As the disease progresses, there is exophthalmos, chemosis of the conjunctiva, and progressive immobility of the eye. There also may be some interference with the vision. At this point the patient is usually quite ill and has a high fever and severe pain. X rays of the sinuses should be taken to determine the origin of infection. Although the ethmoid sinus is the most common site of origin, the infection may stem from any of the other sinuses. Treatment should be vigorous because of the danger of extension of the infection into the intracranial spaces, producing such complications as meningitis and cavernous sinus thrombosis.

It is often difficult to determine whether or not an orbital abscess is present unless obvious fluctuation can be palpated. As a general rule, if the condition is not responding to intensive therapy, an exploratory operation should be performed in which the orbit is approached through a frontoethmoidectomy incision. The orbital periosteum is carefully elevated posteriorly, superiorly, and laterally. Since many orbital abscesses are extensions from a chronic ethmoiditis or acute exacerbation thereof, a point of breakthrough may be found in the lamina papyracea. In such cases, it is wise to perform an external ethmoidectomy simultaneously with exploration of the orbit and drainage of the orbital abscess. If an abscess is found, it should be drained for at least four days.

Cavernous Sinus Thrombosis. Cavernous sinus thrombosis can be a fatal disease, even when all modern therapeutic tools are utilized. It is sometimes difficult to differentiate between cavernous sinus thrombosis and orbital cellulitis or abscess. In addition to the signs for orbital cellulitis described above, a dilation of the retinal veins and edema of the optic disk may be found with cavernous sinus thrombosis. Intermittent rises of temperature to 104° or 105°F following a chill should make one suspicious of this complication. A blood culture and examination of the spinal fluid are indicated. The physician should be on the lookout for signs of meningitis.

Involvement of Optic Nerve. Approximately 15% of cases of retrobulbar neuritis are said to be caused by sinus disease. This is not surprising since the optic nerve may be in close relationship to the sphenoid, ethmoid, and maxillary sinuses, depending on their degree of pneumatization. The inflammatory process may spread directly through the sinus wall or by phlebitis. The loss of vision may be of sudden or gradual onset. The therapy consists in administration of antibiotics and specific surgery of the involved sinus. Benign and malignant tumors of the sinuses, as well as of the pituitary gland, can cause blindness or defects in the visual fields.

Superior Orbital Fissure Syndrome. The third, fourth, and sixth cranial nerves, the first division of the fifth cranial nerve, the ophthalmic vein, and sympathetic nerves from the cavernous plexus may become involved in disease of the sphenoid sinus. The lateral wall of this sinus, if well pneumatized, is in very close proximity to the superior orbital fissure. An acute or chronic inflammatory process may extend from the sphenoid sinus to this region. Cystic lesions, such as a mucocele or a craniopharyngioma, benign neoplasms, and primary or secondary malignant disease of the sphenoid sinus may be complicated by a superior orbital fissure syndrome. Any or all of the structures passing through the superior orbital fissure may be affected by the disease processes. The sixth cranial nerve is usually implicated first, with subsequent involvement of the third, fourth, and fifth nerves. As the disease progresses the fifth cranial nerve is affected, as manifested by pain in the eye and forehead. This is followed by exophthalmos and, finally, total ophthalmoplegia. X rays of the sinuses should include laminography of the sphenoid sinuses. Treatment consists in immediate exploration by means of the transethmoid approach to the sphenoid sinus (see p. 78).

Osteomyelitis of the Frontal Bone

Etiology. In the great majority of the reported cases of osteomyelitis of the frontal bone the organism recovered is the Staphylococcus aureus. The streptococcus, pneumococcus, and anaerobic streptococcus are found in a few instances. The degree of involvement depends to a certain extent upon the virulence of the organism and the resistance or immunity of the patient to the particular bacteria present.

In children the origin of osteomyelitis of the frontal bone is almost always hematogenous; in adults the disease is more likely to result from trauma during an episode of acute frontal sinusitis. The majority of the patients are under 30 years of age. The disease is more common in females than in males and in many instances follows swimming. Chronic infection of the sinuses, especially an acute exacerbation of the infection, may predispose to osteomyelitis. Trauma in the region of the frontal sinus or an operation upon the frontal sinus frequently precedes the advent of the osteomyelitis.

Symptoms. The clinical course may be acute or chronic.

In the acute fulminating type, fever, headache, and edema of the upper eyelid on the affected side are present. The soft, doughy swelling (Pott's puffy tumor) or pericranial abscess is pathognomonic of osteomyelitis of the underlying bone. This type frequently follows swimming. Spread to the intracranial structures is not unusual. As a rule, however, osteomyelitis is a slowly progressive disease, even in the acute stage.

The chronic localized form of frontal bone osteomyelitis, without perforation of the internal table, is usually characterized by an insidious onset, a low-grade fever, local pain or tenderness, doughy swelling of the forehead, general malaise, and, occasionally, chills. Fistulas may form, and sequestra may separate from the bone during cyclic exacerbations.

Diagnosis. The diagnosis is made by means of roentgenogram combined with the signs and symptoms of fluctuating swellings, advancing edema, persistent low-grade temperature, leukocytosis, and pain and headache with cyclic exacerbation.

According to Mosher and Judd, the edema of the soft tissue of the forehead is the first sign of infection of the periosteum and the medulla of the frontal bone. This edema, in the past, was a practical guide to the extent of bone to be removed. X rays do not show positive change until necrosis is present and this is not apparent until 7 to 10 days after forehead edema appears. If antibiotics have been administered the clinical correlation just described does not hold true, for the edema of the forehead is no longer an index of the degree of osteomyelitis and, in fact, may not be present.

Treatment. Antibiotics, selected in accordance with bacteriologic sensitivity tests, should be given intravenously in large doses. Any localized abscess should be drained. If x rays show that the frontal sinus(es) contains pus, a trephine operation of the frontal sinus(es) should be carried out, both for inspection of the interior of the sinus(es) and to obtain purulent secretions for culture and antibiotic sensitivity tests. Usually the antibiotic of choice is penicillin. This should be administered intravenously and local therapy, such as application of heat, nasal spray, and systemic decongestants, should be instituted.

If there is not rapid reversal of the osteomyelitic process or if there is any question regarding involvement of the posterior wall of the frontal sinus, surgical intervention in the early course of therapy is indicated. If, on the other hand, the patient continues to show improvement, manifested both clinically and radiologically, the antibiotic therapy is continued for approximately 10 days.

After the osteomyelitis has been controlled by surgical drainage and antibiotic therapy, attention should then be directed more specifically to the frontal sinuses. If there is any question of persistent or chronic frontal sinusitis, a bilateral osteoplastic adipose obliteration operation (see p. 141) should be carried out. A more conservative approach is contraindicated, for a complication such as an extradural abscess could subsequently result. At the time of the osteoplastic operation any diseased bone is removed, and the sinus(es) is obliterated by insertion of subcutaneous abdominal adipose tissue. Antibiotic therapy is continued for at least 10 days following this operation.

The radical procedures which were most often necessary in the past for the treatment of osteomyelitis of the frontal bone are, for the most part, no longer necessary, if the proper antibiotics are administered in adequate doses. The operations advocated by Mosher and Judd are now procedures of the past.

On occasion it is necessary to remove a portion of devitalized bone. The resulting defect can be repaired by using an autogenous osseous autograft or a plastic implant. Since regeneration of bone is often a very slow process, this reconstructive procedure should not be attempted for many months following removal of the devitalized bone.

Osteomyelitis of the Superior Maxilla

Acute osteomyelitis of the superior maxilla is usually secondary to an infection of dental origin. In infants, it is occasionally secondary to a buccal infection. Involvement of the dental sac follows with extension of the necrotic process to the walls of the maxillary antrum, resulting in a purulent discharge into the nose and mouth. Lederer believes that the associated acute osteomyelitis is a result of the venous infection. He bases his opinion upon carefully studied serial sections from an infant in whom a nasal infection and sinusitis were found to be the primary cause of the osteomyelitis of the maxilla.

Osteomyelitis of the maxilla in nurslings and infants may occur from the first week following birth up to the ninth month. The highest incidence is during the first three weeks. The portal of entry and the manner of spreading of the primary infection may vary.

As shown by Lederer a sinusitis may produce a periosteitis and osteitis with a fistulous tract formation which extends in any one of three ways: (1) to the facial surface with swelling of the soft parts of the cheek, breaking down of Bichat's pad, and abscess formation; (2) to the palatine and alveolar process with a fistula into the roof of the mouth; (3) to the zygomatic process with a necrosis of the zygomatic arch and extension into the pterygoid fossa with abscess formation. Extension along the fascial planes to the mandibular foramen may occur. An ethmoiditis may result in a periosteitis, osteitis, and periorbital cellulitis which may extend in one or both of two ways: (1) thrombophlebitis of the venous channels, with extension to the cavernous sinus and the production of a thrombosis; (2) a periorbital abscess, with an occasional complicating external fistula.

Symptoms. The signs and symptoms are those of a sinusitis accompanied by marked swelling and chemosis of the cheek. Exophthalmos with limitation of movement of the eye may be present.

The first or septicemic stage may last for about 10 days with the formation of fistulas in the infraorbital regions, palate, and, in rare instances, into the nose. This is followed by a chronic indolent stage with persistent fistulas and sequestration of dead bone. This second stage is not seen if antibiotics, proper drainage, and local therapy are instituted early in the course of the disease.

Treatment. Treatment consists of administration of large doses of specific antibiotics, surgical establishment of free drainage, and local application of heat. On occasion there is considerable loss of bone from osteomyelitis of the superior maxilla and a resultant large oroantral fistula, which can be repaired by using the various techniques outlined in Chapter 6 (pp. 219–227).

Osteomyelitis of the Sphenoid Bone

Osteomyelitis of the sphenoid bone is quite rare. Many of the reported cases have been associated with osteomyelitis of the base of the skull or secondary to an infection of the petrous portion of the temporal bone. Eagleton attributes the rarity of infection of the base of the sphenoid to the preponderance of red cellular bone marrow found throughout life in this bone.

The organisms usually recovered are hemolytic streptococcus and beta hemolytic Staphylococcus aureus. The early symptoms consist in a rather profuse postnasal discharge and a deep-seated headache described as being either in the center of the head or behind the eyes, which on occasion radiates to the temporal or occipital regions. Infection may spread laterally to the retrobulbar region, producing any of the various manifestations described in this chapter under the heading "Superior Orbital Fissure Syndrome."

Later, as the body of the sphenoid becomes more extensively invaded, symptoms of sepsis ensue, although the temperature may be low and the toxemia not marked. The retro-orbital and temporal pain becomes especially severe. There may be, at this time, bacterial invasion of the meninges and bloodstream. Cavernous sinus thrombosis, brain abscess, encephalitis, and intracranial hemorrhage may result.

Treatment. Osteomyelitis of the sphenoid bone is frequently not diagnosed until severe complications, which can be fatal, have developed. Careful x-ray examination of the sphenoid bone, including laminography, is imperative. The patient should also be followed closely by an ophthalmologist and neurologist. Treatment is essentially that of antibiotic therapy and surgical drainage.

Intracranial Complications of Sinus Disease

The modern otolaryngologist should be constantly on the lookout for intracranial complications of sinus disease. Most of these complications are readily apparent by their clinical manifestations. On the other hand, others have a slow, insidious onset which makes the diagnosis quite difficult.

The possible intracranial complications from disease of the nasal passages and sinuses are meningitis, extradural and subdural abscess, dural fistula, the various types of brain abscesses, and septic thrombosis of the cavernous or superior longitudinal sinus (the other venous sinuses are rarely involved in infections of the nasal sinuses). Meningitis which has its origin from sinusitis is more frequently observed than thrombosis of the venous sinuses.

Intracranial complications are more apt to result from acute infections of the sinuses than from chronic infections. These complications are more common in males than in females (4 to 1).

All infected sinuses may give rise to an intracranial complication, but an extension from a maxillary sinusitis is rare. Courville and Rosenvold state that a maxillary sinusitis of dental origin is more apt to provoke intracranial suppurative lesions than is maxillary sinusitis of any other type.

Infections from the nose or sinuses may invade the intracranial structures (1) after trauma; (2) through congenital dehiscences or nonclosure of fetal defects; (3) by a direct pathway through the sinus wall; (4) along the sheaths of the olfactory nerves; (5) by way of the communicating veins; (6) by means of septic thrombi along the diploetic veins with a retrograde thrombophlebitis or periphlebitis to the cavernous sinus; (7) by way of the angular or ethmoid veins to the cavernous sinus; or (8) by way of the orbit. There has been some question as to the possibility of a direct extension of an infection of the sinuses to the intracranial structures by way of the lymphatic vessels.

Temporal lobe abscesses most commonly originate from infection in the temporal bone and lateral dural sinus. A temporal lobe abscess can originate from the sphenoid sinus or indirectly from the other sinuses by way of the cavernous sinus. Frontal lobe abscesses may complicate acute or chronic frontal sinusitis or tumors of the frontal sinus (such as osteoma), following surgical treatment of frontal or ethmoid sinus or trauma to the forehead.

Frontal Sinus Pneumocele

A pneumocele (pneumatocele) is a collection of air, under pressure, in the tissues. The air usually escapes from a defect in the bony wall of the frontal sinus and collects adjacent to the sinus. If the defect is on the forehead, an external pneumocele results. If the defect is in the posterior wall of the frontal sinus, an internal or intracranial pneumocele is present.

A pneumocele may follow fracture, trauma, operation, congenital cleft, dehiscence, or necrosis of the bone. The latter may be due to syphilis, osteomyelitis, or sinusitis. Cases have been reported as secondary to, or associated with, an osteoma of the frontal sinus.

The sinus mucous membrane or frontal periosteum is intact over the bony defect, so that a ballooning of the mucosa or periosteum occurs; this forms an air sac when under pressure from blowing the nose, coughing, or sneezing. A pneumocele may occur in connection with a mucocele of the frontal sinus if air takes the place of the fluid contents and there is a connection from the nasal cavity to a defect in the mucocele.

In addition to the external and internal pneumoceles, a third type, characterized by an excessive dilation of the sinus (pneumosinus dilatans), may occur. Dilation of the sinus is usually associated with acromegaly or localized osteitis, or follows fractures in the region of the sinuses. Enlargement of the sinus is more apt to result if the bone changes occur before the sinuses are fully developed. Any of the sinuses may be involved on one or both sides. The exact mechanism by which the dilation occurs is not understood.

REFERENCES

Courville, C. B., and Rosenvold, L. K.: Intracranial Complications of Infections of the Nasal Cavities and Accessory Sinuses. Arch Otolaryng. *27*:692–731 (June) 1938.

Eagleton, W. P.: Meningitis—the Result of Disease of the Petrous Apex and Sphenoidal Base. Surg. Gynec. Obstet. *60*:586–587 (Feb. 15) 1935.

Furstenberg, A. C.: Osteomyelitis of the Skull: Osteogenetic Processes in the Repair of Cranial Defects. Ann. Otol. *40*:996–1012 (Dec.) 1931.

Johnson, C. I.: Osteomyelitis of the frontal bone of rhinogenic origin. *Ann. Otol. 63*:180–188 (March) 1954.

Lederer, F. L.: *Diseases of the Ear, Nose, and Throat,* 6th ed. Philadelphia, F. A. Davis Co., 1953, p. 611.

Montgomery, W. W.: Mucocele of the Maxillary Sinus Causing Enophthalmos. EENT Monthly *43*:41–44 (May) 1964.

Mosher, H. P., and Judd, D. K.: An Analysis of Seven Cases of Osteomyelitis of the Frontal Bone Complicating Frontal Sinusitis. Laryngoscope *43*:3:153–212 (March) 1933.

Reinecke, R. D., and Montgomery, W. W.: Oculomotor Nerve Palsy Associated with Mucocele of the Sphenoid Sinus. Arch Ophthal. *71*:50–51 (Jan.) 1964.

3

Surgery of the Ethmoid and Sphenoid Sinuses

ETHMOIDECTOMY

Surgical Anatomy

The ethmoid bone is situated in the anterior cranium between the two orbits and the upper half of the nasal cavities. The lower two thirds of the lateral nasal wall is the medial wall of the maxillary sinus. The ethmoid bone appears to consist of crossed vertical and horizontal plates with the bony capsule of the labyrinthine cells attached to the inferior and lateral portion of the horizontal plate. The vertical plate rises slightly over the horizontal to form the crista galli, while the inferior vertical portion forms the perpendicular plate of the nasal septum (Fig. 3.1). The ethmoid bone articulates anteriorly with the frontal bone, posteriorly with the sphenoid bone, and inferiorly with the quadrangular septal cartilage and perpendicular plate of the vomer bone. The horizontal plate of the ethmoid bone, adjacent to the midline, is perforated by many foramina for the passage of the olfactory nerve endings. The cribriform plate (lamina cribrosa) articulates with the frontal bone laterally and anteriorly. Posteriorly, it is in contact with the sphenoid bone (Fig. 3.2a).

The ethmoid cells lie between the upper third of the lateral nasal wall and the medial wall of the orbit (Fig. 3.1). The number of cells varies according to the size of the cells. The attachment of the middle turbinate roughly divides the ethmoid cells into anterior and posterior groups. Thus, the ostia of the anterior

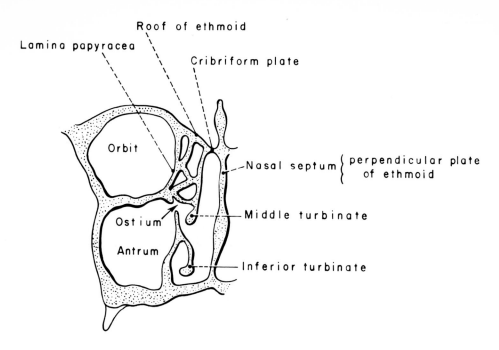

FIGURE 3.1. *Diagrammatic representation of the relationships of the orbit, maxillary antrum, ethmoid labyrinth, and nasal cavity.*

Note particularly that the medial wall of the ethmoid labyrinth is an upper extension of the attachment of the middle turbinate. The upper extension separates the roof of the ethmoid and the cribriform plate.

ethmoid cells communicate with the middle meatus, while those of the posterior ethmoid cells communicate with the superior meatus.

The ethmoid labyrinth is pyramidal in shape; it is wider posteriorly than anteriorly and wider above than below. The anterior width of the labyrinth is 0.5 to 1 cm. The posterior width is approximately 1.5 cm. The anteroposterior dimension, or length of the labyrinth, is 4 to 5 cm. The height is 2 to 2.5 cm.

The lacrimal bone forms the lateral wall of the anterior ethmoid cells, and the os planum (lamina papyracea) forms the lateral wall of the posterior ethmoid cells (Fig. 3.3). As a general rule, the outer half of the front face of the sphenoid sinus is the posterior limit of the ethmoid labyrinth.

The cribriform plate is the roof of the olfactory slit in the anterior superior nasal cavity. It is attached to the roof of the ethmoid labyrinth, which in turn joins the orbital plate of the frontal bone. The plane of the cribriform plate and roof of the ethmoid labyrinth correspond to a horizontal plane at the level of the pupils. The superior prolongation of the attachment of the middle turbinate, which forms the superolateral nasal wall, is the division between the cribriform plate and the roof of the ethmoid labyrinth (Figs. 3.1 and 3.4).

The anterior half of the ethmoid labyrinth is made up of cells which are overlaid medially by the upper anterior part of the middle turbinate (the agger nasi cells, lacrimal cells, infundibular cells, and cells of the ethmoid bulla). The posterior half of the ethmoid labyrinth is made up of cells which are overlaid medially by the upper extension of the attachment of the middle turbinate and the superior turbinate (Fig. 3.2b). The most important surgical relationships of the anterior ethmoid cells are: (1) the lacrimal bone, (2) the floor of the frontal sinus, (3) the semilunar hiatus, (4) the unciform groove, (5) the nasofrontal orifice, and (6) the

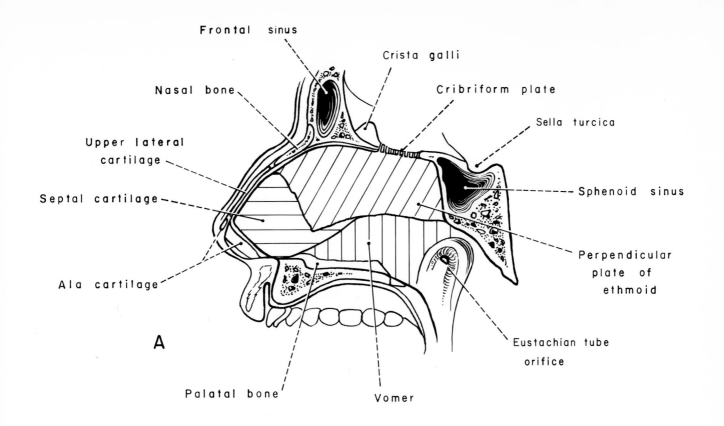

Frontal sinus

Crista galli

Nasal bone

Cribriform plate

Upper lateral cartilage

Sella turcica

Septal cartilage

Sphenoid sinus

Ala cartilage

Perpendicular plate of ethmoid

Eustachian tube orifice

Palatal bone

Vomer

A

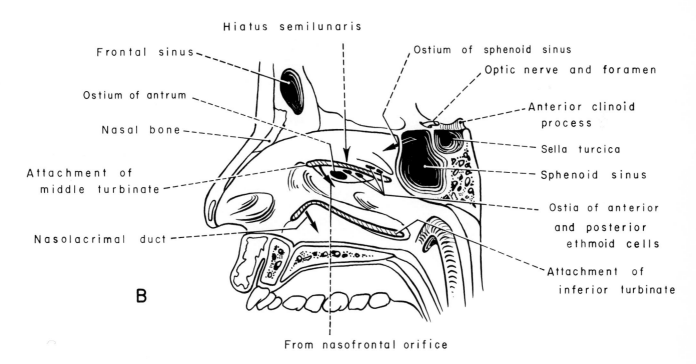

Hiatus semilunaris

Ostium of sphenoid sinus

Frontal sinus

Optic nerve and foramen

Ostium of antrum

Anterior clinoid process

Nasal bone

Sella turcica

Attachment of middle turbinate

Sphenoid sinus

Ostia of anterior and posterior ethmoid cells

Nasolacrimal duct

Attachment of inferior turbinate

B

From nasofrontal orifice

FIGURE 3.2

A. Midsagittal section showing the various components of the nasal septum, the relationship of the sphenoid sinus to the sella turcica, the cribriform plate, and crista galli.

B. The lateral wall of the nose and the middle and inferior turbinates have been removed. The nasofrontal orifice is shown in the anterior aspect of the hiatus semilunaris as are the ostia for the antrum and the anterior ethmoid cells. The posterior ethmoid cell orifices are located in the superior meatus. The nasolacrimal duct orifice is situated in the anterosuperior aspect of the inferior meatus. The sphenoid ostium is usually found in the spheno-ethmoidal recess. Also, note the relationship between the sphenoid sinus, sella turcica, anterior clinoid process, and optic foramen.

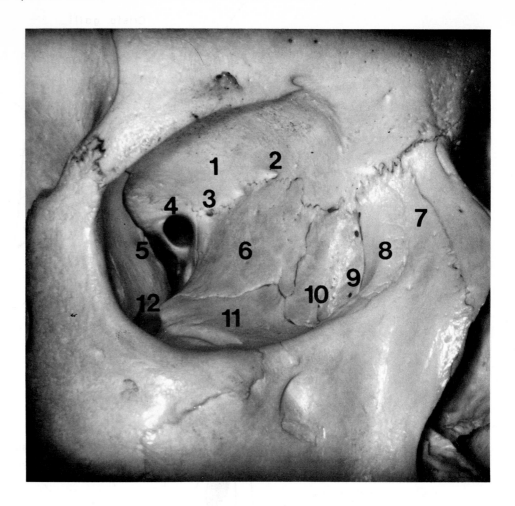

FIGURE 3.3. *The relationships of the medial wall of the orbit (also the lateral wall of the ethmoid labyrinth).*

The anterior ethmoid cells are medial to the lacrimal bone, and the posterior ethmoid cells are medial to the lamina papyracea.

The anterior and posterior ethmoid foramina indicate the level of the roof of the ethmoid and the cribriform plate fairly accurately.

1. Orbital plate of frontal bone
2 and 3. Anterior and posterior ethmoid foramina
4. Optic foramen
5. Superior orbital fissure
6. Lamina papyracea
7. Ascending process of the maxillary bone
8. Anterior lacrimal crest
9. Lacrimal fossa
10. Posterior lacrimal crest
11. Orbital plate of the maxillary bone
12. Inferior orbital fissure.

ostium of the antrum. The most important relationships of the posterior ethmoid cells are: (1) the outer half of the front wall of the sphenoid sinus, (2) the posterior half of the inner wall of the orbit (lamina papyracea), and (3) the optic nerve. The thickness of bone between the optic nerve and the posterior ethmoid cells varies between 1 mm and 5 mm. On occasion, the nerve may mound into the posterior ethmoid cells (Figs. 3.4 and 3.5).

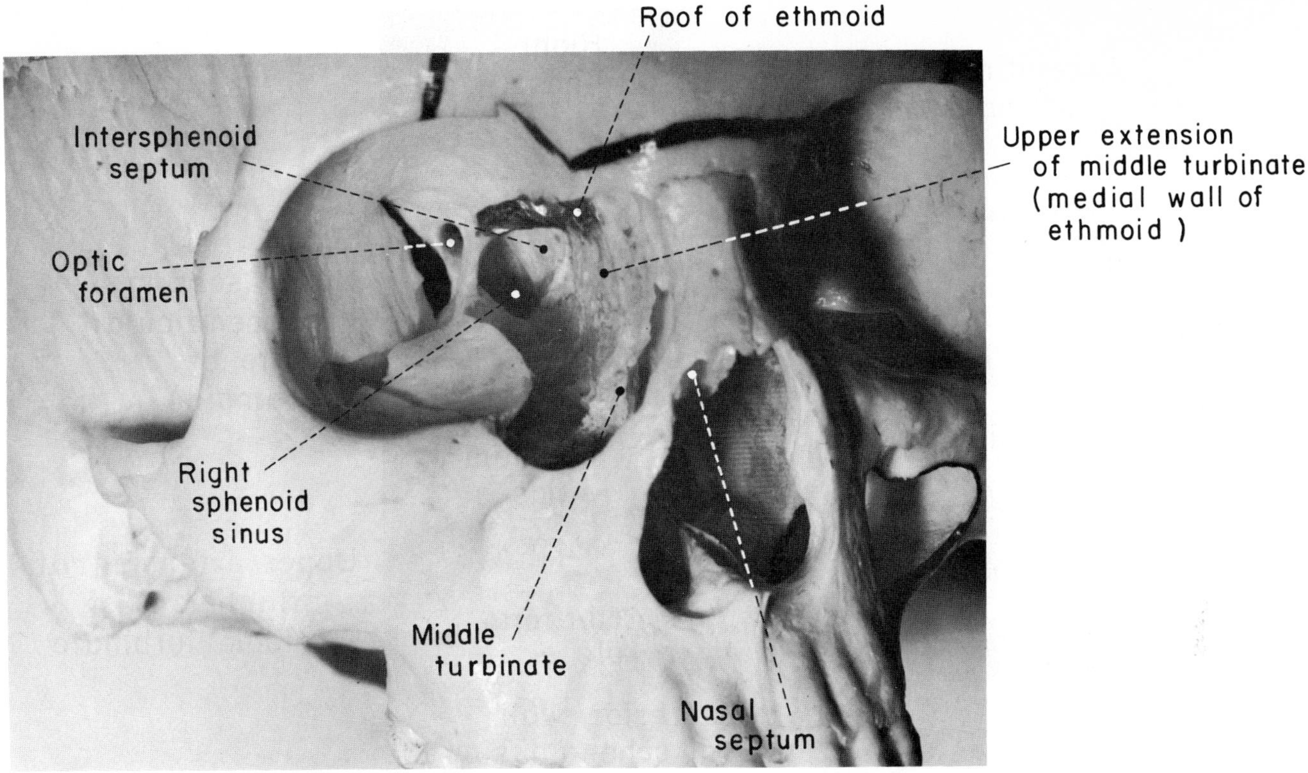

FIGURE 3.4. *The right orbit.*

A portion of the ascending process of the maxilla, the lacrimal bone, lamina papyracea, and anterior and posterior ethmoid cells have been removed. The middle turbinate and its upper extension, which forms the medial wall of the ethmoid labyrinth, remain intact. The roof of the ethmoid has been painted. The cribriform plate is not seen, for it is medial to the attachment of the upper extension of the middle turbinate and at the same level as the roof of the ethmoid. Note the close relationship between the posterior ethmoid and the optic foramen. The anterior wall of the sphenoid sinus has been removed, exposing the intersphenoid septum.

There are common extensions of both the anterior and posterior ethmoid cells. The anterior cells may extend anteriorly, upward and outward, to the inside of the ascending process of the maxilla, making a cell series with the frontal sinus (the fronto-ethmoidal cell), and medially into the turbinate, producing a cellular turbinate. The common extensions of the posterior ethmoid cells are over, or to the side of, the sphenoid sinus posteriorly, and into the antrum and the pterygoid process inferiorly.

The arterial blood supply of the ethmoid cells is through the lateral branches of the sphenopalatine artery and the anterior and posterior ethmoid arteries. The ethmoid sinus thus receives blood from both the external and internal carotid systems. The venous drainage is by way of the ophthalmic vein or pterygoid plexus. The lymphatic vessels related to the ethmoid sinuses are few in number. Most of these pass directly to the nasal mucosa.

Intranasal Ethmoidectomy

Indications. Intranasal surgery of the ethmoid labyrinth is quite effective when indicated, but has been neglected by many otolaryngologists. Chronic polypoid ethmoiditis, with or without nasal polyps, is a positive indication for this type of

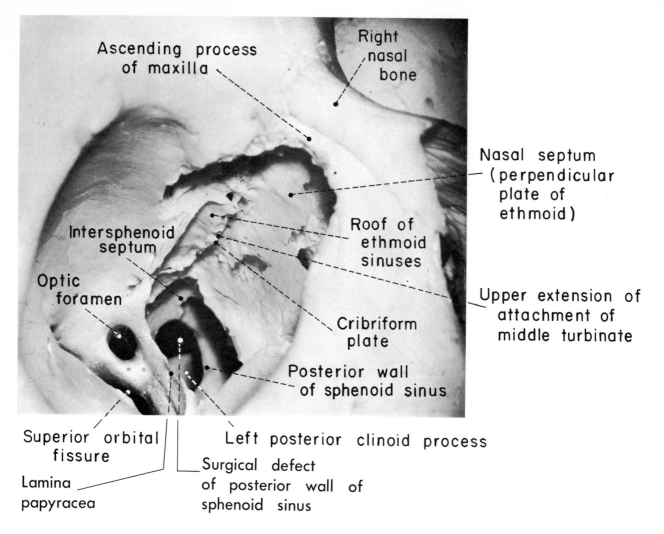

Ascending process
of maxilla

Right
nasal
bone

Nasal septum
(perpendicular
plate of
ethmoid)

Intersphenoid
septum

Roof of
ethmoid
sinuses

Optic
foramen

Upper extension of
attachment of
middle turbinate

Cribriform
plate

Posterior wall
of sphenoid sinus

Superior orbital
fissure

Left posterior clinoid process

Surgical defect
of posterior wall of
sphenoid sinus

Lamina
papyracea

FIGURE 3.5. *Completed intranasal ethmoidectomy.*

The upper extension of the attachment of the middle turbinate has been removed, leaving only a small ridge between the roof of the ethmoid and the cribriform plate. In this specimen the anterior and posterior walls of the sphenoid sinus have been removed giving a view of the left posterior clinoid process. It is important to avoid injury to the nasal mucous membrane in order to prevent postoperative synechiae in the superior nasal cavity.

operation. The eradication of chronic ethmoid infection is often sufficient to bring about a cure of chronic frontal and sphenoid infection. Even though the external ethmoidectomy provides a safer and a more thorough method of approaching the entire ethmoid labyrinth, a skillfully performed intranasal ethmoidectomy is perfectly adequate to bring about resolution of chronic polypoid ethmoiditis.

Technique of Surgery. Since the intranasal ethmoidectomy is used for the treatment of chronic polypoid ethmoid sinusitis, which almost invariably involves both ethmoid labyrinths, it is usually a bilateral procedure.

A submucous resection of the nasal septum facilitates the intranasal ethmoidectomy and is performed as a routine part of this operation by many surgeons. Each nasal cavity is packed with cotton or cottonoid strips impregnated with 1:1000 epinephrine or 4% cocaine solution. This assists in hemostasis and in providing a better view of the area to be operated upon. Polyps projecting into the nasal cavities are removed.

The patient is placed in a position of slight extension so that the middle meatus and anterior ethmoid region may be seen. The bulla and infundibulum can also be viewed unless the anatomic relationships have been distorted by disease. A sharp curette is used for penetration into the anterior ethmoid labyrinth in the region of the bulla. Sharp, angulated, looped curettes are employed to remove the anterior ethmoid cells; if the bleeding is troublesome, the anterior ethmoid labyrinth is packed with epinephrine-impregnated gauze strips. The anterior ethmoid cells on the contralateral side are then removed in like manner.

The anterior one half or two thirds of the middle turbinate must be removed in order to gain access to the posterior ethmoid cells. The attachment of the middle turbinate is cut with turbinate scissors (or straight or slightly curved scissors). The turbinate is then transected, at the desired location, with a wire snare or a right-angled scissors. If bleeding is profuse, epinephrine-impregnated gauze strips are inserted for its control.

The posterior ethmoid cells lie behind the attachment of the middle turbinate. At times, the middle turbinate cannot be recognized as such, having been chewed away during repeated intranasal polypectomies. In such cases, the posterior ethmoid cells must be dissected with extreme care. On occasion, after the middle turbinate or a portion thereof has been removed, the attachment cannot be identified because of destruction by disease. In such cases, the relative position of the posterior ethmoid cells can be fairly well judged, since the anterior portion of the turbinate has just been removed. A ring curette is inserted into the posterior ethmoid cells. By gentle curettage and with a knowledge of the approximate dimensions of the area, the limits of the posterior ethmoid cells can be precisely outlined. Debris (bone, polyps, etc.) is best removed with either Brownie* or Takahashi forceps. Bleeding may be profuse at this point. It is well to remember that it can be controlled by repeated packing accompanied by patience. The posterior limit of the ethmoid labyrinth is the anterior wall of the sphenoid sinus. If indicated, the sphenoid sinus can be entered, diseased tissue removed, and a portion of the anterior wall resected in order to establish drainage. The close relationship of the optic canal to the lateral aspect of the posterior ethmoid cells must be clearly kept in mind during this dissection.

Packing. Bleeding is usually well controlled by the time all ethmoid cells have been removed. On the other hand, there is a somewhat significant incidence of postoperative epistaxis following intranasal ethmoidectomy. Some surgeons prefer not to use packing until bleeding becomes apparent. Others pack the ethmoid area routinely. A favorite packing is 1-inch iodoform gauze impregnated with Aureomycin ointment. Approximately 24 inches of this packing are inserted into each ethmoid defect and held in place by a finger-cot packing inserted into each nasal cavity.

Postoperative Care. The finger-cot packing is removed on the first postoperative day. The ethmoid packing remains in place for from 3 to 5 days. Systemic antibiotic therapy, as prescribed by laboratory sensitivity tests, is usually instituted following intranasal ethmoidectomy.

Usually the patient can be discharged from the hospital on the fifth or sixth postoperative day. The intranasal spaces are not disturbed during the first postoperative week except for possible gentle cleansing executed with suction or forceps. A medicated oily spray may be used during the first few postoperative weeks in

---

*Manufactured by Richards Mfg. Co.

order to soften the crusts. It is most important that the patient be examined two weeks following this operation in order that any intranasal synechiae which may have formed will be detected and treated. When synechiae are present they are anesthetized with topical anesthesia and disrupted. A small piece of double-faced Telfa gauze can be inserted to prevent their re-formation. The patient will experience dryness and repeated crust formation for a number of weeks following the intranasal ethmoidectomy. If he is warned of this, he will be more ready to accept the discomfort as due to the normal process of healing.

External Ethmoidectomy

Indications. External ethmoidectomy is indicated for those patients with acute ethmoiditis who do not respond to antibiotic therapy and have redness, swelling, and fluctuation over the ethmoid sinuses, as well as chronic ethmoid infection. Extension of the purulent infection into the orbital cavity with a resultant orbital abscess is also an indication for this operation. Mucocele, pyocele, and tumors of the ethmoid must be approached by way of the external route.

With the presence of pain in the region of the ethmoid sinus and a palpable mass in the region of the medial aspect of the orbit and/or ptosis, mucocele of the ethmoid sinus should be considered with the differential diagnosis. Routine sinus x rays will most often confirm this diagnosis (Fig. 3.6a).

A mucocele of the ethmoid sinus can be a difficult diagnostic problem. There may be a history of pain, tenderness, and a swelling in the medial aspect of the orbit. If these signs and symptoms are intermittent, they may not be present at the time of examination by the physician. Routine x rays of the sinuses can be normal with the presence of a fairly large ethmoidal mucocele (Fig. 3.7a). Polytomography of the ethmoid sinus is an essential part of this workup, both to make the diagnosis and to outline the extent of an ethmoidal mucocele (Figs. 3.6b, 3.7b). Ultrasonography will demonstrate an orbital mass if the lamina papyracea has been displaced laterally. CT body scanning will show the presence of an ethmoidal mucocele (Fig. 3.8).

Mucocele of the ethmoid sinus is removed using the external ethmoid operation (Fig. 3.9). The entire ethmoid labyrinth should be resected along with the middle turbinate and its upper extension (medial wall of the ethmoid). Otherwise there is a significant chance for recurrence of the mucocele. The external ethmoidectomy also provides the route for external frontal sinus surgery (the Lynch procedure) and an approach to the sphenoid sinus and to the pituitary gland.

Technique of Surgery. Proper positioning of the patient's head for an external ethmoidectomy is imperative. The plane of the patient's face should be facing and exactly parallel to the ceiling, while the back of the head rests in a donut-type head support. The patient's entire face, including the eyelids, is prepared using povidone-iodine soap and povidone-iodine solution. The face is scrubbed twice with this soap and each time is rinsed thoroughly using sterile water. Following the last rinse, the skin is dried diligently using sponges. The face is then carefully painted with povidone-iodine solution. After this solution dries, three towels are placed so as to leave exposed both eyes and nose (Fig. 3.10). The towels are stitched together using #3-0 silk suture on a straight Keith needle. The lids of both eyes are sutured together using #5-0 monofilament polyethylene suture material. The area to be used for the external ethmoidectomy incision is carefully infiltrated with 1%

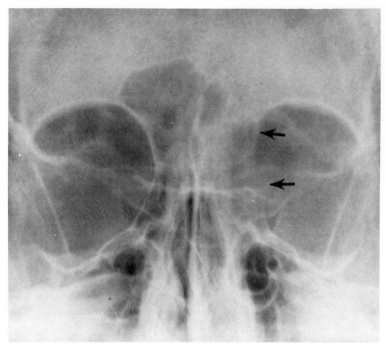

a

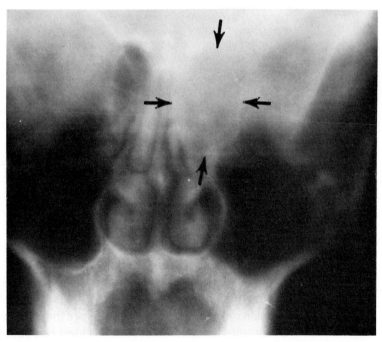

b

FIGURE 3.6.

a. A 36-year-old female presented with left exophthalmos of 7 months' duration. There was no history of pain. A non-tender smooth mass could be palpated in the medial aspect of the left orbit. Visual acuity was normal. The left eye was myopic by 3 mm as compared to the right. Routine sinus x rays clearly show the presence of a mucocele (arrows).

b. A polytome cut through the left ethmoid sinus is also consistent with the diagnosis of ethmoidal mucocele.

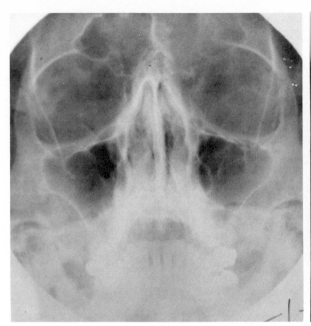

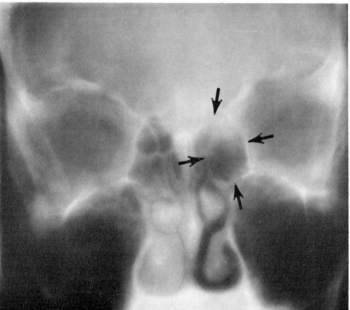

a   b

FIGURE 3.7.

　　a. Repeated routine sinus x rays are normal in this case of a 33-year-old male with 14 years' history of intermittent pain and proptosis of the left eye. He remained sign and symptom free between these exacerbations.

　　b. Polytomography demonstrates lateral displacement of the medial wall of the orbit (arrow) and evidence of a mucocele of the left ethmoid sinus.

Xylocaine with added epinephrine. A half-sheet is applied over the upper chest such that the long ends cover each side of the table. An A-sheet is used as a second layer to cover the entire patient with the exception of the exposed portion of the face (Fig. 3.10). Several half-inch strips of cottonoid or cotton, impregnated with 4% cocaine solution, are used to pack the entire nasal cavity on the side of surgery. The purpose of this packing is to decongest the nasal mucous membrane and reduce its vascularity. The number of cottonoid, cotton, and gauze strips must be counted before, during, and after surgery.

　　There should be an interval of at least 10 minutes between the Xylocaine-epinephrine infiltration and the skin incision. A slightly curved vertical incision approximately 2 to 3 cm in length is made halfway between the inner canthus and the dorsum of the nose (Fig. 3.11). Care is taken to make the initial incision through the skin only. Subcutaneous tissues are then carefully dissected layer by layer using a mosquito-type hemostat so that vessels can be identified, divided, and cauterized. Bipolar cautery is preferred in order to avoid the postoperative subcutaneous thickening that occurs when more than a few catgut ligatures are applied.

　　The periosteum should be exposed along the entire length of the incision before it is incised. The periosteum is elevated in an antromedial direction exposing the ascending process of the maxilla and the suture line between this structure and the nasal bone using a sharp, flat-end periosteal elevator such as is used during mastoidectomy surgery. This same instrument is used to elevate the periosteum in a posterolateral direction until the anterior crest of the lacrimal bone is identified.

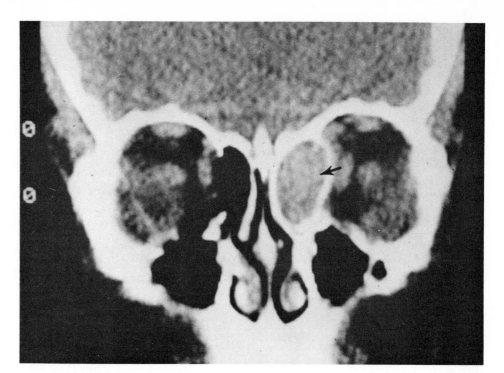

a

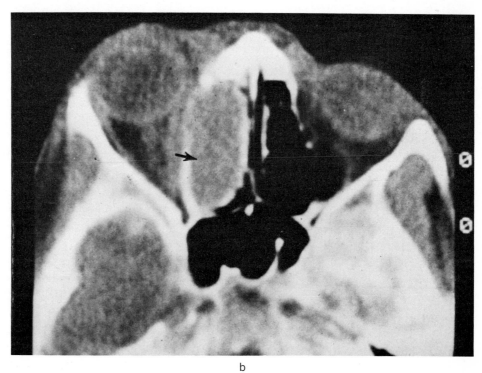

b

FIGURE 3.8. *A CT body scan demonstrating the outline of an ethmoid mucocele (arrows).*

a. Coronal plane
b. Horizontal plane

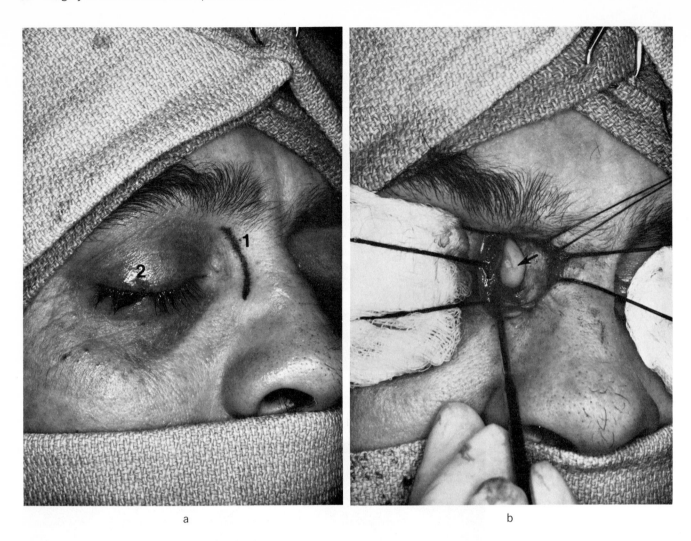

a   b

FIGURE 3.9.

   a. The incision used to approach the mucocele of the ethmoid is identical to that for the external ethmoidectomy operation.
   1. Incision for external ethmoidectomy
   2. Eyelid suture
   b. A mucocele (arrow) has been dissected from the ethmoid sinus and is being removed intact.

Retraction of the incision is necessary at this point. Many self-retaining retractors designed for this purpose are, in my opinion, bulky and cumbersome. Excellent retraction can be accomplished by using three #00 chromic catgut sutures on a taper needle on each side (Fig. 3.12). The needle is introduced in the subcutaneous tissues and then through the margin of the periosteum, which has been elevated. These sutures are weighted by using heavy hemostats and, to protect the eyes, are placed over a folded four-by-four sponge or eyepad. The hemostats are allowed to hang so that they exert traction.

A more blunt and curve-ended periosteal elevator (such as a McKenty or Freer) is used to elevate the periosteum over the anterior lacrimal crest, lacrimal fossa, and posterior lacrimal crest. In so doing, the lacrimal sac, which is in continuity with the orbital periosteum, is carefully dissected laterally. The nasal

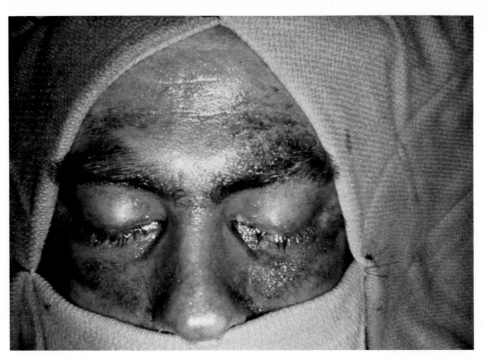

a

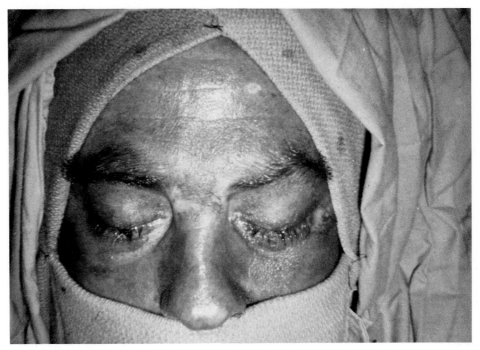

b

FIGURE 3.10.

    a. Three towels are placed so as to leave exposed the lower forehead, both eyes, and the nose.

    b. A large A-sheet is used as the second layer to cover the entire patient with the exception of the exposed portion of the face.

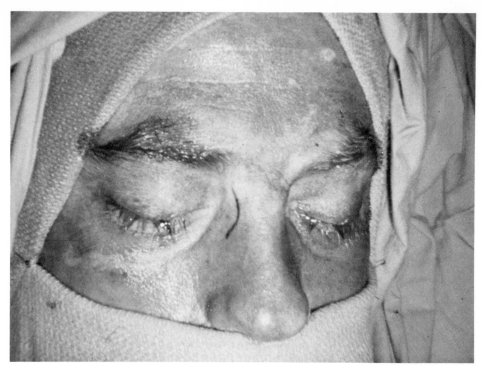

a

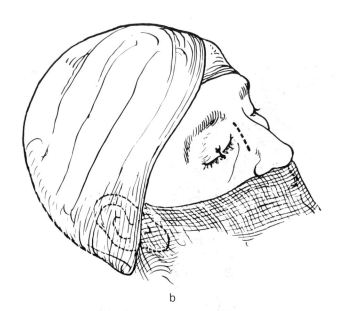

b

FIGURE 3.11. *External ethmoidectomy.*

a. The slightly curved vertical incision (also see Fig. 3.9a) is approximately 2 to 3 cm in length and placed halfway between the inner canthus and the dorsum of the nose.

b. The patient has been prepared, draped, and the eyelids have been sutured together. The external ethmoid incision is indicated.

lacrimal duct is identified so that it will not be injured. The periosteum superior to the lacrimal fossa is elevated by sweeping superiorly with the flat surface of a Ballenger periosteal elevator. This maneuver detaches the medial canthal ligament. The periosteum over the remainder of the medial wall of the orbit is very easily elevated using a Ballenger periosteal elevator aided by a short periorbital retractor.

The anterior and posterior ethmoid arteries are identified. These vessels are cauterized and transected. In so doing, the suture line between the lacrimal bone, lamina papyracea, and the orbital process of the frontal bone is identified. By identifying this suture line, the surgeon learns the level and direction of the roof of the ethmoid and cribriform plate (Fig. 3.13).

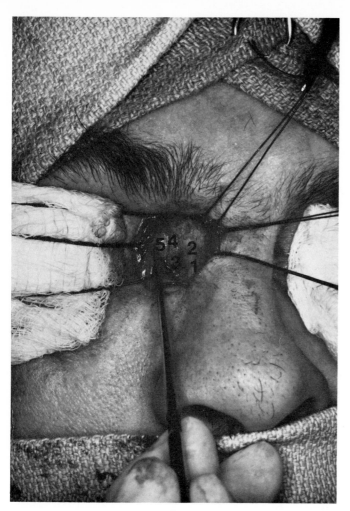

a

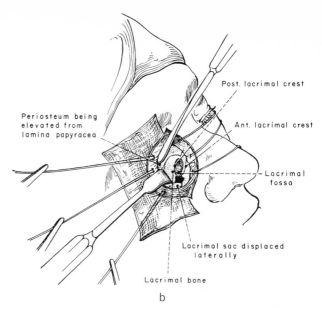

b

FIGURE 3.12. *External ethmoidectomy.*

a. The incision has been carried through the periosteum. #0-0 chromic catgut sutures are placed subcutaneously and through the periosteum on each side of the incision in order to serve for retraction.
1. Ascending process of the maxilla
2. Anterior lacrimal crest
3. Lacrimal fossa
4. Posterior lacrimal crest
5. Lacrimal plate.

b. The incision has been carried through the periosteum Chromic catgut (#0-0) sutures are used for retraction. The periosteum and lacrimal sac have been dissected and are retracted laterally. The ascending process of the maxilla, lacrimal fossa, lacrimal bone, and a portion of the lamina papyracea can be seen.

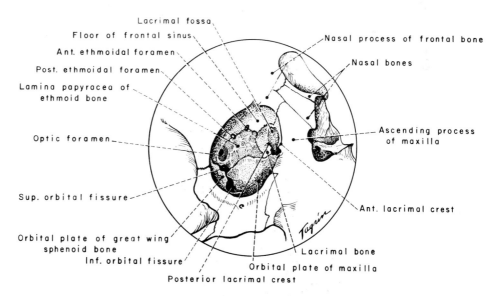

FIGURE 3.13. *Anatomy of the medial wall of the orbit.*

The anterior and posterior ethmoid foramina and suture line between the orbital plate of the frontal bone and the lamina papyracea are at the level of both the cribriform plate and the roof of the ethmoid. Note the proximity between the posterior ethmoid cells and the optic foramen.

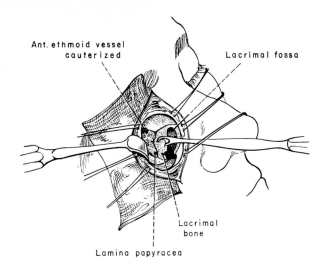

FIGURE 3.14. *External ethmoidectomy.*

The ethmoid labyrinth is entered by curetting away a portion of the lacrimal bone just behind the posterior lacrimal crest. The anterior ethmoid artery has been cauterized.

The anterior ethmoid cells are located medial to the lacrimal bone and lateral to the upper lateral wall. These cells are entered by way of the lacrimal plate or fossa, depending on which bone is thinner. A mastoid curette is best suited for this dissection (Fig. 3.14). The opening is enlarged sufficiently so a Kerrison rongeur can be used to remove the entire lacrimal bone and at least a portion of the ascending process of the maxilla (Fig. 3.15). The entire ascending process of the maxilla in this region can be removed without any resulting cosmetic deformity. The membranous and bony anterior ethmoid cells are removed using a Brownie or Takahashi forceps and a mastoid curette. The bone medial to the anterior ethmoid cells is carefully elevated from the lateral aspect of the mucous membrane of the upper anterior lateral nasal wall which is anterior to the anterior tip of the middle turbinate. Once the lateral aspect of this mucous membrane is exposed in its entirety, a U-shaped incision is made so as to fashion a posteriorly based mucous membrane flap (Fig. 3.16).

The intranasal packing is visualized and removed. The strips are counted so that none remain behind. When this flap is reflected in a posterolateral direction, the mucous membrane of the nasal septum and the anterior tip of the middle turbinate can be visualized. The purpose of this maneuver is to avoid misdirected

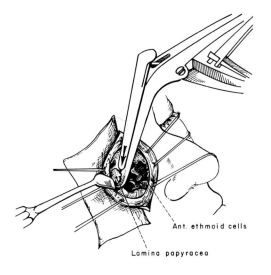

FIGURE 3.15. *External ethmoidectomy.*

Kerrison forceps are used to remove the lateral wall of the ethmoid labyrinth.

FIGURE 3.16. *External ethmoidectomy.*

An incision is made in the mucous membrane of the lateral nasal wall as indicated. The posteriorly based flap thus created is reflected laterally, exposing the superior nasal cavity, nasal septum, and anterior tip of the middle turbinate. When the above-named structures have been positively identified, the flap is removed.

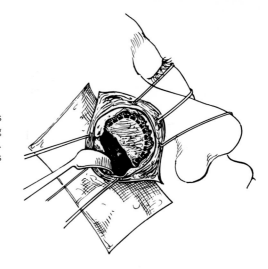

surgery and injury to the mucous membrane of the nasal septum. The mucosal flap is of no further value at this point and can be resected.

At this stage, the middle turbinate and its upper extension, which form the medial wall of the ethmoid labyrinth (Fig. 3.17), and the lamina papyracea, which forms the lateral wall of the posterior ethmoid labyrinth, remain intact. Knowing this situation, and also having determined the level and direction of the roof of the ethmoid by identifying the ethmoid arteries (this information can be double checked by examining the lateral view sinus x ray), the surgeon can remove the remaining ethmoid cells without fear of misdirected surgery. It is usually necessary to remove approximately one half of the lamina papyracea during this latter dissection. The orbital periosteum is protected during this dissection by using periorbital retractors of varying lengths.

The anterior tip of the middle turbinate and the entire medial wall of the ethmoid labyrinth is now in view. The upper extension of the attachment of the middle turbinate is cut using turbinate scissors. If these scissors are not available, Mayo scissors can be used. The upper attachment of the middle turbinate is cut to the level of the front face of the sphenoid sinus. If there is any doubt about the position of the front face of the sphenoid, it can be easily identified by palpating the rostrum of the sphenoid bone intranasally with any probe-like instrument.

The middle turbinate can be transected posteriorly using a nasal polyp snare or the turbinate scissors. On occasion, it is necessary to remove the turbinate piecemeal. As the turbinate is resected, there is most often rather brisk bleeding from the nasal branches of the sphenopalatine artery. This bleeding is controlled using cautery applied with an insulated suction tip or packing with gauze strips.

At the completion of the ethmoidectomy, the nasal septum, intranasal and ethmoid portions of the anterior face of the sphenoid sinus, the olfactory region, the entire roof of the ethmoid, the ostium of the sphenoid sinus, the communication to the frontal sinus, and the remaining portion of the lamina papyracea should be identified (Fig. 3.18).

The entire front face of the sphenoid sinus is resected in order to determine whether disease exists within the sphenoid sinus (Fig. 3.19).

I believe that I get better results by using packing following an ethmoidectomy. One-inch iodoform gauze which has been impregnated with Aureomycin ointment is quite satisfactory for this packing. The iodoform gauze is introduced

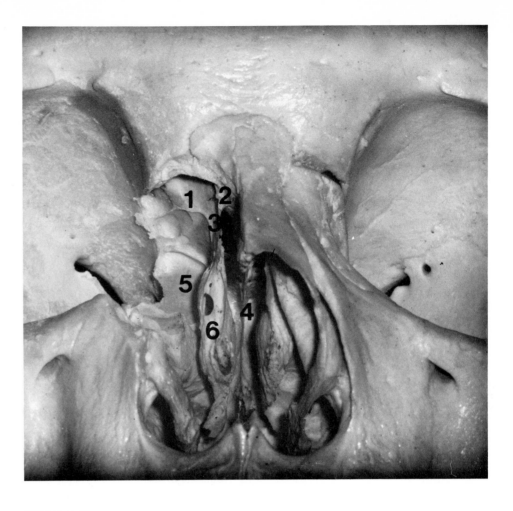

FIGURE 3.17.

Anterior and posterior ethmoid cells have been removed. The middle turbinate with its upper attachment separates the roof of the ethmoid from the cribriform plate.

1. Roof of ethmoid
2. Cribriform plate
3. Upper extension of attachment of middle turbinate
4. Nasal septum
5. Anterior wall of sphenoid sinus
6. Middle turbinate.

into the ethmoidectomy defect by way of the nostril after the roof of the ethmoid has been surfaced with compressed Gelfoam. The upper half of the nasal cavity is also packed with this gauze and is supported by inserting one or two finger-cot packs into the lower half of the nasal cavity.

The retraction sutures and those used to approximate the eyelids are removed. A circular piece of compressed Gelfoam is applied over the packing, which can be visualized from the operative field. This layer of Gelfoam prevents the iodoform packing from adhering to the margins of the bony dissection or periosteum. The periosteum is sutured with two or three #4-0 chromic catgut sutures.

Subcutaneous sutures are undesirable in this area. The skin is approximated with #5-0 or 6-0 dermal suture.

A moderate-pressure dressing will prevent troublesome postoperative edema and ecchymosis about the eye. A small strip of Telfa gauze is placed over the incision. An eyepad is covered with three or four fluffed 4 x 4 inch gauze sponges. The skin of the forehead and lateral cheek is painted with tincture of benzoin. The dressing is secured in place with three 6-inch strips of 2-inch elastic adhesive.

Postoperatively, the head should remain elevated for at least 24 hours. The finger-cot packing is removed on the first postoperative day and the dressing is

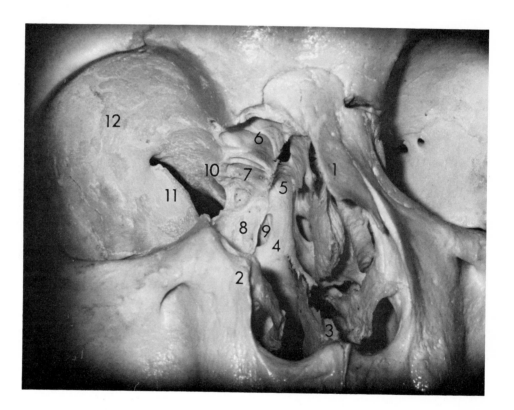

FIGURE 3.18. *Dissection showing result of a complete external ethmoidectomy.*

In addition to the dissection to show the results of an ethmoidectomy, a portion of the ascending process of the maxilla has been resected to permit a better view of the nasal septum and cribriform plate. Note the ridge of bone between the roof of the ethmoid and the cribriform plate. This ridge represents the attachment of the upper extension of the middle turbinate.

1. Nasal bone
2. Ascending process of maxilla
3. Anterior margin of bony nasal septum
4. Nasal septum
5. Cribriform plate
6. Roof of anterior ethmoid sinuses
7. Roof of posterior ethmoid sinuses
8. Anterior wall of the sphenoid sinus
9. Ostium of the sphenoid sinus
10. Optic foramen
11. Superior orbital fissure
12. Orbital plate of frontal bone (roof of orbit)

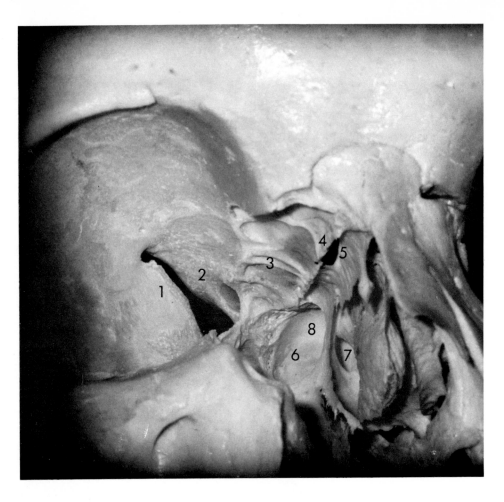

FIGURE 3.19.

Having completed the external ethmoidectomy, the front face of the right sphenoid sinus is removed in order to determine whether disease exists within the sphenoid sinus.
1. Superior orbital fissure
2. Optic foramen
3. Roof of ethmoid
4. Attachment of the upper extension of the middle turbinate
5. Defect in the right cribriform plate
6. Posterior wall of the right sphenoid sinus
7. Ostium of the left sphenoid sinus
8. Bulge made by the anterior sella turcica

removed on the second. The iodoform packing is removed from the third to fifth postoperative day depending on the degree of its adherence to intranasal structures. The patient can usually be discharged from the hospital on the fifth or sixth postoperative day. He should be evaluated 2 weeks following discharge from the hospital to detect excessive intranasal crusting or intranasal adhesions. Excessive crusting is treated using a lubricant nasal spray and intranasal irrigation with alcohol solution which is diluted with an equal part of warm water. Intranasal adhesions are disrupted using 4% cocaine solution for topical anesthesia if necessary. An oval-shaped piece of Telfa or silicone sheeting is placed intranasally for approximately 5 days to prevent further synechiae.

DACRYOCYSTORHINOSTOMY

Anatomy

The superior and inferior puncta are situated at the apex of the papillae. The papillae are found on the posteromedial aspect of the lids, about 4 mm lateral to the inner canthus. The puncta are about 0.3 mm in diameter and point in a posterosuperior and posteroinferior direction respectively (Fig. 3.20).

The canaliculi pass from the puncta to the lacrimal sac and are about 10 mm in length. The course of the canaliculi is at first vertical (2 mm superiorly or inferiorly and then 8 mm horizontally). In most cases the canaliculi join to form the common canaliculus just before entering the lacrimal sac. The common canaliculus enters the lacrimal sac at a point 3 mm from its apex.

The lacrimal sac is about 12 mm in height and 5 mm in diameter. Its size roughly corresponds to the outline of the lacrimal fossa (see Fig. 3.3). The nasolacrimal duct is simply a continuation of the lacrimal sac in an inferior and slightly posterior direction. It is approximately 20 mm in length and 3 mm in diameter and empties into the anterior aspect of the inferior meatus of the nose. The most common site of obstruction is in the upper portion of the duct.

Indications for Dacryocystorhinostomy

As a general rule, dacryocystorhinostomy is indicated in patients with chronic stenosis of the nasolacrimal duct when manifestations (epiphora, repeated infections, mucocele) are of sufficient severity to be annoying. A fistula from the lacrimal sac to the surface is certainly an indication. Age is not a contraindication, and the operation may be performed on children as well as elderly persons. On the other

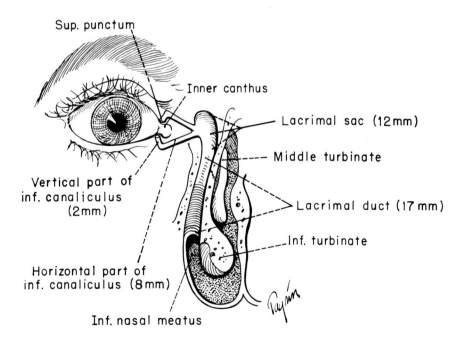

FIGURE 3.20. *Anatomy of the lacrimal system.*

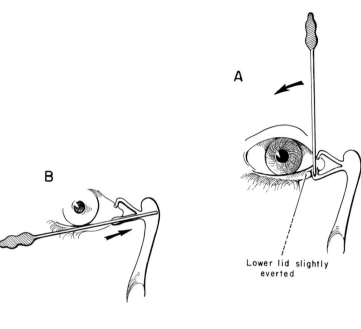

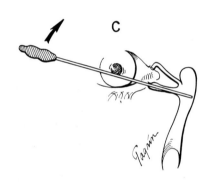

Lower lid slightly
everted

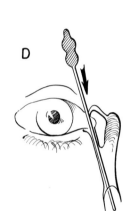

FIGURE 3.21. *Technique for probing the nasolacrimal system.*

A. The lacrimal probe is inserted into the
punctum in an inferior direction after it has been
rendered patent with a punctum dilator.

B. As soon as the probe has entered the canaliculus it is rotated 90° so that it is parallel with the
lid margin.

C. The probe is inserted medially for nearly
1 cm until it strikes the medial wall of the lacrimal
sac.

D. The probe is rotated 90° back to its original
direction as it is inserted into the nasolacrimal duct.

hand, in older individuals in poor health and with minimal infection and only
moderate epiphora the operation can be deferred. Definite contraindications are
the presence of acute dacryocystitis, carcinoma or tuberculosis of the lacrimal sac,
or a severe chronic dacryocystitis that has repeatedly failed to respond to surgical
treatment (a dacryocystectomy is indicated for the latter condition).

Many patients who are presented for consideration of dacryocystorhinostomy
have had repeated probings and irrigations of the nasolacrimal system, both for
diagnosis and treatment.

Diagnosis

Patency of the nasolacrimal system can be tested by probing and by application of fluorescein to the eye. X-ray examination is employed to determine the
site of stenosis and whether or not a fistula is present, and to demonstrate the
general anatomy of the system.

Technique for Probing the Nasolacrimal System (Fig. 3.21). In order to probe the nasolacrimal ducts of infants and children, a general anesthetic is necessary. For adults, a topical agent, such as 2% Pontocaine, applied directly to the punctum with a cotton swab, may be used.

The lower lid is slightly everted and a punctum dilator is inserted, in a vertical direction, for approximately 2 mm. This will allow a #0 or #1 lacrimal probe to enter the canaliculus. The probe is passed inferiorly for 1 or 2 mm and then turned to a 90-degree horizontal medial direction. As the probe reaches the medial wall of the lacrimal sac, it will encounter the solid obstruction of the lacrimal fossa. It is again redirected so that it becomes vertical, and thus enters the nasolacrimal duct.

Fluorescein Test. A simple test to determine the patency of the nasolacrimal system consists in placing a drop of fluorescein in the eye. After a few minutes the mucous membrane of the floor of the nose and of the nasopharynx will have a yellow tinge if the system is patent. A piece of cotton placed in the inferior meatus and subsequently observed under ultraviolet illumination is an even more accurate method of obtaining the endpoint in this test.

X-ray Examination of the Nasolacrimal System. The punctum is dilated as described for probing the nasolacrimal system. A more satisfactory outline of the lacrimal sac will be obtained if the sac is irrigated with normal saline solution and then evacuated by pressure over the sac prior to injection of contrast medium. Pantopaque, or Lipiodol, is injected into the canaliculus with a 2-cc syringe and a lacrimal cannula. Anteroposterior and lateral x rays are taken immediately (Figs. 3.22, 3.23, and 3.24).

Technique of Dacryocystorhinostomy

Anesthesia. General anesthesia is preferable for the operation unless there is some contraindication to its use.

The technique for local anesthesia is as follows (Fig. 3.25):
1. Premedication, consisting of Nembutal, Demerol, and atropine, is given.
2. Intranasal packing (4% cocaine-impregnated cotton strips) is placed in the superior nasal cavity to anesthetize the mucous membrane innervated by the anterior ethmoid nerves and to reduce the size of the middle turbinate. This packing is also placed posteriorly to anesthetize the distribution of the sphenopalatine nerve.
3. With a 27-gauge needle, 2 cc of procaine with epinephrine (1:100,000) are infiltrated along the line of incision.

A needle is inserted 1 cm above the inner canthus, to a depth of 3 cm, while being kept in contact with bone medially, to anesthetize the nasociliary branch of the ophthalmic nerve (2 cc of the procaine-epinephrine solution are used).

The infraorbital foramen can usually be palpated. A needle is inserted below this level and directed upward to locate the foramen. Two cubic centimeters of solution are injected just inside the foramen to anesthetize the infraorbital nerve.

The eyelids are sutured with #5-0 plastic or silk material. One suture through the center of each tarsal plate is usually sufficient.

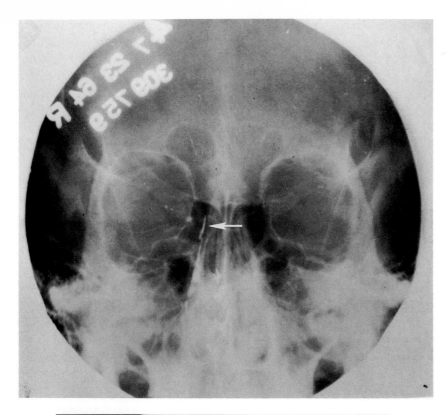

FIGURE 3.22. *X-ray appearance of normal lacrimal system.*

a. Contrast radiographic study of the normal right nasolacrimal system, antero-posterior view. The arrow indicates the contrast material.

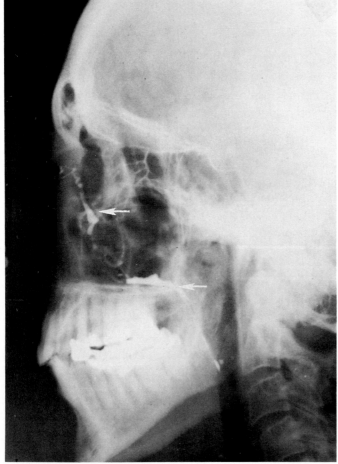

b. A lateral view of the normal lacrimal system. Note the contrast medium on floor of nose and in nasopharynx.

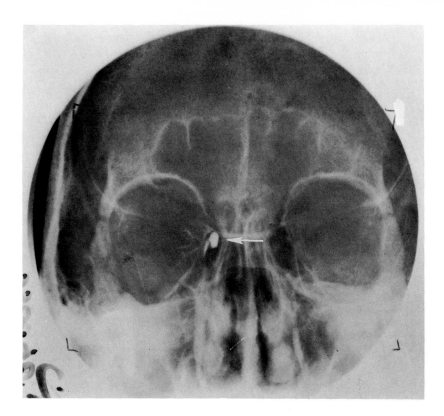

FIGURE 3.23. *X-ray appearance of obstructed nasolacrimal duct.*

a. Obstructed right nasolacrimal duct,
anteroposterior view. The arrow points to the
contrast material in the lacrimal sac.

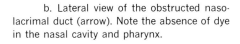

b. Lateral view of the obstructed nasolacrimal duct (arrow). Note the absence of dye
in the nasal cavity and pharynx.

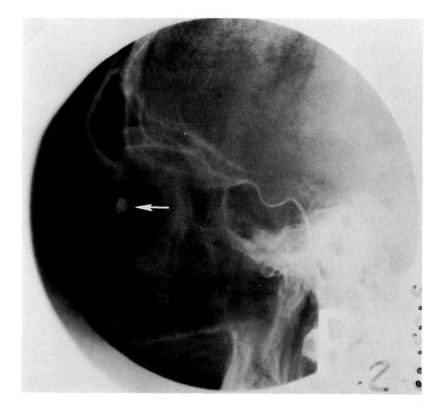

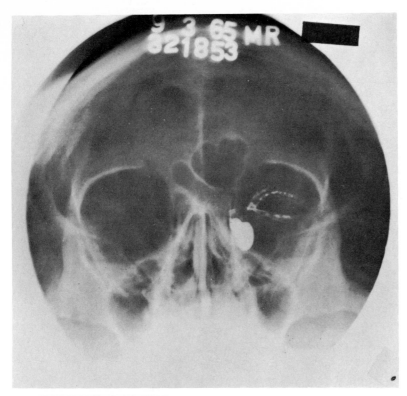

FIGURE 3.24. *X-ray appearance of obstruction of nasolacrimal duct by a mucocele.*

a. A rather large mucocele of the left lacrimal sac and obstruction of the nasolacrimal duct.

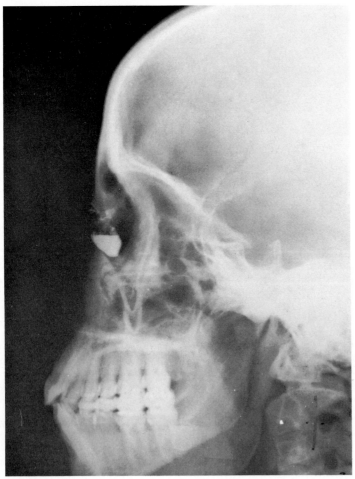

b. A lateral view of the enlarged lacrimal sac. Note the fluid level.

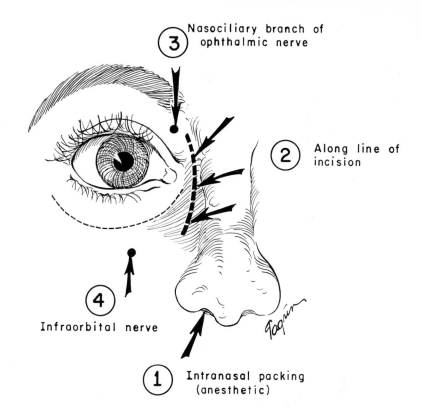

FIGURE 3.25. *Technique for local anesthesia.*

1. Cotton strips impregnated with a topical anesthetic agent such as 4% cocaine are inserted into the superior nasal cavity and middle meatus.

2. The line of incision is infiltrated with a 2% local anesthetic agent (procaine, Xylocaine, etc.) with added epinephrine. The anesthetic agent is placed only in the subcutaneous layer in order to avoid formation of a hematoma resulting from puncturing the large angular vessels in this area.

3. The nasociliary branch of the ophthalmic nerve (see text).

4. The infraorbital nerve can be injected through the skin of the cheek or through the gingivobuccal sulcus in the canine fossa.

Incision. The incision for a dacryocystorhinostomy is identical to that for an external ethmoidectomy, i.e., a 2- to 3-cm, vertical, slightly curved incision, halfway between the inner canthus and the midline of the nasal dorsum (Fig. 3.26. Some surgeons prefer to start the incision 3 mm medial to, and 3 mm above, the inner canthus. The upper half of the incision is vertical, while the lower half curves laterally along Langer's lines. Skin hooks are used for retraction while the skin is undermined along the incision. The incision is then carried in layers through the periosteum. The subcutaneous and periosteal layers are elevated as a unit, both medially and laterally so as to expose the anterior lacrimal crest, the ascending process of the maxilla, and a portion of the nasal bone.

Troublesome vessels are either cauterized or ligated. Insulated suction tips are of value here when cautery is used. The medial palpebral ligament is avoided by careful elevation of the periosteum.

For retraction, two or three #00 chromic catgut sutures are placed through the subcutaneous and periosteal layers on each side of the incision. A square-edged periosteal elevator or chisel is the instrument of choice for the initial elevation of the periosteum. After the anterior lacrimal crest has been exposed, a small, sharp, curved-end periosteal elevator is used to elevate the periosteum away from the posterior aspect of this crest, as well as from the lacrimal fossa and the posterior lacrimal crest. A smooth orbital retractor is then inserted, reflecting the lacrimal sac laterally; the periosteum is then readily elevated from the anterior aspect of the lamina papyracea. It is important that the inferior aspect of the sac and the beginning of the nasolacrimal duct are freed and retracted laterally.

A curette is used to provide entrance into the ethmoid labyrinth just behind the posterior lacrimal crest. A few anterior ethmoid cells will be encountered and

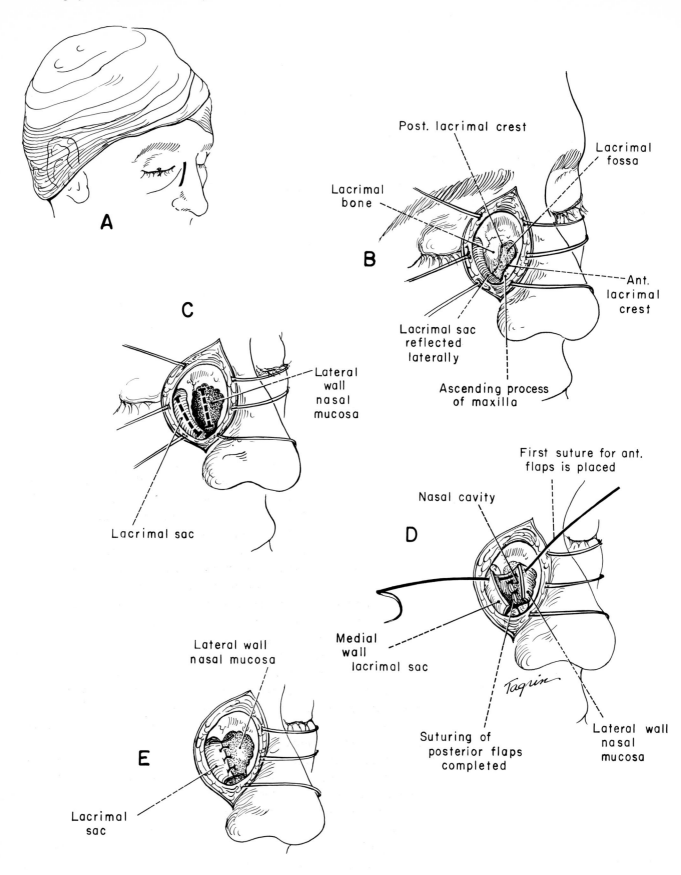

A

B

Post. lacrimal crest

Lacrimal fossa

Lacrimal bone

Ant. lacrimal crest

Lacrimal sac reflected laterally

Ascending process of maxilla

C

Lateral wall nasal mucosa

Lacrimal sac

D

First suture for ant. flaps is placed

Nasal cavity

Medial wall lacrimal sac

Suturing of posterior flaps completed

Lateral wall nasal mucosa

Tagrin

E

Lateral wall nasal mucosa

Lacrimal sac

FIGURE 3.26. *Dacryocystorhinostomy—double "I" method.*

A. The external ethmoid incision is used.

B. Exposure is acquired by employing traction sutures through the subcutaneous and periosteal layers. The sutures are weighted by heavy hemostats. The lacrimal sac has been reflected laterally, exposing the lacrimal fossa and the anterior and posterior lacrimal crests.

C. Bone approximately 2 x 2 cm has been removed along with anterior ethmoid cells in order to expose the mucosa of the lateral nasal wall adequately. The bone dissection includes a portion of the lamina papyracea, the anterior and posterior lacrimal crests, the lacrimal fossa, and a portion of the ascending process of the maxilla and the nasal bone. The "I" incision has been made in the medial wall of the lacrimal sac and also in the mucous membrane of the lateral wall of the nose. This provides anterior and posterior flaps. It is most important to insert a probe by way of the canaliculus into the lacrimal sac, thus tenting out the medial wall of the sac prior to making the initial incision in this wall.

D. The posterior flaps are approximated with two or three #4-0 chromic catgut sutures.

E. The anterior flaps are approximated with two or three #4-0 chromic catgut sutures. It is best to place all necessary sutures prior to tying any of them so that the lacrimal sac may be displaced medially while the tying is being done.

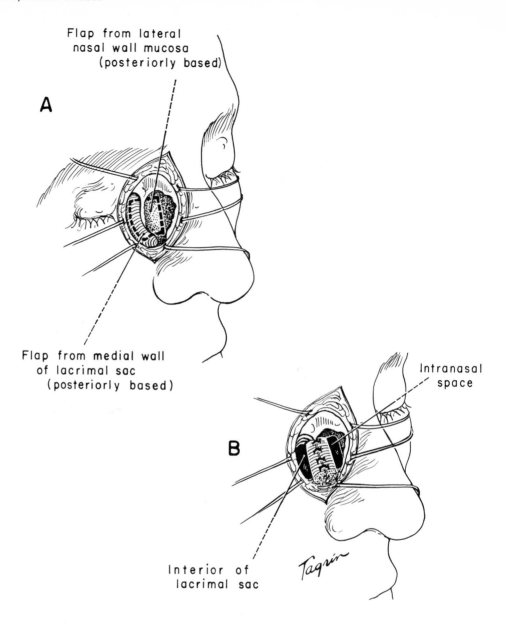

Flap from lateral
nasal wall mucosa
(posteriorly based)

A

Flap from medial wall
of lacrimal sac
(posteriorly based)

B

Intranasal
space

Interior of
lacrimal sac

Tagrin

FIGURE 3.27. *Dacryocystorhinostomy—posteriorly based flap method.*

A. Incisions for the posteriorly based flap, in both the medial wall of the lacrimal sac and the lateral wall of the nasal mucous membrane, are outlined.

B. These flaps are more easily constructed and sutured than are the flaps employed in the double "I" method. The technique ensures mucosal communication between the lacrimal sac and the nose.

should be removed. The opening is enlarged with various-sized Kerrison forceps. In order to properly expose the mucous membrane of the upper lateral nasal wall, it is essential to make a bony fenestra at least 2 cm in diameter (Fig. 3.26). To accomplish this, a small portion of the anterior aspect of the lamina papyracea, the anterior and the posterior lacrimal crests, the lacrimal fossa, and a portion of the ascending process of the maxilla and of the nasal bones must be removed. Anterior ethmoid cells in this area can be easily removed with Brownie or Takahashi forceps. The identity of the lateral wall mucous membrane is ascertained by inserting a cotton applicator stick, or periosteal elevator, intranasally and testing to determine whether or not the nasal mucosa bulges laterally.

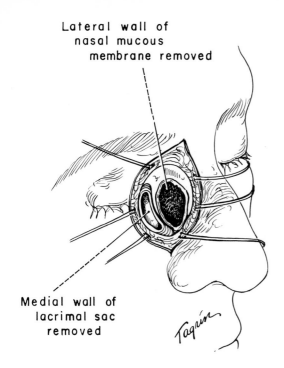

Lateral wall of
nasal mucous
membrane removed

Medial wall of
lacrimal sac
removed

FIGURE 3.27c. *Dacryocystorhinostomy—technique without mucosal flaps.*

This is a good technique for use by one not skilled in construction and suturing of mucosal flaps. It is essential to construct as near as is possible a 2 x 2.5-cm bony or mucous membrane opening in the lateral nasal wall. The entire medial wall of the lacrimal sac is removed after it has been tented medially by inserting a probe into the sac by way of the canaliculus.

Mucosal Anastomosis. There are many variations of technique for constructing mucosal flaps in order to prevent recurrent stenosis. The "I"-shaped incision, both in the nasal mucous membrane and on the medial wall of the sac, seems to be most popular (Fig. 3.26).

A vertical incision is made in the center of the medial wall of the lacrimal sac with a knife (#11 blade) and scissors, along with small skin hooks or grasping forceps. Horizontal incisions are made at each end of the vertical incision, completing the "I" incision and thus fashioning an anteriorly and posteriorly based flap. A similar incision producing identical flaps is made in the lateral nasal mucous membrane wall. It is almost never necessary to remove the anterior tip of the middle turbinate.

The posterior flaps are sutured together with two or three #4-0 chromic catgut sutures (Fig. 3.26d). Relaxation of the traction sutures will facilitate the suturing of the anterior flaps (Fig. 3.26e). The subcutaneous layers are approximated with #4-0 catgut sutures. The skin incision is closed with interrupted stitches of #5-0 suture material or a continuous subcuticular suture. The dressing is identical to that described for the external ethmoid operation. Intranasal packing is usually not necessary. The dressing is removed at the end of 24 or 48 hours, at which time the patient may be discharged from the hospital.

An alternate and somewhat simpler technique is that involving the construction of posteriorly based mucosal flaps from both the medial wall of the lacrimal sac and the lateral wall of the nose (Fig. 3.27a and b). The anterior margins of these flaps are easily approximated with #4-0 chromic catgut suture material on a small non-cutting curved needle.

Some surgeons prefer to remove the medial wall of the lacrimal sac and the mucous membrane of the lateral nasal wall without attempting to fashion mucosal flaps (Fig. 3.27c). Prior to making the vertical incision in the lacrimal sac, a lacrimal probe is inserted into the sac by way of the inferior canaliculus. This tents the medial wall of the lacrimal sac, allowing for positive identification of the sac and facilitating removal of the medial wall of the lacrimal sac. This is the ideal technique for surgeons not skilled in constructing and suturing mucosal flaps. It enjoys nearly as good results as those procedures in which lacrimal sac mucosa is sutured to nasal mucosa.

SURGICAL TREATMENT OF MALIGNANT EXOPHTHALMOS

Malignant exophthalmos is of endocrine origin. The exophthalmos produced by increase in the orbital contents is due mainly to an increased bulk of the extraocular muscles and orbital adipose tissue. As proptosis increases the eyelids become unable to cover the globes adequately, thus corneal ulceration may ensue. Also, with increasing proptosis, there is impairment of the venous return from the orbit, which results in chemosis and edema of the conjunctiva and eyelids. With the fullness of the eyelids, epiphora becomes a problem. Diplopia and finally ophthalmoplegia occur with progression of the disease. The circulatory embarrassment of the retina results in papilledema and, finally, a loss of vision.

Indications for Surgical Treatment

An indication for immediate operation is an impending loss of vision and/or ophthalmoplegia. Severe exophthalmos with complicating corneal exposure, chemosis of the conjunctiva and lids, and unsightly appearance due to increasing exophthalmos are also indications for surgical treatment.

Techniques in Surgical Treatment (Fig. 3.28)

Naffziger Technique. This operation consists in creating two frontal flaps by means of which the orbital roof is exposed and removed as far back as the optic foramen. The optic foramen may be decompressed if edema of the nerve is noted during the operative procedure. The superior orbital rim is preserved in order to maintain the contour of the forehead. The nasal sinuses are not entered. The direction of expansion of the orbital contents is into the anterior cranial fossa. The dura, lateral to the frontal sinuses, and the anterior cranial fossa are exposed. It is obvious that careful study of the preoperative x-ray films is necessary in order to determine the degree of lateral extension of both the ethmoid and frontal sinuses. If the frontal sinus is entered the hazard of complicating frontal sinusitis and/or mucocele formation is increased. On occasion the Naffziger operation is impractical because of lateral extension of the frontal sinus. Sometimes, following this operation, the pulsations of the cerebral vessels are transmitted to the eye and are notable.

Sewall's Method. Sewall, in 1926, utilized the paranasal sinuses to decompress the orbit in the treatment of malignant exophthalmos. The Sewall decompression consists of a complete ethmoidectomy and removal of the entire floor of the frontal sinus. This operation is less disfiguring and formidable than the Naffziger procedure. An actual, rather than potential, space is created. There

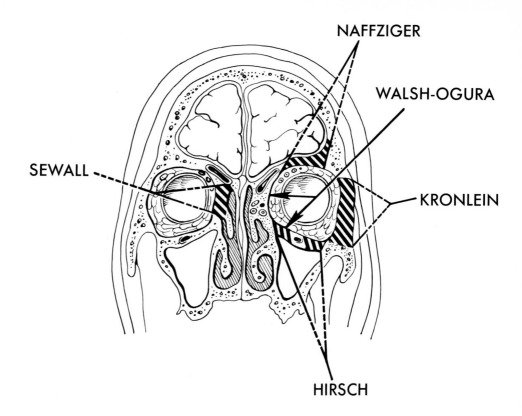

FIGURE 3.28. *The various operative procedures for relief of malignant exophthalmos.*

Naffziger—removal of orbital roof lateral to frontal sinus.
Sewall—ethmoidectomy and removal of floor of frontal sinus.
Hirsch—removal of roof of maxillary sinus with preservation of bony infraorbital canal.
Kronlein—resection of lateral orbital wall.
Combined technique (Walsh-Ogura)—ethmoidectomy and resection of roof of maxillary sinus.

is no subjective or objective evidence of pulsations of the orbit following the operation.

Hirsch Technique. This operation consists in removal of the orbital floor. The maxillary sinus is entered by the Caldwell-Luc approach. Its roof is removed on both sides of the infraorbital nerve. A narrow bony ridge is left in place for support of the infraorbital nerve. The periorbital fascia is incised. Orbital fat then prolapses into the maxillary sinus. A portion of this adipose tissue can be removed. A large fenestration is made in the nasoantral wall of the inferior meatus. Hirsch indicates that this operation is a simple procedure, leaving no external scar and attended with minimal danger of infection. A fairly large potential space for decompression is provided with an orbital recession of from 3 to 7 mm depending on the size of the maxillary sinus.

Swift or Kronlein Operation. The lateral wall of the orbit is removed by way of an incision over the lateral orbital rim. The bony defect is covered with orbital periosteum and temporalis muscle. This procedure provides limited space for decompression, although many satisfactory recessions have been secured by its use. There is an external scar and absence of the lateral orbital rim exposes the orbit to injury.

Combined Technique (Walsh-Ogura). In this procedure, both the floor and medial walls of the orbit are removed. The maxillary sinus is entered by way of the Caldwell-Luc incision. As much of the anterior wall of the antrum as possible is removed for exposure. The ethmoid sinuses are entered through the transantral route. As complete an ethmoidectomy as possible is carried out with removal of the lamina papyracea. Both the anterior and the posterior cells of the ethmoid sinuses are removed, exposing the anterior wall of the sphenoid sinus. The floor of the orbit is removed by using various rongeurs. The infraorbital nerve is preserved. Several anteroposterior incisions are made in the orbital periosteum. The orbital fat herniates into both the ethmoid and maxillary sinuses. A large nasoantral window is fashioned, and the gingivobuccal incision is closed.

This certainly is a more formidable operation for severe exophthalmos than those previously described. As with the Sewall operation there is a risk of postoperative emphysema, but this is not a severe complication and it can be avoided by the patient's refraining from nose blowing, sneezing, etc. When performing the combined ethmoid and antral decompression, it is probably wise for one not experienced with the transantral ethmoidectomy to use both the external ethmoidectomy and Caldwell-Luc incisions.

SPHENOIDOTOMY

Surgical Anatomy

The sphenoid sinus is situated posterior to both the upper nasal cavity and the ethmoid labyrinth. The site of the ostium is variable according to the degree and direction of sinus pneumatization. Usually the ostium is found in the sphenoethmoidal recess which is located above and behind the posterior aspect of the middle turbinate and just lateral to the nasal septum. The sinus may be contained entirely within the body of the sphenoid bone or may extend into the pterygoid process, rostrum of the sphenoid, greater wing of the sphenoid, or basilar process of the occipital bone. Whereas the posterior aspect of the nasal septum is usually in the midline, the intersphenoidal septum is rarely so. On occasion, the intersphenoid septum is oblique and can even be horizontal.

The sphenoid sinus has a number of important anatomic relations with which the surgeon must be very familiar. An easily recognized superolateral ridge formed by the optic canal into the sphenoid sinus is quite often present (Fig. 3.29A). Other structures which may indent the lateral wall are the carotid artery and the maxillary nerve. A ridge on the floor of the sphenoid sinus may represent the vidian canal. The posterior superior wall of the sphenoid sinus is almost invariably in close contact with the sella turcica (Fig. 3.2a and b). This is especially true when the anterior and posterior clinoid processes are pneumatized.

There are a number of important structures to be found in a coronal plane through the sella turcica. These include the cavernous sinus, the internal carotid artery, all three divisions of the trigeminal nerve, and the third, fourth, and sixth motor nerves to the orbit (Fig. 3.29b). The intracranial relation of the sphenoid sinus and its association with the ethmoid sinuses must be familiar to the surgeon who is operating in the vicinity of the sphenoid sinus and sella turcica (Fig. 3.30).

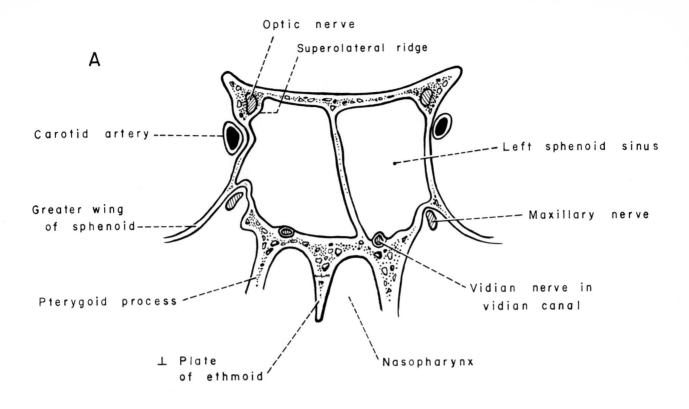

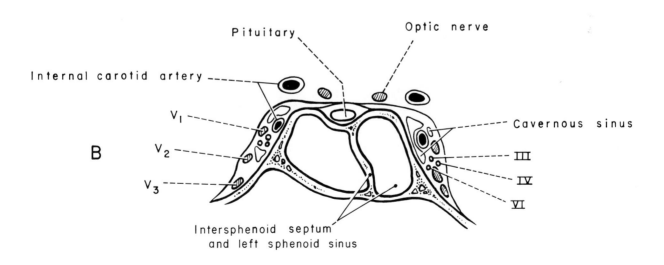

FIGURE 3.29

A. Coronal section through the mid-sphenoid sinus.
B. Coronal section of the posterior aspect of the sphenoid sinus and hypophyseal fossa.

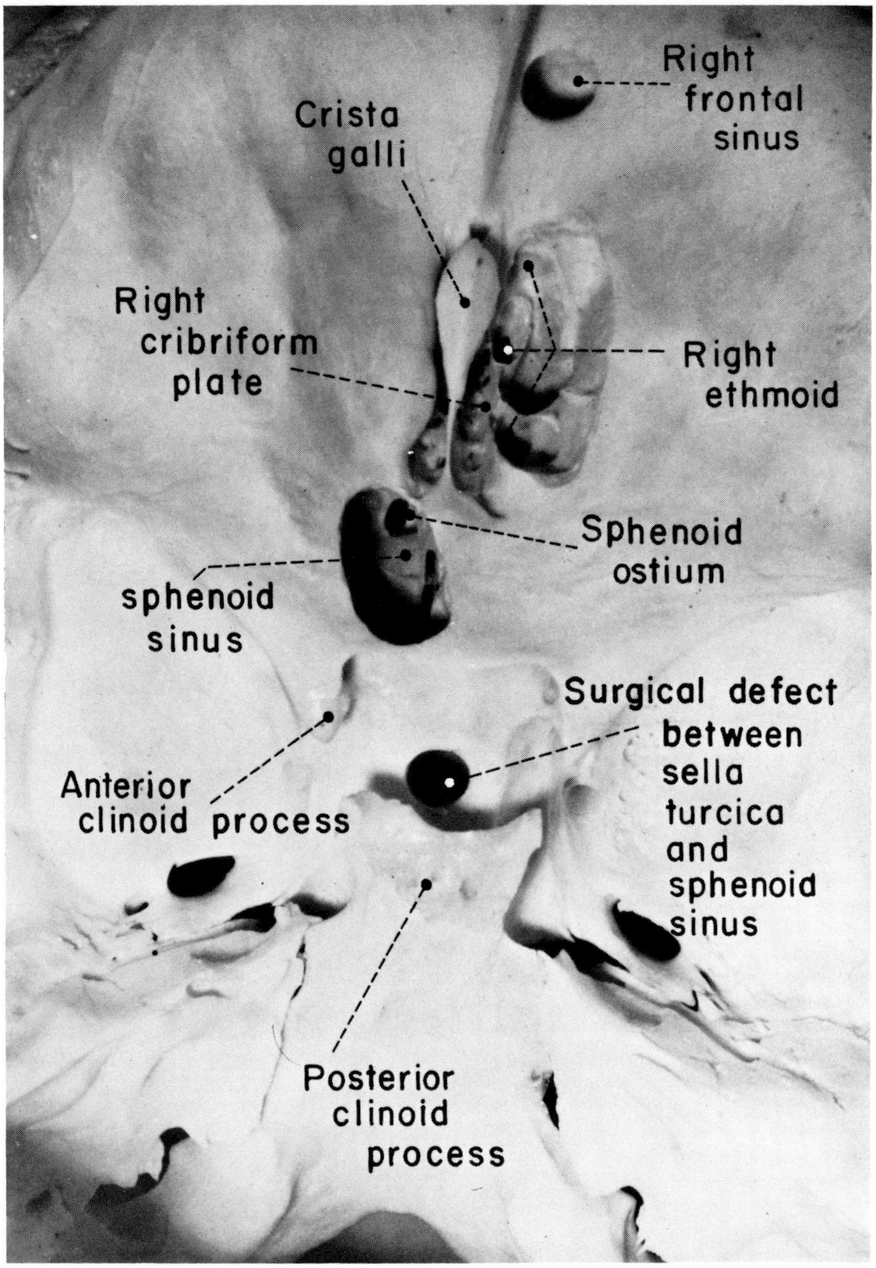

FIGURE 3.30. *Intracranial view of the sinuses and sella turcica.*

A photograph of the middle and anterior cranial fossae. The anterior and posterior clinoid processes are seen in relation to the sella turcica where there is a defect in the anterior wall, giving a view into the sphenoid sinus. The roof of the sphenoid sinus has been removed on the left side. The sphenoid ostium can be seen in the spheno-ethmoidal recess. The roof of the ethmoid has been removed on the right side showing a number of ethmoid cells in relation to the cribriform plate and crista galli. The anterior defect enters the right frontal sinus.

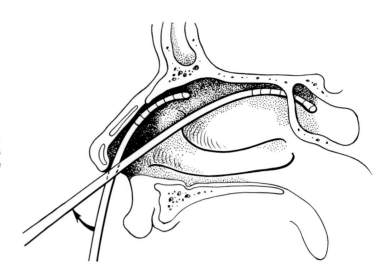

FIGURE 3.31. *Technique for cannulation of the sphenoid sinus.*

The cannula is introduced along the roof of the nasal cavity adjacent to the nasal septum and then directed towards the posterior tip of the middle turbinate. The ostium of the sphenoid will usually be found at this point.

Intranasal Surgery of the Sphenoid Sinus

Irrigation of the Sphenoid Sinus. On occasion, irrigation of the sphenoid sinus is indicated for diagnosis and treatment of subacute and chronic sphenoid sinusitis. The sphenoid ostium can usually be seen after reducing the size of the turbinates with intranasal cotton packing impregnated with 4% cocaine solution. The mucous membrane over the anterior wall of the sphenoid sinus should also be treated with 4% cocaine solution to produce anesthesia and effect decongestion of edematous mucous membrane in the region of the sphenoid sinus ostium. As indicated under "Surgical Anatomy" (p. 74), the site of the ostium is variable as are the direction and degree of sinus pneumatization. The sphenoid cannula (Fig. 3.31) is 10 cm in length and slightly curved at its tip. It is introduced along the roof of the nasal cavity, adjacent to the nasal septum in the direction of the posterior tip of the middle turbinate, making approximately a 30-degree angle with the floor of the nose. If the sphenoid sinus cannot be viewed directly, it is located by gentle manipulation. As soon as the sinus has been entered, aspiration is used to determine the presence of fluid. The sinus is then slowly irrigated with warm saline solution.

If cannulation of the sphenoid ostium is not possible, a Hajek sphenoid hook with a Trumbel guard is introduced into the sphenoid sinus just lateral to the nasal septum at the level of the posterior tip of the middle turbinate. Hajek forceps are used to enlarge this opening. The sphenoid sinusotomy should be made as inferior on the anterior wall of the sphenoid sinus as is possible. The purpose of the intranasal sphenoidotomy is to obtain material for culture and antibiotic sensitivity tests and also to effect drainage. In addition to antibiotic therapy, the follow-up care should include use of nasal decongestants.

External Sphenoidotomy

Diagnosis of Sphenoid Disease. The one symptom typical of sphenoid disease is constant headache described as severe and located in the center of the head. The pain may radiate to the suboccipital region or penetrate deep behind the eye.

Other symptoms of sphenoid disease are the result of its extension to surrounding structures rather than emanating from the sinus itself. The important neighbors of the sphenoid sinus are:

Dura mater	Oculomotor nerve
Pituitary gland	Ophthalmic nerve
Cavernous sinus	Trochlear nerve
Internal carotid artery	Maxillary nerve
Pterygoid canal	Sphenopalatine nerve
Abducens nerve	Ophthalmic artery
Optic nerve chiasma	

X rays should include routine sinus views plus laminograms. Usually sagittal plane laminograms are sufficient. At times it is impossible to differentiate radiologically between infection and tumor of the sphenoid sinus or to determine whether the lesion originates in the sinus or is an extension from a neighboring area.

Lesions involving the sphenoid sinus are:

Infection, acute and chronic	Secondary invaders:
Polypoid sinusitis	Craniopharyngioma
Mucocele or pyocele	Chordoma
Fracture	Pituitary tumor
Aneurysm	Nasopharyngeal angiofibroma
Cholesteatoma	Meningioma
Eosinophilic granuloma	Adamantinoma
Primary tumors:	Malignant lesions from the maxillary
Squamous cell carcinoma	and ethmoid sinuses
Adenocarcinoma	Metastatic tumors such as adeno-
Cylindroma	carcinoma and thyroid carcinoma
Giant cell tumors	
Sarcoma	

Exploratory sphenoidotomy is in order when there is clinical or radiological evidence of sphenoid disease which has not responded to conservative therapy. Too many lesions of the sphenoid sinus are missed. The sphenoid sinus is approached by the transethmoid route when chronic inflammatory, benign, and malignant lesions are to be treated. The malignant lesions are approached to obtain biopsy specimens and to establish adequate drainage and decompression.

Technique of Operation. A complete ethmoidectomy is carried out as has been described (see Figs. 3.5 and 3.18). It is essential that the posterior aspect of the lamina papyracea, anterior and posterior ethmoid foramina, roof of the ethmoid, and olfactory slit be identified.

The ostium of the sphenoid sinus is usually quite large and can be readily recognized. The front face of the sphenoid sinus is entered by using a sharp curette and the anterior wall is removed with various side-biting bone forceps. Diseased tissue is removed from the sinus. When treating chronic inflammatory disease, it is best to remove the amount of the anterior wall required to provide adequate drainage. A wide-open sphenoid sinus can, on occasion, cause a very troublesome headache.

The intranasal packing and postoperative care are identical to those procedures outlined under "External Ethmoidectomy."

HYPOPHYSECTOMY

The transsphenoid approach to the pituitary gland is attended with lower morbidity and mortality rates than is the anterior craniotomy route. It provides less chance for injury to the optic chiasm. Postoperative complications, such as seizures, extradural hematoma, brain damage, and cerebral edema, are rare. The convalescent period is usually quite short.

There are a number of routes and modifications for the transsphenoidal hypophysectomy.

Types of Procedures

Transseptal-sphenoidal Hypophysectomy. This operation was pioneered by Oscar Hirsch in 1910. Cushing later used a sublabial modification of this route. Heck and associates were the first in this country to use the transseptal approach for the treatment of advanced carcinoma of the breast. The main objection to this route is that it provides a long narrow approach. Two instruments cannot be used simultaneously, and the dissecting microscope cannot be employed. It is, however, still employed by many surgeons, because it is a direct midline dissection.

Transantro-ethmoidosphenoidal Hypophysectomy. Hamberger and associates used this approach in a large series of patients with remarkable success. For most surgeons, however, this is a long oblique route to the hypophyseal fossa. It also has the disadvantage of an increased hazard of postoperative infection, for the oral route in some patients traverses a potentially septic area.

Transnasal Osteoplastic Hypophysectomy. Macbeth and Hall have devised a unique direct midline approach using an osteoplastic skin flap based at the root of the nose. The only disadvantage of this procedure is that it leaves undesirable scarring of the nasal bridge. Those who perform this operation point out that this is not a factor when treating patients with advanced carcinoma of the breast.

Transethmoidosphenoidal Hypophysectomy. This technique for hypophysectomy has been used since the turn of the century. Chiari, in 1912, described this method for the removal of a pituitary adenoma. A few of the otolaryngologists who deserve credit for improving the techniques for this approach are Bateman, James, and Nager, who have used this operation because it provides the shortest route to the hypophysis that affords a wide field, permitting easy manipulation of instruments and use of more than one instrument simultaneously. One instrument may be inserted by way of the nasal cavity and another by way of the operative field. The advent of the surgical microscope has also increased the popularity of the transethmoidosphenoidal hypophysectomy.

The transethmoidosphenoidal approach has been used for removal of solid and cystic pituitary tumors (Figs. 3.32, 3.33, and 3.34), and hypophysectomy for palliative therapy in patients with advanced breast carcinoma, patients with diabetic retinopathy, and those with advanced prostatic carcinoma. Cystic tumors can easily be marsupialized. Solid tumors can be resected and/or decompressed. Most authors, Riskaer and Bateman, for example, report 60% to 80% transient remissions when employing hypophysectomy in treating patients having generalized metastases from carcinoma of the breast.

Hypophysectomy for metastatic carcinoma of the breast is a palliative opera-

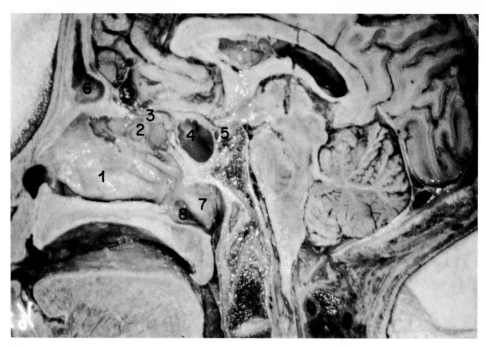

Ethmoidectomy completed

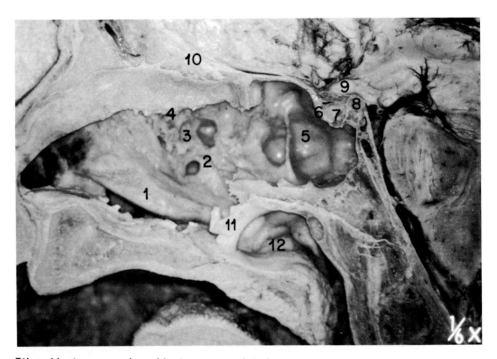

Ethmoidectomy — sphenoidectomy completed

tion. The transsphenoidal hypophysectomy is the ideal operation, for it is minimal in nature and more acceptable to a patient with terminal disease than are other procedures. Best results can be expected in those patients in the premenopausal group who have had a good response to castration and in postmenopausal patients who have responded well to estrogenic or androgenic hormone therapy.

FIGURE 3.32. *Transethmoidosphenoidal approach for hypophysectomy.*

a. A sagittal section just to the right of the midline. The middle turbinate, its upper extension, and the ethmoid cells have been removed. The lateral wall of the ethmoid labyrinth (i.e., the lacrimal bone and lamina papyracea) remains intact. The sphenoid sinus has been entered. The front wall, however, has not been removed. In this specimen the anterior wall of the sella turcica does not produce a convexity of the posterior sphenoid sinus wall, but is still easily accessible by the transsphenoidal route.

1. Inferior turbinate
2. Lateral wall of the ethmoid
3. Roof of ethmoid
4. Sphenoid sinus
5. Pituitary gland
6. Frontal sinus
7. Torus tubarius
8. Eustachian tube orifice

b. A midsagittal section demonstrating the transethmoidosphenoidal approach to the sella turcica and pituitary gland. Portions of the nasal septum remain intact for orientation. All ethmoid cells and the front wall of the sphenoid sinus have been removed. The sella turcica in this specimen is easily identified because of the convexity of the posterior wall of the sphenoid sinus.

1. Inferior turbinate
2. Ostium of right antrum
3. Ethmoid
4. Perpendicular plate of ethmoid obscuring view of cribriform plate and roof of ethmoid
5. Sphenoid sinus
6. Anterior wall of sella turcica
7. Pituitary gland
8. Posterior clinoid process
9. Optic chiasm
10. Crista galli
11. Posterior nasal septum
12. Eustachian tube orifice

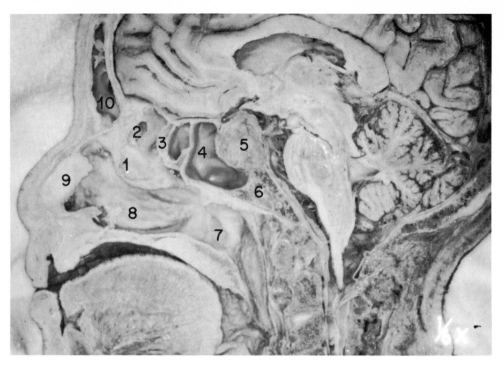

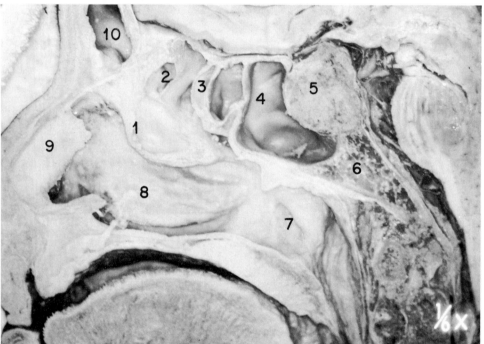

Painful bony metastatic lesions respond best to hypophysectomy. Skin and pulmonary metastases often regress. The operation is not advised for liver or brain metastases.

Patients with breast carcinomatosis, who have been so weak that they could hardly turn in bed, have had dramatic results following hypophysectomy. In 65% of patients with diabetic retinopathy treated by hypophysectomy there has been improvement in vision or cessation of progression of the disease.

FIGURE 3.33. *Pituitary tumor.*

a. A midsagittal section through a specimen with a moderate-sized pituitary chromophobe adenoma. The patient was an African who succumbed to carcinoma of the esophagus. There was a history of visual abnormality.

1. The middle turbinate remains intact except for removal of the medial wall of a large turbinate cell and its upper extension which forms the medial wall of the ethmoid.
2. Anterior ethmoid cells
3. Posterior ethmoid cell
4. Sphenoid sinus
5. Pituitary tumor
6. Body of sphenoid bone
7. Eustachian tube orifice
8. Inferior turbinate
9. Portion of anterior nasal septum
10. Frontal sinus

b. A close-up view of (a) to demonstrate more detail in the region of the sphenoid sinus and pituitary tumor. The anterior clinoid process is not present. The posterior clinoid process remains intact and does not appear to have been displaced posteriorly (see Fig. 3.39). The anterior wall of the sella turcica is displaced anteriorly markedly thinning the posterior sphenoid sinus wall. It is obvious that this tumor could be easily approached and removed by the transsphenoid route.

Pituitary tumor depressed

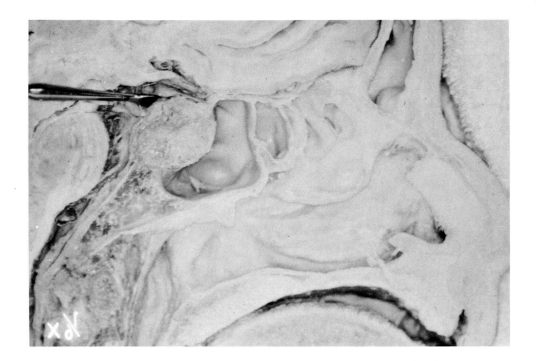

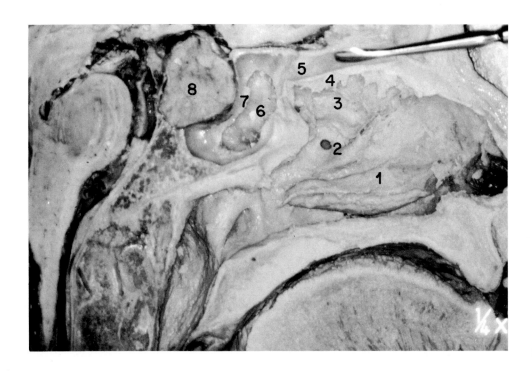

FIGURE 3.34. *Pituitary tumor.*

a. This tumor is similar to that shown in Figure 3.33. An elevator has been placed between the tumor and the right half of the optic chiasm. This produces orbitotemporal hemianopia and decreased visual acuity, which can progress into an increasing loss of visual field and blindness.

b. The opposite half of the specimen shown in a. The ethmoid and anterior wall of the left sphenoid sinus have been removed.

The specimen is tilted slightly to show the roof of the ethmoid (elevator). The posterior portion of the nasal septum and a small segment of the intersphenoid septum has been left in place for orientation.

1. Inferior turbinate
2. Ostium of left antrum
3. Ethmoid
4. Perpendicular plate of ethmoid
5. Roof of ethmoid
6. Opening into the left sphenoid sinus
7. Posterior wall of sphenoid sinus
8. Pituitary tumor

Preoperative Management in Transethmoidosphenoidal Hypophysectomy

A team consisting of a neurologist, ophthalmologist, endocrinologist, and surgeon is essential for the proper management of the patient during the preoperative and postoperative periods. A rhinologist who attempts a hypophysectomy without the assistance of these specialties is only inviting disaster. If neurologic and endocrinologic work-ups have not been carried out prior to the patient's admission to the hospital, the patient should be admitted several days prior to surgery so that these may be executed.

The neurologist's careful survey, in the patient with a pituitary tumor, should include radioactive scanning, pneumoencephalogram, and arteriograms. The endocrinologist determines the preoperative endocrine balance and prescribes the necessary hormones during the preoperative, operative, and postoperative periods. Patients with bony metastases from carcinoma of the breast should be thoroughly investigated for blood dyscrasia. A complete ophthalmologic examination should also be made prior to operation. A careful examination of the nasal cavities and the nasopharyngeal space is important to rule out the possibility of sepsis and other disease and also to orient the surgeon as to the exact anatomy of the nasal septum.

Preoperative X rays (Sinus Series)

Complete sinus x rays are taken to rule out the possibility of septic or other sinus disease. The lateral view will demonstrate the size and relationship of the sella turcica. This view, however, is misleading as to the exact pneumatization of the sphenoid sinuses because of the densities cast by the greater wings of the sphenoid bone.

Lateral planograms of the sphenoid sinuses will give a detailed anatomy of these structures and also show their relationship to the sella turcica.

A submental vertical view will show the lateral extent of the sphenoid sinuses and the position of the sphenoid septum which is most often not in the midline.

Operative Technique

The anatomy of the sphenoid and sella turcica should be reviewed (Figs. 3.35, 3.36, and 3.37).

The objectives of this operation are: (1) to obtain a wide field so that a surgical microscope can be used to illuminate and outline the posterior wall of the sphenoid sinus properly (when this is accomplished, more than one instrument can be used simultaneously); (2) to define the midline with accuracy at all times during the procedure; (3) to control all bleeding and cerebrospinal fluid leakage at the completion of the operation.

An external ethmoidectomy is carried out, as is outlined on pages 48–60. It is most important that the patient's head be secured in a supine position with

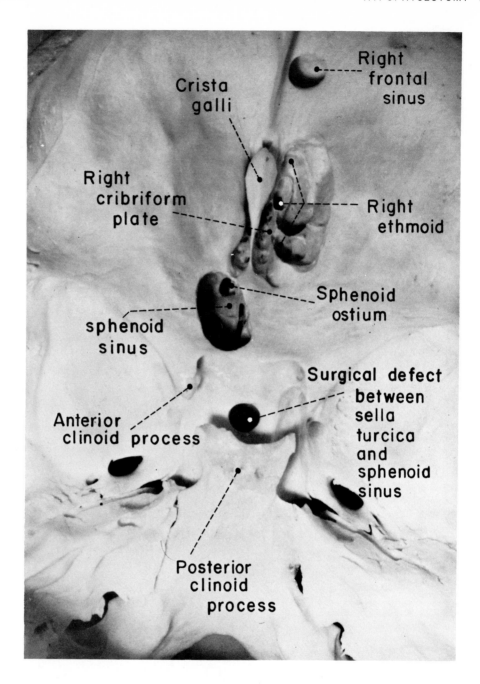

FIGURE 3.35. *Osteology of completed hypophysectomy, intracranial view.*

Anteriorly, there is a small opening in the posterior wall of the right frontal sinus. The crista galli is rather thick and partially obscures a view of the cribriform plate. The roof of the right ethmoid cells has been removed. Through an opening in the roof of the left sphenoid sinus can be seen its natural ostium which enters into the spheno-ethmoidal recess. An opening has been made into the sella turcica from the sphenoid sinus in the midline. Note the relations of the anterior and posterior clinoid processes and the beginning of the optic canals.

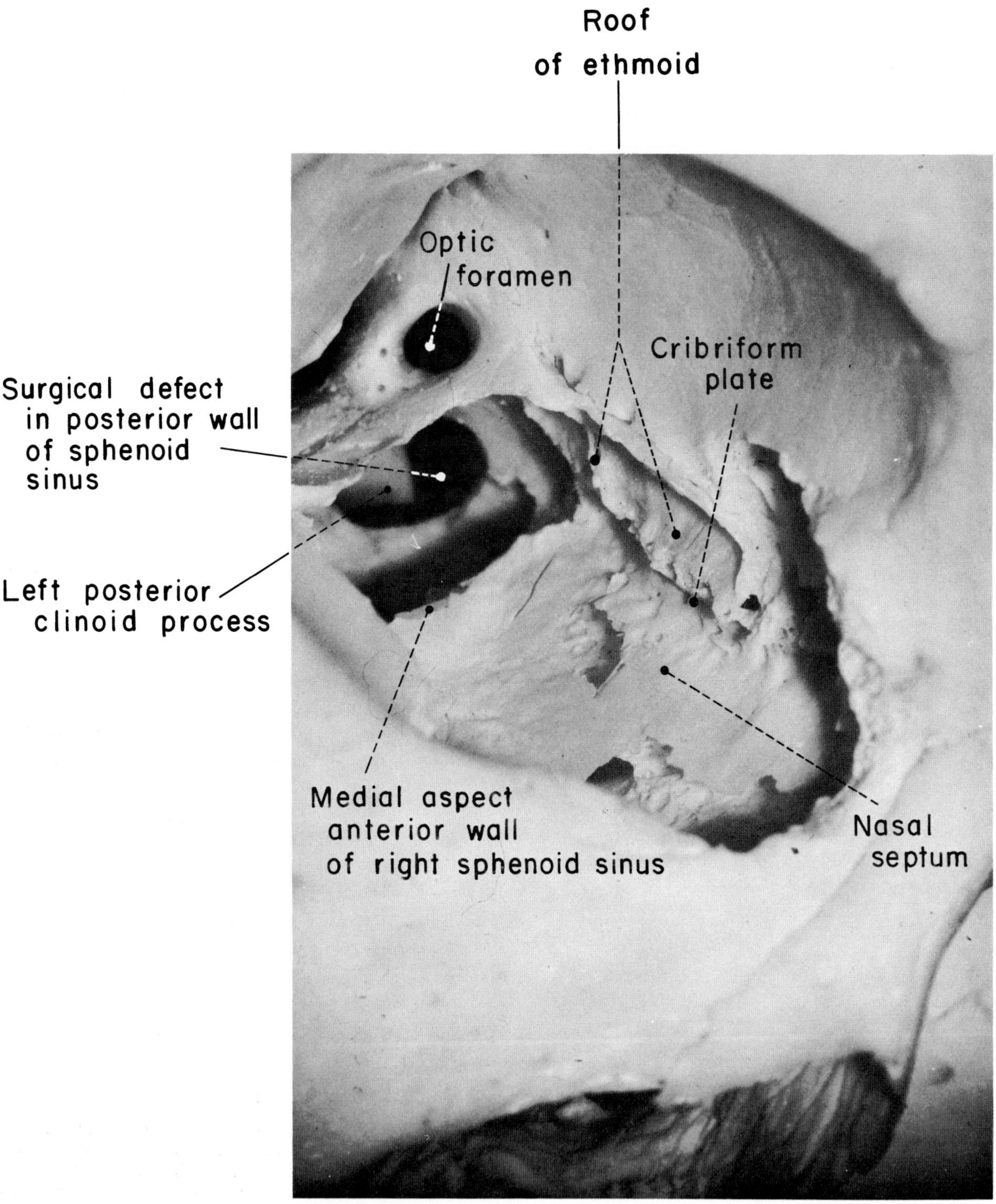

FIGURE 3.36. *Completed transethmoidosphenoidal hypophysectomy, extracranial view.*
Note the superior orbital fissure, optic foramen, anterior and posterior ethmoid foramina, roof of the ethmoid, upper extension of the attachment of the middle turbinate, cribriform area, and nasal septum. The anterior wall of the right sphenoid sinus has been removed as well as a portion of the posterior wall (anterior wall of the sella turcica). The left posterior clinoid process can be viewed through this latter surgical dehiscence.

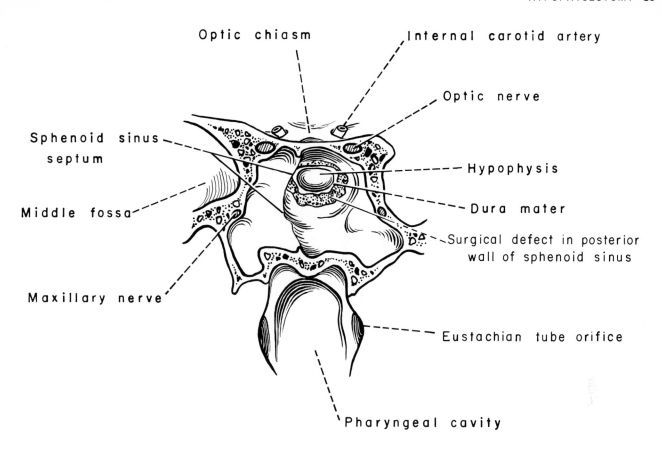

Optic chiasm

Internal carotid artery

Optic nerve

Sphenoid sinus
septum

Hypophysis

Middle fossa

Dura mater

Surgical defect in posterior
wall of sphenoid sinus

Maxillary nerve

Eustachian tube orifice

Pharyngeal cavity

FIGURE 3.37. *A coronal section through the sphenoid sinuses.*

The intersphenoid septum, which is most often not in the midline, and a portion of the posterior wall of the sinus (anterior wall of the sella turcica) have been removed.

The pituitary gland can be seen through an opening in the dura.

the aid of sandbags. After the ethmoidectomy has been performed, incisions for construction of a septal mucosal flap are made as shown in Figure 3.38. The purpose of the mucosal flap is to reduce the incidence of postoperative hemorrhage, cerebrospinal rhinorrhea, and meningitis.

A vertical incision (1) is made through the mucosa of the nasal septum at a point approximately half-way between the nasal orifice and the anterior wall of the sphenoid. Since this incision determines the length of the septal mucosal flap, it may be varied according to the demands of the pneumatization of the sphenoid sinus. Mucosal incisions are then carried posteriorly from the superior (2) and inferior (3) end of the vertical incision. The superior incision extends along the nasal septum just inferior to the cribriform plate to the front face of the sphenoid sinus. It is carried laterally across the superior aspect (4) of the front face of the sphenoid sinus and then inferiorly. (5) The inferior septal incision is carried posteriorly to the front face of the sphenoid sinus in the region of the sphenoid rostrum. The mucosal flap is carefully elevated and reflected into the nasopharynx until the hypophysectomy has been completed.

The right sphenoid sinus is entered, and the entire anterior wall is removed. The bony nasal septum is usually left intact as an accurate guide to the midline.

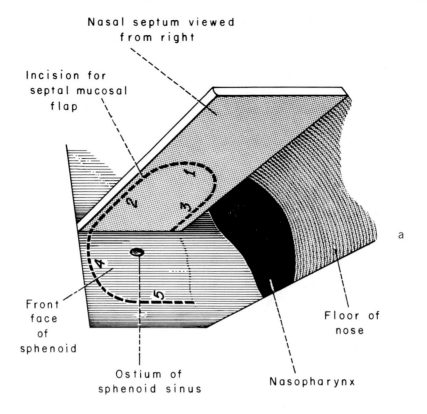

Nasal septum viewed
from right

Incision for
septal mucosal
flap

Front
face
of
sphenoid

Ostium of
sphenoid sinus

Floor of
nose

Nasopharynx

a

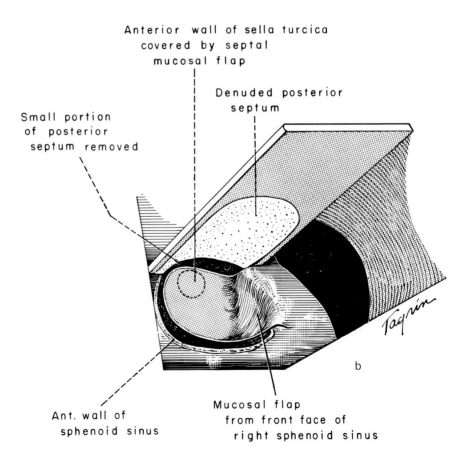

Anterior wall of sella turcica
covered by septal
mucosal flap

Denuded posterior
septum

Small portion
of posterior
septum removed

Ant. wall of
sphenoid sinus

Mucosal flap
from front face of
right sphenoid sinus

b

FIGURE 3.38. *Construction of septal mucosal flap.*

a. A schematic outline showing the incisions for construction of the flap. This is based in the region of the sphenoid rostrum at the inferior aspect of the anterior wall of the sphenoid sinus.

b. The septal mucosal flap is reflected into the sphenoid sinus, covering the defect in the posterior wall.

However, a small portion of the posterior nasal septum may be removed for a wider exposure without destroying the septum's usefulness as a midline guide.

The dissecting microscope is employed for the remainder of the operation. The bulge of the sella turcica can be seen on the posterior wall of the sphenoid sinus. The midline is again checked by using the posterior aspect of the nasal septum as a guide. If the anatomic relationships are doubtful, x rays may be taken with a portable machine, metallic probes or lead-shot attached to suture material being used as pointers (Fig. 3.39). This step becomes decreasingly necessary as the number of patients operated upon increases. A small opening is made in the posterior wall of the sphenoid sinus (anterior wall of the sella turcica) with a diamond rotating bur (Fig. 3.40). This is enlarged by using various rongeurs. It is important to remove the entire anterior wall of the sella turcica in order to define accurately the limits of the hypophyseal fossa (Fig. 3.36). Either a vertical or a cruciate incision is made in the dura; the pituitary gland or tumor thereof is then removed by using suction and various dissectors.

Following the completion of the pituitary surgery, the fossa is packed with Gelfoam saturated with thrombin solution if there is any bleeding or spinal fluid leakage. Fascia or adipose tissue may also be used to control bleeding or leakage. The septal mucosal flap is elevated from the nasopharynx and reflected into the sphenoid sinus. The flap is placed over the defect in the posterior wall of the sphenoid sinus, covered with a layer of Gelfoam, and then packed in place with iodoform gauze treated with petroleum jelly (Fig. 3.38b). When dealing with a cystic tumor, the septal mucosal flap is reflected into the hypophyseal fossa rather than used to cover the defect. This is done to ensure marsupialization of the cyst. The end of the iodoform gauze is placed in the nasal cavity so that it can be easily removed on the fifth postoperative day. The external ethmoid incision is closed subcutaneously with # 4-0 chromic catgut; # 5-0 Dermalene is used for the subcuticular sutures. A dry external pressure dressing is applied over the eye and lateral nasal bridge.

Postoperative Treatment

Cortisone and other supportive hormonal therapy are prescribed by the endocrinologist. Hydrocortisone (100 mg on the average) is administered the evening before the operation, with the preoperative medication, during the operation, and postoperatively. The amount is variable and must be adjusted in accordance with the patient's basic hormonal balance. As a general rule, partial or complete removal of the pituitary gland is not as disturbing to the general glandular metabolism as one would suppose. Symptoms of thyroid insufficiency are not common and usually do not appear until one to three months postoperatively. One and one-half grain of thyroid extract or 0.1 and 0.2 mg of Thyroxine is administered daily when indicated.

Occasionally, estrogens or androgens are necessary following hypophysectomy. Sex hormones are withheld from cancer patients. Three hundred milligrams of Depo-Testosterone are administered every month to maintain potential improved strength and well-being in male patients. In female patients, the administration of estrogens is of similar value.

The use of prophylactic antibiotic therapy is questionable. Six hundred thousand units of procaine penicillin may be administered intramuscularly twice a day.

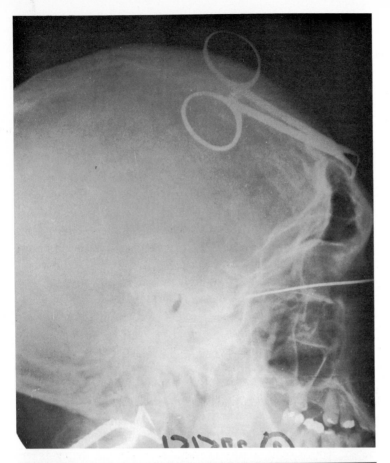

FIGURE 3.39. *X rays illustrating the use of metallic probes and lead shot attached to suture material to aid in demonstrating the anatomic relationships.*

a. As with many lateral views of the paranasal sinuses the outline of the sphenoid sinus is poorly delineated. A probe has been placed against the anterior wall of the sphenoid sinus.

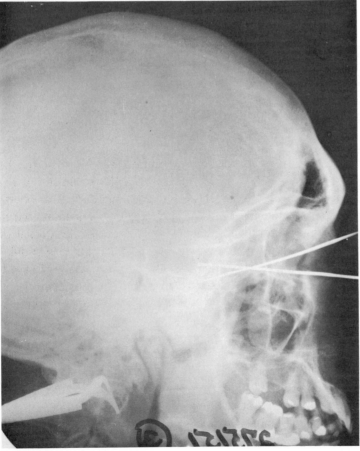

b. The anterior wall of the frontal sinus has been resected and a probe is placed against the anterior and inferior walls of the sella turcica.

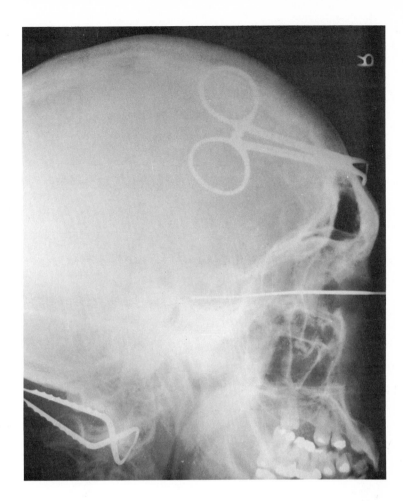

FIGURE 3.39. (Continued)

c. The tumor has been removed from the sella turcica and a probe introduced.

d. A rather large pituitary tumor has been removed. Lead shot attached to suture material is introduced into the sella turcica for identification purposes. Either metallic probes or lead shot can be inserted anytime during the hypophysectomy and the midline identified by taking an anteroposterior x ray.

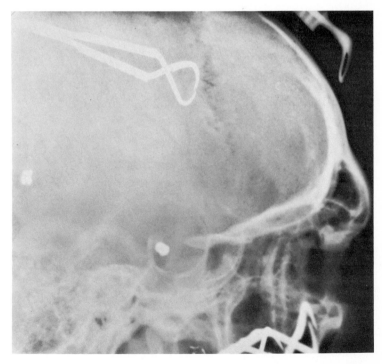

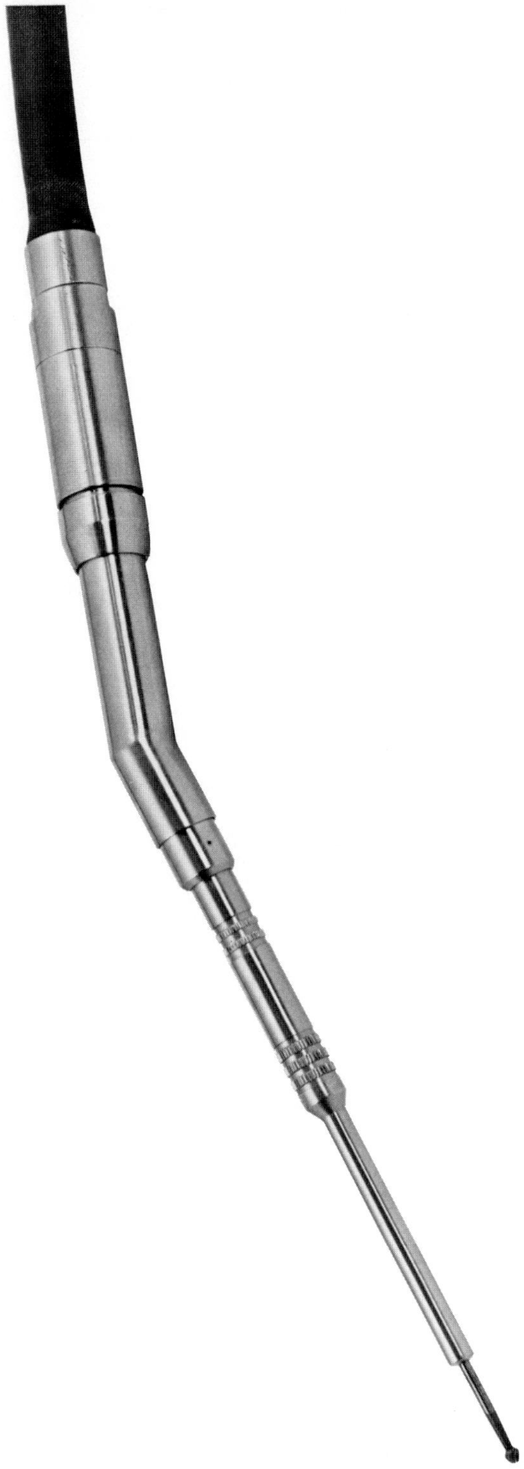

FIGURE 3.40.

Stryker drill used to resect the posterior wall of the sphenoid sinus (anterior wall of sella turcica). This drill is strong, smooth running, and slender. It has proven to be very useful in transsphenoid as well as posterior fossa surgical procedures.

Diabetes insipidus may occur. This is easily controlled by administering vasopressin (Pitressin) in oil. The fluid intake and output chart will demonstrate the onset of diabetes insipidus. Disturbances in the metabolism of glucose will be demonstrated by sugar in the urine and abnormal quantities of sugar in the blood.

The pressure dressing over the eye and lateral nasal bridge is removed on the second postoperative day, and the patient is allowed full activity at this time.

The iodoform-gauze packing and subcuticular sutures are removed on the fifth postoperative day. The patient is discharged from the hospital on the sixth or seventh postoperative day.

Postoperative Complications

Hemorrhage. The potential hazard of hemorrhage from the ethmoidal artery, sphenopalatine artery, and dural sinuses is fairly well eliminated by the use of the septal mucosal flap and the iodoform-gauze pack treated with petroleum jelly.

Cerebrospinal Fluid Rhinorrhea. Leakage of spinal fluid may occur in the immediate postoperative period or several weeks later. The patient complains of lightheadedness, headache, and soaking of his pillow and clothing from the cerebrospinal rhinorrhea. This, for the most part, is self-limiting, but on occasion can be a very troublesome complication. The septal mucosal flap, used to cover the posterior wall of the sphenoid sinus, seems to eliminate this complication.

Meningitis. It would seem that meningitis would be a fairly common complication, since the hypophyseal fossa has been exposed to the upper respiratory tract. It is, however, surprisingly rare, although its occurrence has been reported in the immediate postoperative period or weeks and months later. The septal mucosal flap may be the barrier needed to prevent this complication.

Damage to the Eye. Bateman states: "It has been suspected that wide exposure of the sphenoid through an orbital incision would be likely to cause blindness because of stretching of the optical nerve. This has not been reported."

Intracranial Hemorrhage. Subarachnoid hemorrhage has on occasion been reported and has been attributed to anatomic anomalies and misdirected surgery.

Case Reports

Four case reports are presented to exemplify the advantages of the septal mucosal flap. The first two cases demonstrate complications which can occur when a defect in the posterior wall of the sphenoid sinus is not covered. The septal mucosal flap was used in the third and fourth cases and has been used in all subsequent cases to date.

Case I. A 52-year-old right-handed construction inspector was first examined on October 1, 1957. A history of intermittent right epistaxis, decreased visual acuity on the left side, and intermittent right-sided occipital headaches was obtained. The patient had noted a decrease in his sexual desires during the past year, but there had been no change in his body hair. He had also noted increasing nervousness.

The past history was negative except for a right petrosal nerve section in 1947 as treatment for tic douloureux.

X rays of the sinuses showed an old surgical defect in the right temporal fossa. The sinuses were entirely within normal limits. The sella turcica was enlarged.

Ophthalmologic examination demonstrated normal globes. The pupils were round and reacted normally to light. Extraocular motion was within normal limits. There was no nystagmus. Examination of the fundi

CASE I

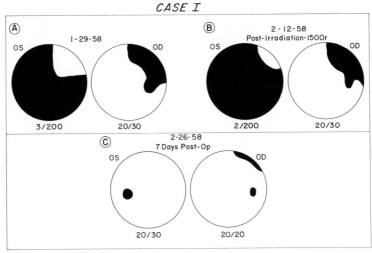

CASE II

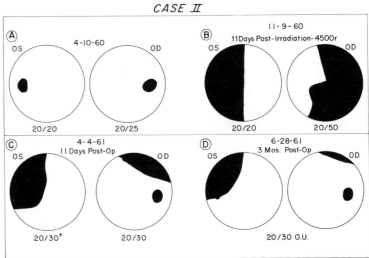

FIGURE 3.41. *Pituitary tumor.*

Cases I and II: Eye data.

showed no abnormality. The corneal reflexes were active and equal. The visual acuity in the right eye was 20/30 and in the left eye 3/200. There was a visual defect on the left involving the entire field with the exception of a portion of the upper medial field. There was an upper temporal quadrant defect on the right side (Fig. 3.41).

A general neurologic examination showed all reactions to be within normal limits. On lumbar puncture the initial spinal fluid pressure was 280 mm and the final pressure, 220 mm. Spinal fluid studies demonstrated no abnormality except for a protein content of 180 mg%. The basal metabolic rate was − 14. Encephalograms demonstrated many α and β frequencies at less than 50μ and poorly defined θ- and δ- frequencies at 50μ or less. Most of the activity was normal. Arteriograms were within normal limits except for evidence of an enlarged sella turcica. A pneumoencephalogram demonstrated a moderately dilated ventricular system; there was a very good delineation of a large mass occupying the sella turcica and projecting into the sphenoid sinus.

A diagnosis of pituitary tumor was established and, after consultation, radiation therapy was recommended. Biopsy study of the pituitary region was not made. Radiation therapy was begun on February 8, 1958. By February 18, a total dose of 1500r had been administered. The patient had almost no vision in the left eye and decreasing visual activity in the right eye. His headaches had become unbearable. On February 19, a transethmoidosphenoidal hypophysectomy was performed with the patient under general endotracheal anesthesia. The sphenoid sinus was found to be well pneumatized. The anterior wall of the sella turcica could be seen bulging into the sphenoid sinus. The tumor was removed with hypophyseal forceps and aspiration.

Postoperatively, the patient's headaches disappeared, and his visual acuity and field defect gradually improved. By February 26, his visual fields were within normal limits, and his vision was 20/20 on the right and 20/30 on the left (Fig. 3.41). The final pathologic diagnosis was chromophobe pituitary adenoma. Radiation therapy was reinstituted as soon as the visual fields were normal. A total dose of 4000r was administered.

On March 21, the patient was readmitted to the hospital after having had an upper respiratory infection for a week and severe occipital headaches, nausea, vomiting, and chills for 24 hours. His meningitis responded dramatically to high doses of penicillin, chloramphenicol (Chloromycetin), and sulfadiazine. The patient was discharged from the hospital on March 29. He has remained well since this admission and has had no endocrine disturbance.

COMMENT. This case demonstrates a fairly rapidly expanding pituitary chromophobe adenoma resulting in visual field defects. The additional swelling produced an ophthalmologic emergency. Removal of the tumor by the transethmoidosphenoidal approach resulted in a dramatic improvement in the patient's vision. Meningitis occured one month postoperatively. This might have been prevented if an adequate barrier had been established between the hypophyseal fossa and the upper respiratory tract.

Case II. A 45-year-old white-haired lady was first examined at the Massachusetts General Hospital in April of 1960. She was described as a typical acromegalic with large hands, feet, and facial features. Her voice was deep and coarse. Her complaints were limited to intermittent headache and pain in the eyes, without visual difficulties, of several years' duration.

A thorough ophthalmologic examination revealed no ocular involvement (Fig. 3.41). X rays of the skull showed a marked expansion of the sella turcica which measured 22 x 26 mm. A pneumoencephalogram demonstrated that the intrasellar tumor displaced the chiasmatic and interpeduncular cisterns superiorly. There was a slight concave indentation of the anterior portion of the third ventricle, indicating pressure from a suprasellar extension of the tumor. Cerebrospinal fluid studies showed no evidence of increased intracranial pressure. The total protein in the cerebrospinal fluid was 72 mg%. Studies indicated a slight hypopituitarism.

Because of the size of the pituitary tumor and the suprasellar extension, it was decided to institute radiation therapy. A total of 4500r was administered from April 22 to May 16.

The patient was readmitted to the hospital on November 15, 1960, complaining of failing vision of four months' duration. Ophthalmologic work-up showed a bitemporal hemianopia (Fig. 3.41) and decreased vision in the right eye (to 20/50). The fundi were normal.

On November 23 the patient was prepared for a transethmoidosphenoidal hypophysectomy. During anesthesia induction, intubation by either the oral or nasal route was impossible because of the presence of tremendous macroglossia. A tracheotomy was rapidly performed, and the anesthetic was administered through the incision into the trachea. The sphenoid area was explored, but the patient's general condition did not allow sufficient time for either adequate decompression or removal of the tumor. There was no postoperative improvement in the visual fields. A cerebrospinal fluid rhinorrhea persisted until December 6.

On March 20, 1961, the patient was readmitted to the hospital for a second attempt at hypophysectomy. The tracheotomy incision was reopened prior to anesthesia induction. The pituitary tumor was resected and a good decompression of the area was accomplished. A septal mucosal flap was used to cover the defect in the posterior wall of the sphenoid sinus. The postoperative course was uneventful. The visual fields gradually improved (Fig. 3.41). The patient has remained well while receiving some supportive endocrine therapy. A photograph of the patient on her fifth postoperative day is shown in Figure 3.42.

COMMENT. This was our first attempt to intubate a patient with marked macroglossia. A rapidly performed tracheotomy rectified the situation. A troublesome cerebrospinal fluid rhinorrhea followed the first attempt at hypophysectomy, in which neither adequate decompression of the area nor removal of the tumor were accomplished. The operation was successfully undertaken at a later date. A septal mucosal flap was used to cover the defect in the posterior wall of the sphenoid sinus to prevent the recurrence of the cerebrospinal fluid rhinorrhea.

Case III. A 59-year-old white, obese caterer was admitted to the hospital on July 4, 1961, with the chief complaint, "I can't walk downstairs." For the past eight years, she had been struggling unsuccessfully to wear bifocals. Two years prior to this hospital admission, her family doctor found that her lateral vision was blurred. X rays of the skull were taken because the patient had severe headaches. These demonstrated an enlargement of the sella turcica. The past history was otherwise not significant.

General physical examination revealed no abnormality except for obesity and a blood pressure of 190/110. Complete neurologic examination yielded findings within normal limits.

The pressure and dynamics of the spinal fluid were normal. The spinal fluid protein content was 64 mg%. The complete blood cell count gave normal values. The electroencephalogram and the blood studies, which included those for determination of protein-bound iodine, blood urea nitrogen, fasting blood sugar, and calcium content, showed no

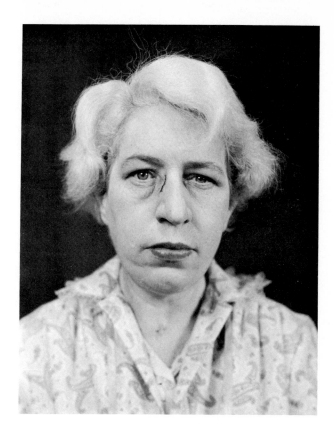

FIGURE 3.42. *Pituitary tumor.*

Case II: A photograph taken on the fifth postoperative day. A dye has been used to accentuate the scar.

abnormality. The x rays of the skull demonstrated marked enlargement of the sella turcica. The posterior clinoid processes were destroyed. The pineal body was calcified and in the midline. The pneumoencephalogram demonstrated a pituitary tumor of 3.5-cm diameter. The electrocardiogram showed no abnormality.

Ophthalmologic examinations demonstrated a complete bitemporal hemianopia (Fig. 3.41). The globes were white and in normal position. The extraocular motion was normal. The pupils were equal (4 mm) and reacted well to light. There was no nystagmus or red lens diplopia. The fundi were normal. The visual acuity was 20/30 in both eyes.

On July 13, a transethmoidosphenoidal hypophysectomy was performed. The sphenoid sinus was found to be normal except for an anterior convexity of the posterior wall. The substance of the tumor mass was soft and granular. The tumor was easily removed with hypophyseal forceps and suction. A posterior septal mucosal flap was used to cover the defect in the posterior wall of the sphenoid sinus.

The postoperative course was uneventful except for epistaxis of brief duration occurring on the eighth day. The patient was discharged on the twelfth postoperative day. Her headache was absent. She noted a definite improvement in her vision (Fig. 3.43). Her visual fields were normal one month postoperatively. Hydrocortisone was administered for four months following the operation. The final diagnosis was chromophobe pituitary adenoma.

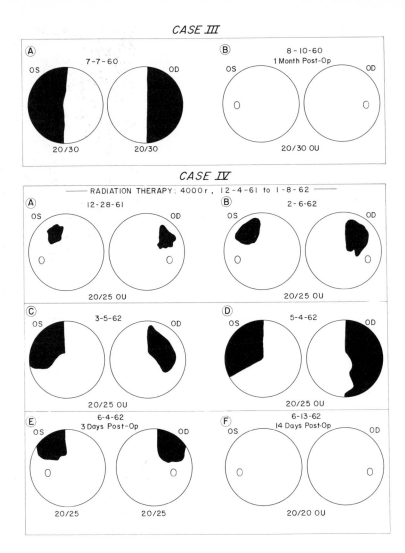

FIGURE 3.43. *Pituitary tumor.*

Cases III and IV: Eye data.

Case IV. A 61-year-old salesman was admitted to the Massachusetts General Hospital on November 27, 1961, with a six months' history of intermittent blurring of vision while reading, and occasional diplopia. During the two months prior to admission these symptoms increased in frequency, and the patient had the feeling that "things were closing in" on him. He also complained of bitemporal headaches which were readily relieved by taking aspirin.

On examination a definite left temporal field defect to a 3-mm white object and a similar but less apparent defect in the right temporal field were noted (Fig. 3.43). There was no defect on finger confrontation. The red glass test revealed a variable diplopia. It was crossed on forward gaze, homonymous on looking to the right, and not present on looking to the left. The optic disks were normal and other cranial nerves intact. The reflexes were active and equal. The motor nerves and sensation were normal.

As demonstrated by x rays of the skull, the pituitary fossa was enlarged and the dorsum sellae and the right anterior clinoid process were eroded.

An electroencephalogram showed no abnormality. The spinal fluid protein content was 90 mg%. The pneumoencephalogram gave evidence of a suprasellar expansion of an intrasellar mass. Routine blood and endocrine studies yielded values within normal limits.

Radiation therapy (total of 4000r) was delivered to the sellar region from December 4, 1961, to January 8, 1962.

There was no improvement in the patient's symptoms after the radiation therapy. He admitted to a mild loss of energy, decreased libido and potentia, and increasing constipation. Repeated field examinations indicated an increasing bitemporal hemianopia (Fig. 3.43).

On May 29, the patient was admitted to the Massachusetts Eye and Ear Infirmary. X rays showed the sella turcica to measure 18 mm in its anteroposterior dimension and the posterior clinoid processes to be decalcified. A neuromedical and endocrine evaluation revealed no changes since the previous hospital admission other than the increasing defects in the visual fields.

On June 1, a transethmoidosphenoidal hypophysectomy was performed from the right side. The fluid center of a dark-brown tumor was aspirated. The lesion was then removed, but its capsule was left in place. The dural incision was covered with a septal mucous membrane flap. This was covered with Gelfoam and packed in place with petrolatum-impregnated iodoform gauze. Cortisone therapy was given both pre- and postoperatively. The pathologic diagnosis was "chromophobe adenoma."

Examination of the visual fields made three days postoperatively showed an improvement (Fig. 3.43). The subcuticular sutures were removed on the fourth postoperative day. The patient was discharged from the hospital on June 7, 1962. His visual fields were normal on June 15 (Fig. 3.43).

COMMENT. Cases III and IV demonstrate a rapid return to normal visual fields and relief of other symptoms produced by pituitary tumors. In both of the patients the septal mucosal flap was used to cover the defect in the posterior wall of the sphenoid sinus. The postoperative courses were short and benign.

TRANSETHMOIDOSPHENOIDAL APPROACH TO THE OPTIC NERVE

Injury to the optic nerve by intracanular compression can result from (1) hemorrhage complicating surgery of the ethmoid or trauma, (2) misdirected surgery to the region of the optic canal, and (3) fractures resulting from a blunt trauma to the face. If the loss of vision is sudden and complete following compression injury of the optic nerve, a decompression procedure is rather pointless. On the other hand, if the loss of vision is gradual and incomplete, then immediate surgical intervention is indicated. As a general rule, the optic canal has been explored by way of an anterior craniotomy. Anterior exploration of the optic canal by way of the ethmoid and sphenoid may prove to be a much more practical and effective method.

Technique of Surgery

The operation is performed by the external ethmoidectomy route which is described beginning on page 48. A complete ethmoidectomy is accomplished making certain to expose the entire roof of the ethmoid. The optic canal is in approximately the same plane as the roof of the ethmoid. As can be seen in Figures 3.44 and 3.45, the posterior wall of the optic foramen is directly behind the posterosuperior aspect of the lamina papyracea. Having established these landmarks, the anterior wall of the sphenoid sinus is completely removed so as to obtain a good view of the lateral wall of the sphenoid sinus. The indentation made by the carotid artery can be visualized. The medial wall of the optic canal above the

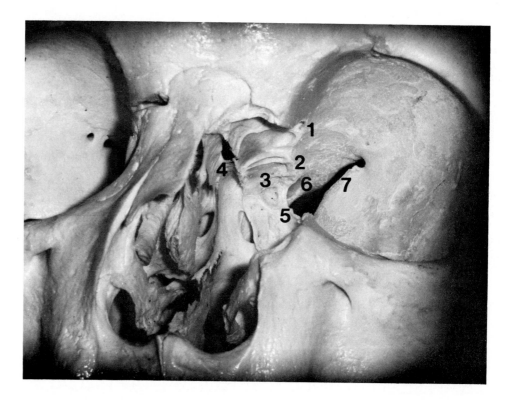

FIGURE 3.44.

A complete left ethmoidectomy has been accomplished. The anterior and posterior ethmoid foramina, roof of the ethmoid, cribriform plate, and lamina papyracea are shown in their relation to the optic foramen. Note that the posterosuperior aspect of the lamina papyracea is continuous with the medial wall of the optic canal.

1. Anterior ethmoid foramen
2. Posterior ethmoid foramen
3. Roof of left ethmoid
4. Left cribriform plate
5. Posterior aspect of left lamina papyracea
6. Optic foramen
7. Superior orbital fissure

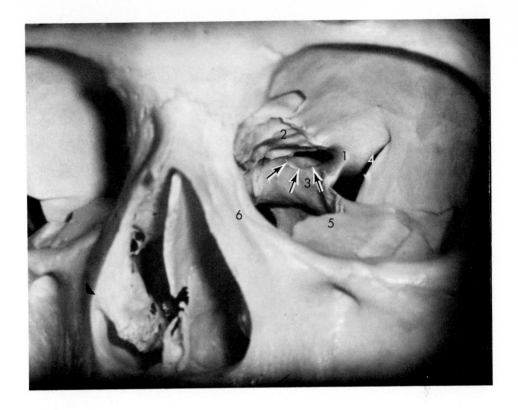

FIGURE 3.45.

The medial wall of the left optic canal (arrows) has been removed to the level of the dura.
1. Lateral rim of left optic foramen
2. Roof of left ethmoid sinus
3. Lateral aspect of left sphenoid sinus
4. Superior orbital fissure
5. Floor of left orbit
6. Ascending process of maxilla

level of the carotid artery is removed using a large diamond bur with constant suction irrigation. Packing, closure, and dressing are as described with the external ethmoidectomy operation.

TRANSSPHENOID APPROACH TO CYSTIC LESIONS OF THE PETROUS APEX

The transsphenoid approach to cystic lesions of the petrous tip has been made possible by advances in techniques for diagnosis as well as improved surgical instruments. The advances in diagnostic techniques include polytomography, angiography, and CT brain scanning. The extent of bone destruction and the size, shape, and position of a cystic lesion of the petrous apex can be determined by polytomography (Fig. 3.46). The CT brain scan indicates whether the lesion is cystic and to some degree the thickness of the capsule (Fig. 3.47). By angiography, the position and size of the lesion are confirmed as well as whether the lesion is avascular (Fig. 3.48).

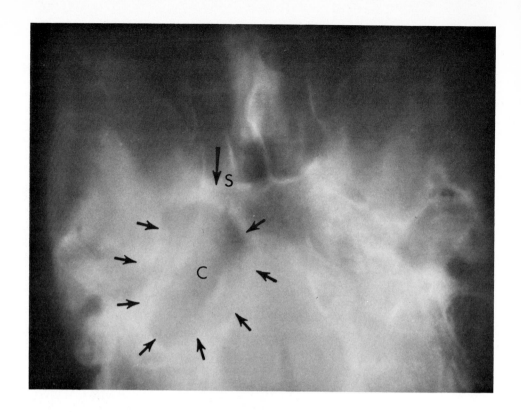

FIGURE 3.46.

This horizontal polytome is seen through a cystic lesion of the petrous apex and also the sphenoid sinuses. The arrows point to the destruction in the right, middle, and posterior cranial fossae. The large arrow is in the right sphenoid sinus (S). This arrow points to the posterior wall of the right sphenoid sinus and also indicates the direction of the surgical approach to the anterior wall of the cyst (C) (Montgomery, 1977).

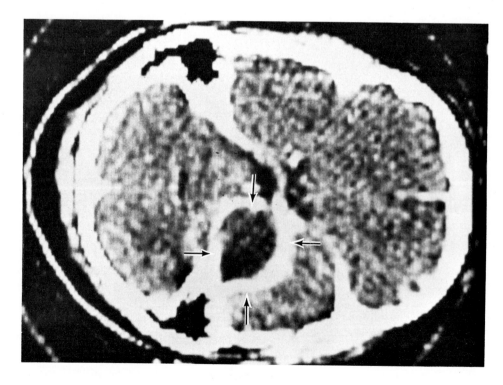

FIGURE 3.47. *A CT scan demonstrating the lesion (arrows) in the region of the right petrous tip (Montgomery, 1977).*

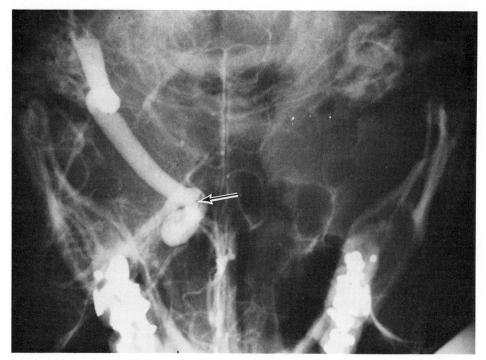

a

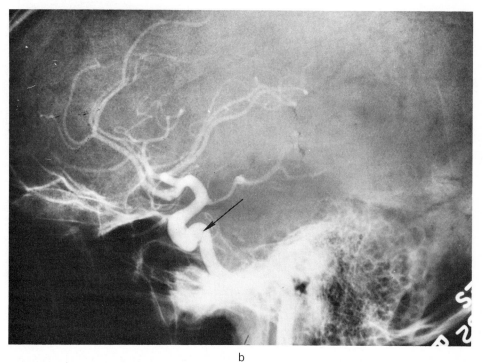

b

FIGURE 3.48.

A right transfemoral bilateral carotid (a) and right vertebral (b) arteriogram demonstrate upward and medial displacement of the right superior cerebellar artery. The basilar artery is displaced slightly posteriorly. There is downward and forward displacement of the petrous portion of the internal carotid artery (Montgomery, 1977).

The primary epidermoid of the petrous apex can produce a variety of signs and symptoms. Pain may be present in the form of a unilateral headache or that evoked by pressure against the fifth cranial nerve. This headache and pain can be quite severe and disabling. Diplopia may result from pressure against the sixth cranial nerve with resulting paresis or paralysis of this nerve. Hearing loss can be either conductive or neural in type. The neural type of hearing loss is caused by pressure against the cochlear nerve, whereas the conductive hearing loss is the result of an obstructed eustachian tube. Pressure against the vestibular nerves can lead to varying degrees of vertigo. A facial weakness or paralysis can also result from pressure exerted by this expanding cystic lesion.

A number of surgical approaches have been used to reach the cystic lesion of the petrous apex. Since it is impossible to resect these lesions, the goal of the surgeon should be the diagnostic exploration and externalization of the expanding cyst. The middle fossa extradural craniotomy can be used to approach the petrous tip. A biopsy can be obtained and the cyst evacuated. Permanent drainage of the

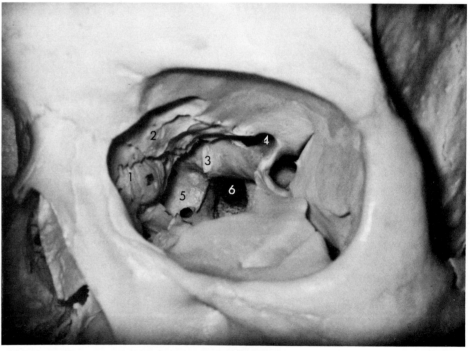

a

FIGURE 3.49.

a. A complete left ethmoidectomy and sphenoidectomy have been performed in this specimen. The bulge in the posterolateral wall of the right sphenoid sinus is identified, and an opening has been made through the posteroinferior wall of the right sphenoid sinus.
1. Nasal septum
2. Roof of ethmoid
3. Roof of sphenoid
4. Optic canal
5. Bulge made by right internal carotid artery
6. Surgical defect in the posteroinferior wall of the right sphenoid sinus (Montgomery, 1977)

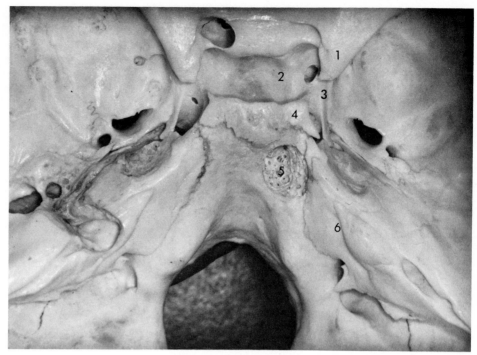

b

FIGURE 3.49. (Continued)

    b. This view of the posterior and middle cranial fossae shows the surgical defect in the posterior wall of the right sphenoid sinus, which approaches the petrous apex.
    1. Right anterior clinoid process
    2. Sella turcica
    3. Groove for right internal carotid artery
    4. Posterior clinoid process
    5. Surgical defect
    6. Petrous apex. (Montgomery, 1977)

cyst, however, is not possible by this route. The posterior fossa craniotomy has also been used to approach the epidermoid cyst of the petrous apex. Again, a biopsy can be performed and the contents of the cyst evacuated, but permanent drainage cannot be established by the posterior route.

    The translabyrinthine approach to the petrous tip has been the operation of choice for the epidermoid cyst of the petrous apex. Wide access to the petrous tip is accomplished. The cyst is permanently exteriorized by skin graft in the bony fistula between the mastoid and the petrous apex. The obvious disadvantage to the translabyrinthine approach is the loss of cochlear and vestibular functions.

    The transsphenoid approach to the cystic lesion of the petrous apex by way of a contralateral external ethmoidectomy should be the ideal operation providing the anterior aspect of the cyst abuts against the posterior wall of the sphenoid sinus (Fig. 3.49). A pedicled septal mucosal flap is reflected into the cyst by way of the surgical defect in the posterior wall of the sphenoid sinus to create permanent fistulization. A silicone drainage device (Fig. 3.50) is inserted to ensure against closure of the communication between the sphenoid sinus and the epidermoid cyst (Fig. 3.51).

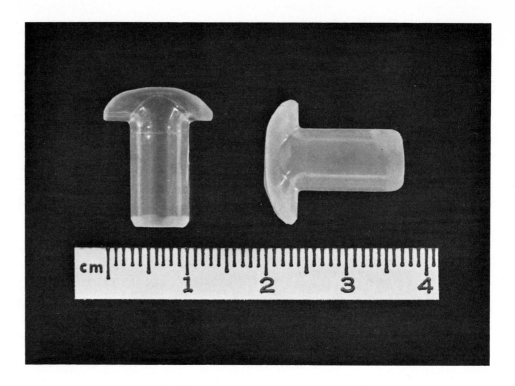

FIGURE 3.50. *The silicone drainage device.*

It can be constructed from a silicone tracheal T-tube or purchased* (Montgomery, 1977).

*E. Benson Hood
 211 Vine Street
 Duxbury, Mass. 02332

Technique of Surgery

A complete external ethmoidectomy is performed on the side opposite the cystic lesion of the petrous apex (Fig. 3.52). The anterior wall of the sphenoid sinus is removed and the intersphenoid septum identified (Fig. 3.53). The intersphenoid septum is removed giving a good view of the entire sphenoid sinus complex which includes identification of the bulge in the posterior superior wall by the anterior sella turcica and also the bulge on the opposite lateral wall made by the internal carotid artery. This view of the lateral wall of the sphenoid sinus can be accomplished only by approaching the sphenoid sinus by way of the ethmoid sinus opposite to the side of the cystic lesion of the petrous apex (Fig. 3.54).

Intraoperative x rays are taken with a metal probe in place in order to determine the position and direction of the surgery (Fig. 3.55). Both anteroposterior and lateral x rays are necessary.

An opening in the posterior wall of the sphenoid sinus anterior to the cystic lesion and below the level of the indentation made by the carotid artery is made using a large diamond bur. If there is any doubt as to the position of the internal carotid artery, the lateral wall of the sphenoid sinus is also removed in this region and a small caliber spinal needle inserted into the carotid artery. The anterior wall of the cyst can also be positively identified by inserting a needle into the cyst and aspirating the typical watery, golden-brown material.

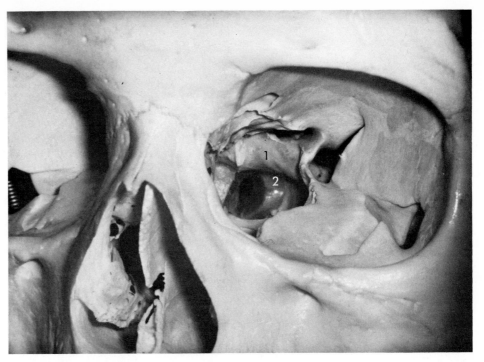

a

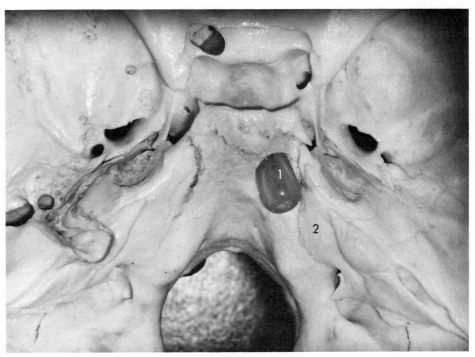

b

FIGURE 3.51.

a. The silicone drainage device has been inserted through the defect in the right sphenoid sinus.

1. Roof of sphenoid
2. Extracranial or intrasphenoid portion of the drainage device (Montgomery, 1977)

b. A view of the intracranial portion of the silicone drainage device (1), and the petrous apex (2) (Montgomery, 1977)

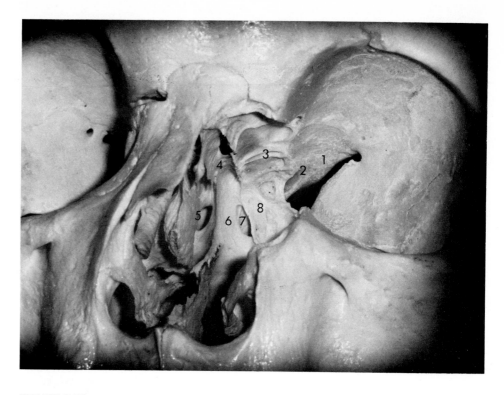

FIGURE 3.52.

A complete ethmoidectomy has been accomplished on the left side in this specimen. The left nasal bone and the ascending process of the maxilla have been removed for a better view.

1. Left superior orbital fissure
2. Optic foramen
3. Roof of ethmoid
4. Cribriform plate
5. Right sphenoid sinus
6. Nasal septum
7. Left sphenoid ostium
8. Anterior wall of the left sphenoid sinus
(Montgomery, 1977)

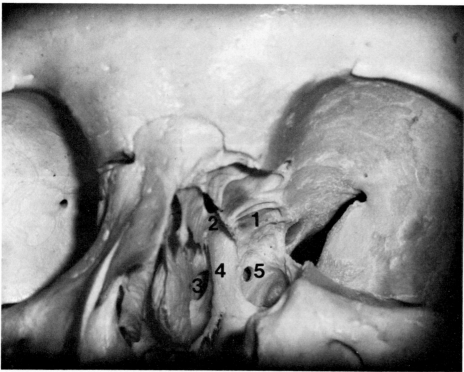

FIGURE 3.53.

The anterior wall of the left sphenoid sinus has been removed and a small opening made in the intersphenoid septum.

1. Roof of left ethmoid
2. Left cribriform plate
3. Right sphenoid ostium
4. Nasal septum
5. Intersphenoid septum
(Montgomery, 1977)

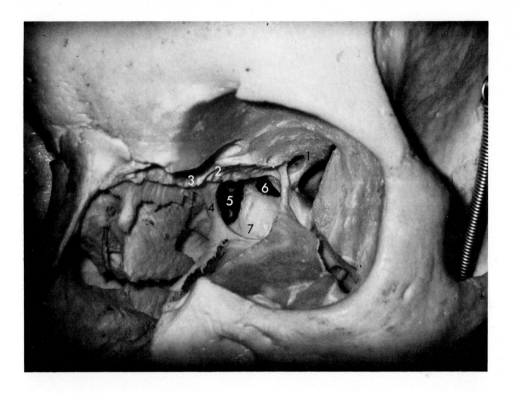

FIGURE 3.54.

The intersphenoid septum and a small portion of the posterior aspect of the nasal septum have been resected. The position of the anterior wall of the sella turcica and the bulge made by the right internal carotid artery are indicated. In order to approach the right petrous apex, the bone of the posterolateral right sphenoid sinus is removed below the level of the indentation made by the carotid artery.

1. Optic foramen
2. Roof of the ethmoid
3. Attachment of the upper extension of the middle turbinate, which separates the roof of the ethmoid and the cribriform plate
4. Posterior aspect of the nasal septum
5. Bulge made by the carotid artery
6. Anterior wall of the sella turcica
7. Direction of approach to the right petrous apex (Montgomery, 1977)

After the communication between the posterior wall of the sphenoid sinus and the anterior wall of the cyst has been enlarged as much as possible and the cyst completely evacuated, tantalum powder is dusted into the cyst cavity. The purpose of the tantalum powder is to obtain postoperative x rays that will demonstrate the size of the deflated cyst which can be used for future reference (Fig. 3.56a).

In order to ensure against closure of the communication between the sphenoid sinus and the cyst, a septal mucosal flap is constructed as described and illustrated with the technique for hypophysectomy. The septal mucosal flap is inserted through the opening between the sphenoid sinus and the cyst. A silicone drainage device, which can be constructed from a tracheal tube stent or obtained commercially,* is also inserted into this opening (Fig. 3.56b). The remainder of the operation is identical to that described with the external ethmoidectomy or hypophysectomy.

*E. Benson Hood, 211 Vine Street, Duxbury, Massachusetts 02332

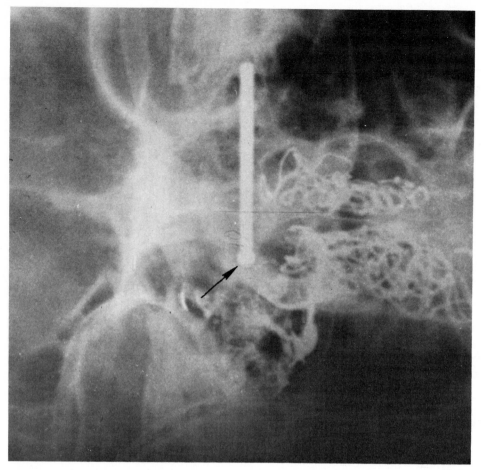

a

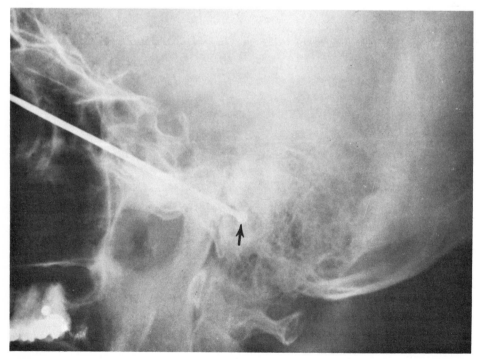

b

FIGURE 3.55.

Anteroposterior (*a*) and lateral (*b*) intraoperative x ray.

The x rays show the end of the probe (arrow) inside the cystic lesion of the right petrous apex (Montgomery, 1977).

FIGURE 3.56.

a. A basal x ray showing the outline of the tantalum powder inside the collapsed primary epidermoid cyst of the petrous apex (Montgomery, 1977).

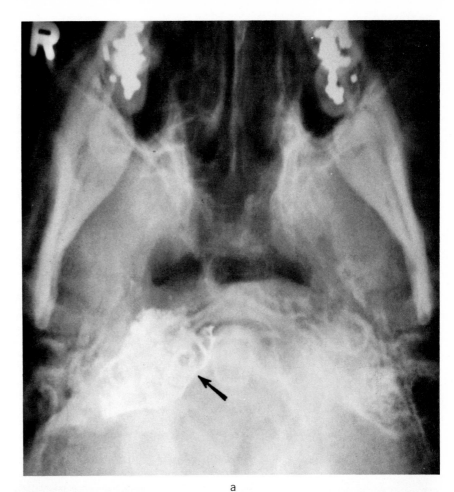

a

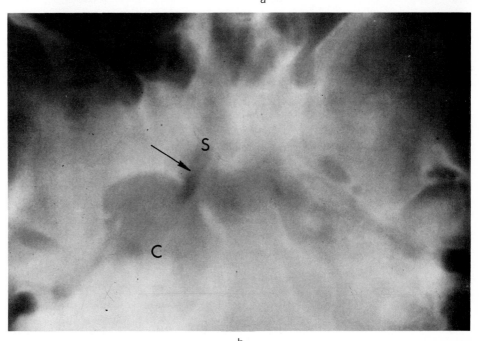

b

b. A horizontal polytome cut through the cystic lesion of the petrous apex and the sphenoid sinus similar to Figure 3.46. The arrow points to the position of the silicone drainage device between the sphenoid sinus and the cyst. S = right sphenoid sinus; C = cyst (Montgomery, 1977)

REFERENCES

Alexander, F. W.: Primary Tumors of the Sphenoid Sinus. Laryngoscope *73*:537–546 (May) 1963.

Arslan, M.: Ultrasonic Selective Hypophysectomy. Ann. Otol. *75*:3:798–807 (Sept.) 1966.

Ballenger, J. (Ed.): *Diseases of the Ear, Nose and Throat,* 11th ed. Philadelphia, Lea & Febiger, 1969, p. 165.

Bateman, G. H.: Trans-sphenoidal Hypophysectomy: a Review of 70 Cases Treated in the Past Two Years. Trans. Amer. Acad. Ophthal. Otolaryng. *66*:103–110, 1962.

Beard, C.: Lacrimal Sac Surgery. Trans. Amer. Acad. Ophthal. Otolaryng. *69*:970–976 (Sept.–Oct.) 1965.

Berris, R. F.: Preoperative and Postoperative Management of Hypophysectomy Patients. Arch. Otolaryng. *86*:282–286 (Sept.) 1967.

Burian, K.: Transsphenoidal Operation for Tumors of the Pituitary Gland. Arch. Otolaryng. *86*:4:449–452 (Oct.) 1967.

Chandler, P. A.: Dacryocystorhinostomy. Trans. Amer. Ophthal. Soc. *34*:240–263, 1936.

Chiari, O.: Zur Kasuistik der Erkrankungen der Unterkieferspeicheldrüse. Wien Klin. Wschr. *25*:1562–1567, 1912.

Cushing, H.: The Pituitary Body and Its Disorders. Philadelphia, J. B. Lippincott Co., 1912.

deLima, E. E.: Fundamentos anatomo-fisiologicos transmaxilar na cirurgia dos sejos da face. Rev. Brasil. Med. *6*:249–253 (April) 1949.

Diamant, M.: Hypophysectomy in a Nonpneumatized Sphenoid. Arch. Otolaryng. *74*:9–10, 1961.

Hamberger, C. A., Hammer, G., Norlen, G., and Sjogren, B.: Transantrosphenoidal Hypophysectomy. Arch. Otolaryng. *74*:2–8, 1961.

Heck, W. E., McNaught, R. C., Dobson, L. G., and Greenspan, F. S.: Palliation for Advanced Cancer of the Breast, Trans-septal-sphenoid Subtotal Hypophysectomy. Calif. Med. *92*:201–203, 1960.

Hirsch, O.: Ueber Methoden der operativen Behandlung von Hypophysistumoren auf endonasalem Wege. Arch. f. Laryng. u. Rhinol. *24*:129–177, 1910.

Hirsch, O.: Surgical Decompression of Malignant Exophthalmos. Arch. Otolaryng. *51*:325–334, 1950.

James, J. A.: Transethmoidosphenoidal Hypophysectomy. Arch. Otolaryng. *86*:256–264 (Sept.) 1967.

Kasper, K. A.: Dacryocystorhinostomy. Survey Ophthal. *6*:2:95–107 (April) 1961.

Loré, J. M., Jr.: Transseptal Transsphenoidal Hypophysectomy. Amer. J. Surg. *112*:4:577–582 (Oct.) 1966.

Macbeth, R., and Hall, M.: Hypophysectomy as a Rhinological Procedure. Arch. Otolaryng. *75*:440–450, 1962.

Montgomery, W. W.: Transethmoidosphenoidal Hypophysectomy with Septal Mucosal Flap. Arch. Otolaryng. *78*:68–77 (July) 1963.

Montgomery, W. W.: Transsphenoid Approach to the Cystic Lesions of the Petrous Apex. Ann. Otol. Rhinol. Laryngol. *86*:429–435, 1977.

Mosher, H. P.: The Combined Intranasal and External Operation on the Lacrimal Sac (Mosher-Toti). Ann. Otol. *32*:1:1–14 (Mar.) 1923.

Mosher, H. P.: The Surgical Anatomy of the Ethmoidal Labyrinth. Trans. Amer. Acad. Ophthal. Otolaryng. *34*:376–410, 1929.

Nager, F. R.: Paranasal Approach to Intrasellar Tumours. J. Laryng. *55*:361–381, 1940.

Netzer, H. R., and McCoy, E. G.: Transseptal Transsphenoidal Hypophysectomy. Arch. Otolaryng. *86*:252–255 (Sept.) 1967.

Noguera, J. T., and Haase, F. R.: Transsphenoidal Hypophysectomy for Metastatic Carcinoma of the Breast. EENT Digest (Mar.) 1965, p. 87.

Ogura, J. H., and Walsh, T. E.: The Transantral Orbital Decompression Operation for Progressive Exophthalmos. Laryngoscope *72*:8:1078–1096 (Aug.) 1962.

Pico, G.: Dacryocystorhinostomy, Trans. Amer. Acad. Ophthal. Otolaryng. *62*:709–711 (Sept.–Oct.) 1958.

Poppen, J. L.: Exophthalmos; Diagnosis and Surgical Treatment of Intractable Cases. Amer. J. Surg. *64*:64–79 (April) 1944.

Proetz, A. W.: Operation on the Sphenoid. Trans. Amer. Acad. Ophthal. Otolaryng. *53*:538–545 (May–June) 1949.

Raiford, M., Ackerly, E., and Vidal, F.: New Operative Technique in Naso-lacrimal Surgery. EENT Monthly *42*:37 (July) 1963.

Rand, R. W.: Cryohypophysectomy and Transfrontosphenoidal Craniotomy in Pituitary Tumors. Arch. Otolaryng. *86*:265–267 (Sept.) 1967.

Riskaer, N., Munthe Fog, C. V., and Hommelgaard, T.: Transsphenoidal Hypophysectomy in Metastatic Cancer of the Breast. Arch. Otolaryng. *74*:483–493, 1961.

Saunders, W. H., and Miglets, A.: Surgical Techniques for Eradicating Far Advanced Carcinoma of the Orbital-ethmoid and Maxillary Areas. Trans. Amer. Acad. Ophthal. Otolaryng. *71*:426–431 (May–June) 1967.

Schimek, R. A.: Pituitary Ablation in Progressive Diabetic Retinopathy. Arch. Otolaryng. *86:*274–281 (Sept.) 1967.

Scott, J. K.: Transsphenoidal Hypophysectomy for Diabetic Retinopathy. Arch. Otolaryng. *84:*77–81 (July) 1966.

Sewall, E. C.: External Operation on the Ethmoidosphenoid-frontal Group of Sinuses under Local Anesthesia. Arch. Otolaryng. *4:*377–411 (Nov.) 1926.

Sewall, E. C.: Operative Control of Progressive Exophthalmos. Arch. Otolaryng. *24:*621–623 (Nov.) 1936.

Spaeth, E. B.: The Mosher-Toti Dacryocystorhinostomy. Arch. Ophthal. *4:*4:487–496 (Oct.) 1930.

Sutaria, S. N.: Dacryocystography, J. All-India Ophthal. Soc. 6:64, 1958.

Turnbull, F. M.: An Antro-ethmoidosphenoidal Operation. Arch. Otolaryng. 9:271–281 (Mar.) 1929.

Van Buren, J. M.: Studies in Human Hypophyseal Ablative Procedures. Arch. Otolaryng. *86:*268–273 (Sept.) 1967.

Veirs, E. R.: The Lacrimal System in Clinical Practice. A manual prepared by the Amer. Acad. Ophthal. Otolaryng., Rochester, Minn., 1963.

Walsh, T. E., and Ogura, J. H.: Transantral Orbital Decompression for Malignant Exophthalmos. Laryngoscope *67:*544–568 (June) 1957.

Weille, F. L.: A Practical Technique for Intranasal Ethmoidectomy and an Evaluation of its Usefulness. Laryngoscope *69:*4:449–462 (April) 1959.

Willson, J. T.: Anatomical Considerations in Transsphenoidal Hypophysectomy. Arch. Otolaryng. *86:*245–251 (Sept.) 1967.

4

Surgery of the Frontal Sinus

FRONTAL SINUS ANATOMY

The frontal bone consists of two portions: (1) a squamous or vertical portion which forms the forehead and houses the frontal sinuses, and (2) an orbital or horizontal portion which serves as the roof of the orbital cavity and floor of the anterior cranial fossa. The nasal process of the frontal bone articulates with the two nasal bones and the ascending process of the maxilla. Along with the zygomatic bone, the frontal bone makes up the supraorbital margin. Laterally, in the temporal fossa, the frontal bone articulates with the greater wing of the sphenoid bone. Posteriorly, it articulates with the parietal bone to form the coronal suture. In the orbital cavity, the frontal bone articulates with the lacrimal, ethmoid, and sphenoid bones.

Each frontal sinus is usually somewhat pyramidal in shape and lies between the inner and outer table of the vertical portion of the frontal bone. The roof of the orbital cavity forms its base. There are usually two frontal sinuses, but there may be three or even more. If additional frontal sinuses are present, they may lie lateral or posterior to one another. Quite frequently a frontal sinus is partially subdivided by septa. These septa can be so placed as to interfere with proper drainage. The two frontal sinuses are frequently asymmetrical. In about 10% of persons, one frontal sinus does not develop above the level of the supraorbital rim. The important relations of the frontal sinus are the anterior cranial fossa and the orbit. The bony plate separating the frontal sinus from these neighbors can be quite thin and is potentially the direction for extension of disease.

Drainage from the frontal sinus into the nasal cavity is variable. In most persons the nasofrontal duct is absent and drainage takes place directly from the

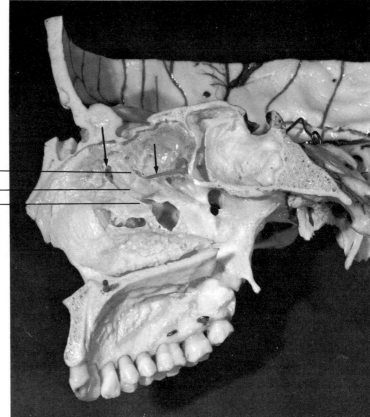

Ethmoid bulla ———————
Hiatus semilunaris ———
Uncinate process ———

a

FIGURE 4.1. *Right lateral nasal wall.*

a. The anterior wall of the frontal sinus and the middle turbinate have been removed. The long arrow points to the opening of the nasofrontal duct in the upper hiatus semilunaris. Usually the frontal sinus drains directly into this area. The shorter arrow points to a straw in the right sphenoidal ostium.

b. The arrow points to a straw which has been placed in the nasofrontal orifice. In approximately 15% of individuals the sinus does not drain directly into the nasofrontal recess, and there is a true nasofrontal duct which empties into the infundibulum.

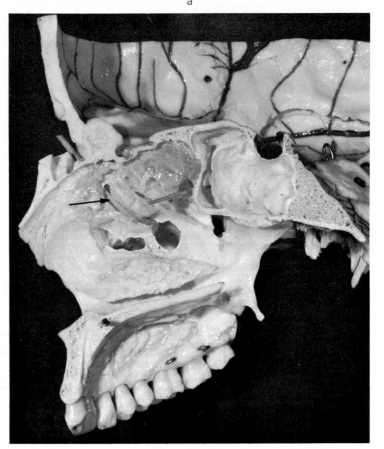

b

frontal sinus into the frontal recess of the nasal cavity (Fig. 4.1). In approximately 15%, the drainage from the frontal sinuses is by way of a nasofrontal duct into the infundibulum ethmoidale. Probably the most common cause for blockage of drainage and maintenance of a chronic infection of the frontal sinus is impingement of the nasofrontal orifice in the middle meatus. This can be caused by abnormally large ethmoid cells in this region, a cystic or cellular middle turbinate, a deviated nasal septum, or a chronic edematous inflammatory process of the middle turbinate. In some persons, an anterior ethmoid cell may extend superiorly and interfere with the patency of the nasofrontal orifice or duct.

The blood supply to the frontal sinus is from the internal carotid artery by way of the supraorbital branch of the ophthalmic artery. On occasion there may be a branch of the anterior ethmoid artery supplying the frontal sinus. Externally, blood is drained from the sinus into the facial vein; posteriorly, venous drainage takes place through emissary vessels passing into the dura, and internally, by way of the orbit.

The frontal sinus is innervated by the supraorbital branch of the ophthalmic nerve. Most of the sensory nerve endings are found in the region of the nasofrontal orifice; thus an increase or decrease of intrasinus pressure can produce severe frontal pain.

DIAGNOSIS OF FRONTAL SINUS DISEASE

Acute frontal sinusitis is manifest clinically by history of a recent upper respiratory infection or such activity as diving into or swimming underwater. An airplane ride or a drive to the mountains with an upper respiratory infection is not an uncommon history preceding acute frontal sinusitis.

The pain associated with acute frontal sinusitis is almost invariably directly over the sinus on the forehead. There may also be pain in the orbit, especially superiorly. Tenderness elicited by palpation of the floor of the frontal sinus just posterior to the medial aspect of the supraorbital rim is typical of acute frontal sinusitis. The pain associated with acute frontal sinusitis is severe. It often begins at eight or nine o'clock in the morning and gradually increases in intensity until its departure at about four o'clock in the afternoon. It is thus often referred to as "union headache."

Since the inflammatory process of acute frontal sinusitis extends into the orbit, the lids swell. A complicating orbital cellulitis or orbital abcess may be manifest by proptosis. This type of extension of infection into the orbit, however, is much less frequent with acute frontal sinusitis disease than it is with acute ethmoiditis.

X-ray diagnosis of acute frontal sinusitis can be difficult. Thickened mucous membrane accompanied by a fluid level and the absence of bony sclerosis around the frontal sinus are typical of acute frontal sinusitis. The x-ray findings, however, may not be typical and are often behind the current disease process, making serial x rays mandatory for proper diagnosis, treatment, and prognosis. It must be remembered that the x-ray findings of acute frontal sinusitis may persist even after months of therapy and are not by themselves an indication for surgical intervention. This is especially true of acute osteomyelitis of the frontal bone which has complicated acute frontal sinusitis. In such cases the antibiotic therapy is continued for at least 2 months, and x-ray findings of resolution of disease may not be in evidence for 2 additional months.

A submucosal hemorrhage in the frontal sinuses must not be misinterpreted as acute frontal sinusitis. This condition results from acute pressure change, such as rapid descent in an airplane.

Chronic frontal sinus disease often remains undiagnosed for a long time, especially when an orbital manifestation of chronic frontal sinus disease (page 32) is being treated by an ophthalmologist or a frontal bone defect (by x ray) is diagnosed by a neurosurgeon.

Today much less supposition is associated with the diagnosis of chronic frontal sinus disease compared with a decade ago. The introduction of polytomography, ultrasonography, CT scanning, and EMI body scanning have accounted for this change. The diagnosis of a large osteoma (Fig. 4.2a, b, c) is obvious by routine sinus x rays and, as a rule, additional studies are not necessary. An example of such is a 60-year-old male, who gives a history of a right frontal sinus trephine operation at the age of 14 years as treatment for acute frontal sinusitis. He remained symptom free for 30 years and then began having progressively worsening intermittent right forehead pain. The symptom of right tearing has been present during the past 2 years. One year ago he noted diplopia and downward and outward displacement of the right eye without change in his pain pattern (Fig. 4.3a). Routine sinus x rays demonstrated a large mass in the frontal sinuses, which was presumed to be a mucocele or pyocele. The outline of the frontal sinuses was not lost and there was no evidence of sclerosis around the frontal sinuses. By routine sinus x rays a defect was noted in the medial aspect of the floor of the right frontal sinus (Fig. 4.3b-arrow). This defect may have resulted from the previous frontal sinus trephine operation. Polytomes of the sinuses and orbit did not demonstrate a mass in the orbit (Figs. 4.3c, d). As a general rule polytomes will not demonstrate a soft tissue mass, such as a mucocele which has extended into the orbit, for there is little or no contrast difference between a mucocele and the orbital contents.

CT scanning did not demonstrate a mass in the orbit. EMI body scanning, however, clearly outlined the orbital mass in both the coronal and horizontal planes (Fig. 4.3e, f).

Ultrasonography showed a very large mass along the orbital wall medially. The lesion is well circumscribed and ovoid; it measured 35 mm in the anteroposterior dimension. The low amplitude echoes suggest a cystic lesion (Fig. 4.3g).

The patient's signs and symptoms disappeared following a bilateral osteoplastic frontal sinus operation with adipose obliteration.

TREPHINATION OF THE FRONTAL SINUS

Indications

Most episodes of acute frontal sinusitis clear spontaneously or following local intranasal therapy (decongestant sprays), intermittent packing with 4% cocaine-impregnated cotton pledgets in the region of the middle meatus, and/or local application of heat combined with systemic treatment (antibiotics and systemic decongestants).

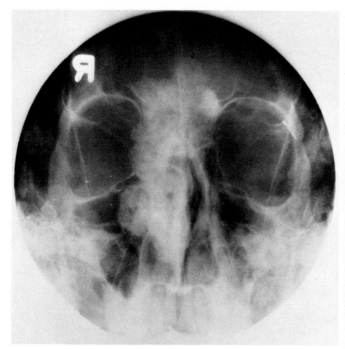

a

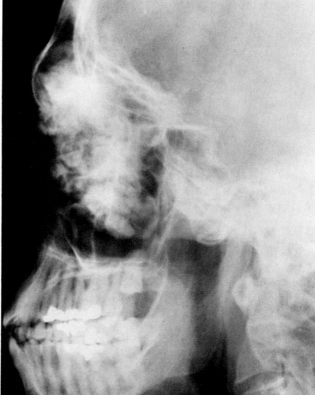

b

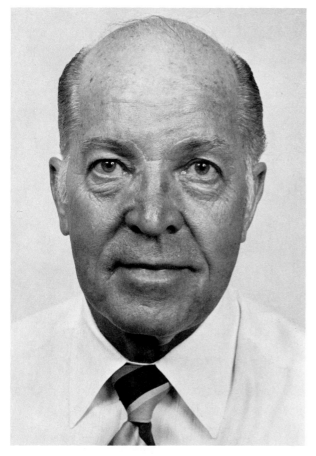

c

FIGURE 4.2.

a. A large osteoma involving both frontal sinuses, extending to both ethmoid sinuses and into the nasal cavity and maxillary sinus on the right side.

b. A lateral x ray demonstrating this large osteoma. Routine sinus x rays are sufficient for preoperative evaluation in such cases. This osteoma was removed by performing a bilateral osteoplastic frontal sinus adipose obliteration operation along with a right lateral rhinotomy.

c. A photograph taken 1 year following the above surgery demonstrates the good cosmetic results of the above operation.

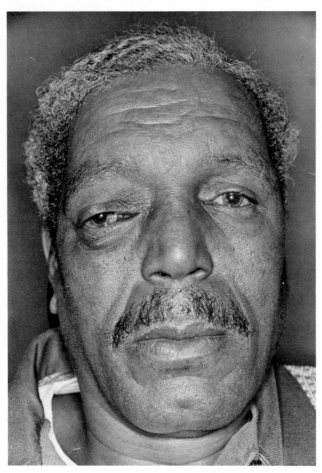

a

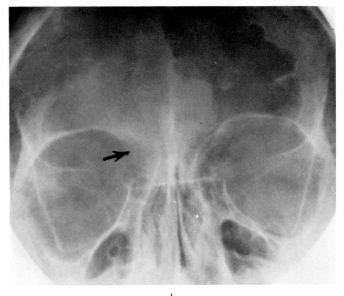

b

FIGURE 4.3.

a. A 60-year-old man with a history of a frontal trephine operation at the age of 14 years, right frontal pain of 15 years' duration, tearing of 2 years' duration, downward and outward displacement of right eye with diplopia of 1-year duration.

b. Routine sinus x rays demonstrated a mass in the frontal sinuses and a defect in the medial aspect of the floor of the right frontal sinus (arrow), which may have resulted from his previous frontal sinus trephine operation.

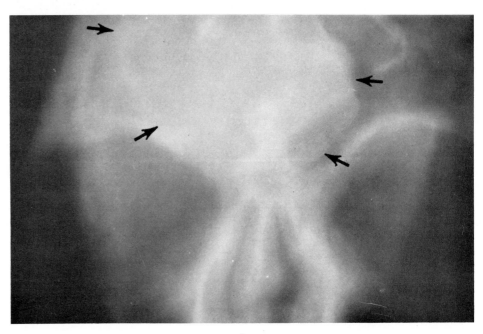

c

c. A coronal polytome of the sinuses and orbit demonstrate the mass (arrow) in the frontal sinuses but no mass in the right orbit.

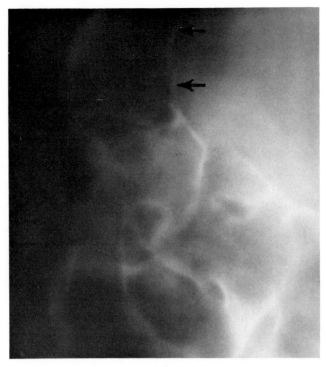

d

d. A lateral polytome of the frontal sinus proves that the posterior wall (arrow) of the frontal sinuses was intact.

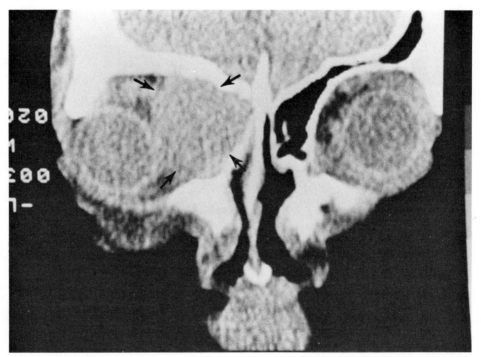

e

e. Body scanning in the coronal plane clearly demonstrates the mass in the right orbit.

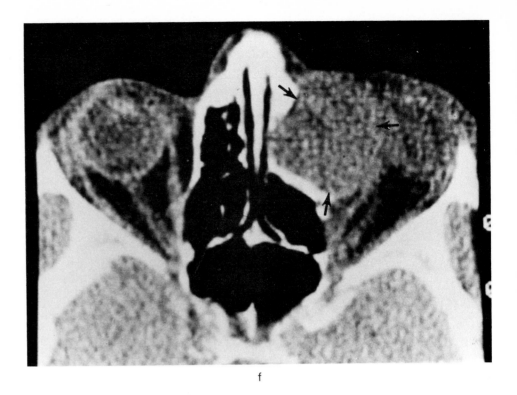

f

FIGURE 4.3. (Continued)

f. The right orbital mass is again demonstrated by EMI body scanning in the horizontal plane.

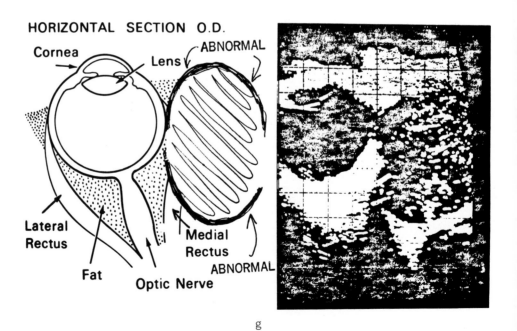

g

g. Ultrasonography demonstrates a 35-mm well-circumscribed ovoid mass in the medial aspect of the right orbit. Low amplitude echoes suggest a cystic lesion.

If pain is not present, a 10-day to 2-week period of local and systemic therapy should be prescribed. X rays of the sinuses should be taken (upright Waters' views) at 2- to 4-week intervals until the sinuses appear normal. X-ray evidence of fluid and/or swelling of the mucosal lining of the frontal sinus is not positive indication for the trephine operation unless the patient has persistent pain.

If, on the other hand, the acute frontal sinusitis is accompanied by persistent pain in the region of the sinus and edema of the upper eyelid and there is lack of response to conservative measures, it will be necessary to obtain drainage in order to prevent complications.

In addition to its use in the treatment of acute frontal sinusitis, the trephine operation may be employed as an exploratory procedure, to determine the nature of chronic frontal-sinus disease and/or to obtain a biopsy specimen.

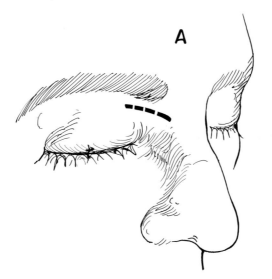

A

FIGURE 4.4. *Trephination of frontal sinus.*

A. The incision for trephination of the frontal sinus is made in the superomedial aspect of the orbit, immediately below the eyebrow and supraorbital rim. It is carried through all layers including the periosteum over the floor of the frontal sinus.

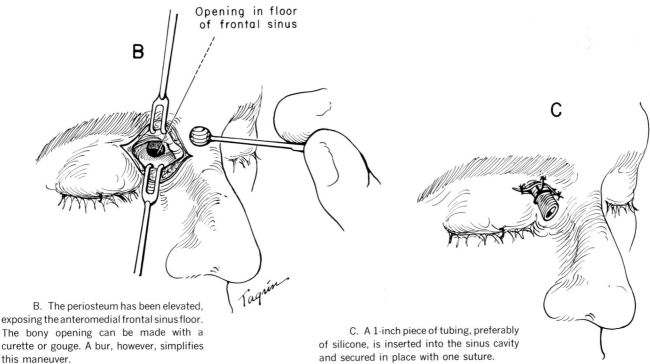

Opening in floor of frontal sinus

B

C

B. The periosteum has been elevated, exposing the anteromedial frontal sinus floor. The bony opening can be made with a curette or gouge. A bur, however, simplifies this maneuver.

C. A 1-inch piece of tubing, preferably of silicone, is inserted into the sinus cavity and secured in place with one suture.

Technique

Trephination of the frontal sinus can be carried out with the patient under either local or general anesthesia. A ¾-inch horizontal incision is made in the superomedial aspect of the orbit just below the eyebrow, through skin, subcutaneous tissue, and the periosteum over the floor of the frontal sinus (Fig. 4.4a). The periosteum is then elevated above and below this incision, exposing the floor of the frontal sinus. The floor, rather than the anterior wall, is penetrated, for the floor consists of laminar bone containing no marrow, whereas the bone of the anterior wall is cancellous and contains marrow. If cancellous bone becomes contaminated by the purulent secretions from the frontal sinus there is danger of complicating osteomyelitis. A curette, or, preferably, a rotating cutting bur is used to penetrate the bone (Fig. 4.4b) and make an opening in the floor 6 to 8 mm in diameter. Material for a culture is then taken.

Some idea of the status of the interior of the sinus can be obtained by direct vision and also by inspection with an instrument, such as a nasopharyngoscope, inserted into the sinus through the trephine opening. Following inspection of the sinus, a rubber or plastic drainage tube, approximately 1 inch in length, is inserted and sutured in place (Fig. 4.4c).

Following the release of pus, the edema of the mucous membrane in the region of the nasofrontal orifice soon subsides, and normal drainage is reestablished. Irrigation of the sinus through the drainage tube with warm normal saline solution is of value, and should be executed at least four times a day. Specific antibiotics, prescribed according to results of sensitivity tests, may be added to the irrigation solution. In addition to local treatment the patient is given systemic antibiotics. The patency of the nasofrontal communication may be determined by inserting a dilute dye solution (methylene blue) into the sinus through the trephine tubing. If the nasofrontal orifice is patent the dye should appear in the nasal cavity almost immediately. The trephine tube is removed as soon as drainage by the natural route has been reestablished.

INTRANASAL SURGERY FOR CHRONIC FRONTAL SINUSITIS

The treatment of chronic frontal sinusitis has been a frustrating problem for the rhinologist. Antibiotics alone are often of little value but should be given during the subacute and early chronic stages, along with local and systemic nasal decongestants.

In many instances, chronic frontal sinusitis can be cured by correcting the intranasal situations which either interfere with proper drainage by way of the nasofrontal passage or initiate re-infection of the sinus. The establishment of adequate drainage with ultimate resolution of the infection can often be accomplished by an intranasal operation. A careful submucous resection of the nasal septum, removal of intranasal polyps and/or the anterior portion of the middle turbinate, and an anterior ethmoidectomy are the procedures used to reestablish this drainage. If chronic ethmoiditis seems to be the offender, a complete external ethmoidectomy is indicated.

Intranasal probing and attempted enlargement or cannulization of the naso-frontal orifice are mentioned only to be condemned. Once the virginity of the nasofrontal passage is violated, scarring and stenosis are inevitable. If conservative intranasal surgery is not successful, then radical frontal sinus surgery is indicated.

EXTERNAL SURGERY OF THE FRONTAL SINUS

Indications

Chronic frontal sinusitis, complicated with persistent pain, external fistula, internal fistula, intracranial extension, bone necrosis, orbital complications, and/or a mucocele or pyocele, and benign and malignant tumors of the frontal sinuses are positive indications for external frontal sinus surgery.

Various Techniques

There are numerous external frontal sinus operations, each having many variations. Those currently popular in the United States and the anatomic changes effected by each are shown in Figure 4.5.

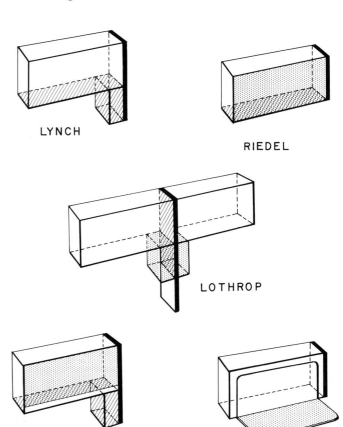

FIGURE 4.5. *Various frontal sinus operations.*

Box sketches indicating the anatomic changes effected by the various frontal sinus operations currently popular in the United States.

LYNCH

RIEDEL

LOTHROP

KILLIAN

OSTEOPLASTIC

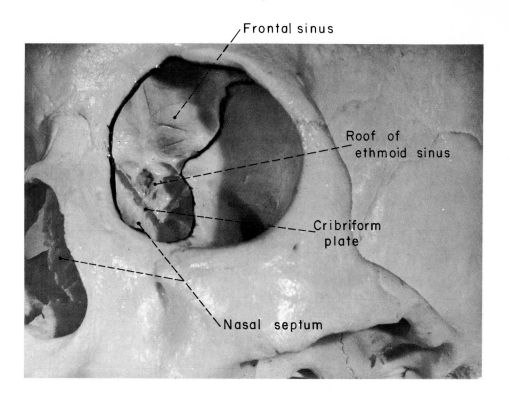

Frontal sinus

Roof of
ethmoid sinus

Cribriform
plate

Nasal septum

FIGURE 4.6. *Skull demonstrating the osteology of a Lynch operation on the left frontal sinus.*

A complete ethmoidectomy has been performed and the entire floor of the frontal sinus has been removed. The roof of the ethmoid sinus and the cribriform area can be seen as well as the nasal septum. Note that the upper extension of the attachment of the middle turbinate separates the roof of the ethmoid sinus from the cribriform plate.

Lynch Frontal Sinus Operation (1920). In the United States, this is probably the most frequently employed procedure for the treatment of chronic frontal sinus disease (Fig. 4.6). An ethmoidectomy, removal of the middle turbinate, and resection of the entire floor of the frontal sinus are included in this operation. A rubber or plastic tube is placed between the frontal sinus and the nasal cavity by way of the ethmoid labyrinth. This tube is left in place from one to three months following the operation and, at times, requires considerable care. As a general rule, the Lynch frontal approach has been highly effective in the control of chronic frontal sinus disease; on the other hand, its failure rate is sufficient to warrant the search for a better operation. Incomplete removal of the mucous membrane of the sinus can result in mucocele and pyocele formation. A stenosis of the reconstructed nasofrontal passage may lead to recurrent chronic frontal sinusitis.

Riedel Operation (1898). This consists of removing the anterior wall and floor of the frontal sinus, thus offering wide exposure of the sinus. The sinus cannot be completely obliterated in many cases, especially when its anteroposterior dimensions are large. Mosher modified the Riedel operation by removing the posterior wall of the sinus also. As a general rule, the Riedel procedure is disfiguring and offers a percentage of cure no higher than that of the Lynch operation.

Lothrop Frontal Sinus Operation (1914). This procedure entails a unilateral or bilateral anterior ethmoidectomy and middle turbinectomy. The interfrontal septum is removed. A large opening from the frontal sinuses into the nasal cavity is made by connecting the two nasofrontal ducts and resecting a portion of the superior nasal septum. The operation may be technically difficult, but it is quite effective in a patient with bilateral frontal sinus disease and in frontal sinuses with wide anteroposterior dimensions.

Killian Operation (1904). This is a modification of the Riedel procedure. In the Killian operation also, an anterior ethmoidectomy and middle turbinectomy are performed. However, a bridge of bone 10 mm wide is left in place at the supraorbital rim. This functions, of course, to prevent postoperative disfigurement. This operation is attended with much less alteration of the forehead contour than is the Riedel procedure; on the other hand, the bridge prevents obliteration of the sinus. Actually, the end result of the Killian operation is quite similar to that of the Lynch operation.

Anterior Osteoplastic Frontal Sinus Operation. This operation, described in the late nineteenth century literature, has been revived during the past decade. In this operation an inferiorly hinged "trapdoor" of bone is fashioned from the anterior wall of the frontal sinus. This affords direct access to the entire contents of the frontal sinus and an excellent view of the nasofrontal orifice from above. The intrasinus disease can be removed with ease. Revisions of previous frontal sinus surgery can be performed. Adequate drainage from the frontal sinus to the intranasal space can be established, or the frontal sinus can be obliterated completely by the implantation of adipose tissue.

The modification of the osteoplastic adipose obliterative frontal sinus operation is basically similar to that outlined by Bergara and Itoiz and by Tato and associates. It has been very successful in the treatment of chronic frontal sinus disease. The advantages of this technique are:

1. It is a direct approach. The entire sinus, including the orifice of the nasofrontal duct, can be seen. The intrafrontal disease can be eradicated entirely. The dissecting microscope may be employed, if necessary, to accomplish this task. A decision whether or not to obliterate the sinus can be made readily. For example, when revising a Lynch frontal operation, the surgeon has the choice of revising the approach from above or obliterating the sinus with adipose tissue.
2. There is rarely facial deformity following the operation. All other radical frontal sinus operations do produce orbital or forehead defects (Fig. 4.7).
3. The operation is relatively atraumatic and its morbidity is low. Postoperative care is negligible. We have found follow-up care to be unnecessary other than for the purpose of clinical research.
4. The two frontal sinuses may be operated upon simultaneously.

Adipose Obliteration. Experimental evidence has shown that adipose tissue seems to be the ideal implantation substance for long-term obliteration of the frontal sinus. Adipose obliteration of the feline frontal sinus has led to the following observations and conclusions:

1. Varying amounts of adipose tissue survive. The remaining portion is replaced by fibrous tissue to complete the obliteration.
2. Time is not a factor, for both one-week and one-year experiments showed 95% survival of adipose tissue, while other experiments (Fig. 4.8a) showed only 50% survival of the adipose tissue.
3. Revascularization of the adipose implant from the blood supply available in the osseous sinus wall occurs during the first few days by ingrowth of blood vessels and direct blood-vessel anastomosis.

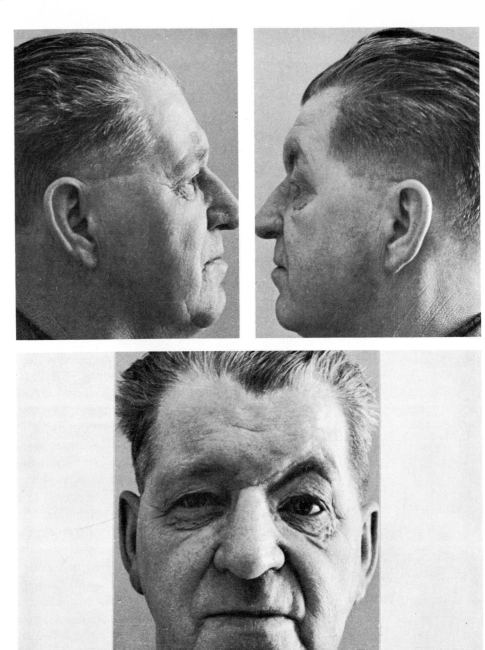

FIGURE 4.7. *Comparison of deformity following Lynch operation with the result of an osteoplastic frontal sinus procedure.*

In this patient the deformity resulting from a Lynch frontal sinus operation on the left side may be compared with the result of an osteoplastic frontal sinus operation on the right. The Lynch frontal sinus operation was performed in 1939 for treatment of left pansinusitis. The right osteoplastic frontal sinus operation was performed in 1960 for removal of a mucocele.

4. Traumatized adipose implants do not survive well and are for the most part replaced by fibrous tissue.

5. Adipose tissue seems to resist infection. Clinical results demonstrate that cartilaginous adipose implants have not been affected by the presence

of pathogenic organisms. None of our experimental adipose implants became infected.

6. There was complete obliteration of the frontal sinus in all experiments when adipose tissue implants were used.

7. There was no regeneration of mucous membrane. It is apparent that the rapid revascularization of the implant prevents ingrowth of mucous membrane into the frontal sinus or into the nasofrontal region.

8. The evidence obtained from the experiments as well as clinical experience strongly emphasizes the fact that the removal of both the mucosal and inner cortical linings (Fig. 4.8b) of the frontal sinus is absolutely necessary for a successful obliteration.

Case Report. A 39-year-old man was admitted to the Massachusetts Eye and Ear Infirmary with a history of a left exophthalmos of 1-year duration. Intermittent pain in the region of the left eye and forehead had also been present during this period. The osteoma was quite large, nearly filling the left frontal sinus and extending down into the ethmoid (Fig. 4.9). The osteoma (Fig. 4.10) was removed using a unilateral osteoplastic flap. Since the sinus was otherwise normal, it was not obliterated using adipose tissue. The resulting cosmesis was very good (Fig. 4.11). The patient remained asymptomatic until 1972 (15 years later) when he returned with recurrence of this exophthalmos and forward displacement of the osteoplastic flap caused this time by a mucocele of the left frontal sinus (Fig. 4.12). He has remained asymptomatic following revision of the operation and obliteration of the frontal sinuses with adipose tissue. Had an adipose obliteration been added to his original operation in 1957, a second operation for mucocele would most likely not have been necessary.

Technique of Unilateral Osteoplastic Operation

Preoperative Preparation. Preoperative bacteriologic cultures from the nose should be obtained for antibiotic sensitivity tests. Cultures must be made well in advance so that appropriate antibiotic therapy may be instituted prior to surgery. Pathogenic organisms are often not found in cultures of intranasal material obtained prior to operation, and therefore it is important that additional material for culture be taken from the frontal sinus at the time of the operation.

An x-ray cutout (template) is made preoperatively from the Caldwell view of the x rays of the sinus. This is done by placing an exposed transparent x-ray film over the Caldwell view and outlining the sinuses with a glass-marking pencil. The cutout may be made slightly smaller than the actual dimensions of the sinus to ensure that the cut will lie within the sinus limits. However, with careful cutting this is not essential. The cutout is placed in sterilizing solution prior to surgery.

The abdomen should be prepared so that an adipose autograft may be obtained from the subcutaneous layer of the left abdominal wall (a right rectus incision is avoided so that the scar will not at a later date be interpreted as one resulting from an appendectomy).

The Operation. The forehead and face are prepared and draped in the manner appropriate for any frontal sinus procedure. The patient lies on the table in the supine position with his head slightly raised and inclined forward. The patient's eyelids are sewed together with #5-0 dermal sutures to prevent injury to the eyes during the operation. The eyebrows are not shaved.

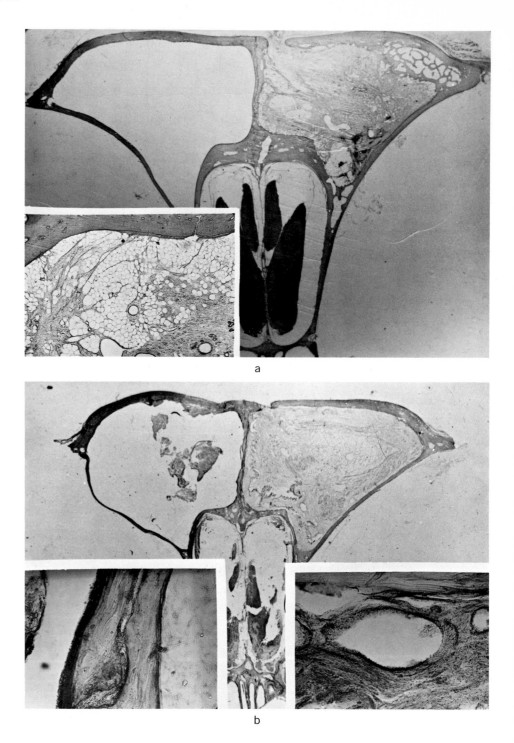

a

b

FIGURE 4.8.

a. The left frontal sinus was implanted with adipose tissue after removal of the mucosal and inner cortical linings. The right frontal sinus was unaltered and used as a control. The animal was perfused with formalin at the end of 1 year. The left frontal sinus is well obliterated and there has been no mucous membrane regeneration. Seventy-five percent of this 1-year implant (insert) survived as adipose tissue.

b. The left frontal sinus was implanted with adipose tissue after the mucous membrane and inner cortical lining had been removed with curettes and forceps. The inner cortical lining of the right sinus was not removed. The animal was perfused with formalin solution at the end of 3 months.

The left frontal sinus is completely obliterated. No mucous membrane regeneration has occurred. Approximately 55% of the implant has survived as adipose tissue.

The right frontal sinus has been completely obliterated. The adipose tissue has been completely lost and remains as a small amount of fibrous tissue attached to the anterior sinus wall. The entire frontal sinus is relined with mucous membrane. It is obvious that the adipose implant was not revascularized with the presence of an intact inner cortical lining.

The lower left insert is a photomicrograph of the right frontal sinus, inner frontal septum, and left frontal sinus. The right frontal sinus is not obliterated and there is regeneration of mucous membrane. The left frontal sinus is completely obliterated without mucous membrane regeneration. The lower right insert is a photomicrograph from the anterior aspect of the right frontal sinus. The adipose tissue has been replaced by fibrous tissue. The mucous membrane-lined cysts that have formed in this area may well represent early mucoceles.

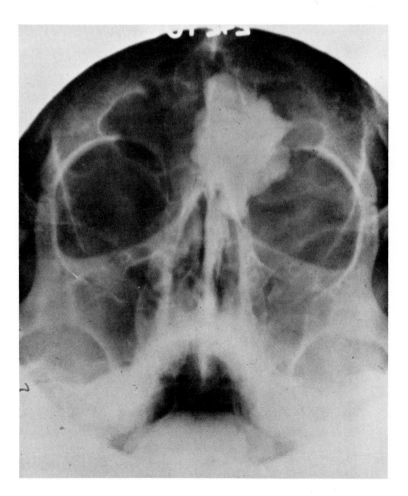

FIGURE 4.9. *X ray of an osteoma.*

This osteoma was located in the left frontal sinus in a 39-year-old man who presented with left exophthalmos in 1957.

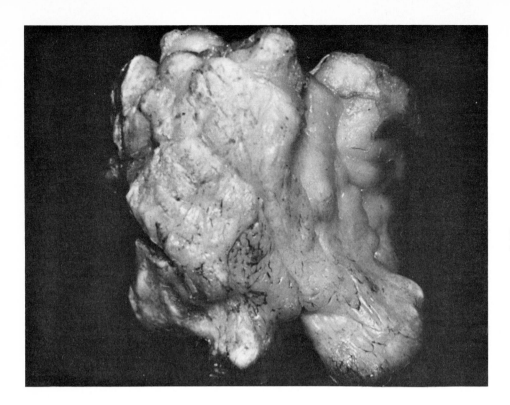

FIGURE 4.10. *The osteoma, which was removed intact.*

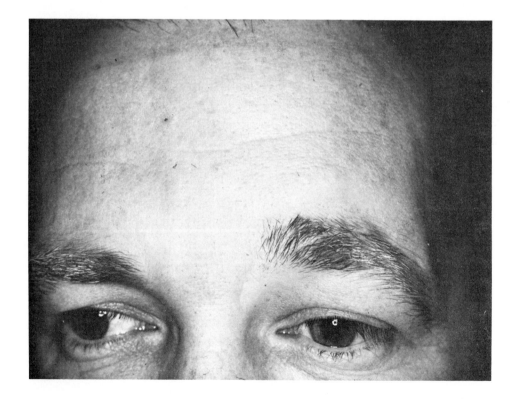

FIGURE 4.11.
This postoperative photograph shows the good cosmetic result following removal of the osteoma by way of a left osteoplastic frontal sinus operation. The sinus was not obliterated with adipose.

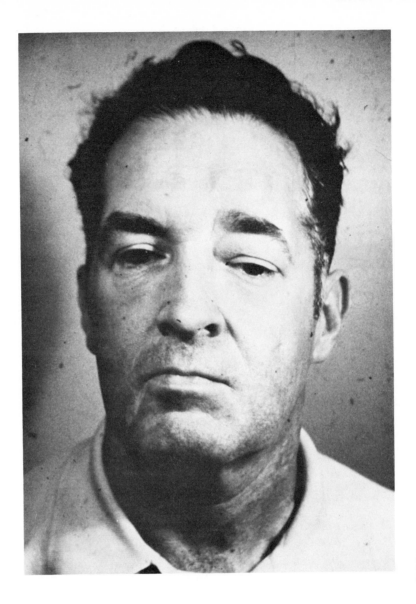

FIGURE 4.12.

This photograph of the patient was taken 15 years (1972) following removal of the osteoma. Recurrent exophthalmos is now caused by a mucocele of the left frontal sinus. It is speculated that this mucocele would not have formed had the original operation included adipose obliteration.

Procaine or Xylocaine (2%), with added epinephrine, is infiltrated along the upper margin of the eyebrow, both to reduce the amount of bleeding and to supplement the general anesthetic.

In the unilateral procedure the first incision is made along the entire length of the upper margin of the eyebrow (Fig. 4.13). The incision is carried through the subcutaneous tissues and the frontalis muscle to the periosteum covering the frontal bone. It is essential not to extend the incision into the periosteum in order that the blood supply to the osteoplastic flap be preserved.

With scissors and blunt dissection a plane of cleavage is easily established between the frontalis muscle and the frontal periosteum (Fig. 4.13b). It is important

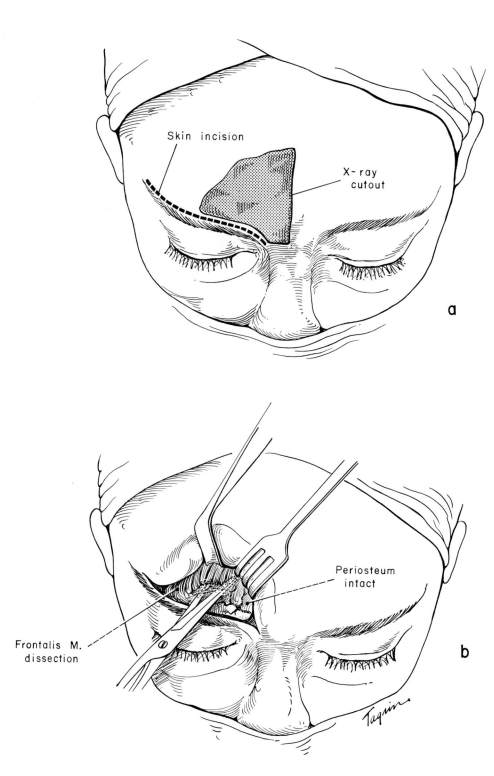

FIGURE 4.13. *Unilateral osteoplastic operation.*

    a. The skin incision is made along the upper margin of the eyebrow. For adequate exposure it is best to extend this incision along the entire length of the eyebrow.

    The x-ray cutout, which is traced around the Caldwell x-ray view of the frontal sinus, is used to outline the periosteal incision.

    b. The periosteum over the frontal bone is exposed with dissection in the plane deep to the frontalis muscle.

to make this exposure wide enough so that the x-ray cutout may be applied to the periosteum to outline the periosteal incision (Fig. 4.13a).

The periosteal incision is made around the x-ray cutout (template). This incision should include the periosteum over the supraorbital rim medially and laterally (Fig. 4.14). The periosteum along the supraorbital rim between the above incisions is not disturbed so as to ensure an adequate blood supply for the osteoplastic flap. The periosteum above the incision is then elevated a few millimeters in order to obtain adequate space for a clean bone cut.

The bone incision is made along the outline of the periosteal incision with a Stryker saw blade which has been especially designed for this purpose (Fig. 4.15). The saw is slightly angulated so that it is directed towards the cavity of the frontal sinus (Fig. 4.14b). Beveling of this bone incision accomplishes two purposes: it ensures that the incision is within the limits of the frontal sinus and it allows for accurate replacement of the osteoplastic flap. Following the outline of the periosteal incision, the bone incision is extended so as to include the supraorbital rim medially and laterally (Fig. 4.16). This step is essential to provide for a fracture which hinges the osteoplastic flap across the floor of the frontal sinus, just posterior to the supraorbital rim.

A mallet and chisel are used to inspect the completeness of the bone incision (Fig. 4.14c). Inspection is accomplished by inserting the chisel, tapping lightly, and prying around the entire bone incision. The chisel is then placed superiorly and, with a prying maneuver, the osteoplastic flap is elevated downward and forward (Fig. 4.14d).

The interior of the frontal sinus can now be inspected (Fig. 4.14e). A sample is taken for culture. It is at this point that the surgeon makes his final decision as to the extent of the operation. If a benign tumor, such as an osteoma, is present, it is removed and no further surgery is necessary, providing the mucous membrane lining is not diseased and the nasofrontal orifice is adequate. If the mucous membrane lining of the frontal sinus is so extensively diseased that there is no possibility of its recovery, it is removed and the surgeon should proceed with an obliterative procedure. The entire inner cortical bony lining of the sinus, including that on the inner aspect of the osteoplastic flap, is removed with a rotating cutting bur (Fig. 4.17a). This step must be systematically and carefully accomplished. The dissecting microscope may be used if necessary. The removal of the inner cortical lining is essential both to ensure a complete removal of the mucosal sinus and to establish a blood supply to nourish the adipose autograft. The removal of mucous membrane and inner cortical lining is carried up to, but not into, the nasofrontal orifice. Revascularization of the adipose implant, during the first few postoperative days, creates a barrier between the nasofrontal orifice and the sinus cavity.

Subcutaneous adipose tissue is obtained from the left abdominal wall by way of a left rectus incision. Subcutaneous catgut sutures are used to eliminate the dead space resulting from the removal of this tissue. Blood vessels are carefully ligated to prevent formation of a hematoma. A drain should remain in place for 48 hours.

The adipose tissue autograft is then fashioned so as to fill the frontal sinus completely (Fig. 4.17b). The osteoplastic flap is then returned to its original position. The periosteum is sutured with #4-0 chromic catgut (Fig. 4.17c). The wound is then closed subcutaneously with #4-0 chromic catgut sutures and the skin with #5-0 dermal sutures.

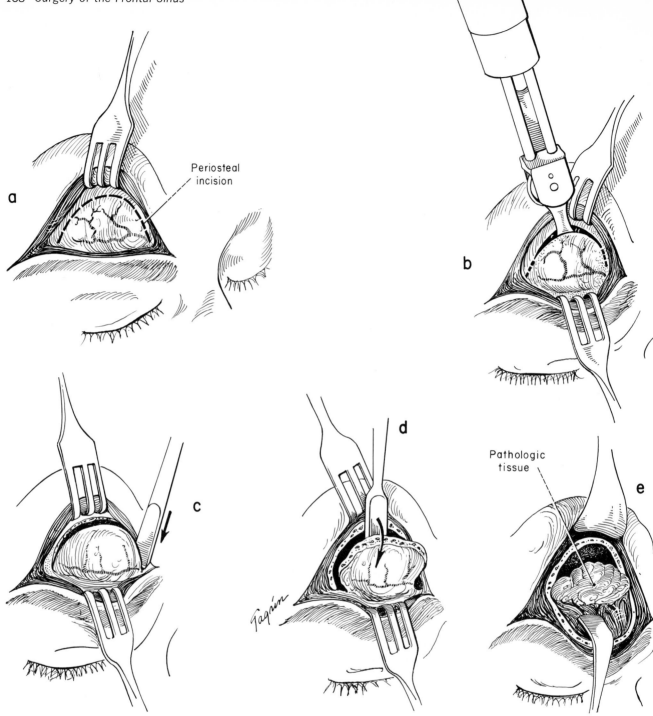

FIGURE 4.14. *Unilateral osteoplastic operation.*

a. The periosteal incision is made according to the outline of the x-ray film template. It is important to extend the periosteal incision medially and laterally so as to include the supraorbital rim.

b. A Stryker saw of special design (see Fig. 4.15) is used to cut the bone flap. The bone incision is beveled, at least superiorly, to facilitate replacement of the bone flap and prevent its inward displacement.

c. A chisel is used to inspect the entire bone incision before the osteoplastic flap is elevated. A few taps with the mallet are usually necessary to complete the bone incision.

d. The flap is elevated by placing a chisel superiorly and prying in an anterior direction.

e. The osteoplastic flap has been reflected inferiorly for inspection of the interior of the frontal sinus.

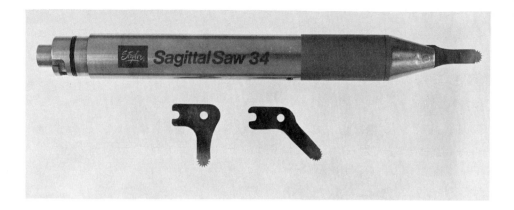

FIGURE 4.15.

The new tangential Stryker saw 34 is used for frontal sinus and other facial bone surgery. Blades directed straight ahead, at 45- and 90-degree angles, are available with this oscillating saw.

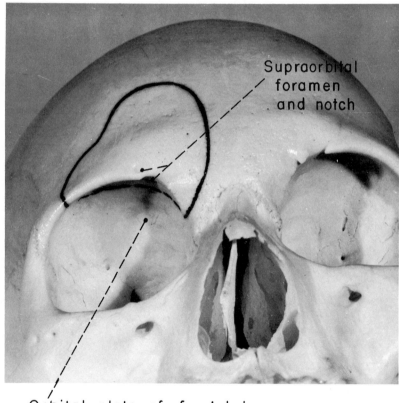

FIGURE 4.16. *Outline of the unilateral osteoplastic flap.*

The indicated periosteal and bone incision is made around the outline of the frontal sinus and just lateral to the interfrontal septum (or midline). This incision must be extended medially and laterally through the supraorbital rim. At least the superior portion of the bone incision should be beveled so as to facilitate replacement of the bone flap and prevent its being displaced into the sinus. As the flap is elevated a fracture occurs across the floor of the frontal sinus, just posterior to the supraorbital rim. The periosteum in the region of the supraorbital rim remains intact, thus ensuring a blood supply to the osteoplastic flap.

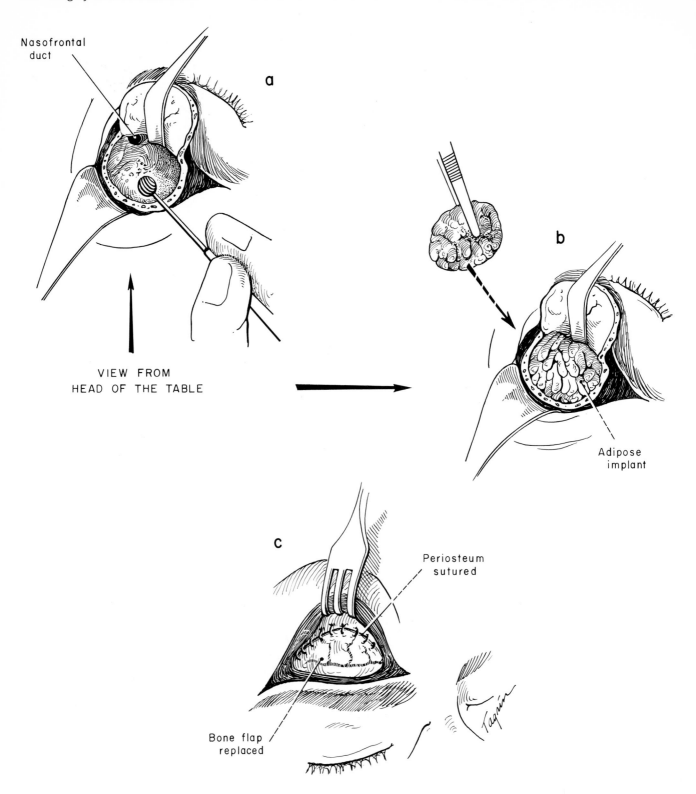

FIGURE 4.17. *Unilateral osteoplastic operation.*

     a. Rotating cutting bur is used to remove any remaining fragments of the lining of the mucous membrane and also the inner cortical lining of the frontal sinus. The latter is removed to ensure an adequate blood supply for the adipose implant.

     b. Subcutaneous abdominal adipose tissue is fashioned so as to fill the frontal sinus completely.

     c. The osteoplastic flap has been replaced and the periosteum sutured.

The forehead dressing consists of Telfa gauze, placed over the incision, an eye pad, fluffed 4- x 4-inch sponges and three strips of Elastoplast adhesive. An elastic bandage is placed over this dressing.

The elastic bandage is removed at the end of 24 hours. The remainder of the dressing is removed at the end of 48 hours. No further postoperative care is necessary other than administration of antibiotics, if prescribed, and removal of the skin sutures on the fifth and sixth postoperative day.

Techniques of Bilateral Osteoplastic Operation

Preoperative Preparation. X rays of the sinuses are taken within a few weeks prior to the operation in order to determine the extent of disease. It is of particular interest to note: (1) the depth of the sinuses; (2) whether or not the anterior and posterior walls are intact; and (3) if the interfrontal septum has been perforated or destroyed by disease. A pattern (template) of the outline of the frontal sinuses is obtained from the Caldwell x-ray view. The template is made by placing a transparent exposed piece of x-ray film over the Caldwell view and tracing the outline of the sinus with a glass-marking pencil. The template, of course, must be sterilized prior to surgery.

A culture of the nasal cavity should be obtained at least one week before the operation. If pathogens are found, sensitivity tests should be carried out and the proper antibiotic administered during the immediate postoperative period.

If the coronal incision is to be used the patient is given a thorough shampoo with hexachlorophene solution the evening before the operation. The abdomen is shaved and prepared for the removal of the subcutaneous abdominal adipose tissue that is to be used to obliterate the frontal sinuses.

The Operation. Either the eyebrow or the coronal incision can be used for the bilateral osteoplastic frontal sinus operation (Fig. 4.18). The eyebrow incision should be made along the entire length of the upper margin of the eyebrow and extended horizontally over the nasal process of the frontal bone. If the coronal incision is employed the hair is saturated with undiluted hexachlorophene solution, combed back, and shaved approximately 1½ inches behind the anterior hairline. The incision is made approximately 1 inch behind the anterior hairline as is shown in Figure 4.18. Drapes are carefully sutured in place in order to maintain a sterile field during the operative procedure. The eyelids are closed with # 5-0 polyethylene or silk suture material when using the eyebrow incision. This is not necessary when the coronal incision is employed. The bilateral eyebrow flap is elevated superiorly in a plane between the frontalis muscle and the periosteum over the frontal bone (Fig. 4.18). The coronal flap is elevated in the same plane and reflected inferiorly (Fig. 4.19). Since bleeding is much more of a problem with the coronal incision, 1% Xylocaine or procaine solution, with added epinephrine, is infiltrated into the line of the incision. Hemostatic clips much facilitate the control of this bleeding.

The bilateral eyebrow flap is elevated superiorly, exposing the nasal process of the frontal bone. The coronal flap is reflected inferiorly over the face, exposing both supraorbital rims and the nasal process of the frontal bone.

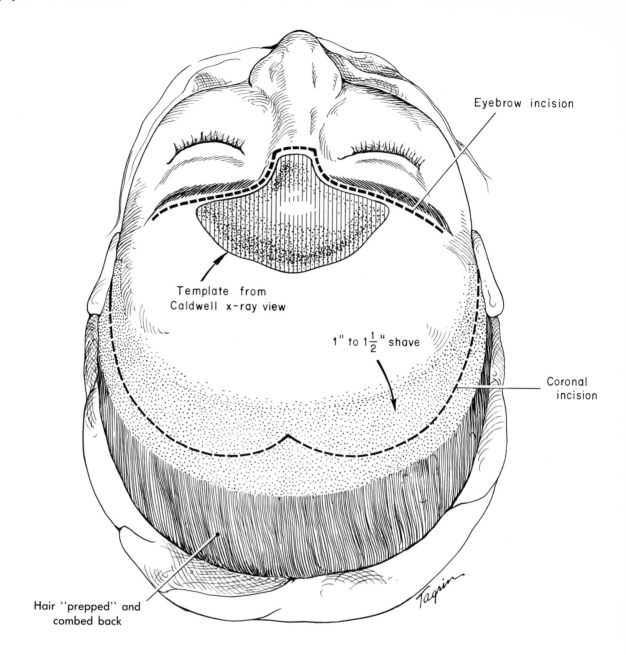

Eyebrow incision

Template from
Caldwell x-ray view

1" to 1½" shave

Coronal
incision

Hair "prepped" and
combed back

FIGURE 4.18.   *Incisions for the bilateral osteoplastic operation.*

The coronal incision is made approximately 1 inch posterior to the anterior hairline. This is most suitable for female patients but can also be used for males.

The bilateral eyebrow incision is made along the entire length of the upper margin of both eyebrows and straight across the nasal process of the frontal bone.

Both flaps are elevated in a plane between the frontalis muscle and the pericranium. A pattern for the periosteal incision is obtained from the Caldwell x-ray view.

The x-ray template is taken from the sterilizing solution, rinsed with saline solution, and placed over the frontal periosteum. The inferior aspect of the template is cut across horizontally at a level just above the cribriform plate. A notch placed in the superior aspect of the template to indicate the midline or position of the interfrontal septum is quite helpful. The template is positioned so that it

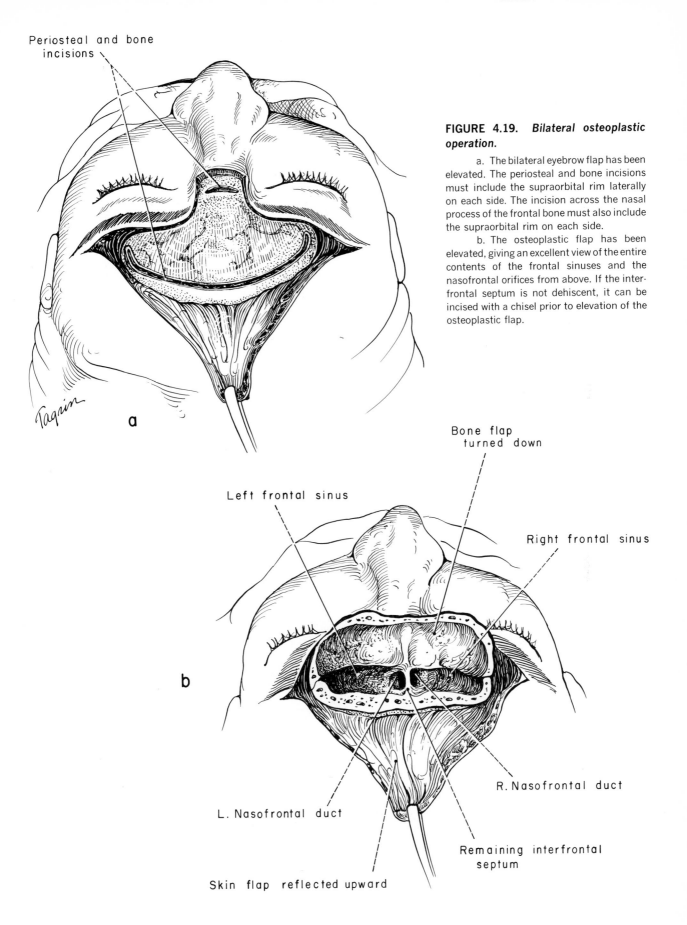

Periosteal and bone
incisions

FIGURE 4.19. *Bilateral osteoplastic operation.*

a. The bilateral eyebrow flap has been elevated. The periosteal and bone incisions must include the supraorbital rim laterally on each side. The incision across the nasal process of the frontal bone must also include the supraorbital rim on each side.

b. The osteoplastic flap has been elevated, giving an excellent view of the entire contents of the frontal sinuses and the nasofrontal orifices from above. If the interfrontal septum is not dehiscent, it can be incised with a chisel prior to elevation of the osteoplastic flap.

a

Bone flap
turned down

Left frontal sinus

Right frontal sinus

b

L. Nasofrontal duct

R. Nasofrontal duct

Remaining interfrontal
septum

Skin flap reflected upward

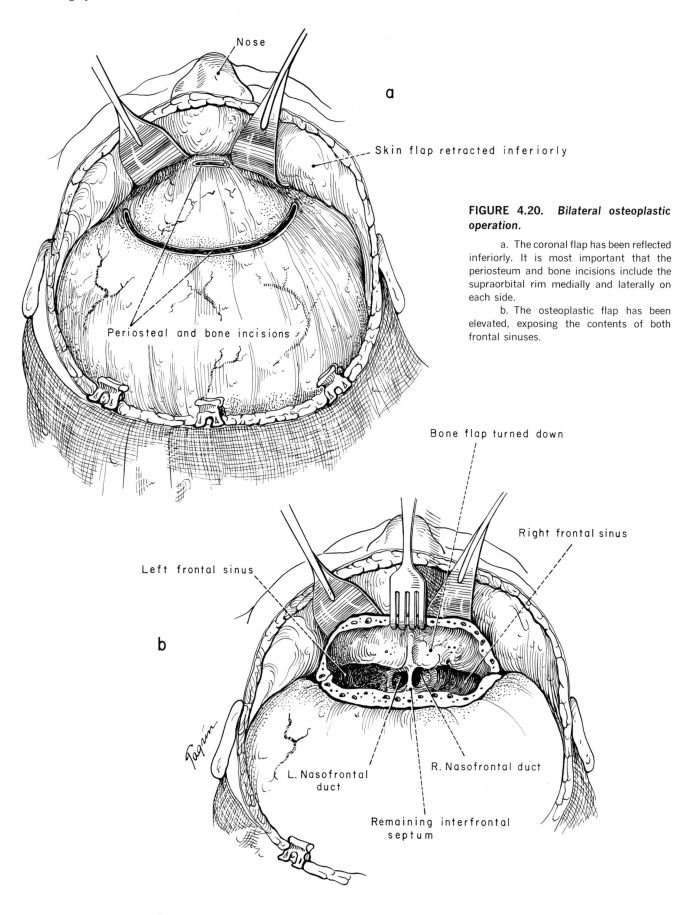

Nose

a

Skin flap retracted inferiorly

FIGURE 4.20.   *Bilateral osteoplastic operation.*

a. The coronal flap has been reflected inferiorly. It is most important that the periosteum and bone incisions include the supraorbital rim medially and laterally on each side.

b. The osteoplastic flap has been elevated, exposing the contents of both frontal sinuses.

Periosteal and bone incisions

Bone flap turned down

Left frontal sinus

Right frontal sinus

b

L. Nasofrontal duct

R. Nasofrontal duct

Remaining interfrontal septum

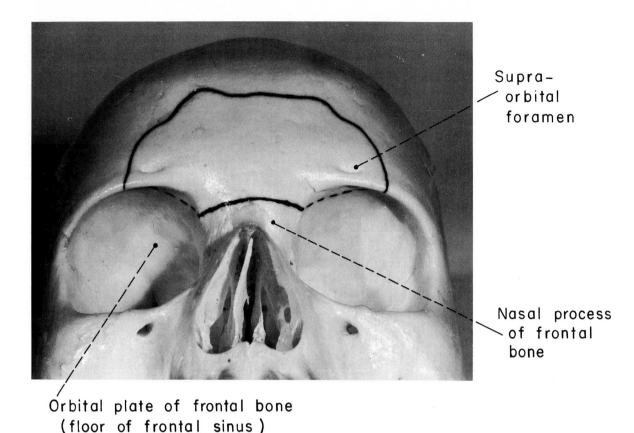

Supra-
orbital
foramen

Nasal process
of frontal
bone

Orbital plate of frontal bone
(floor of frontal sinus)

FIGURE 4.21. *Outline for the bilateral osteoplastic flap.*

The periosteal and bone incision around the outline of the frontal sinus must include the supraorbital rim laterally on each side. The periosteal and bone incision across the nasal process of the frontal bone must include the supraorbital rim medially on each side. The bone incision superiorly must be beveled so as to facilitate replacement of the flap and prevent it from being displaced into the sinuses. As the flap is elevated, a fracture occurs across the floor of both frontal sinuses, just posterior to the supraorbital rim. The periosteum in the region of both supraorbital rims remains intact to ensure a blood supply for the osteoplastic flap.

accurately approximates the supraorbital rims on each side. It is held in place by any sharp object, such as a needle or knife, by stabbing through the template, periosteum, and against the frontal bone. A #15 scalpel blade is used to incise the periosteum around the outline of the template. A horizontal incision is made in the periosteum over the nasal process of the frontal bone (Figs. 4.18a and 4.19a). It is important to include the periosteum over the supraorbital rims, both medially and laterally (Fig. 4.21). Superiorly, the bone incision is made on a bevel so as to make certain that it enters the frontal sinus and to ensure an accurate reapproximation of the osteoplastic flap.

The osteoplastic flap is then elevated by prying with a chisel or an elevator at the superior aspect of the bone incision. As the flap reflects downward and forward there is a fracture across the floor of the frontal sinuses just behind the supraorbital rims where the bone is invariably quite thin (Fig. 4.20). If the inter-frontal septum is present, it will interfere with the elevation of the osteoplastic

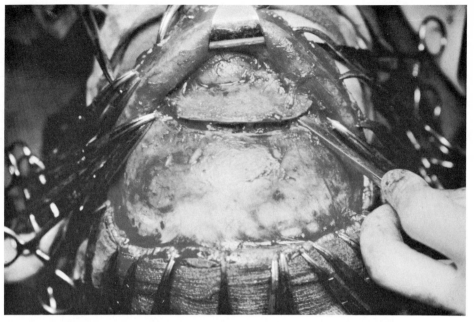

a

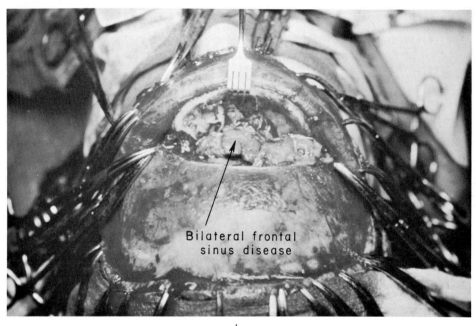

b

FIGURE 4.22. *Bilateral osteoplastic operation (coronal incision).*

a. Photograph of the bilateral osteoplastic flap being elevated in a patient who had a downward and outward displacement of the right orbital contents and diplopia as a result of extensive bilateral polypoid sinusitis. A coronal flap has been reflected inferiorly.

b. The osteoplastic flap has been elevated and reflected inferiorly. The frontal sinus is filled with purulent material and diseased mucous membrane.

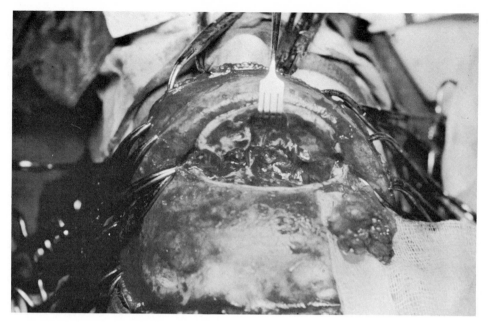

a

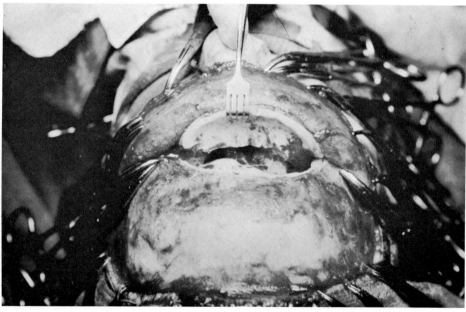

b

FIGURE 4.23. *Bilateral osteoplastic operation.*

a. The diseased mucous membrane has been grossly removed from both frontal sinuses. The interfrontal septum is found to have been destroyed by disease. The pathologic tissue can be seen on a sponge to the right.

b. The remaining mucosal and entire inner cortical lining of both frontal sinuses has been removed with a rotating cutting bur. The superior aspect of both nasofrontal orifices can be seen.

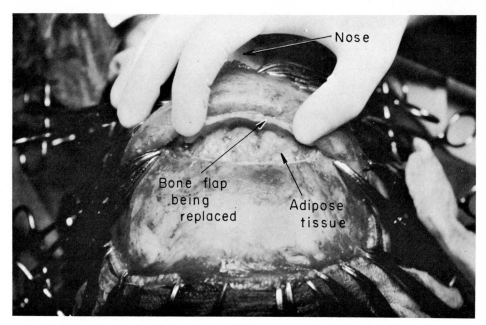

a

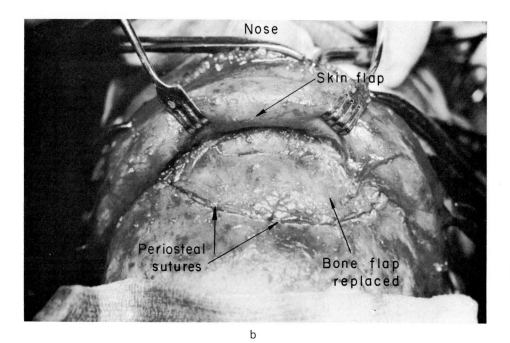

b

FIGURE 4.24. *Bilateral osteoplastic operation.*

a. The frontal sinus complex has been filled with subcutaneous abdominal adipose tissue, and the osteoplastic flap is being replaced.

b. The osteoplastic flap has been replaced and the periosteum sutured.

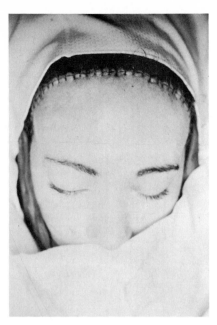

a

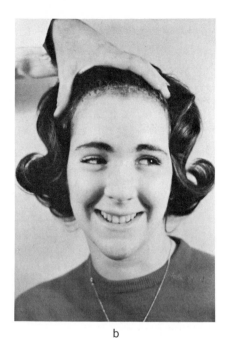

b

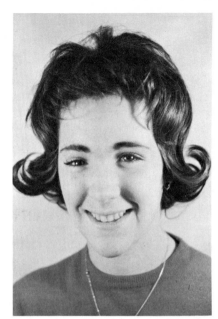

c

FIGURE 4.25. *Bilateral osteoplastic operation (coronal incision).*

    a. The coronal incision has been sutured, thus completing the operation.

    b. The patient is shown one week after surgery. The sutures are to be removed at this time.

    c. One week following operation. The suture line is hidden by a temporary revision of the hair style.

flap. This septum must be incised by inserting a chisel from above before attempting to elevate the flap.

After the osteoplastic flap has been reflected inferiorly, the interior of the sinuses is inspected (Figs. 4.19b, 4.20b, and 4.22b). The diseased tissue and mucous membrane are removed from the frontal sinus and the superior margin of the nasofrontal orifice. The interfrontal septum is removed. A rotating cutting bur is then used to remove the remnants of mucous membrane and also the inner cortical lining of the sinuses. The inner cortical lining of the inner aspect of the osteoplastic flap should also be removed to ensure complete removal of the mucosal lining and to establish an adequate blood supply to nourish the adipose implant (Fig. 4.23b).

Subcutaneous adipose tissue is taken by way of either a vertical or a horizontal left rectus incision and fashioned so that it completely fills both frontal sinuses and obstructs the superior aspect of both nasofrontal ducts (Fig. 4.24). It is not important to attempt placing adipose tissue into the nasofrontal ducts, for they will be sealed from the sinuses by revascularization of the adipose implant within a few days after the operation. The osteoplastic flap is returned to its original position, and the periosteum sutured with #3-0 chromic catgut or Dexon sutures (Fig. 4.24). If the osteoplastic flap is not stable following application of the periosteal sutures, two small holes are drilled on each side of the osteoplastic incision so that wires may be applied (Fig. 4.26). The coronal incision is sutured as a single layer, using #3-0 polyethylene sutures (Fig. 4.25). A pressure dressing, to remain in place for 24 to 48 hours, is placed over both eyes and the forehead. Antibiotic therapy is continued for at least 7 days postoperatively.

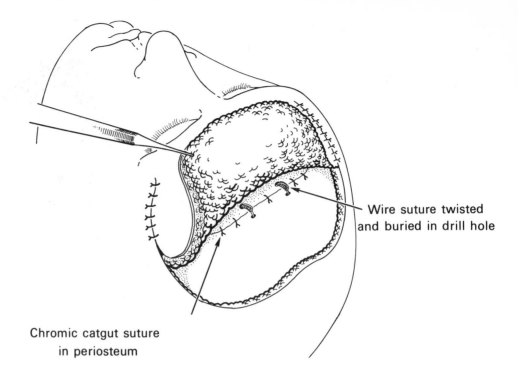

Wire suture twisted
and buried in drill hole

Chromic catgut suture
in periosteum

FIGURE 4.26.

Two wire sutures are used to stabilize the osteoplastic flap when suturing of the periosteum is ineffective. These sutures prevent the osteoplastic flap from becoming displaced forward and the resultant forehead deformity (Montgomery, 1973).

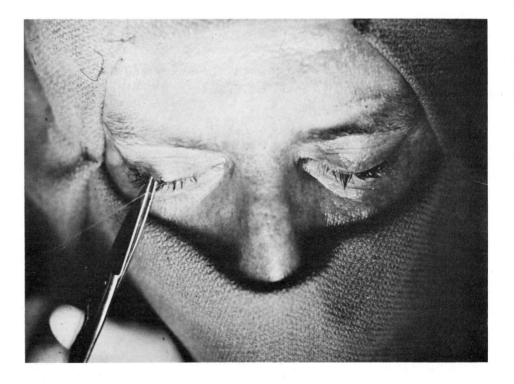

FIGURE 4.27.

The eyelids have been closed using one suture of #5-0 polyethylene suture material.

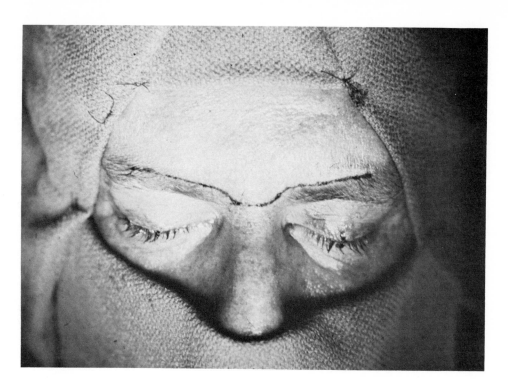

FIGURE 4.28.

The incision is made along the entire length of the upper margin of both eyebrows. These two incisions are connected by an incision in the skin over the nasal process of the frontal bone.

Bilateral Osteoplastic Operation (Eyebrow Incision)

The bilateral osteoplastic operation using the eyebrow incision is demonstrated in Figures 4.27 through 4.37.

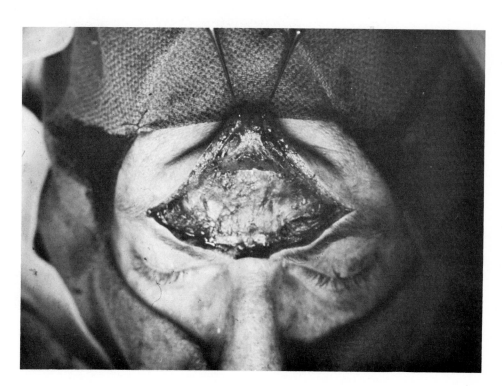

FIGURE 4.29.

The superiorly based flap is elevated between the frontalis muscle and the periosteum over the frontal bone.

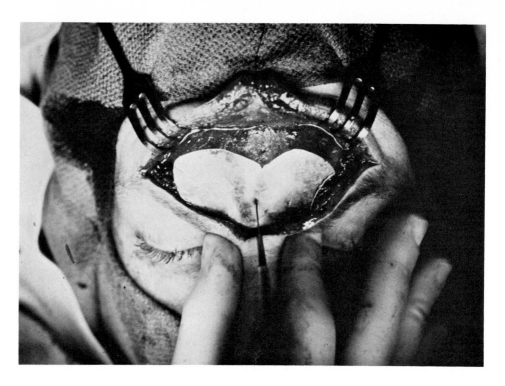

FIGURE 4.30.

A template made from the Caldwell x ray is placed over the frontal bone. This template is directed inferiorly against the thumb and index finger of the right hand, which are placed against the supraorbital rim. This maneuver is imperative to avoid a misdirected bone incision.

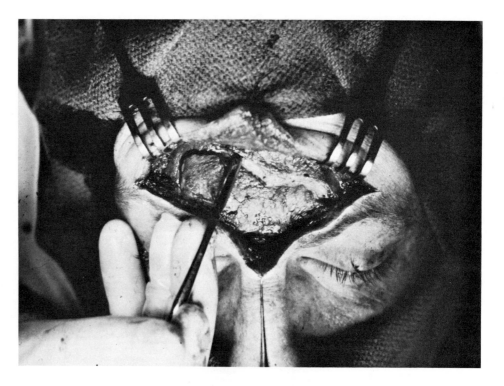

FIGURE 4.31.

The periosteum is elevated superiorly so that it will not be injured when the bone cut is made. The periosteum is not elevated inferiorly.

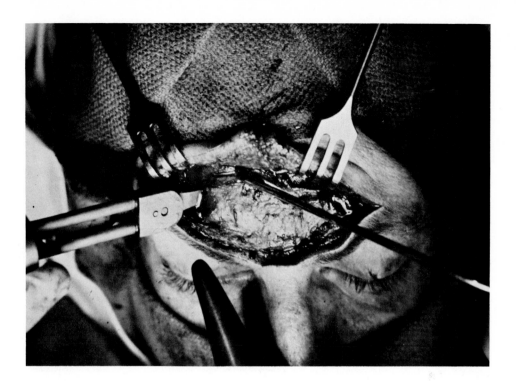

FIGURE 4.32.

The bone cut is beveled as is shown so that the osteoplastic flap can be accurately approximated following obliteration with adipose tissue.

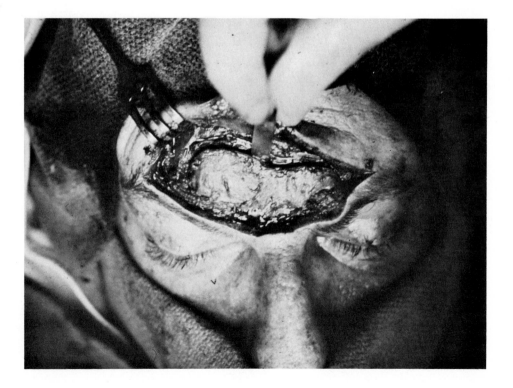

FIGURE 4.33.

The interfrontal septum is being incised with an osteotome.

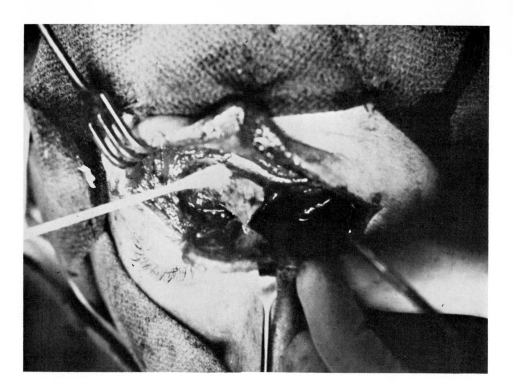

FIGURE 4.34.

The osteoplastic flap is elevated exposing the disease in the frontal sinuses.

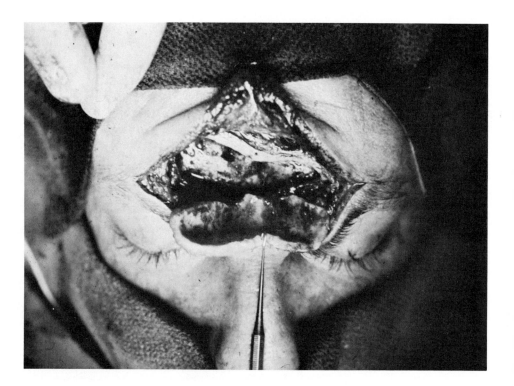

FIGURE 4.35.

The disease, mucosal and inner cortical lining have been removed from the *entire* frontal sinus complex.

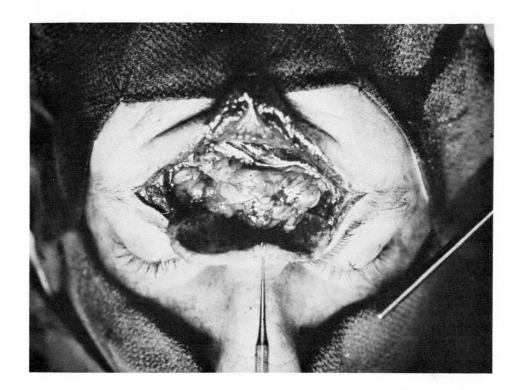

FIGURE 4.36.

Adipose tissue obtained from the subcutaneous abdomen (left) is used to obliterate the frontal sinus complex.

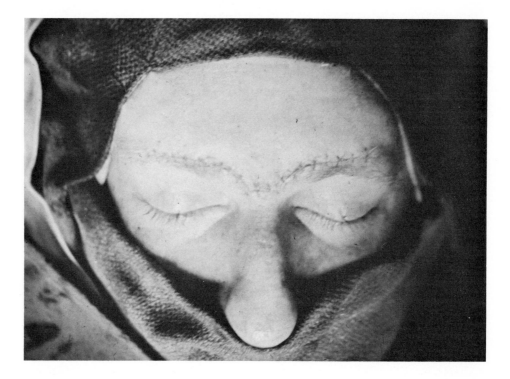

FIGURE 4.37.

The incision has been repaired in three layers, using #3-0 chromic catgut and #5-0 polyethylene suture material.

Osteoplastic Frontal Sinusotomy: An Analysis of 250 Operations

Twenty years' experience with the osteoplastic frontal sinusotomy operation has been accumulated at the Massachusetts Eye and Ear Infirmary, and 250 consecutive operations performed from 1956 through 1972 were reviewed. Of these, 62% were male; 38% female. Ages ranged from 10 to 84 years. A follow-up of 83% of the patients was obtained by examination or questionnaire. Median follow-up was 8 years but ranged from 3 to 19 years (Table 4.1).

TABLE 4.1
Osteoplastic Frontal Sinusotomy

1956–1972	250 consecutive operations
62%	male
38%	female
Ages	10 to 84
Follow-up	83% from 3 to 19 years

The causes of frontal sinus disease leading to surgery are broken down into four categories: chronic infection, osteoma, trauma, and miscellaneous (Table 4.2).

TABLE 4.2
Etiologies for Osteoplastic Frontal Sinusotomy

Chronic Infection	190 patients (76%)
Osteoma	25 patients (10%)
With infection (13 patients)	
Without infection (12 patients)	
Trauma	25 patients (10%)
With infection (15 patients)	
Acute without infection (10 patients)	
Miscellaneous	10 patients (4%)
	Total: 250 patients

190 patients (76%) had chronic infection as the cause for surgery. Of these patients 61% had mucoceles or pyoceles, and 19% had chronic infection without mucocele or pyocele. In this group of 250, 25 patients (10%) were operated on for osteoma, 13 of whom had secondary chronic infection, while 25 patients (10%) had surgery due to trauma or its sequelae in the frontal sinus. Associated infection was present in 15 of these patients, and cerebrospinal fluid leak in 3. Ten patients (4%) had miscellaneous indications for sinusotomy, including chronic infection secondary to nasal inverted papilloma or to fibrous dysplasia of the frontal sinus.

Analysis. 42% of the 250 patients had had previous frontal surgery including 46 Lynch operations, 37 trephines, 8 duct probings, 6 Riedel procedures, and 5 osteoplastic sinusotomies performed at other institutions. Several patients had histories of multiple frontal procedures. These operations were performed from 4 days to 43 years prior to the definitive surgery (Table 4.3).

Frontal pain or headache was the chief complaint in 61% of all 250 patients, forehead or periorbital swelling in 27%, draining fistulae in 5%, and diplopia in 4%.

TABLE 4.3
Previous Frontal Surgery

(42% of 250 patients)	
Lynch	46
Trephine	37
Duct probe	8
Riedel	6
Osteoplastic	5

TABLE 4.4
Chief Complaint in 250 Patients

Frontal pain or headache	61%
Forehead or periorbital swelling	27%
Draining fistula	5%
Diplopia	4%
Duration	1 day to 40 years

Symptoms had been present from 1 day to 40 years, but were present an average of 7 years in 40% of all patients (Table 4.4).

Signs of chronic infection on physical examination in order of decreasing frequency were: proptosis, masses in the medial canthus, frontal or lid edema, tenderness, purulent rhinorrhea, Pott's puffy tumor, and decreased extraocular movement (EOM) on transillumination (Table 4.5).

TABLE 4.5
Physical Examination Findings

Proptosis	45 patients
Medial canthal mass	43 patients
Frontal or lid edema	42 patients
Tenderness	31 patients
Purulent rhinorrhea	16 patients
Pott's puffy tumor	13 patients
Decreased EOM	6 patients
Normal	78 patients

Of special interest are 28 patients who had painless mass of the forehead or upper lid or had painless proptosis as their only presenting symptom or sign. This group included patients of all etiologies except acute trauma. All but 2 of these patients had erosion of the bony walls of the sinus, including 6 with erosion of the posterior wall with exposure of dura. Thus, these patients had rather frighteningly extensive disease in light of the paucity of symptoms.

Regional complications of frontal sinusitis were present in 12% of the 250 patients, and included meningitis, brain abscess, periorbital cellulitis, periorbital abscess, and osteomyelitis of the frontal bone (Table 4.6). These patients rarely had a past history of symptoms compatible with frontal sinus disease, and the presenting picture was most often that of the complication rather than of the primary chronic frontal sinus disease. The brain and the periorbital abscesses were drained 4 to 6 weeks before the sinusotomy.

TABLE 4.6
Regional Complications of Frontal Sinus Disease

(12% of 250 patients)	
Meningitis	4
Brain abscess	6
Periorbital cellulitis	9
Periorbital abscess	4
Osteomyelitis of frontal bone	8

TABLE 4.7
Incisions

		Average Blood Loss
Brow	187	
Unilateral	(60%)	250 cc
Bilateral	(40%)	350 cc
Coronal	60	650 cc
Previous scar	3	

In the group of 250 patients, 187 had operative approach via brow incisions, 60% of these being unilateral. Sixty had coronal incisions and 3 had incisions via previous scar. Average blood loss was 250 cc for unilateral brow incision, 350 cc for bilateral brow incision, and 650 cc for coronal incision (Table 4.7).

Among these 250, 50% of patients had unilateral osteoplastic bone flaps for approach to unilateral sinus disease, 13% had bilateral bone flaps for approach to unilateral disease, and 37% had bilateral bone flaps for approach to bilateral disease (Table 4.8). One osteoplastic flap was fractured into three pieces during elevation. The periosteum was kept intact between the pieces and the final cosmesis was good. There were no instances of necrosis or osteomyelitis of a bone flap.

TABLE 4.8
Osteoplastic Bone Flap

Unilateral	124 patients
Bilateral	126 patients
For unilateral disease	32 patients
For bilateral disease	94 patients

Bony wall erosion of the frontal sinus occurred in 118 patients. Of these, 70 had exposed periorbita, 51 had exposed dura, 20 had interfrontal septum erosion, and 13 had front wall erosion. Eight of the 51 patients with exposed dura had a history of meningitis or frontal lobe brain abscess (Table 4.9).

TABLE 4.9
Bony Wall Erosion of Frontal Sinus

118 of 250 patients (47%)	
Floor (periorbita)	70 patients
Posterior (dura)	51 patients
8 with CNS applications	
Septum	20 patients
Anterior	12 patients

In the patients who had pathogens isolated by operative culture of the frontal sinus, 64% revealed Staphylococcus aureus. Other organisms in order of decreasing frequency were Pneumococcus, Beta streptococcus, E. coli, B. proteus, Pseudomonas, Klebsiella and Bacteroides.

Eighty-three percent of the frontal sinuses were obliterated with subcutaneous abdominal adipose tissue after meticulous removal of all mucous membrane and the inner cortical lining of the sinus. Seventeen percent did not have fat obliteration, most of these being performed in the early years of experience with this procedure.

Supraorbital ethmoid cells located between the floor of the frontal sinus and the roof of the orbit were recognized in 19 patients. In 22 patients the cells were obliterated with fat after converting them into a common cavity with the frontal sinus, and none required revision. Of the 7 patients in which the supraorbital ethmoid was not obliterated, 1 had an unrecognized pyocele which led to revision operation.

Eleven patients had deep posterior extensions of the frontal sinus, often reaching as a slit-like pseudopod for 2 or more centimeters posteriorly between the roof of the orbit and the anterior cranial fossa. Nine were obliterated with fat and remained uncomplicated. There has been 1 revision of the 2 cases not obliterated.

47 patients (18%) had early complications related to the frontal sinus surgery. 13 patients had abdominal wound complications of hematoma, seroma, or abscess. In the frontal wound, 6 patients had hematoma or seroma, and 8 patients had abscess. Of the 8 with abscess, 6 required revision surgery. In 8 patients the osteoplastic flap was made outside the confines of the frontal sinus. In 7 of these dura was exposed, but no brain injury occurred. In 7 patients, inadvertent dura laceration occurred, 3 due to bone cuts outside the frontal sinus whereas 4 occurred while mucous membrane was being stripped from dura which had been exposed by disease.

Of these lacerations 5 were small and were controlled by the adipose obliteration. In 2 the lacerations were large: 1 was an avulsion which required fascia for repair and 1 was repaired with silk sutures. There were no central nervous system sequelae and all of these patients with dural lacerations remain asymptomatic. Skin necrosis of the nasal dorsum developed in 2 patients due to the pressure dressing. Other complications included total anosmia, temporary ptosis, and temporary loss of unilateral frontalis muscle function.

TABLE 4.10
Follow-up Symptoms

(208 patients)	
No significant symptoms	93%
Persistent postoperative pain	6%
Persistent neuralgia	1%

Analysis of follow-up symptoms revealed that 93% of patients had no significant symptoms, after median follow-up of 8 years (Table 4.10); 12 patients had persistent moderate or severe frontal pain or headache which did not have the characteristics of neuralgia. The only significant relationship to coexistent factors is the presence of chronic preoperative pain or headache. Of these 12 patients, 11 had such preoperative symptoms, and in 8 the symptoms had been present more than 2 years. All of these patients had extensive negative work-up, including neurologic and serial radiologic evaluation. Of these patients, 4 had revision sinusotomies and no evidence of frontal disease was found. An additional 3 patients had persistent frontal neuralgia for up to 10 years postoperatively. All had brow incisions with the necessary severance of the supraorbital nerves, which probably is causative.

Cosmesis after the osteoplastic procedure is generally considered superior to other frontal operations. Of all operative scars, 88% were considered to have excellent cosmesis. Unsatisfactory coronal scars were due to exposure of the scar by natural balding in 2 males. Unsatisfactory brow scars occurred when the incision was too high above the brow, when the incisions from previous surgery were reincised, or when the incision between the brows did not extend to the deepest recess of the glabella. In 6% of patients bony contour of the forehead was considered unsatisfactory due to depression or elevation of the osteoplastic flap. This deformity can usually be avoided by beveling the bone cuts and by meticulous closure of periosteum. Drill holes and wiring are indicated if there is any question concerning the stability of the bone flap.

Of the 208 with follow-up 20 patients have had revision frontal surgery from 4 days to 14 years after the initial procedure. In 6, revisions were done in the first few days or months after the original surgery because of persistent purulent drainage via a fistula following acute wound infection. The operative findings in each was acute infection with fat necrosis. In 1 of these patients the persistent infection was due to an unrecognized supraorbital ethmoid pyocele. In 14 patients there was revision a median of 5 years after the original surgery. Of these 14 patients, 6 had negative reexplorations for persistent postoperative pain and 2 others developed frontal bone osteomyelitis at sites of previous trauma outside the sinus. Of the 8 patients with recurrent chronic infection within the frontal sinus, the probable reasons for failure were evident in all but 1 of them: 3 did not have removal of all the mucous membrane, 3 were not obliterated with fat, and 1 patient had recurrent fibrous dysplasia. It should be mentioned that all the patients with recurrent chronic infection presented with gross physical or radiologic findings of complicated chronic disease. This finding is in marked contrast to no evidence of disease on physical examination or x-ray evaluation in the 4 patients reexplored for persistent postoperative pain. Of the 20 patients who required revision, there were thus 13, or 6% of those with follow-up, who had revision due to acute infection or recurrent chronic infection within the frontal sinus (Table 4.11). It is of note that only 4% who had adipose obliteration were later revised versus 10% of those who were not obliterated with fat. Likewise, 13 patients had adipose obliteration at revision surgery and none have evidence of disease to date. Conversely, 4 of 7 patients with no fat obliteration subsequently had a second revision.

TABLE 4.11
Revision Due to Recurrent Sinus Infection

Acute infection	6 (3% of 208 with follow-up)
Chronic infection	7 (3% of 208 with follow-up)
Total	13 (6% of 208 with follow-up)

Conclusions

1. Osteoplastic frontal sinusotomy with adipose obliteration is the procedure of choice for treating all chronic complicated diseases of the frontal sinus except malignant disease.

2. Subcutaneous fat should be obtained with atraumatic technique just before insertion into the prepared sinus. In 2 patients with acute postoperative wound infection and fat necrosis, fat was obtained at the beginning of the procedure, possibly allowing drying and necrosis before insertion into the sinus.

3. Preoperative antibiotic coverage for Staphylococcus aureus should be instituted. Antibiotic coverage is changed according to operative culture and sensitivity.

4. The coronal incision offers better cosmesis and exposure than the brow incision at the expense of increased blood loss. The coronal incision is ideal for females and for males who have demonstrated no tendency for balding. No patient with the coronal incision had postoperative neuralgia.

5. Supraorbital ethmoid cells should be converted into a common cavity with the frontal sinuses and obliterated with fat. Likewise, deep posterior extensions of the frontal sinus should be included with fat obliteration. Removal of the inner cortical lining from these extensions often requires the smallest diamond bur, and an operating microscope may be necessary.

6. Treatment of osteomyelitis associated with chronic frontal sinus disease should include preoperative antibiotics, osteoplastic adipose obliteration and debridement of necrotic bone, and postoperative antibiotics for up to 6 weeks.

7. Operative and postoperative complications of osteoplastic sinusotomy have been minor and of no major consequence.

8. Since 13 patients had revision due to recurrent frontal sinus infection, the failure rate is 6%. In 6 patients, or 3%, revision was needed due to acute postoperative wound infection and fat necrosis. Such patients should be treated aggressively with specific antibiotics and drainage. If infection persists, the sinus should be reexplored, the necrotic fat removed, and fresh adipose obliteration accomplished. In 7 patients, or 3%, revisions were due to recurrent chronic infection. This complication can be avoided by strict adherence to the principles of osteoplastic sinusotomy with adipose obliteration.

9. In contrast with most other radical frontal sinus procedures, postoperative follow-up and patient discomfort are minimal after the osteoplastic operation. Patients should have postoperative x rays 3 weeks after surgery, after 1 year, and serially thereafter if symptomatic.

10. Of the patients 6% had significant persistent frontal pain or headache postoperatively with no evidence of recurrent disease. Those with chronic severe preoperative pain or headache seemed most likely to develop this distressing symptom. Reexploration was rarely indicated if extensive otolaryngologic, neurologic, and serial radiologic workup is negative.

11. While it is believed that the osteoplastic sinusotomy with adipose obliteration is far superior to other frontal sinus operations in regard to disease eradication, cosmesis, postoperative care, and patient discomfort, it must be reiterated that frontal sinus disease can be insidious. Follow-up in this study is up to 19 years whereas recurrent disease has become evident up to 43 years after other types of frontal sinus surgery.

External Frontoethmoidectomy (Lynch Frontal Sinus) Operation

The classic incision is made along the inferior margin of the eyebrow extending downward, halfway between the inner canthus and the anterior aspect of the nasal bones, well down onto the lateral aspect of the nose (Fig. 4.38a). This incision is extended through skin, subcutaneous tissue, and periosteum. Troublesome bleeding is usually encountered from the angular vessels. Before proceeding further it is best to control all bleeding either by ligation or electrodesiccation.

The periosteum is elevated from the medial wall of the orbit, exposing the lacrimal crests and fossa (Fig. 4.38b). The lacrimal sac is displaced laterally, thus allowing exposure of the cribriform lacrimal bone and, more posteriorly, the lamina papyracea. The anterior ethmoid artery is encountered during the elevation of the periosteum from the lamina papyracea. The bleeding from this vessel can be troublesome and is controlled by cautery and by packing for a short period. The posterior ethmoid artery, found further back along the suture line between the orbital plate of the frontal bone and the lamina papyracea, is similarly treated. Some surgeons prefer to ligate both the anterior and the posterior ethmoid arteries.

The periosteum is elevated from the floor of the frontal sinus. This elevation is most easily begun at the junction of the superior and medial orbital walls. The periosteal dissection is then carried laterally until the floor of the frontal sinus has been completely exposed.

The frontal sinus is approached by way of the ethmoid sinus (Fig. 4.39a). Entrance into the ethmoid sinus is accomplished by removing the lacrimal bone with a sharp curette; it is important not to disturb the underlying nasal mucous membrane anteriorly. The opening is enlarged with various-sized Kerrison forceps and rongeurs. The anterior ethmoid cells are removed with Brownie or Takahashi forceps. If a mucous membrane flap is to be used, it is fashioned at this time. A superiorly based mucosal flap, 1 to 2 cm wide and 2 to 3 cm long, is made in the upper lateral nasal wall. This flap is later turned upward for epithelialization of the reconstructed nasofrontal communication.

With Kerrison forceps, bone is removed from the upper medial orbital wall to the beginning of the osseous floor of the frontal sinus. At this point the frontal sinus cavity is encountered. The entire floor of the frontal sinus is resected (Fig. 4.39b). The mucous membrane lining of this sinus is removed by means of periosteal elevators, curettes, and forceps. This is often quite difficult if the sinus has lateral or superior projections and this step in the procedure represents one of the shortcomings of this approach. If the mucous membrane lining is not entirely removed, a mucocele may form at a later date.

The remainder of the anterior and posterior ethmoid cells are removed as well as the lamina papyracea and as much of the middle turbinate as is necessary to establish an adequate opening into the nasal cavity. The relative position of the cribriform plate must be kept in mind at all times. Cerebrospinal fluid leakage will not be a complication if the surgeon's work has been performed carefully. Lynch marked the position of the cribriform plate by means of a probe inserted through the nostril with its tip in contact with the roof of the olfactory slit. The anterior wall of the sphenoid is encountered at the posterior limit of the ethmoid labyrinth. If indicated, the sphenoid sinus is entered with a sharp curette. This

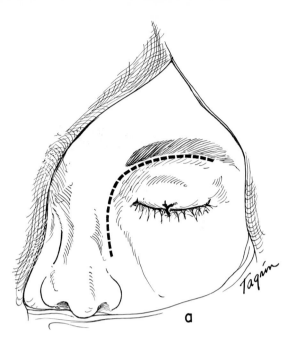

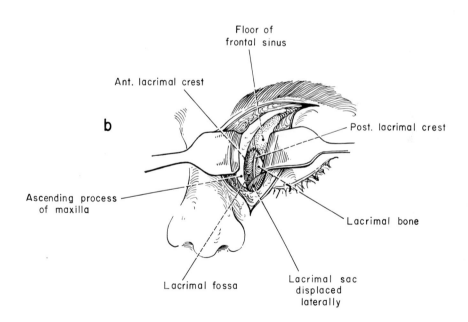

FIGURE 4.38. *External frontoethmoidectomy (Lynch frontal sinus operation).*

a. The incision is made along the inferior margin of the eyebrow, extending downward, and midway between the inner canthus and dorsum of the nose. Bleeding from the angular vessels can be troublesome. This should be well controlled before beginning elevation of the periosteum.

b. The periosteum is elevated so as to expose the ascending process of the maxilla, lacrimal fossa, anterior and posterior lacrimal crests, lacrimal bone, lamina papyracea, and orbital plate of the frontal bone. The anterior ethmoid artery is carefully approached and cauterized before being transected.

Floor of frontal sinus

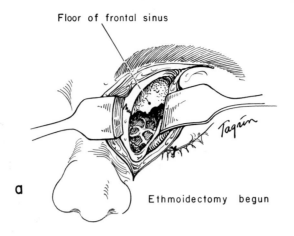

a

Ethmoidectomy begun

Floor of frontal sinus
completely removed

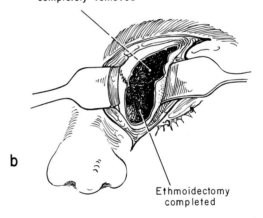

b

Ethmoidectomy
completed

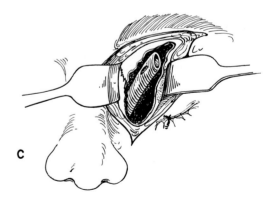

c

FIGURE 4.39. *External frontoethmoidectomy (Lynch frontal sinus operation).*

a. An anterior and posterior ethmoidectomy has been completed with removal of the middle turbinate and exposure of the roof of the ethmoid sinuses.

b. The entire floor of the frontal sinus is removed so that the diseased tissue and mucous membrane can be removed from the sinus cavity.

c. The frontoethmoidectomy has been completed. A tube is in place extending from the frontal sinus through the ethmoid sinus into the nasal cavity.

opening is enlarged with Kerrison or Hajek forceps, and the diseased tissue is removed.

The mucous membrane flap which has been fashioned from the upper lateral nasal wall is turned upward to line the medial wall of the newly formed nasofrontal opening. This is kept in place by petrolatum gauze, a "cigarette" drain, or a rubber or plastic tube (Fig. 4.39c). The support for this mucosal flap is removed on the sixth postoperative day.

Other supports for maintaining the patency of the reconstructed nasofrontal passage include split-thickness skin grafts or Cargile membrane-covered tubes, uncovered plastic or rubber tubing, and tantalum foil. It is necessary that these supports remain in place from 1 to 3 months following the operation.

The success of external frontoethmoidectomy is dependent upon: (1) removal of the entire bony floor of the frontal sinus; (2) removal of the entire mucous membrane lining; (3) a complete ethmoidectomy; and (4) establishing an adequate opening into the intranasal cavity. Even after these requirements have been met, there is a significant incidence of subsequent stenosis of the nasofrontal passage, recurrent sinusitis, and mucocele formation. (Fig. 4.6).

The one positive indication for the Lynch frontal sinus operation is carcinoma of the frontal sinus. The operation is usually followed by a full course of radiation therapy.

FRACTURES OF THE FRONTAL SINUS

Etiology. The most common cause of fracture of the frontal sinus today is an automobile accident in which the victim's forehead strikes against the steering wheel or dashboard. Falls and missile injuries are also relatively common causes. A fracture into the frontal sinus may also occur during a frontal craniotomy; a bur-hole disk may enter the periphery of a frontal sinus (Fig. 4.40).

Diagnosis. Routine x rays of the sinuses usually demonstrate fractures of the anterior and posterior walls of the frontal sinuses and any degree of displacement that may be present (Fig. 4.41). Laminograms may be necessary to more clearly outline the contour of the posterior wall of the frontal sinus. The most common deformity results from posterior displacement of the anterior wall (Fig. 4.42). The nasal process of the frontal bone may be posteriorly displaced (Fig. 4.43). This fracture is quite frequently associated with a cerebrospinal fluid rhinorrhea, with the fluid escaping by way of the cribriform plate. Superior displacement of the floor of the frontal sinus may be associated with a fracture of a supraorbital rim. Air in the orbit is diagnostic of fracture of the floor of the frontal sinus (Fig. 4.44), while air in the anterior cranial fossa behind the frontal bone signifies fracture of the posterior wall of the sinus. A degree of enophthalmos may be found to be associated with a fracture of the posterior wall.

Complications. The most common sequela of fracture of the frontal sinus is a mucocele or pyocele. The lesion usually does not occur for several years following the fracture. As has been mentioned, cerebrospinal fluid leakage may be associated with fracture of the posterior wall of the frontal sinus or with posterior displacement of the nasal process of the frontal bone. Secondary infection may occur with a compound fracture. Delayed secondary infection may appear with a subsequent upper respiratory infection and may extend from the frontal sinus to the extradural spaces (Fig. 4.45).

Treatment. A history of the circumstances of the injury is most important. Immediate unconsciousness is usually the result of a concussion or intracranial hemorrhage. On the other hand, increasing unconsciousness after the injury may be the result of cerebral edema. Unconsciousness occurring days or weeks after the injury may be due to secondary infection.

Patients with simple fractures without displacement are treated expectantly. Antibiotics are administered when there is air in the orbit, or behind the posterior wall of the frontal sinus, in order to prevent any potential infection.

The patient should have carefully executed local and neurologic examinations. Neurosurgical consultation is requested when any sign of brain damage is present.

A depressed fracture of the frontal bone should be explored whether or not it is compounded. This is done to prevent deformity, to determine the presence of a hematoma, and to detect splintering of the posterior wall with a resultant laceration of the dura of the frontal lobe which may lead to cerebrospinal fluid leakage.

The depressed fracture of the frontal bone is often compounded, and thus repair can be accomplished through the wound. If this is impossible, the area is exposed by turning down a coronal flap or by making an incision along the upper margin of the eyebrow.

A trephine opening through healthy bone is useful for both inspection of the sinus and for insertion of instruments for elevation of the bony fragments. Usually the displaced fragments can be elevated through the fracture lines. A steel hook is inserted in the fracture line and turned 90 degrees for elevation in the direction of the loose fragments. The hook is then rotated to the position of its insertion and removed. If this is not possible, a small trephine opening is made at the margin of the fracture line to allow for instrument insertion. Small or soiled fragments of bone should be removed. Hooks, elevators, and chisels are the most useful instruments for repair of depressed fragments.

A cerebrospinal fluid rhinorrhea caused by laceration of the dura of the frontal lobe is positive indication for exploration of the frontal sinus. If comminution and displacement of the anterior wall of the frontal sinus is not extensive, an osteoplastic approach is ideal for management of the spinal fluid leakage. As indicated, either a unilateral or bilateral osteoplastic flap is elevated (see Figs. 4.16 and 4.19b), providing an excellent view of the entire posterior wall and the site of leakage. A portion of the posterior wall in the vicinity of the dural defect is removed, and the dura is repaired by primary suture if possible. If this method of repair is not satisfactory, the entire mucosal and inner cortical lining of the frontal sinus is removed, and the sinus is obliterated with adipose tissue. The adipose tissue is placed directly against the dural defect.

A mucocele or pyocele not uncommonly follows a fracture of the frontal sinus. It may occur several months or many years following the injury. It can be treated by using the osteoplastic adipose obliteration procedure.

If secondary infection complicates a frontal sinus fracture and extends into the extradural space, the first line of therapy should be the administration of antibiotics according to culture and sensitivity tests. Surgical intervention, such as an anterior craniotomy by a neurosurgeon or a trephination of the frontal sinus by an otolaryngologist, may be necessary. As soon as the infection is under control, the sinuses should be obliterated with adipose tissue. Usually ten days to two weeks of antibiotic therapy are required prior to the osteoplastic obliteration operation.

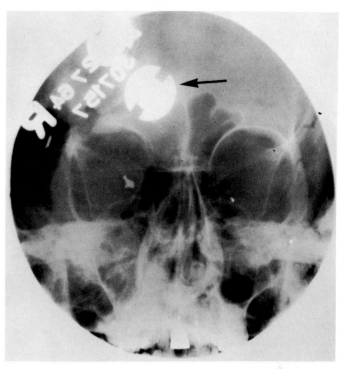

a

FIGURE 4.40. *Frontal sinus fracture—injury to the frontal sinus during frontal craniotomy.*

a and b. A 46-year-old woman underwent an emergency craniotomy for a berry aneurysm. Two years later she noted a 2-cm fluctuant swelling in the right side of her forehead. X rays showed a tantalum bur-hole disk (arrows) infringing upon the boundary of the right frontal sinus and increased density in that sinus. At operation a mucocele was found filling the right frontal sinus. This extended posteriorly to the tantalum disk and was attached to the dura of the frontal lobe. The mucocele was resected and the frontal sinus obliterated with adipose tissue.

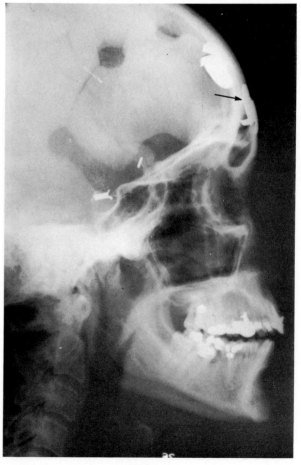

b

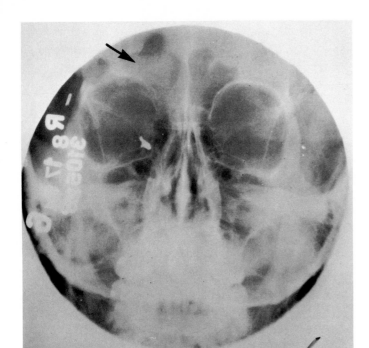

c

FIGURE 4.40. (Continued)

    c. Anteroposterior view of the same patient. The tantalum disk and mucocele have been removed. The arrow points to the right frontal sinus which has been obliterated with adipose tissue.

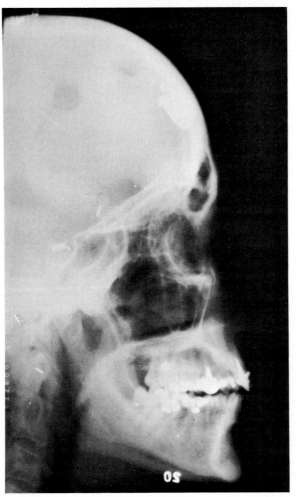

d

    d. Lateral view. The patient has remained well and free from symptoms for 12 years.

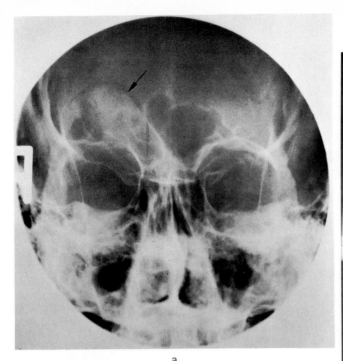

a

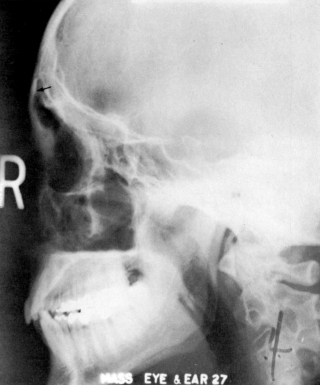

c

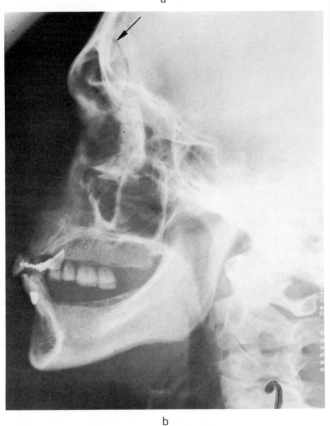

b

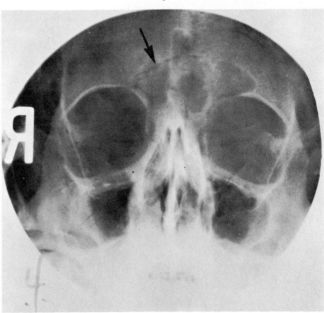

d

FIGURE 4.41. *Frontal sinus fracture without displacement.*

a and b. A 33-year-old man received direct trauma to the right side of his forehead. There was some bleeding from the right nasal cavity but no deformity other than soft-tissue swelling of the forehead. X-ray films showed a linear fracture (arrow) extending into the right frontal sinus without displacement. The right frontal sinus was filled with blood. The patient had no symptoms from the time of the injury up to the time of examination, a few days following.

c and d. A 27-year-old man received trauma to his mid-forehead without resultant deformity. He had moderate epistaxis following the injury but no other symptoms. X rays showed a fracture (arrow) of the anterior wall over both frontal sinuses without appreciable displacement. Blood filled both frontal sinuses. This patient also experienced no symptoms from the time of his injury up to the time of the examination, a few days following.

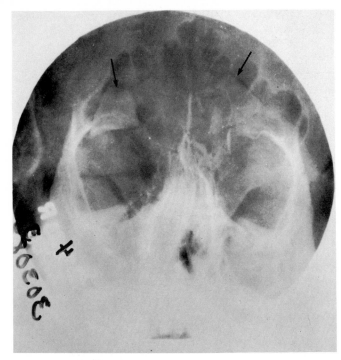

a

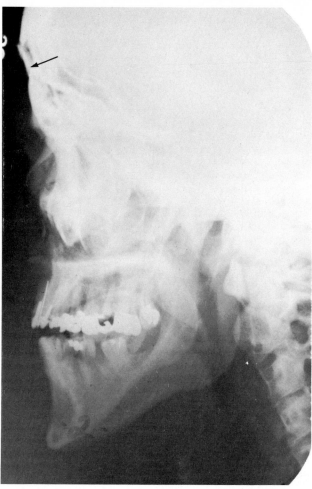

b

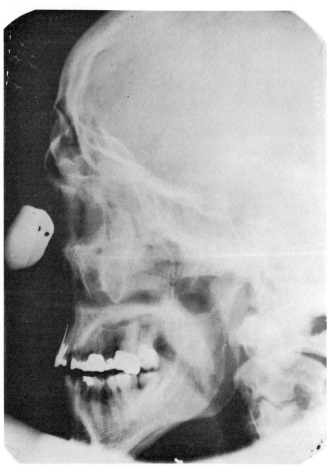

c

FIGURE 4.42. Comminuted and depressed fracture of the frontal sinus.

The patient, a 46-year-old man, received severe trauma to his forehead, nose, and right orbit during an automobile accident.

a and b. Anteroposterior and lateral x rays showed a depressed comminuted fracture of the anterior wall of both frontal sinuses and of the right orbit.

c. The anterior wall of the frontal sinuses has been reconstituted by elevating the multiple fragments in an anterior direction. A metal nasal splint has been employed.

The patient shows no deformity nor has he had any complications following surgical repair up to the time of this report, nine years following the accident.

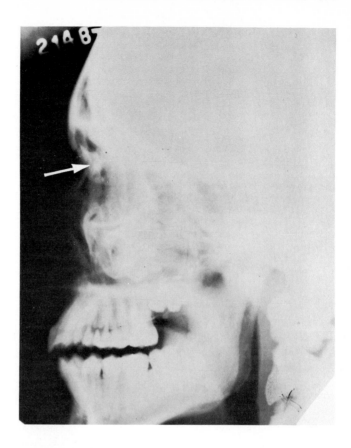

FIGURE 4.43. *Fracture with posterior displacement of the nasal process of the frontal bone.*

Lateral x-ray views of two patients, each of whom struck the lower forehead against the steering wheel in an automobile accident. Each x ray shows a depressed fracture (arrow) of the nasal process of the frontal bone. This type of fracture is likely to be complicated by cerebrospinal fluid leakage from the cribriform area.

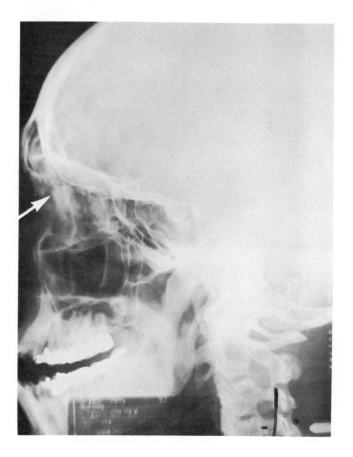

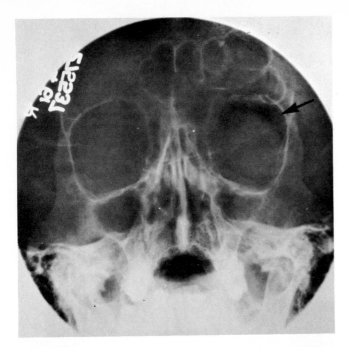

FIGURE 4.44. *Fracture with displacement and air in the orbit.*

A 40-year-old man received a severe blow over his left eye. There was rather marked swelling of the left side of the forehead and moderate proptosis of the left eye which subsided after one week. Crepitus could be palpated in the upper lid. The x ray shows comminuted fracture of the anterior wall of the left frontal sinus with air (arrow) in the left orbit. The patient was placed on antibiotic therapy and advised against nose-blowing. He has remained free of symptoms for 12 years.

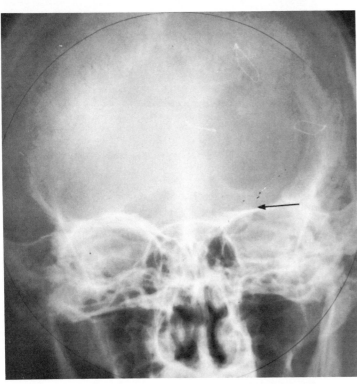

a

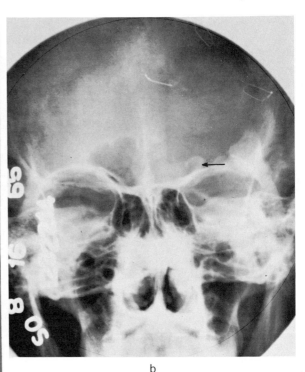

b

FIGURE 4.45. *Fracture of the frontal sinus with secondary infection of the extradural space.*

a. The patient, a 28-year-old metal worker, was admitted to the hospital as an emergency patient after being struck on the left side of his forehead by a grinding wheel which flew off its mounting. At operation, it was necessary to resect a portion of the left frontal lobe as well as numerous comminuted bone fragments. These fragments included the lateral aspect of the left frontal sinus (arrow). The dura was repaired with a fascia lata graft.

The postoperative course was complicated by episodes of left frontal extradural abscess. A collection of air in the abscessed area led to the conclusion that the extradural space was being contaminated by way of the nasal route.

The left frontal sinus was exposed, an anterior osteoplastic flap technique having been used. The sinus walls were found to be absent superiorly and laterally. The remainder of the sinus was filled with a markedly thickened mucous membrane and polypoid tissue. The mucous membrane was removed as well as the inner cortical lining.

b. The sinus was obliterated with adipose tissue (arrow).

The patient has remained well for the 10 years that have elapsed following the sinus operation.

REFERENCES

Alford, B. R.: Osteoplastic Approach to the Frontal Sinus for Osteoma. Arch. Otolaryng. *80*:16–21 (July) 1964.

Antoniuk, M. R.: The Trephine-Puncture Method in Diagnosis and Therapy of Diseases of the Frontal Sinuses. Acta Otolaryng. *54*:111–123 (Feb.) 1962.

Beck, J. C.: A New Method of External Frontal Sinus Operation without Deformity. J.A.M.A. *51*:451–455 (Aug. 8) 1908.

Bergara, A. R., and Bergara, C.: Chronic Frontoethmoidal Sinusitis: Osteoplastic Method According to Author's Technique. Ann Oto-Rhino-Laryng. Uruguay 5:192, 1955.

Bergara, A. R., and Itoiz, A. O.: Present Status of Surgical Treatment of Chronic Frontal Sinusitis. Arch. Otolaryng. *61*:616–628, 1955.

Brieger: cited *in:* A. Denker and O. Kahler (Eds.): *Handbuch der Hals-Nasen-Ohren-Heilkunde.* Berlin, J. Springer, 1926, Vol. 2, p. 804.

Dawes, J. D. K.: The Management of Frontal Sinusitis and Its Complications. J. Laryng. *75*:297–344 (April) 1961.

Gibson, T., and Walker, F. M.: Large Osteoma of Frontal Sinus: Method of Removal to Minimize Scarring and Prevent Deformity. Brit. J. Plast. Surg. *4*:210 1951.

Gibson, T., and Walker, F. M.: The Osteoplastic Flap Approach to the Frontal Sinuses. J. Laryng. *68*:2:92–100 (Feb.) 1954.

Goodale, R. L., and Montgomery, W. W.: Experiences with Osteoplastic Anterior Wall Approach to Frontal Sinus. Arch. Otolaryng. *68*:271–285, 1958.

Goodale, R. L., and Montgomery, W. W.: Anterior Osteoplastic Frontal Sinus Operation. Ann. Otol. *70*:860–880, 1961.

Goodale, R. L., and Montgomery, W. W.: Technical Advances in Osteoplastic Frontal Sinusectomy. Arch. Otolaryng. *79*:522–529 (May) 1964.

Hardy, J. M., and Montgomery, W. W.: Osteoplastic Frontal Sinusotomy: An Analysis of 250 Operations. Ann. Otol. Rhinol. Laryngol. *85*:523–532, 1976.

Hoffman, R.: Osteoplastic Operations on the Frontal Sinuses for Chronic Suppuration. Ann. Otol. *13*:598–608, 1904.

Kirchner, F. R., Toledo, P. S., and Robison, J. T.: Modified Osteoplastic Approach to the Frontal Bone, Sinuses and/or the Orbit. Trans. Amer. Acad. Ophthal. Otolaryng. *71*:6:951–955, 1967.

Lovo, G. F.: Esiti di intervento sui seno frontale: riparazione con tessuto adiposo. Minerva Chir. *14*:1141 (Sept.) 1959.

Macbeth, R. G.: The Osteoplastic Operation for Chronic Infection of the Frontal Sinus. J. Laryngol. *68*:465 (July) 1954.

Montgomery, W. W.: Cerebrospinal fluid rhinorrhea. Otol. Clin. N. Amer. 6:657–772, 1973.

Montgomery, W. W.: Osteoplastic Frontal Sinus Operation: Coronal Incision. Ann. Otol. *74*:821–830 (Sept.) 1965.

Podvinec, S., and Savic, D.: Use of Osteoplastic Methods in Surgery of the Frontal Sinuses. Srpski Arh. Celok. Lek., *87*:497–502 (June) 1959.

Schonborn: Cited by A. Willkop: *Ein Beitrag zur Casuistik der Erkrankungen des Sinus Frontalis.* Wurzburg, F. Fromme, 1894.

Soboroff, B. J., and Nykiel, F.: Surgical Treatment of Large Osteomas of the Ethmo-frontal Region. Laryngoscope *76*:1068–1081 (June) 1966.

Winckler: cited *in:* A. Decker and O. Kahler (Eds.): *Handbuch der Hals-Nasen-Ohren-Heilkunde,* Berlin, J. Springer, 1926, Vol. 2, pp. 799, 805.

Work, W. P.: Trauma to the Frontal Sinuses. Arch. Otolaryng. *59*:54–64 (Jan.) 1954.

Tato, J. M., Sibbald, D. W., and Bergaglio, O. E.: Surgical Treatment of the Frontal Sinus by the External Route. Laryngoscope *64*:504–521, 1954.

Zonis, R. D., Montgomery, W. W., and Goodale, R. L.: Frontal Sinus Disease: 100 Cases Treated by Osteoplastic Operation. Laryngoscope *76*:11:1816–1825 (Nov.) 1966.

5

Repair of Dural Defects

This chapter deals with the etiology, diagnosis, and treatment of spinal fluid leakage from the sinuses, cribriform plate, and ear.

Repair for stopping the leakage of cerebrospinal fluid into the nasal and aural spaces can be executed by extracranial operation, with lower morbidity and mortality rates than those attained by an intracranial procedure.

Cerebrospinal fluid rhinorrhea may have its origin in the frontal sinus, sphenoid sinus, ethmoid sinus, or cribriform plate. Cerebrospinal fluid otorhinorrhea may originate in the mastoid or middle ear and reach the nasal space by way of the eustachian tube. It may exit as otorrhea from the mastoid or middle ear by way of the external auditory canal.

The repair for stemming spinal fluid leakage into the frontal sinus can be made by direct suturing of the dura, grafting fascia lata, or by adipose obliteration of the frontal sinuses. The bilateral osteoplastic flap procedure is used for exposure of the defect (see Fig. 4.21).

Spinal fluid otorrhea or otorhinorrhea emanating from the middle or posterior fossa by way of the mastoid can be treated by obliteration, with either a local pedicled connective tissue flap or an adipose autograft. If the spinal fluid leakage is subsequent to a radical mastoidectomy, it may be necessary to use a fascia lata graft. A nasal septal mucoperichondrial pedicled flap is used to stop spinal fluid leakage through the cribriform plate, roof of the ethmoid bone, and sphenoid sinus.

ETIOLOGY

McCoy and Ommaya have simplified the etiologic classification into two groups: (1) traumatic (acute or delayed); and (2) nontraumatic, which would include tumors, congenital anomalies, hydrocephalus infection, and primary or spontaneous cerebrospinal fluid rhinorrhea.

Cerebrospinal fluid rhinorrhea of acute traumatic origin may be caused by a crushing injury in which the skull is fractured. This is most commonly due to a war or automobile injury. Penetrating wounds may also result in cerebrospinal fluid rhinorrhea. Most frequently the penetrating object enters by way of the orbit, ethmoid sinus, cribriform area, otic capsule, or mastoid. On occasion, spinal fluid rhinorrhea is produced by the neurosurgeon or the otolaryngologist. Leakage following neurosurgical procedures is usually through the cribriform area and the frontal sinus. It is possible for the otolaryngological surgeon to produce a cerebrospinal fluid rhinorrhea in any of the following ways: (1) by simply removing an intranasal mass which was actually an encephalocele; (2) by rasping of the nasofrontal duct; (3) during operation upon the frontal sinus; (4) during intranasal or extranasal ethmoid operation or a pituitary operation performed by the sphenoid sinus route; or (5) during mastoid operations, especially when using the translabyrinthine approach for removal of cerebellopontile angle tumors.

Both extracranial and intracranial tumors may produce cerebrospinal fluid rhinorrhea by erosion of the dura mater. The most common tumors causing cerebrospinal fluid leakage are frontal and ethmoid sinus osteomas. Tumors of the olfactory bulb and pituitary gland are common intracranial tumors producing spontaneous leakage. Intracranial tumors in the region of the sphenoid sinus and mastoid may also produce leakage of cerebrospinal fluid.

Congenital defects, with the formation of an encephalocele into the nasal cavity or rupture of a persistent embryonic ventricular lumen of the olfactory tract, can result in spinal fluid rhinorrhea. The discharge in spontaneous, or primary, cerebrospinal fluid rhinorrhea reaches the nasal cavity by way of a prolongation of the subarachnoid space along the filaments of the olfactory nerve. A sudden transient rise in the cerebrospinal fluid pressure, such as with sneezing or coughing, may rupture the membranes which cover a congenitally weak area in the cribriform plate.

DIAGNOSIS

Unless leakage of cerebrospinal fluid is profuse and persistent, the detection of its source is difficult. Thus, the investigation must be systematic and thorough. Leakage should be considered in patients who have had severe trauma to the face, especially in the region of the superior aspect of the nasal bones and the nasal process of the frontal bone. A patient who has had repeated episodes of meningitis should be thoroughly investigated for cerebrospinal fluid rhinorrhea and otorrhea, especially if there is a history of trauma.

Cerebrospinal fluid rhinorrhea may be intermittent. It is most often unilateral. An acceleration in the flow rate with change in position is rather characteristic. If the rate of flow is profuse the patient will swallow frequently when in a recumbent position. The fluid is clear unless there is an associated acute trauma, when it may be sanguinous. It is odorless, salty, and has a specific gravity of about 1.006.

Leakage through the mastoid or middle ear will be attended with a conductive hearing loss and the appearance of fluid or air bubbles behind the tympanic membrane.

The diagnosis and localization of a dural defect may often be made by acquiring from the patient an accurate and detailed past history and present illness description. The interrogation should include the following questions:

1. Has the patient noted a leakage of clear fluid?
2. Which side (ear or nose) is leaking?

3. Is the leakage constant or intermittent?
4. Does the leakage occur unaccompanied by nasal stuffiness or sneezing?
5. Has the patient noticed a salty taste associated with the leakage?
6. Does he notice frequent swallowing when in the recumbent position, or is he aware of excessive liquid entering the pharynx from above?
7. When in the recumbent position, does the rhinorrhea occur only from the dependent side of the nose? An affirmative answer would be consistent with spinal fluid passing from the middle ear by way of the eustachian tube into the nasopharynx and out by way of the dependent nasal cavity.
8. Does the leakage occur in "gushes"? This might indicate that a sinus becomes filled with spinal fluid and then, with a change of position, suddenly evacuates.
9. Is there a history of trauma to or surgery of the nose, nasal cavity, sinuses, or ear or a history of intracranial surgery?
10. Has the patient noticed a hearing loss or a sensation of fluid in the ear?
11. Does the patient report a loss of his sense of smell? This might indicate a fracture defect or tumor in the olfactory region.

Testing of the rhinorrhea fluid for glucose and protein content can add confusion. Spinal fluid contains much more glucose and less protein than nasal secretions. Nasal secretions may contain glucose as a result of lacrimation and may

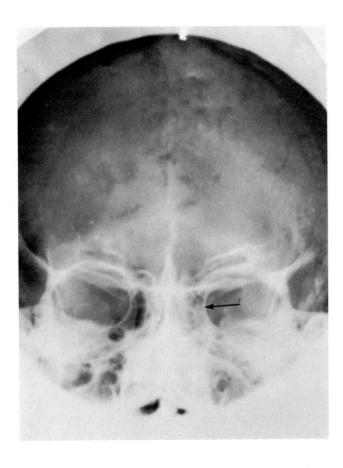

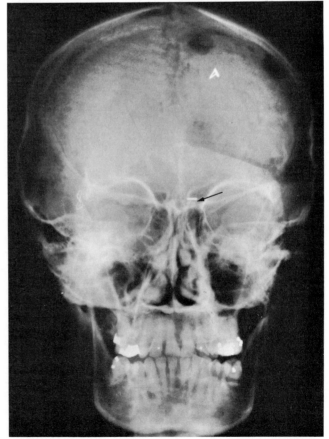

FIGURE 5.1. *Cerebrospinal fluid rhinorrhea.*

a. Rhinorrhea was by way of the left ethmoid (arrow), and resulted from a penetrating wound through the roof of the ethmoid bone and the adjacent dura.

b. Draining was due to a fracture through the left cribriform plate. The silver clip (arrow) is evidence of an unsuccessful repair with fascia lata positioned by way of an anterior craniotomy. The defect was repaired by means of a nasoseptal mucosal flap.

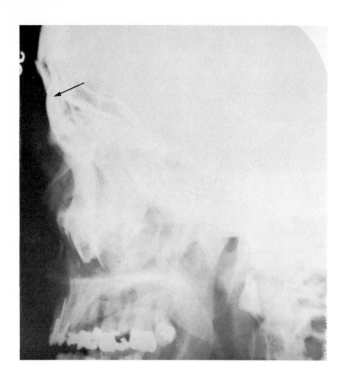

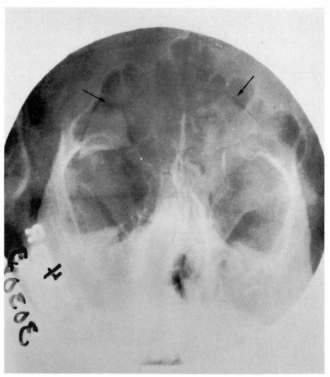

FIGURE 5.2. *Cerebrospinal fluid rhinorrhea due to comminuted fracture of frontal sinus.*

a. A depressed comminuted fracture of the frontal sinus (arrow) can be complicated by cerebrospinal fluid rhinorrhea. The posterior wall of the frontal sinus must, of course, also be fractured. A bone fragment from the posterior wall will lacerate the dura.

b. An anteroposterior view of a depressed comminuted frontal sinus fracture (arrows). This resulted from an automobile accident in which the patient's forehead struck the dashboard.

be "watery" and contain little protein. We have abandoned the testing of the fluid with laboratory paper test strips. The fluid being tested should be allowed to remain in a test tube. After standing, a sediment will be found in a nasal discharge, whereas spinal fluid should remain clear. It is important to culture the fluid.

Routine radiographs of the skull, sinuses, facial bones, and mastoids may demonstrate the presence of a tumor, fluid (Fig. 5.1a), a fracture (Fig. 5.1b, 5.2, 5.3, 5.4), or air in the cranial cavity (Fig. 5.5). Polytomography is a more exacting technique for pinpointing the site of the dural defect. One of the various cavities may be of increased density owing to the presence of cerebrospinal fluid. A small fracture may be demonstrated by laminography or by polytomography (Fig. 5.6). Pneumocephalus is diagnostic of a dural defect and may be positioned so as to indicate the site of leakage (Fig. 5.5).

A fairly accurate method of identifying and localizing the source of cerebrospinal fluid rhinorrhea or otorrhea is a test consisting of intrathecal injection of fluorescein dye solution and subsequent detection of its presence intranasally or by otoscopy. The patient is placed in the sitting position in order to perform the first portion of this examination. After examination of the nasal cavities, nasopharynx, pharynx, and ears for the presence of fluid, both nasal cavities are packed with 4% cocaine impregnated cottonoid strips in order to produce topical anesthesia and shrink the nasal mucous membrane. The cocaine packing is removed after 10 minutes. Next, a separate moist cottonoid strip is inserted into (1) the spheno-

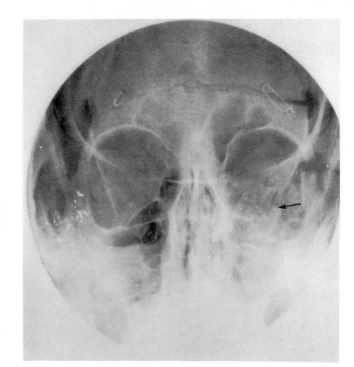

FIGURE 5.3. *Cerebrospinal fluid rhinorrhea.*

a. A cerebrospinal fluid fistula (arrow) which resulted from a large gunshot defect in the left lateral sphenoid wall. The defect was repaired by using both fascia lata and a nasoseptal mucosal flap.

b. Cerebrospinal fluid rhinorrhea can complicate either intracranial or extracranial removal of pituitary tumors. The tumor (arrow) in this patient was removed by way of the transethmoidosphenoidal approach. The defect in the posterior sphenoid sinus wall was repaired using a septomucosal flap.

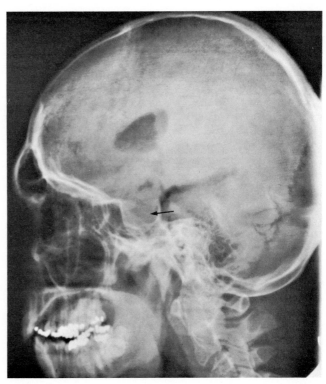

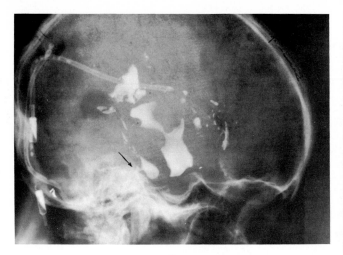

a

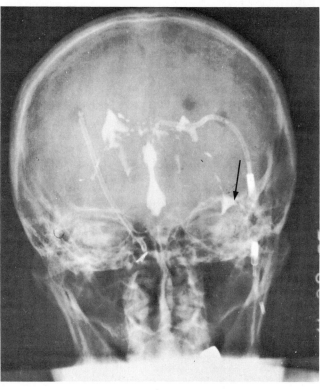

b

FIGURE 5.4.   *Cerebrospinal fluid otorhinorrhea.*

a. A lateral x-ray view of a middle fossa contrast study, demonstrating a dural defect into the left mastoid process (arrow). In this case the tympanic membrane was intact and the cerebrospinal fluid exited by way of the eustachian tube and nasal cavity and was thus termed otorhinorrhea, rather than otorrhea.

b. An anteroposterior view of the contrast study. The arrow points to the communication between the intradural space and the mastoid bone.

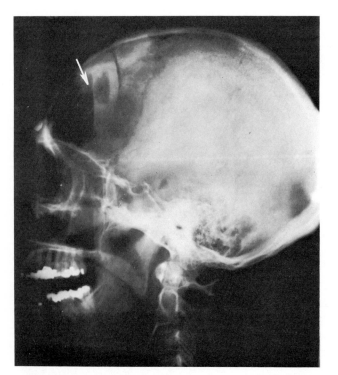

a

FIGURE 5.5.   *Pneumocephalus associated with cerebrospinal fluid rhinorrhea.*

Radiographic evidence of pneumocephalus confirms the diagnosis of a cerebrospinal fistula.

The patient whose x rays are shown in "a" and "b," had a very large defect in the right ethmoid-cribriform area, following intracranial resection of a chondrosarcoma in the anterior cranial fossa. Aphasia and urinary and bowel incontinence resulted from long-standing low or absent spinal fluid pressure. The defect was repaired with both an adipose autograft and a septomucosal pedicled flap.

a. The pneumocephalus (arrow) and fluid level are demonstrated in a lateral view of the skull. The fluid level is verified by lateral radiographic views taken with the patient in the upright, prone, and supine positions.

b. The same findings as in "a" are noted in the anteroposterior view.

The patient, a 21-year-old man, received head injury during an automobile accident. A severe headache, relieved by lying down, along with occasional leakage of fluid from the left nostril, persisted for four months. The patient was referred for diagnosis and treatment following a bout of meningitis. Upon examination he mentioned a peculiar noise in his head when changing from the recumbent to the sitting position. With a stethoscope against the anterior left temporal region, a gurgling followed by a hissing sound could be heard. This was caused by a trapdoor defect in the posterior wall of the frontal sinus and anterior fossa dura.

c. Depressed fracture of the anterior wall of the frontal sinus (white arrow). Pocket of air (pneumocephalus) behind the left frontal sinus (black arrow).

d. Comminuted fracture of frontal sinus and pocket of air (arrow) behind the left frontal sinus.

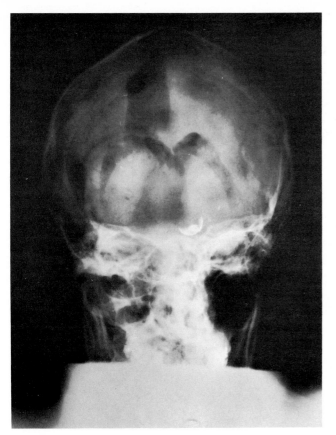

b

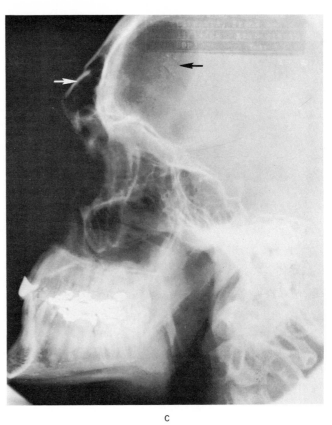

c

FIGURE 5.5. (Continued)

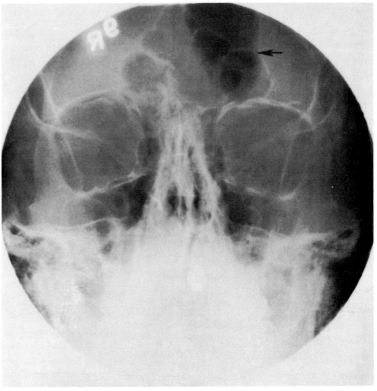

d

ethmoidal recess, (2) the region of the olfactory slit and middle meatus, and (3) the anterosuperior nasal cavity.

A lumbar puncture is accomplished and the spinal fluid pressure recorded. In patients with a large dural defect the spinal fluid pressure is often quite low, making a spinal tap in the recumbent position quite difficult. In these cases the tap is carried out with the patient in the sitting position. Fluorescein (0.5 to 1 ml of a 5% solution) diluted with at least 10 ml of spinal fluid is slowly injected intrathecally. In cases in which 10 ml of spinal fluid cannot be obtained because of low spinal fluid pressure, Hartman's solution may be used to dilute the fluorescein dye.

Following the lumbar puncture the patient is placed in the horizontal supine position. If the leakage has been profuse, the head is elevated on one or two pillows. After a period of 10 minutes to 1 hour, depending on the profuseness of the cerebrospinal fluid leakage, the cotton pledgets are carefully removed and labeled according to their intranasal location. The room is darkened and the pledgets are inspected (using an ultraviolet light source) for the presence of fluorescein dye. The presence of fluorescein dye on the pledget that was placed in the sphenoethmoidal recess most likely indicates leakage by way of a posterior ethmoidal cell or the sphenoidal sinus, or otorhinorrhea. The presence of fluorescein on the pledget placed in the olfactory region and middle meatus indicates a leakage by way of the cribriform plate or anterior ethmoidal cells. If fluorescein is present on the pledget placed in the anterosuperior nasal cavity, the dural defect is probably behind the posterior wall of the frontal sinus.

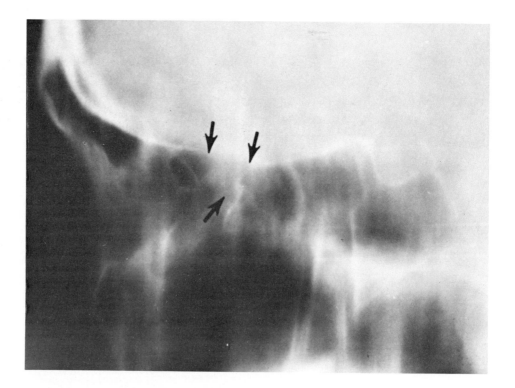

FIGURE 5.6.

This laminogram demonstrates a defect in the ethmoid-cribriform region and the site of cerebrospinal fluid leakage. The density (lower arrow) is an encephalocele, which was resected and the defect repaired using a nasoseptal mucosal flap.

In addition to the foregoing technique, the posterior pharyngeal wall is examined for the presence of fluorescein with an ultraviolet light source. Both tympanic membranes are also examined. If fluorescein dye is present in the middle ear, the yellow-green color will be readily apparent by ordinary otoscopy.

Reactions have been reported following the use of intrathecal fluorescein. However, I have had no incidence of complication in more than 200 cases where 0.5 ml of 5% fluorescein solution diluted with at least 10 ml of spinal fluid have been slowly injected intrathecally.

Cerebrospinal fluid rhinorrhea coming from the middle or posterior fossa and draining into the mastoid antrum and down the eustachian tube may be intermittent even when very active, for when the patient is in the upright or supine position the spinal fluid flows directly into the pharynx. The patient may notice gushes of rhinorrhea with change in head position. The side of the leakage will vary according to the position of the head. Cerebrospinal fluid otorhinorrhea from the mastoid region is best demonstrated by Pantopaque study (Fig. 5.4). Proper positioning and serial x rays, taken for at least 24 hours, may be necessary to demonstrate the point of leakage. Pantopaque will remain in the mastoid cells for many days.

TREATMENT

The early management of post-traumatic cerebrospinal fluid rhinorrhea and otorrhea is conservative (Fig. 5.7). The patient should remain in a semi-sitting position and be given antibiotic therapy. He should avoid nose-blowing, sneezing, and straining. If the leakage persists after 6 weeks, a more aggressive method of therapy should be employed, for sooner or later most of these patients will develop a meningitis which has a very high mortality rate.

Surgical intervention is indicated in the following instances: (1) when the leakage is of more than 6 weeks' duration; (2) when the leakage is intermittent; (3) when pneumoencephalos is present; and (4) when there is a history of recurrent meningitis and cerebrospinal fluid otorrhea.

Leakage of Cerebrospinal Fluid through the Frontal Sinus

The repair occasioned by leakage of spinal fluid through the posterior wall of the frontal sinus may be made by using the exposure acquired by the anterior osteoplastic flap procedure. I have used this technique in the following cases: (1) leakage encountered when dissecting a mucocele of the frontal sinus from the anterior fossa dura (Fig. 5.8), (2) leakage due to traumatic lacerations of the posterior wall of the frontal sinus and adjacent dura (Fig. 5.9), and (3) leakage occurring during removal of an osteoma of the frontal sinus which extended into the anterior cranial fossa and was complicated by a frontal lobe abscess (Fig. 5.10).

The defect in the posterior wall of the frontal sinus and adjacent anterior fossa dura is best exposed by way of the anterior osteoplastic flap, using either the eyebrow or coronal incision. An intrathecal injection of fluorescein dye, as already described, is repeated prior to surgery. This greatly facilitates the pinpointing of the leakage site. After the osteoplastic flap has been retracted inferiorly and both

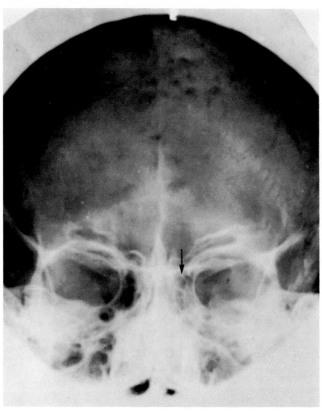

a

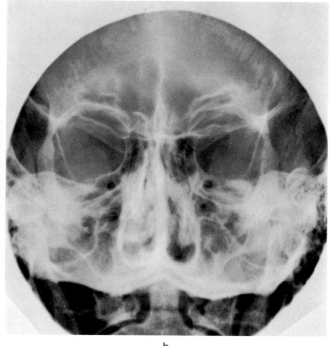

b

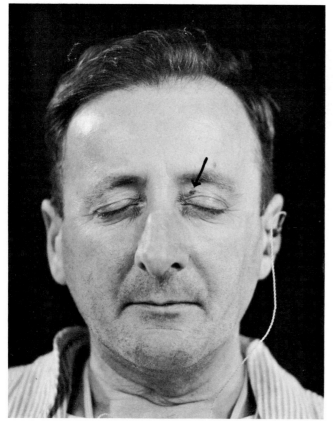

c

FIGURE 5.7.   *Cerebrospinal fluid rhinorrhea following a penetrating wound.*

a. The patient, a 53-year-old lineman, was struck in the left upper eyelid by a recoiling spring wire. A profuse blood-tinged, watery, left rhinorrhea began immediately after he pulled the wire loose. On admission to the hospital a complete examination revealed no abnormality except for the puncture wound in the left eyelid and the left rhinorrhea. Sinus x rays showed a "dense, left ethmoid" (arrow).

b. The patient was placed on antibiotic therapy and given tetanus antitoxin. He was cautioned against nose-blowing, straining, and sneezing. He remained in the semi-sitting position for one week. After three days, no cerebrospinal fluid rhinorrhea was detectable. Sinus x rays showed no abnormality one week following the accident.

c. This photograph shows the puncture wound through which the spring wire perforated the roof of the ethmoid bone and the frontal dura.

frontal sinuses have been exposed, the mucosal lining of the sinus and the interfrontal septum are removed. A fracture or defect in the posterior wall of the frontal sinus is usually present and leads the surgeon to the dural defect (Fig. 5.11a). A sufficient amount of bone is removed from the posterior wall of the linear laceration of the dural defect (Fig. 5.11b). A linear laceration of the dura may be repaired by suturing (Fig. 5.11c). Prior to obliterating the frontal sinuses with adipose tissue, the entire inner cortical lining of the frontal sinus must be removed with a rotating cutting bur. This procedure ensures complete removal of the mucosal lining of the sinus and an adequate blood supply for the adipose implant (Fig. 5.12a).

Subcutaneous adipose tissue is trimmed and implanted so as to completely fill the sinus (Fig. 5.12b). Revascularization of the adipose implant occurs during the first few days by ingrowth of vessels and direct blood vessel anastomosis. The osteoplastic flap is replaced in its anatomic position and secured by multiple periosteal sutures. If there is any question as to the stability of the osteoplastic flap, it should be secured in place with two wire sutures (Fig. 5.12c).

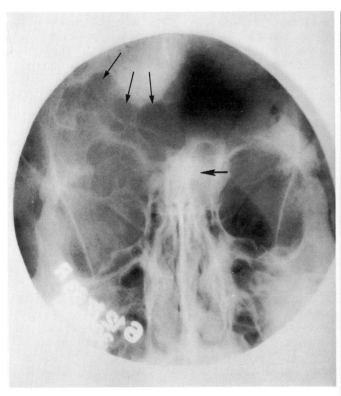
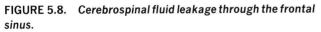
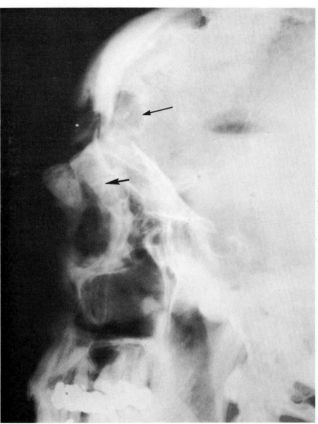

FIGURE 5.8. *Cerebrospinal fluid leakage through the frontal sinus.*

Spinal fluid leakage by way of the frontal sinus occurred in this patient during removal of extensive mucoceles of the right frontal sinus. The patient was first seen in 1928 with exophthalmos due to a large osteoma of the left frontal sinus. The anterior wall of this sinus was resected for exposure and removal of the osteoma. During the subsequent fifteen years, numerous operations were performed for removal of mucoceles of both frontal sinuses.

Anteroposterior and lateral views of the patient when first admitted to the Massachusetts Eye and Ear Infirmary in 1963 with multiple mucoceles (long arrows) which extended into the anterior cranial fossa. Residual osteoma (short arrows) was also present. A spinal fluid leakage was encountered while a mucocele was being dissected from the dura on the right side. Repair was made with #6-0 silk. The osteoma was removed and the entire frontal sinus complex obliterated with an adipose autograft. There has been no recurrence of the mucoceles and no spinal fluid rhinorrhea.

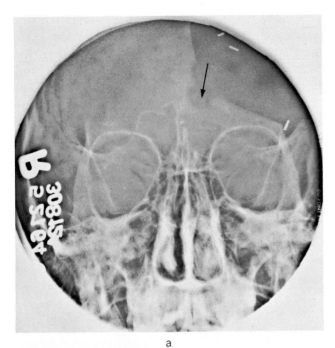

a

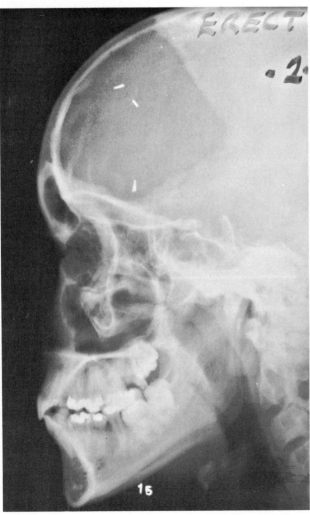

b

FIGURE 5.9. *Cerebrospinal fluid rhinorrhea due to laceration of posterior wall of frontal sinus and adjacent dura.*

a and b. A 20-year-old woman sustained trauma to her forehead which resulted in a compound, depressed, comminuted fracture of the skull. A large portion of the left frontal bone was lost. It was noted at the time of repair that the anterior cranial fossa and a dural defect communicated with the left frontal sinus. A persistent cerebrospinal fluid rhinorrhea complicated the patient's recovery. The anteroposterior and lateral x rays demonstrate the defect in the superior aspect of the left frontal sinus (arrow).

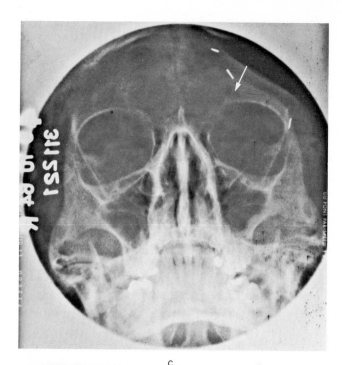

c

FIGURE 5.9. (Continued)

c and d. X rays following osteoplastic adipose obliteration of the frontal sinuses (arrows). The adipose tissue also covered the dural defect. The outline of the osteoplastic flap is difficult to see on the anteroposterior x ray film but is fairly clear on the lateral view.

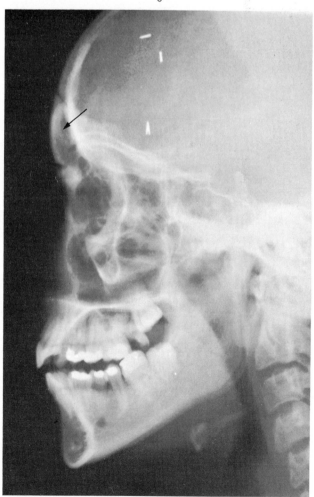

d

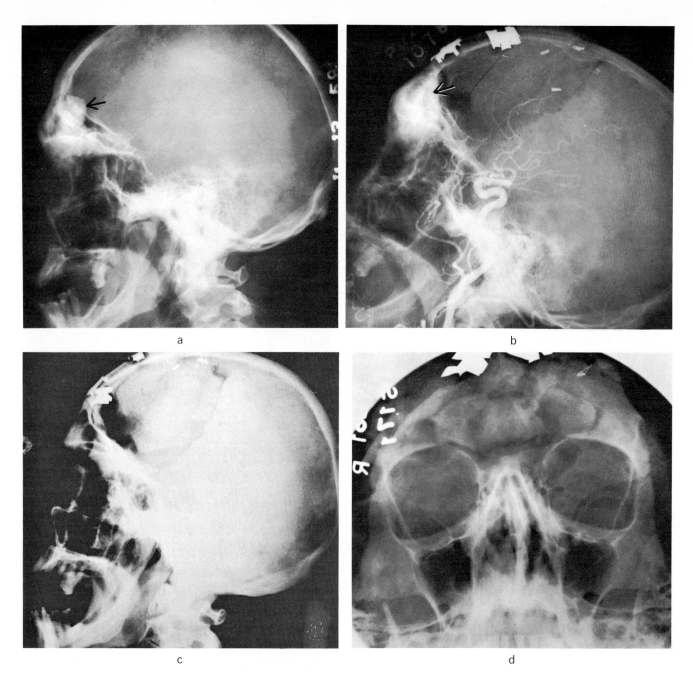

FIGURE 5.10. *Osteoma of frontal sinus with frontal lobe abscess.*

A 54-year old man was first examined one week following a seizure associated with personality change and disorientation. X rays showed a large osteoma in the frontal sinus which had grown through the posterior wall of the sinus and into the frontal lobe, where a large encapsulated abscess had formed.

On November 18, 1959, a large frontal lobe abscess was excised and the portion of the ostium protruding into the frontal lobe was removed by cranioplasty. A polyethylene sheet was placed between the dural defect and the defect in the posterior wall of the frontal sinuses.

On December 30, 1959, the large osteoma was removed by means of a bilateral anterior osteoplastic frontal sinus procedure. The osteoma displaced 33 cc of water. The polyethylene sheeting was removed, exposing a dural defect behind the frontal sinus. The dural defect was covered and the sinuses were obliterated with adipose tissue. The last x ray (d) shows the patient's status one year following this procedure. The patient has not been deformed by this extensive surgery.

a. Preoperative x ray showing a large frontal sinus osteoma extending through the posterior frontal sinus wall and into the anterior cranial fossa (arrow). A frontal lobe abscess was localized behind the osteoma.

b. X ray following craniotomy which involved removal of a frontal lobe abscess and the intracranial portion of the osteoma. The arrow points to the portion of osteoma remaining in the frontal sinus.

c. Postoperative x ray following the bilateral osteoplastic operation for removal of the frontal sinus osteoma and repair of the dural defect by adipose obliteration of both frontal sinuses.

d. An anteroposterior sinus x ray obtained one year following surgery. There had been no cerebrospinal fluid leakage, and there was no external deformity.

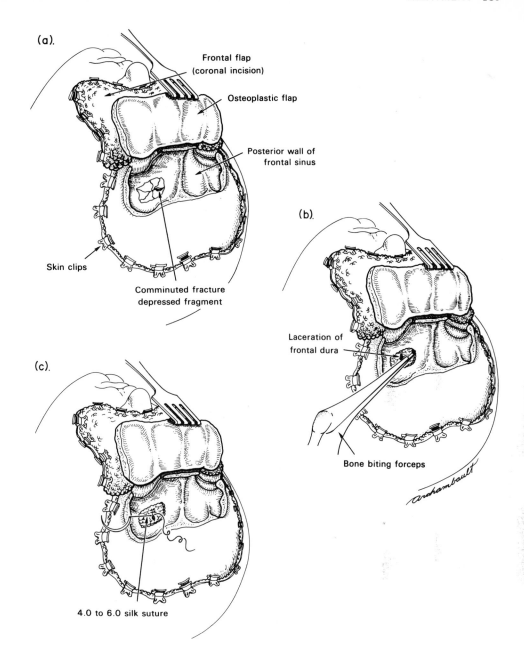

(a).

Frontal flap
(coronal incision)

Osteoplastic flap

Posterior wall of
frontal sinus

Skin clips

Comminuted fracture
depressed fragment

(b).

Laceration of
frontal dura

Bone biting forceps

(c).

4.0 to 6.0 silk suture

FIGURE 5.11.

    a. A defect in the dura behind the posterior wall of the frontal sinus is best approached using the osteoplastic flap. In this illustration the frontal bone and its periosteum have been exposed using the coronal incision and the frontal "scalping" flap. The osteoplastic flap is fashioned using a template from the patient's sinus x ray films as a guide. The Stryker saw is quite suitable for the bone incision around the outline of the frontal sinuses and should include a horizontal incision across the nasal process of the frontal bone and incisions through the supraorbital rim laterally on each side. The osteoplastic flap is being retracted inferiorly, exposing the inner aspect of the flap and a cavity that represents both frontal sinuses. The interfrontal septum has been removed. In this illustration a comminuted fracture of the posterior wall of the left frontal sinus is the obvious site to search for a defect in the frontal lobe dura.

    b. Fragments of bone and portions of the surrounding posterior wall of the left frontal sinus are removed with a Kerrison or other bone biting forceps, in order to adequately expose the laceration in the frontal lobe dura.

    c. A linear laceration of the dura, such as this one, is produced by a sharp spicule of bone and is quite easily repaired by multiple interrupted #4-0 to 6-0 silk sutures (Montgomery, 1973).

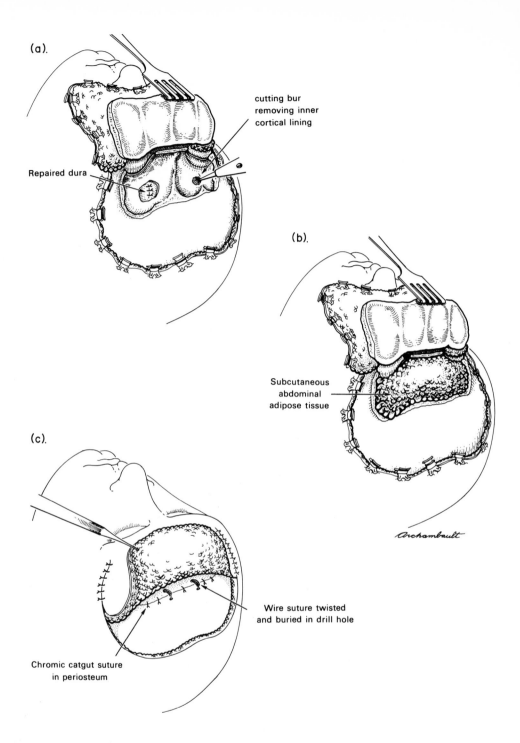

(a).

cutting bur
removing inner
cortical lining

Repaired dura

(b).

Subcutaneous
abdominal
adipose tissue

(c).

Wire suture twisted
and buried in drill hole

Chromic catgut suture
in periosteum

FIGURE 5.12.

a. Reinforcement by fascia is not necessary when linear closure of the dura can be accomplished. It is essential, however, that the mucous membrane and inner cortical lining of the entire frontal sinus complex be removed so that the sinus can be obliterated with adipose tissue.

b. Subcutaneous abdominal adipose tissue has been implanted into the frontal sinuses in order to create a barrier between the intranasal spaces and the dura.

c. As a general rule, the osteoplastic flap can be tightly secured in place by suturing the periosteum with chromic catgut sutures. If, on the other hand, the periosteum is deficient or defective, or there is any question that the osteoplastic flap might become dislodged and migrate forward, four drill holes should be placed as shown and the wire sutures applied. The twisted ends of these wire sutures are buried in a drill hole, as illustrated (Montgomery, 1973).

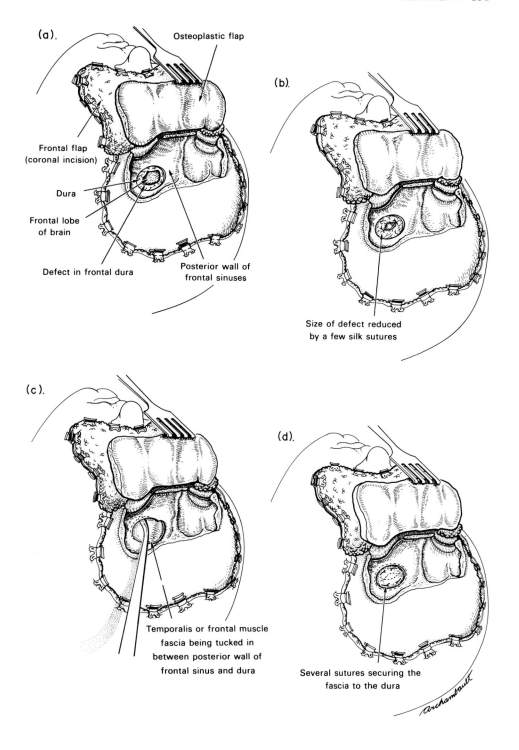

(a). Osteoplastic flap

Frontal flap
(coronal incision)

Dura

Frontal lobe
of brain

Defect in frontal dura

Posterior wall of
frontal sinuses

(b).

Size of defect reduced
by a few silk sutures

(c).

Temporalis or frontal muscle
fascia being tucked in
between posterior wall of
frontal sinus and dura

(d).

Several sutures securing the
fascia to the dura

archambault

FIGURE 5.13.

a. Quite often the defect in the frontal lobe dura cannot be repaired by suturing. Four or five millimeters of normal dura should be exposed around the defect to facilitate the repair.

b. The size of the dural defect can be reduced by applying a few interrupted silk sutures.

c. A section of temporalis or frontal muscle fascia is obtained having a diameter at least 1 cm larger than the bony defect in the posterior wall of the frontal sinus. This fascia is carefully tucked between the posterior wall of the frontal sinus and the frontal lobe dura so as to cover the dural defect.

d. In order to make certain that the fascial graft does not migrate and fits snugly against the dural defect, several interrupted sutures are applied. The repair is continued as shown in Figure 5.12a, b, and c. (Montgomery, 1973).

The defect in the anterior fossa dura is quite often too large for primary closure by suturing (Fig. 5.13a). A few sutures, however, will effect a reduction in the size of the defect (Fig. 5.13b). The remaining defect is closed by a cover of temporalis or frontalis muscle fascia. The fascia should be sufficiently large so that it can be tucked between the posterior wall of the frontal sinus and the dura around the periphery of the bony defect (Fig. 5.13c). The fascia is secured in place with several interrupted sutures (Fig. 5.13d).

Leakage of Cerebrospinal Fluid through the Sphenoid Sinus

The approach to the sphenoid sinus by the intracranial route for the repair occasioned by cerebrospinal fluid leakage through the sphenoid sinus is extremely difficult and, in some instances, impossible because of the anatomic development of this sinus. Hirsch was the first to use a septal flap for repair of spinal fluid rhinorrhea emanating from the sphenoid sinus following hypophysectomy. He removed the mucoperichondrium on one side of the posterior septum and the perpendicular plate of the ethmoid bone in order to rotate a mucoperichondrial flap from the opposite side into the sphenoid sinus. This procedure produces a large posterosuperior perforation of the septum, which is of little consequence. A septomucosal flap is employed routinely in performing hypophysectomies to prevent spinal fluid leakage as well as to create a barrier between the intradural space and the nasal cavity in order to avoid subsequent ascending infection.

A complete ethmoidectomy is carried out. A septal mucosal flap must be fashioned prior to entering the sphenoid sinus, for the mucosa covering the anterior wall of this sinus makes up the base of this flap. The length of the flap can be estimated from a study of anteroposterior and lateral laminograms of the sphenoid sinus. The position of the vertical incision (Fig. 5.14) determines the length of the mucosal flap (i.e., the farther anterior the vertical incision, the longer the septal mucosal flap). Incision number 2 is extended posteriorly from the superior aspect of the vertical incision, along the nasal septum adjacent to the medial aspect of the olfactory slit. This is extended to the front of the sphenoid sinus. Incision number 3 is made parallel to incision number 2 along the inferior aspect of the nasal septum. Incision number 4 is an extension of incision number 2 across the superior aspect of the anterior wall of the sphenoid sinus. Thus, the flap is based at the inferior margin of the front face of the sphenoid sinus. After the mucosal flap has been carefully elevated and reflected into the nasopharynx, the anterior wall of the sphenoid sinus is removed, by using curettes and Kerrison bone-biting forceps (Fig. 5.15).

Usually it is necessary to remove the intersphenoid septum and a small portion of the posterior aspect of the nasal septum in order to provide wide exposure of the sphenoid sinus complex. The mucosal lining of the sphenoid sinuses is removed. The septal mucosal flap is placed over the point of leakage. If the dural defect is large, it may be plugged with adipose tissue or fascia before the septal mucosal flap is reflected in place (Fig. 5.14b). A single layer of Gelfoam is placed over the flap before it is packed in place with a 24-inch strip of 1-inch iodoform gauze which has been impregnated with Aureomycin ointment. A finger-cot packing is inserted into the nasal cavity. The wound closure, dressing, and postoperative care are outlined in the section on ethmoidectomy (Chapter 4).

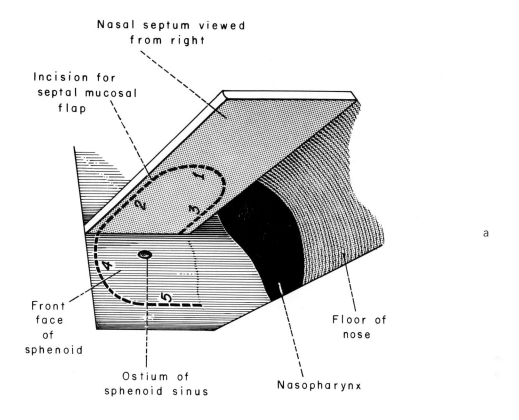

Nasal septum viewed
from right

Incision for
septal mucosal
flap

Front
face
of
sphenoid

Ostium of
sphenoid sinus

Nasopharynx

Floor of
nose

a

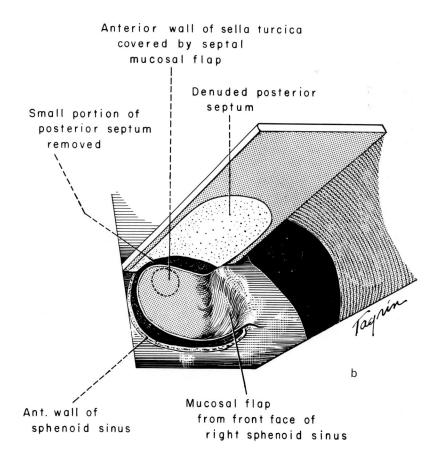

Anterior wall of sella turcica
covered by septal
mucosal flap

Denuded posterior
septum

Small portion of
posterior septum
removed

Ant. wall of
sphenoid sinus

Mucosal flap
from front face of
right sphenoid sinus

b

FIGURE 5.14. *Construction of septal mucosal flap.*

a. Schematic drawing showing incision for the construction of the septal mucosal flap.

b. Sketch demonstrating the mucosal flap reflected into the sphenoid sinus and covering the defect in the posterior wall.

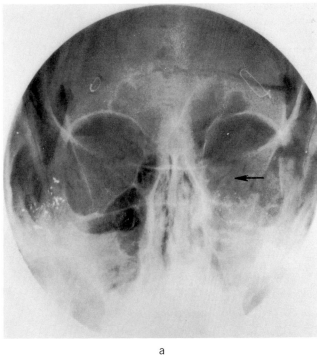

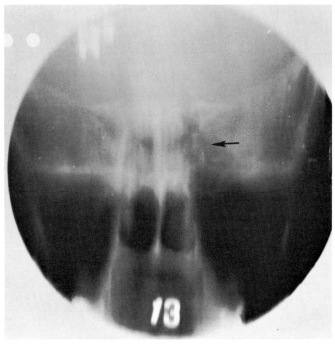

a

b

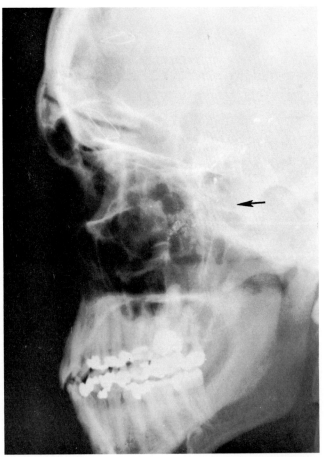

c

FIGURE 5.15. *Treatment of cerebrospinal fluid leakage through sphenoid sinus.*

A 23 year-old, mentally disturbed male was admitted to the hospital after having shot himself with a .38 pistol. The bullet had entered the right temple, transected the ethmoid and sphenoid sinuses, and exited from the left temple. Initial care included débridement of the wounds. Radiographic studies revealed extensive destruction in the region of the left sphenoid (a and b); the sphenoid sinuses were found to contain no air (c).

The recovery period was slow but no cerebrospinal fluid leak was noted and the patient was discharged to a state institution after three weeks. One week later, however, he was readmitted to the hospital for evaluation of a cerebrospinal fluid rhinorrhea. Lumbar puncture with injection of indigo carmine did not reveal any leakage of spinal fluid, but injection of fluorescein on the following day demonstrated leakage through both nostrils. The patient underwent bilateral frontal craniotomy with fascia lata repair of the right cribriform area. However, fluorescein test one week later demonstrated a persistent leakage from the left sphenoid sinus.

The left sphenoid sinus was then approached by way of the ethmoid bone. A large defect in the sphenoid bone and the dura was exposed and repaired with the use of fascia lata and a septo-mucosal flap. Fluorescein tests made one week and one month postoperatively did not show leakage of cerebrospinal fluid.

Leakage of Cerebrospinal Fluid through the Mastoid and Middle Ear

Spinal fluid leakage by way of the mastoid or middle ear can be successfully stopped by the obliterative technique. If the leak enters the mastoid cells or mastoid antrum and the cellular development is not too extensive, an inferiorly pedicled tissue flap will be adequate (Fig. 5.16). On the other hand, if the mastoid area is large, a pedicle flap may not be sufficient to provide an effective seal. In such cases, a free adipose autograft (obtained from the subcutaneous abdominal layer) is used (Fig. 5.17). This latter technique is employed to prevent spinal fluid leakage following the translabyrinthine approach to the cerebellopontile angle. The dura surrounding the defect is widely exposed so that the flap or graft can be packed snugly against the point of leakage. The mastoid incision is tightly closed in layers without drainage. This technique offers closure of the cranial mastoid defect without damage to either the auditory or vestibular function.

If the point of leakage is the anterior aspect of the mastoid antrum or the epitympanic tegmen, a radical mastoidectomy obliteration procedure cannot be employed. The entire mastoid process and middle ear must be obliterated with adipose tissue or muscle (Rambo), thus eliminating the external auditory canal.

An alternate method for repair of cerebrospinal otorrhea is that of grafting fascia lata over the dural defect. This technique was employed in patient M. S., a 19-year-old female college student who was admitted to the Massachusetts Eye and Ear Infirmary on January 6, 1966, complaining of watery otorrhea on the right side of two weeks' duration. Two years before this admission, an endaural radical mastoidectomy had been performed because of longstanding otorrhea and the presence of cholesteatoma. In June of 1965 a mastoidectomy with obliteration and type III tympanoplasty had been undertaken. Following this procedure, there was necrosis of the muscle pedicle flap and the otorrhea continued. Two weeks before the present hospitalization, the patient was admitted for a revision of her mastoidectomy. This procedure was complicated by cerebrospinal fluid otorrhea.

On examination a herniation of tissue in the region of the tegmen mastoideum and a rather profuse spinal fluid leakage were noted. No complicating central nervous system signs or symptoms were present. On January 7, 1966, with a modified Heermann incision with a temporal extension for exposure, a right temporal craniotomy was fashioned in the lower portion of the squamous bone and the temporal dura was exposed (Fig. 5.18). The temporal lobe and dura which had herniated into the mastoid were elevated. These structures were supported and the site of cerebrospinal fluid leakage repaired with a fascia lata graft. Mastoid packing was used to support the graft. The packing was removed on the fourteenth postoperative day. The patient's ear has remained dry.

Leakage of Cerebrospinal Fluid through the Cribriform Plate and Roof of Ethmoid

A dural defect above the cribriform plate or roof of the ethmoidal sinus is by far the most common site of origin of cerebrospinal fluid rhinorrhea. This dural defect is repaired by first performing a complete external ethmoidectomy with removal of the middle turbinate and then covering the dural defect, which has been

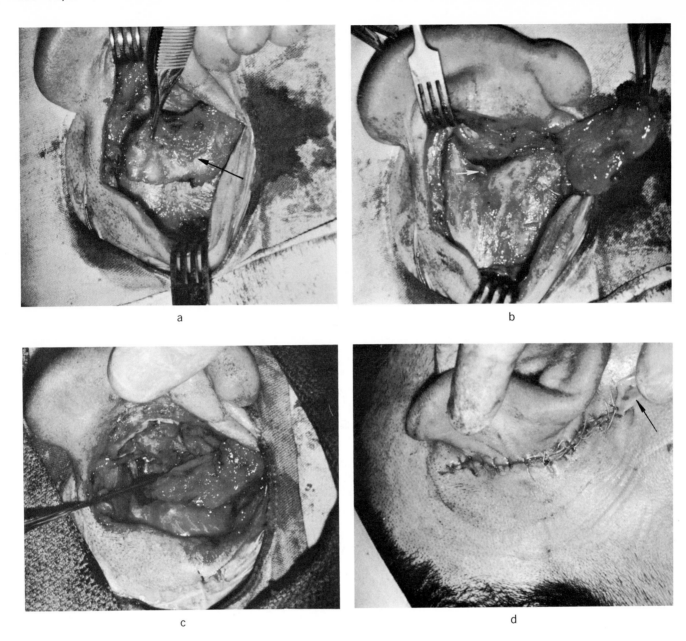

a

b

c

d

FIGURE 5.16. *Treatment of cerebrospinal leakage through the temporal bone (employing pedicled tissue flap).*

a. The inferiorly or superiorly based pedicled tissue flap can be employed to obliterate the mastoid and seal a cerebrospinal fluid leak. The postauricular incision is made in the postauricular crease. Skin flaps are established anteriorly and posteriorly. All subcutaneous adipose tissue and muscle are preserved when exposing the cortex over the mastoid process. An inferiorly based pedicled flap is demonstrated (arrow).

b. The inferiorly based pedicled flap is reflected inferiorly, exposing the cortex over the right mastoid. The bony posterior canal wall and the spine of Henle can be seen (arrow).

c. The mastoid dissection is complete, and the pedicled flap is reflected to obliterate the mastoid and seal the dural defect.

d. The skin flaps have been approximated with #4-0 plastic suture material. A rubber drain (arrow) is placed inferiorly to avoid a hematoma. A pressure mastoid dressing and the rubber drain are removed on the first or second postoperative day.

(Photographs were provided by courtesy of Harold F. Schuknecht, M.D., Chief of Otolaryngology, Massachusetts Eye and Ear Infirmary, Boston.)

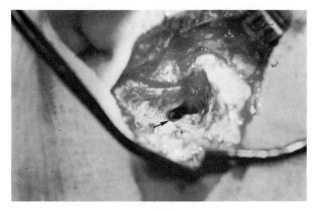

a

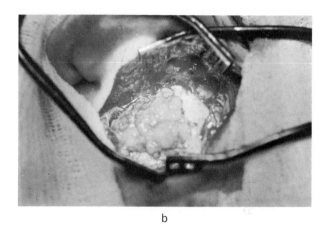

b

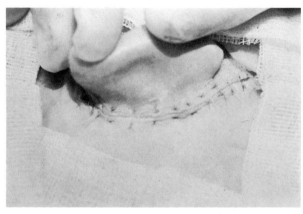

c

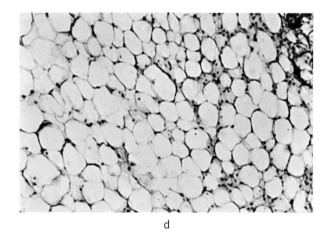

d

FIGURE 5.17.   *Treatment of cerebrospinal leakage through the mastoid bone (employing free adipose autograft).*

a. A photograph showing the dural defect (arrow) resulting from a translabyrinthine resection of a small acoustic neurinoma.

b. The labyrinthine-mastoidectomy defect has been obliterated with abdominal subcutaneous adipose tissue.

c. The skin incision is closed without drainage.

d. A tissue section from an adipose autograft one month after being implanted into the mastoid cavity. There was no loss of adipose tissue and very little fibrous tissue.

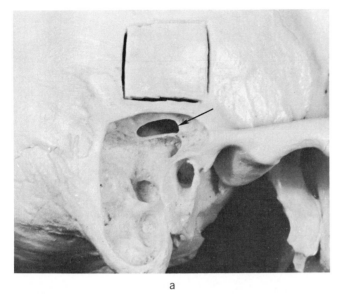

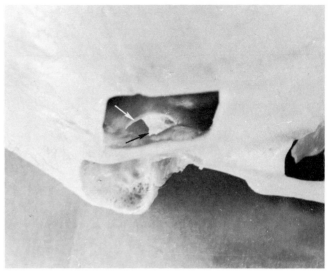

a

b

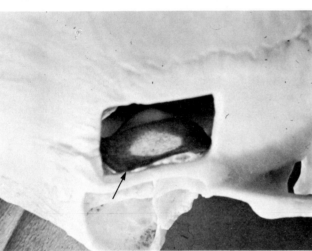

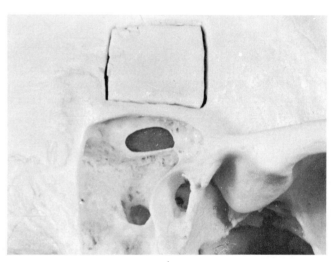

c

d

FIGURE 5.18. *Temporal craniotomy.*

a. This specimen demonstrates a bony defect in the tegmen mastoideum (arrow). When this defect is large the dura and temporal lobe may herniate into the mastoid. A fascia lata repair is indicated when the dural defect occurs in association with a radical mastoidectomy. An adipose obliteration is not practical unless the external auditory canal is also obliterated.

The posterior canal wall has not been removed in this specimen. Landmarks of note are the horizontal semicircular canal, the sigmoid sinus plate, the digastric crest, and the arcuate eminence viewed through the tegmental defect. A rectangular portion of temporal bone above the mastoid is cut, dissected from the dura, and preserved so that it can be replaced following repair of the dural defect.

b. The tegmental defect (white arrow) is viewed from above through the opening provided by the removal of bone in the temporal region. A portion of the horizontal semicircular canal (black arrow) can be seen.

c. The dura is carefully elevated from the cranial surface of the tegmen mastoideum. This is a somewhat difficult procedure when there has been herniation of the temporal lobe into the mastoid. A section of fascia lata (arrow) is placed over the entire tegmen as the dura is retracted. The fascia lata becomes secured in place when the dural retractor is removed.

d. The repaired tegmental defect is viewed from below. The bone is replaced in the temporal region. A split-thickness skin graft may be placed over the tegmen in the mastoid bowl. This serves to support the fascia from below and to line the mastoid bowl with epithelium.

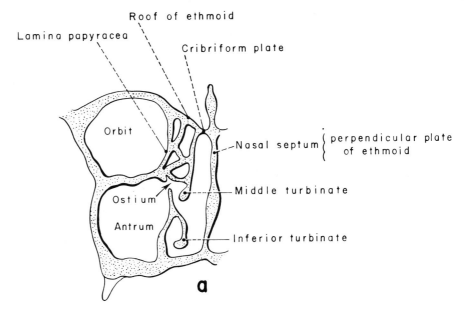

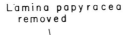

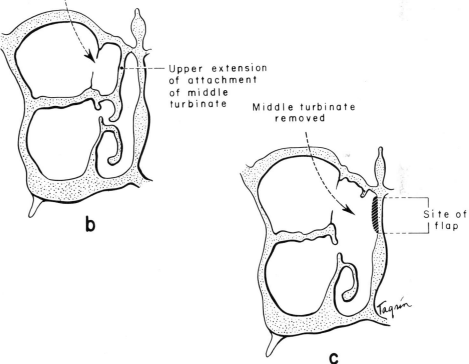

FIGURE 5.19.

a. A sketch showing the relations of the orbit, antrum, ethmoid labyrinth, and nasal cavity. Note particularly that the medial wall of the ethmoid labyrinth is an upper extension of the attachment of the middle turbinate. The latter separates the roof of the ethmoid and the cribriform plate.

b. The ethmoid cells have been removed along with the anterior portion of the lamina papyracea. The medial wall of the ethmoid labyrinth and the middle turbinate still remain intact.

c. The middle turbinate and medial wall of the ethmoid have been removed. This illustrates the wide exposure obtained by the transethmoid approach. The site of the septal mucosal flap, as viewed anteriorly, is shown.

adequately exposed, by a posteriorly based pedicled mucoperiosteal nasoseptal flap. Sketches of coronal sections through the orbit and sinus and nasal cavity in Figure 5.19 illustrate the surgical anatomy of this operation.

Surgical Anatomy. The ethmoid labyrinth is pyramidal in shape, being wider posteriorly than anteriorly and wider above than below. The anterior width of the ethmoid is 0.5 to 1 cm. The posterior width is approximately 1.5 cm. The antero-posterior length of the labyrinth is 3 to 4 cm. The height is 2 to 2.5 cm. The medial wall of the ethmoid is made up of the upper half of the lateral nasal wall (Fig. 5.19a). This is actually an extension of the attachment of the middle turbinate, which also separates the roof of the ethmoid from the olfactory slit in the superior nasal cavity (Fig. 5.20). A prolongation of the orbital plate of the frontal bone is the roof of the ethmoid labyrinth.

The lacrimal bone forms the lateral wall of the anterior ethmoid cells, and the os planum (lamina papyracea) forms the lateral wall of the posterior ethmoid cells. The anterior and posterior ethmoid foramina fairly accurately indicate the level of the roof of the ethmoid and the cribriform plate. The posterior ethmoid cells may be as close to the optic foramen as 1 mm. As a general rule, the outer half of the front face of the sphenoid sinus is the posterior limit of the ethmoid labyrinth.

The number of ethmoid cells varies between four and eight. The most important structures in the proximity of the anterior cells are the lacrimal bone, the floor of the frontal sinus, and the hiatus semilunaris; those in the proximity of the posterior cells are the posterior half of the medial wall of the orbit, the optic nerve, and the lateral half of the front wall of the sphenoid sinus. The plane of the cribriform plate approximately corresponds to: (1) the roof of the ethmoid labyrinth; (2) a horizontal line at the level of the pupils; and (3) the anterior and posterior ethmoid foramina.

Technique of Operation. Cerebrospinal fluid leakage by way of the cribriform plate or roof of the ethmoid is repaired by way of an external ethmoid incision (Fig. 5.21a). The patient's face is prepared with antiseptic solution and draped so as to expose the lower forehead, eyes, cheeks, and nose. The eyelids are fastened together with a single #5-0 suture to prevent injury to the cornea. After infiltration with a 2% local anesthetic agent with added epinephrine, a 1-inch curved incision is made halfway between the inner canthus and the anterior aspect of the nasal ridge (Fig. 5.21a). This incision is extended through the skin, subcutaneous tissue, and periosteum. Troublesome bleeding from the angular vessels and their numerous branches in this area is usually encountered. Before proceeding with the operation it is best to control this bleeding by either ligation or cauterization.

A number of retractors have been devised for exposure, but none of them seems as effective as two or three sutures, weighted with heavy hemostats, placed on each side of the incision (Fig. 5.21b). By elevating the periosteum laterally, the anterior and posterior lacrimal crests and fossae are identified. The lacrimal sac is displaced laterally, exposing the lacrimal bone, and posteriorly, exposing the lamina papyracea (Figs. 5.21b and c). The anterior and posterior ethmoid vessels are encountered during the elevation of the periosteum from the lamina papyracea. As a rule it is necessary to divide these vessels. Should bleeding occur, it can be easily controlled by cautery or by a short period of packing with gauze saturated with epinephrine solution. The ethmoid labyrinth is entered by perforating the thin lacrimal bone just posterior to the posterior lacrimal crest with a sharp curette (Fig. 5.22a). This opening is enlarged with various-sized Kerrison forceps (Fig. 5.22b

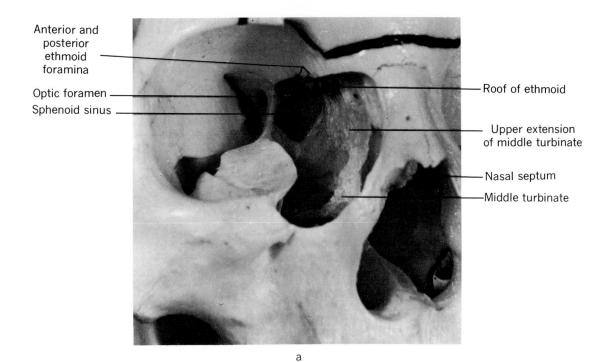

Anterior and posterior ethmoid foramina

Optic foramen

Sphenoid sinus

Roof of ethmoid

Upper extension of middle turbinate

Nasal septum

Middle turbinate

a

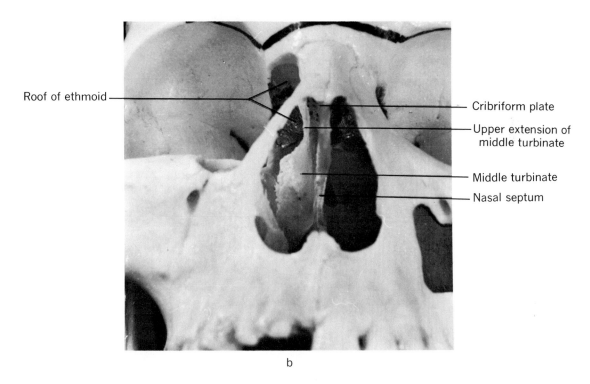

Roof of ethmoid

Cribriform plate

Upper extension of middle turbinate

Middle turbinate

Nasal septum

b

FIGURE 5.20.

a. An anterior and posterior ethmoidectomy has been completed, preserving the middle turbinate and its upper extension. The roof of the ethmoid can be seen. Note its anatomic relationships to the anterior and posterior ethmoid foramina.

b. The same dissection, viewed from below. This clearly demonstrates the upper extension of the middle turbinate attached between the roof of the ethmoid and the cribriform plate.

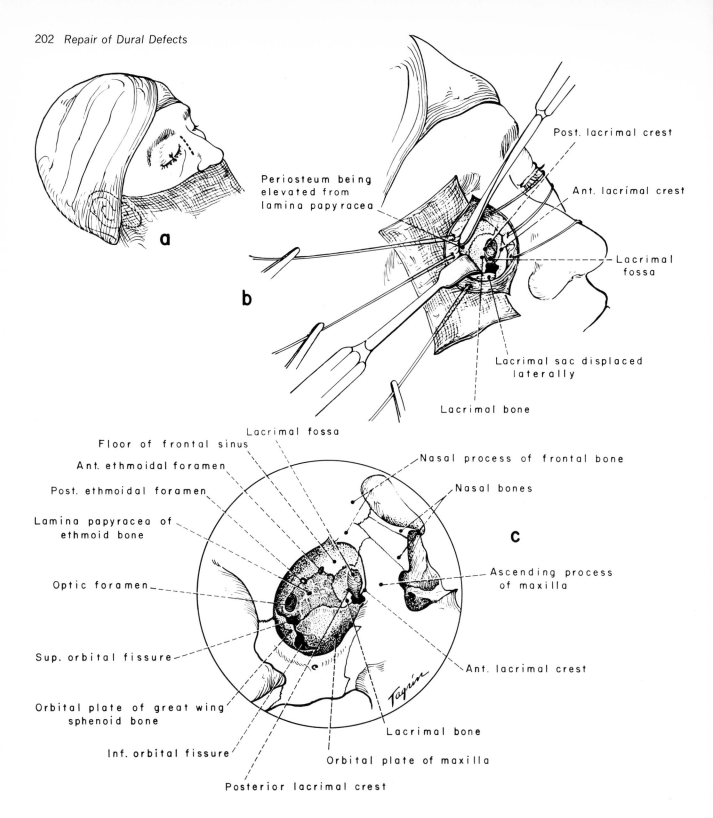

FIGURE 5.21. *Treatment of cerebrospinal fluid leakage through the cribriform plate and roof of ethmoid.*

a. The patient has been prepared, draped, and the eyelids have been sutured together. The external ethmoid incision is indicated.

b. The incision has been carried through the periosteum; #2-0 chromic catgut sutures are used for retraction. The perio-steum and lacrimal sac have been dissected and are retracted laterally. The ascending process of the maxilla, lacrimal fossa, lacrimal bone, and a portion of the lamina papyracea can be seen.

c. The anatomy of the medial wall of the orbit is illustrated. The anterior and posterior ethmoid foramina and suture line between the orbital plate of the frontal bone and the lamina papyracea are at the level of both the cribriform plate and the roof of the ethmoid. Note the close proximity of the posterior ethmoid cells to the optic foramen.

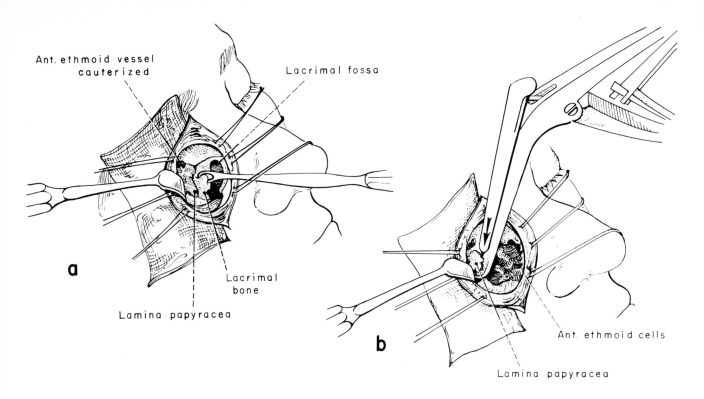

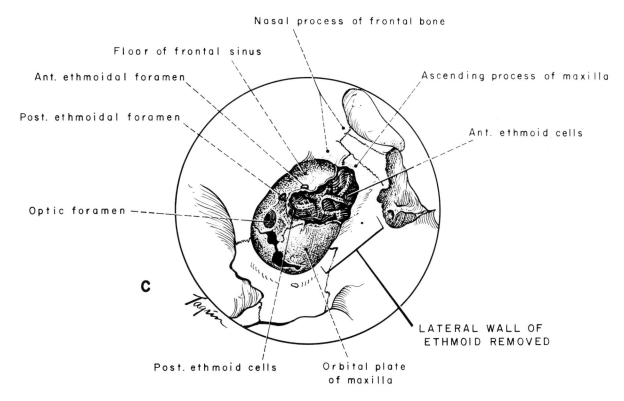

FIGURE 5.22. *Treatment of cerebrospinal fluid leakage through the cribriform plate and roof of the ethmoid.*

a. The ethmoid labyrinth is entered by curetting away a portion of the lacrimal bone just behind the posterior lacrimal crest. The anterior ethmoid artery has been cauterized.

b. A Kerrison forceps is used to remove the lateral wall of the ethmoid labyrinth.

c. A sketch showing the anatomic relationships after the lateral wall of the ethmoid labyrinth has been removed.

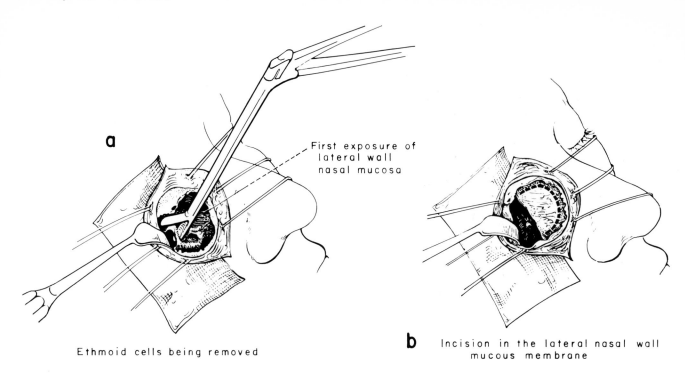

a

First exposure of
lateral wall
nasal mucosa

Ethmoid cells being removed

b Incision in the lateral nasal wall
mucous membrane

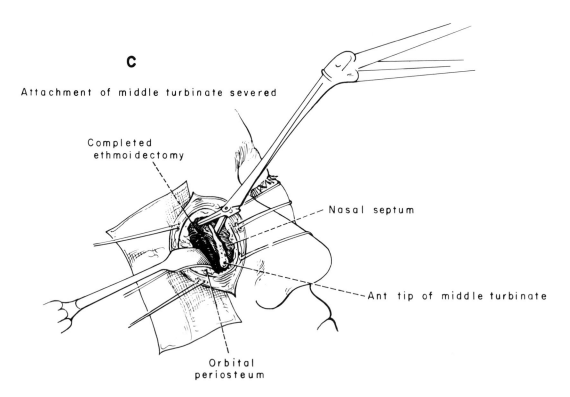

c

Attachment of middle turbinate severed

Completed
ethmoidectomy

Nasal septum

Ant tip of middle turbinate

Orbital
periosteum

FIGURE 5.23. *Treatment of cerebrospinal fluid leakage through the cribriform plate and roof of the ethmoid.*

a. The anterior and posterior ethmoid cells are removed by using curettes, Brownie forceps, and Takahashi forceps. The mucous membrane of the lateral nasal wall anterior to the middle turbinate is exposed as the anterior ethmoid cells are removed.

b. An incision is made in the mucous membrane of the lateral nasal wall, creating a flap which is removed.

c. The mucous membrane flap has been removed, exposing the middle turbinate.

The attachment of the middle turbinate is then incised using scissors designed for this purpose. The middle turbinate is then removed with a wire snare.

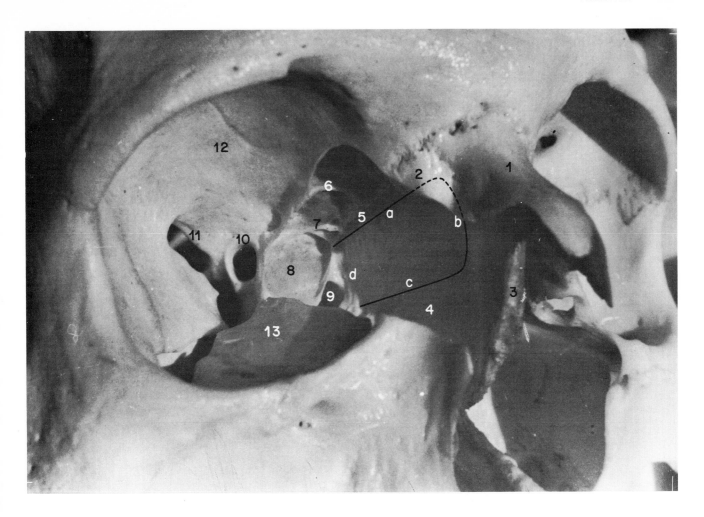

FIGURE 5.24. *Anatomy of the septal mucosal flap.*

1. Nasal bone
2. Ascending process of maxilla
3. Anterior margin of bony nasal septum
4. Posteriorly based septal mucosal flap
   a. An upper anteroposterior incision is made just below the cribriform plate
   b. The anterior vertical incision is made as far forward as possible to ensure adequate length of the flap
   c. The supero-inferior position of this incision determines the width of the mucosal flap
   d. Base of septal mucosal flaps. The blood supply to the flaps is from branches of the sphenopalatine artery
5. Cribriform plate
6. Roof of anterior ethmoid sinuses
7. Roof of posterior ethmoid sinuses
8. Anterior wall of the right sphenoid sinus
9. Ostium of the right sphenoid sinus
10. Optic foramen
11. Superior orbital fissure
12. Orbital plate of frontal bone (roof of orbit)
13. Orbital plate of maxillary bone (floor of orbit)

and c). The anterior ethmoid cells are then removed by using ethmoid curettes and Brownie and Takahashi forceps (Fig. 5.23a).

An instrument such as the periosteal elevator is passed intranasally along the nasal septum and then above the middle turbinate, causing the mucous membrane of the lateral nasal wall to bulge into the field. This membrane is then incised (Fig. 5.23b), affording the operator a view of the middle turbinate. Turbinate scissors are used to sever the attachment of the middle turbinate (Fig. 5.23c); the turbinate is removed with a wire snare. Using the attachment of the middle turbinate as a guide, the posterior ethmoid cells are removed. The upper prolongation of the

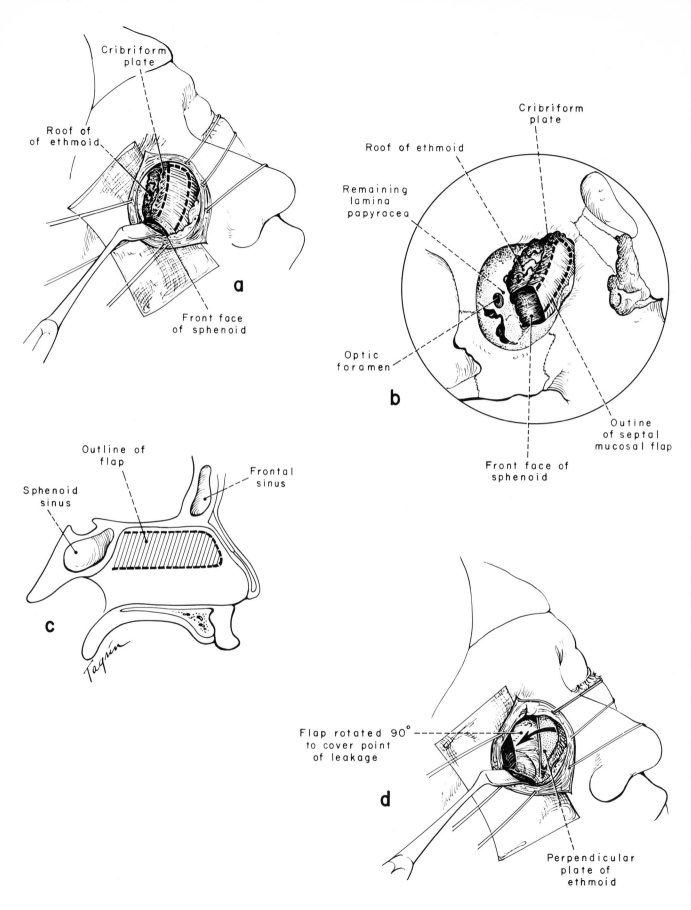

attachment is then removed. The olfactory slit (cribriform plate) thus becomes continuous with the roof of the ethmoid (Figs. 5.24 and 5.25).

The dural defect is usually easily found with the aid of a surgical microscope. The thin bony roof of the ethmoid labyrinth and cribriform plate is carefully removed until the surrounding dura is exposed. After this has been accomplished, a pedicled mucosal flap is obtained from the nasal septum.

Detection of the site of leakage is facilitated by the injection of 1 cc of 5% fluorescein intrathecally prior to the operation. On occasion the dural defect is sufficiently large to reduce the spinal fluid pressure either intermittently or constantly. In such cases it may not be possible to identify the site of leakage, even when fluorescein dye has been injected intrathecally. It is therefore important to measure the spinal fluid pressure preoperatively, prior to the intrathecal injection of fluorescein. If the spinal fluid pressure is low or no pressure is registered, Hartman's solution* is used to elevate the pressure during the operation. A #20 spinal needle is inserted in the lumbar region (the patient is placed in the sitting position, if necessary) and a spinal catheter is inserted. Two cubic centimeters of 5% fluorescein are added to freshly mixed Hartman's solution and the mixture is infused through the spinal catheter.

The Hartman's solution is allowed to flow intrathecally after the area of suspected leakage is exposed. The spinal fluid pressure is determined intermittently by means of a manometer attached to the infusion tubing. The orange-yellow spinal fluid will become obvious as soon as the pressure is raised, especially when the level of the patient's head is slightly below that of his body.

The septomucosal flap used to repair a fistula by way of the cribriform plate and roof of the ethmoid is based posteriorly (Figs. 5.24 and 5.25). The superior incision extends along the anteroposterior dimension of the superior nasal septum at the junction of the septum and the olfactory slit. This incision is carried as far anteriorly as is possible. The lower incision is approximately 1.5 cm below, and parallel to, the superior incision. It may be necessary to obtain a somewhat wider flap if the dural dehiscence involves both the roof of the ethmoid labyrinth and the cribriform area. The anterior incision merely connects the anterior aspect of the superior and inferior mucosal incisions. As the mucosal flap is elevated, the perpendicular plate of the ethmoid bone is exposed. It is quite often necessary

---

*Hartman's solution comes in a two-unit package. The first package contains potassium, sodium, calcium and magnesium chloride and a small amount of hydrochloric acid. The second contains sodium carbonate and phenol red dye. When the two are mixed, a salmon-pink solution having a pH of from 7.2 to 7.5 results.

FIGURE 5.25. *Treatment of cerebrospinal fluid leakage through the cribriform plate and roof of the ethmoid.*

a. The middle turbinate and medial wall of the ethmoid labyrinth have been completely removed. This affords the operator an excellent view of the entire roof of the ethmoid, olfactory slit, front face of the sphenoid, sphenoid ostium, posterior choanae, and the posterior aspect of the lamina papyracea. The outline of the septomucosal flap is shown. The superior incision extends along the anteroposterior dimension of the superior nasal septum at the level of the olfactory slit. The lower incision is parallel to and approximately 1.5 cm inferior to the superior incision. The anterior incision connects the anterior aspects of the above incisions, creating a posteriorly based flap.

b. The outline of the septomucosal flap, roof of the ethmoid, and cribriform plate are illustrated. A leak in either the cribriform plate or the roof of ethmoid area can be easily detected.

c. A midsagittal section, just to the right of the nasal septum, shows the outline of the posteriorly based septal mucosal flap, which is used to repair a spinal fluid leakage by way of the ethmoid labyrinth or cribriform plate.

d. The septal mucosal flap has been rotated 90 degrees upward to cover both the cribriform plate and roof of the ethmoid. The perpendicular plate of the ethmoid becomes denuded.

to remove most of the ascending process of the maxilla in this area to expose the anterosuperior nasal septum.

The septomucosal flap is rotated approximately 90 degrees so as to cover the point of leakage and adjacent dura of the olfactory and ethmoid regions (Fig. 5.25d). The flap is carefully packed in place with a layer of Gelfoam saturated with bacitracin solution. This is covered with 1-inch wide iodoform gauze stripping that has been impregnated with Aureomycin ointment. A finger-cot packing is inserted into the nasal cavity to prevent inferior displacement of the iodoform gauze. A layer of Gelfoam is placed over the iodoform packing in the region of the external ethmoid incision to prevent the packing from adhering to the periosteum. The periosteal incision is then closed with #4-0 catgut and #5-0 silk or plastic suture material. The dressing consists of a layer of Telfa gauze over the suture line, an eye pad, gauze fluffs, and elastic adhesive. After 24 to 48 hours, the entire dressing and finger-cot packing are removed. The iodoform gauze packing, however, must be left in place until the sixth postoperative day.

REFERENCES

Anderson, W. M., Schwartz, G. A., and Gammon, G. D.: Chronic Spontaneous Cerebrospinal Rhinorrhea. Arch. Intern. Med. *107*:723–731, 1961.

Collins, E. W.: Rhinorrhea Following Rasping of the Frontal Sinus. In the Report of Society Transactions, Oct. 19. Arch. Otolaryng. 6:590, 1927.

Goodale, R. L., and Montgomery, W. W.: Technical Advances in Osteoplastic Frontal Sinusectomy. Arch. Otolaryng. 79:522–529 (May) 1964.

Gotham, J. E., et al.: Observations on Cerebrospinal Fluid Rhinorrhea and Pneumocephalus. Ann. Otol. 74:215–233 (March) 1965.

Hall, G. M., Pulec, J. L., and Halberg, O. E.: Persistent Cerebrospinal Fluid Otorrhea. Arch. Otolaryng. 86:4:377–381 (Oct.) 1967.

Hirsch, O.: Successful Closure of Cerebrospinal Rhinorrhea by Endonasal Surgery. Arch. Otolaryng. 56:1–12 (July) 1952.

Jewey, J. W.: Cerebrospinal Rhinorrhea. Trans. Amer. Laryng. Rhinol. Otol. Soc. 38:341, 1932.

Locke, C. F., Jr.: The Spontaneous Escape of Cerebrospinal Fluid through the Nose. Arch. Neurol. Psychiat. 15:309–324, 1926.

McCoy, G.: Cerebrospinal Rhinorrhea: A Comprehensive Review and a Definition of the Responsibility of the Rhinologist in Diagnosis and Treatment. Laryngoscope *73*:1125–1157 (Sept.) 1963.

McKinney, R.: Traumatic Pneumocephalon. Ann. Otol. 41:597–600, 1932.

Montgomery, W. W.: Cerebrospinal Fluid Rhinorrhea in an Accident-Prone Individual. Arch. Otolaryng. 68:493–496 (Oct.) 1958.

Montgomery, W. W., and Pierce, D. L.: Anterior Osteoplastic Fat Obliteration for Frontal Sinus: Clinical Experience and Animal Studies. Trans. Amer. Acad. Ophthal. Otolaryng. 67:46–57 (Jan.–Feb.) 1963.

Montgomery, W. W.: Transethmoidosphenoidal Hypophysectomy with Septal Mucosal Flap. Arch. Otolaryng. 78:68–77 (July) 1963.

Montgomery, W. W.: The Fate of Adipose Implants in a Bony Cavity. Laryngoscope *74*:816–827 (June) 1964.

Montgomery, W. W.: Surgery for Cerebrospinal Fluid Rhinorrhea and Otorrhea. Arch. Otolaryng. 84:538–550 (Nov.) 1966.

Montgomery, W. W.: Cerebrospinal Fluid Rhinorrhea. Otolaryng. Clin. N. Amer. 6:657–772, 1973.

Ommaya, A. K.: Cerebrospinal Fluid Rhinorrhea. Neurology *14*:106–113 (Feb.) 1964.

Rambo, J. H. T.: Musculoplasty: a New Operation for Suppurative Middle Ear Deafness. Trans. Amer. Acad. Ophthal. Otolaryng. 62:166–177 (Mar.–Apr.) 1958.

Schuknecht, H. F., and Olekstuk, S.: Tympanoplasty. Laryngoscope 69:614–643, 1959.

6

Surgery of the Maxillary Sinus

ANTROTOMY

Indications. In maxillary sinusitis, nasoantral irrigations are indicated only after adequate conservative management has failed to effect a cure or in order to obtain material for culture. An adequate trial of conservative therapy is the treatment of choice whether the sinusitis be acute, subacute, or chronic. The appropriate antibiotics are administered along with the use of local and systemic nasal decongestants. If this therapy is properly instituted, nasoantral irrigations are rarely indicated. If medical therapy is not successful, the surgeon should resort to more definitive procedures, in an attempt to establish adequate drainage and remove diseased tissue from the sinus.

Technique of Irrigation. There are two routes for irrigating the maxillary sinus: (1) by way of the natural ostium, and (2) through the inferior meatus. The arguments against the natural route are that irreparable damage to the ciliated respiratory epithelium in the region of the natural ostium is a possibility, and anatomic variations may render this technique extremely difficult or impossible.

Most otolaryngologists prefer to irrigate the maxillary sinus by way of the inferior meatus. For this procedure, the inferior meatus is anesthetized by packing with cotton strips impregnated with 4% cocaine or 2% Pontocaine. Epinephrine (1:1000) or ephedrine (1%) may be added to the Pontocaine. These cotton strips should remain in place for approximately 15 minutes. A straight, thin Lichtwicz needle with a Wolf thumb rest is the instrument of choice for the nasoantral puncture. This is inserted through the nasoantral wall of the inferior meatus, approximately 1 cm behind the anterior tip of the inferior turbinate, and directed toward the lateral canthus. At this point, it is most important not to traverse the sinus cavity completely and enter either the superior or lateral sinus walls. Aspirating before irrigation is essential. Either secretions or air is obtained if the tip of the needle is in the sinus cavity. If the tip is in the sinus cavity and neither secretions nor air is aspirated, then the antrum is filled with a solid material such as that due to polypoid mucositis or to a neoplasm.

The sinus is irrigated with warm normal saline solution. It is not necessary to inject air following this irrigation. There have been some reports of air embolism following injection of air into the maxillary sinus. If the irrigating solution containing the material washed out from the sinus is collected in a black basin, all purulent secretions and debris will be prominent, while the sanguineous material will be invisible and not upsetting to the patient.

ANTROSTOMY (Intranasal Fenestration of the Nasoantral Wall)

A well-constructed nasoantral window is sufficient to cure a chronic purulent maxillary sinusitis, providing the antrum is not filled with polypoid disease and there is no bone necrosis or dental complication. Over the years it has been repeatedly demonstrated that a small nasoantral window closes rapidly and is thus ineffective. A large window is essential.

Technique. The intranasal antrostomy should be performed as an in-patient procedure so that the surgeon can proceed with a radical antrum operation, if indicated, after fenestrating the nasoantral wall of the inferior meatus. Many surgeons perform a radical antrum operation routinely in preference to an intranasal antrostomy. The latter procedure effects a cure in less than 90% of patients, thus necessitating an additional hospitalization and operative procedure for those patients in whom the antrostomy fails to effect a cure.

For the intranasal antrostomy, cotton strips, impregnated with a topical anesthetic agent, are placed in the inferior meatus, medial to and above the inferior turbinate. It is best to leave these packs in place for 15 minutes, even when operating with a patient under general anesthesia, because shrinkage of the mucous membrane affords better visualization of the inferior meatus and better hemostasis than could otherwise be obtained. The topical anesthesia also supplements the general anesthesia.

The inferior turbinate is fractured medially and superiorly with a smooth-edged, flat instrument such as a large periosteal elevator or a tonsil dissector. No portion of the inferior turbinate is removed. The nasoantral wall of the inferior meatus is broken through with a punch or sharp curved hemostat. This opening is first enlarged anteriorly with a Kerrison bone-biting forceps and then posteriorly with side-biting ring forceps. The diameter of the fenestration should be 1.5 to 2 cm. It is obviously important to remove the nasoantral wall down to the level of the floor of the nasal cavity in order to facilitate drainage from the sinus. When the fenestration is of sufficient size, the sinus cavity can be inspected for disease by direct vision. If irreversible disease is found, it is best to enter the antrum by way of the canine fossa and carry out a radical antrum operation.

Usually, it is not necessary to insert packing following the antrostomy. On the other hand, if bleeding is troublesome, the window may be packed with 1-inch petrolatum-impregnated iodoform gauze. The packing is removed on the first or second postoperative day.

EXTERNAL SURGERY OF THE MAXILLARY SINUS
The Caldwell-Luc Operation

Indications. The indications for the Caldwell-Luc procedure are: (1) intractable infection; (2) failure of resolution of a chronic infection following intranasal antrostomy; (3) polypoid tissue filling the antrum; (4) antrochoanal polyp, or cystic disease of the antrum; (5) osteonecrosis; (6) suspicion of maxillary sinus neoplasm; (7) dental cysts; (8) presence of foreign bodies; (9) fractures of the maxilla; (10) the presence of an oroantral fistula.

Technique of Operation. *Anesthesia.* The Caldwell-Luc operation may be performed with the patient under either general or local anesthesia. If local anesthesia is employed, cotton strips impregnated with a topical anesthetic and vasoconstrictor are placed both above and below the inferior turbinate. Two per cent Xylocaine or procaine with added epinephrine is injected along the gingivobuccal sulcus in the region of the canine fossa. The injection is continued superiorly so as to include the infraorbital nerve.

Incision. A horizontal incision is made in the gingivobuccal sulcus well above the roots of the teeth (Fig. 6.1a). The incision extends from the level of the lateral incisor to the second molar and through the mucous membrane and periosteum. The periosteum over the canine fossa is then elevated to the level of the infraorbital canal. The infraorbital nerve is identified and carefully preserved (Fig. 6.1b). The best way to avoid injury to this nerve is to positively identify it. An atraumatic method of elevating the periosteum is to place a bit of gauze ahead of a chisel to provide blunt dissection. Gentle retraction throughout the procedure will also reduce the chance for trauma to the infraorbital nerve as well as to the other soft tissues of the cheek. Two retractors are used to elevate the periosteum. These are placed in a superior medial and superior lateral direction in order to avoid the infraorbital nerve.

Fenestrating the Canine Fossa. The best way to fenestrate the anterior wall of the antrum is with use of a curette (Fig. 6.2a) or a rotating bur (Fig. 6.2b). If a rotating bur is not available, a square window may be made with a sharp chisel (Fig. 6.2c). The four sides of this window are first scored by light tapping in order to avoid fracture. A sharp gouge is another instrument that may be used to fenestrate the anterior wall. Whichever instrument is employed, a fracture must be avoided, for this may extend to, and injure, the infraorbital nerve or a tooth root.

The opening in the anterior wall is enlarged with either a bur or a Kerrison bone-cutting forceps (Fig. 6.2d). Troublesome bleeding may occur from the bone margin. This can be controlled by squeezing tightly with the Kerrison forceps but not hard enough to cut through the bone. It is well to enlarge the sinus opening to a size that will admit the fifth digit (Fig. 6.2e). The entire contents of the antrum can then be viewed.

Cysts and benign tumors can be removed with various elevators and forceps, injury to the normal mucosa being avoided. Removal of the entire mucous membrane lining of the antrum is rarely necessary. However, when the lining seems irreversibly diseased it can be easily removed by first elevating it with a curved blunt dissector and then using various elevators, curettes, and tissue forceps for removal. Dissection in the region of the roof of the antrum must be conducted with care, for the infraorbital nerve may not have a bony covering in this region.

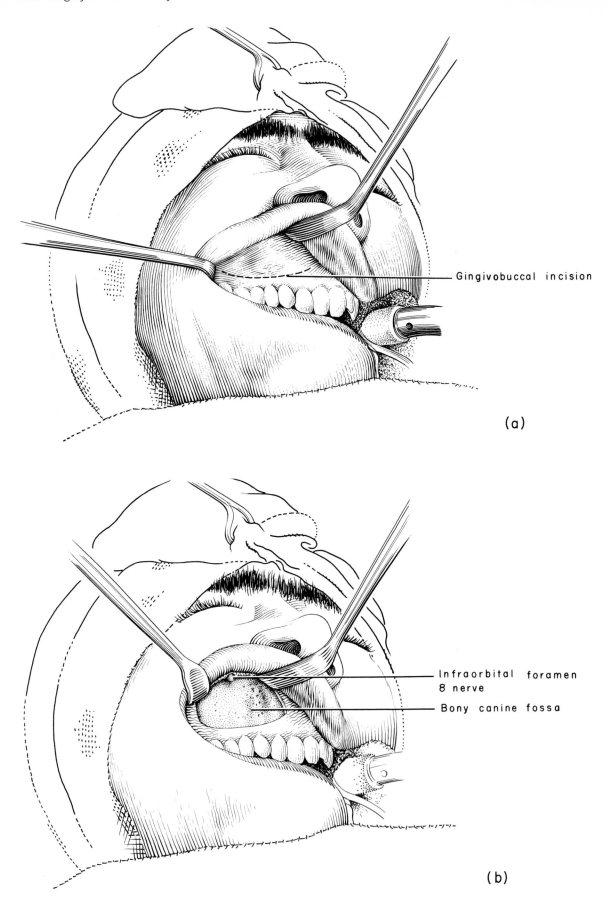

Gingivobuccal incision

(a)

Infraorbital foramen
8 nerve

Bony canine fossa

(b)

FIGURE 6.1. *Caldwell-Luc operation.*

a. The upper lip is retracted superiorly in a direction away from the infraorbital nerve. Stretching of the nerve can cause anesthesia of the upper lip and side of the nose.

The endotracheal tube is directed towards the contralateral angle of the mouth. The pharynx is packed both to assist with a closed system of anesthesia and to prevent blood from entering the pharynx.

An incision is made about 5 mm above the gum margin. It should be slightly "U" shaped, especially when the patient wears an upper denture.

b. The periosteum has been elevated superiorly, exposing the bony front face of the maxillary sinus, known as the canine fossa.

Again, note that the retraction is in a direction away from the infraorbital nerve, which can be seen as it leaves the infraorbital foramen. Bleeding is controlled by packing with epinephrine-impregnated gauze strips or by cautery. A gauze strip pushed ahead of a chisel assists with the elevation of the periosteum.

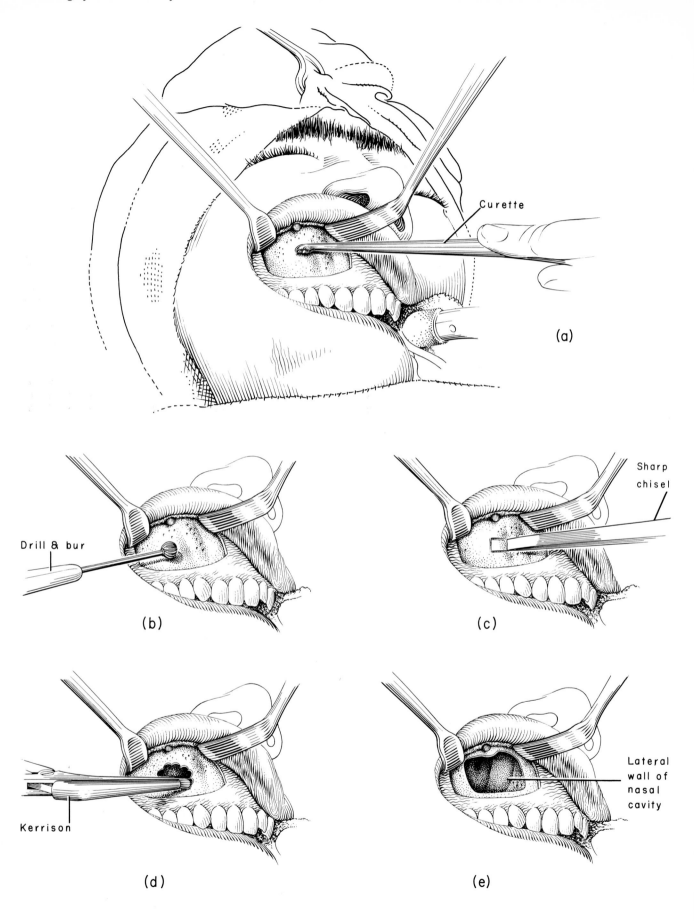

(a)

Curette

(b)

Drill & bur

(c)

Sharp
chisel

(d)

Kerrison

(e)

Lateral
wall of
nasal
cavity

FIGURE 6.2. *Caldwell-Luc operation—methods for entering antrum.*

There are several methods for entering the antrum by way of the anterior wall.

a. A curette can be used if the wall is thin.

b. A cutting "rose" bur can be used both for entrance into the antrum and for removal of the antrum's anterior wall.

c. When a sharp chisel is used, all four sides must be scored with the chisel prior to penetrating into the antrum. This is essential to prevent fracture and possible injury to the infraorbital nerve.

d. The anterior wall of the sinus is being removed with a Kerrison forceps. Troublesome bleeding may occur from the cut edge of bone. This can be controlled by squeezing the bone edge tightly with the Kerrison forceps but not hard enough to cut through.

e. Sufficient amount of anterior wall has now been resected, so that the diseased area can be removed effectively and a nasoantral fenestration fashioned.

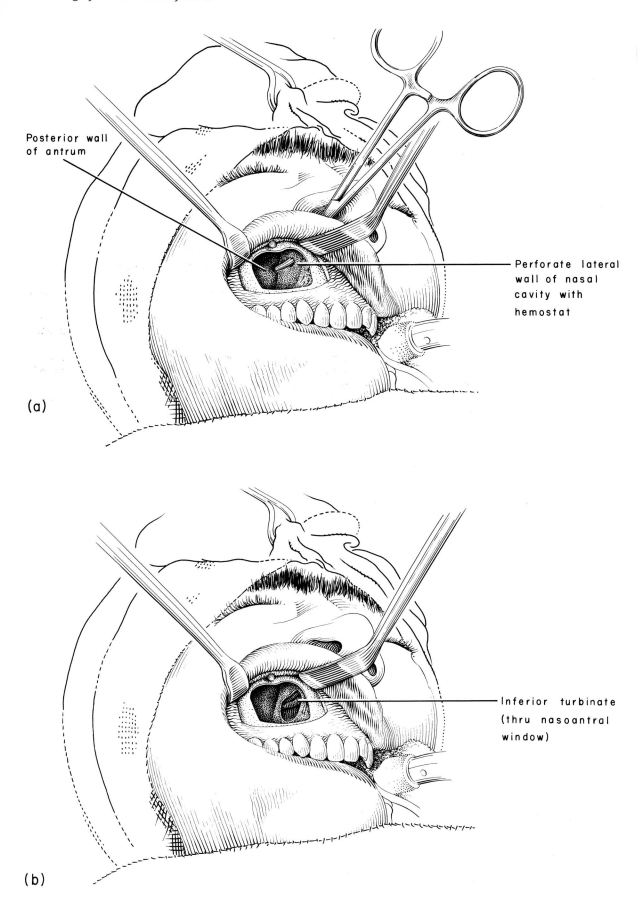

Posterior wall of antrum

Perforate lateral wall of nasal cavity with hemostat

(a)

Inferior turbinate (thru nasoantral window)

(b)

The Nasoantral Window. A curved, sharp hemostat is inserted intranasally into the inferior meatus and, by gentle pressure, an opening is made in the anterior aspect of the nasoantral wall (Fig. 6.3a). The fenestra is enlarged in an anterior direction with Kerrison forceps and posteriorly with a side-biting forceps. This dissection is much more easily carried out by way of the Caldwell-Luc opening in contrast to the intranasal route. The nasoantral window should be at least 1.5 cm in diameter and should include intranasal mucous membrane, sinus mucosa, and the bony nasoantral wall (Figs. 6.3b and 6.4a). Many surgeons hold the opinion that the various mucosal flaps devised for formation of the nasoantral window are not only unnecessary but can, by becoming displaced, close the fenestra.

The Denker modification of the radical antrum operation is preferred by some surgeons (Fig. 6.4b). The opening in the anterior sinus wall is enlarged in a medial direction, thus removing the inferior portion of the ascending process of the maxilla. The anterior half of the lateral nasal wall inferior to the inferior turbinate is resected to serve as the nasoantral communication. The end results of the Caldwell-Luc and Denker operations are quite similar.

Before packing, the sinus cavity is carefully inspected for retained sponges. If there is no bleeding, packing is unnecessary. Petrolatum or Aureomycin ointment-impregnated 1-inch iodoform gauze packing may be inserted into the sinus by way of the nasoantral fenestra in order to control persistent bleeding. The incision in the gingivobuccal sulcus is closed with one or two catgut sutures. Some surgeons prefer not to suture this incision, stating that there is much less postoperative edema if it is not closed.

Postoperative Care. An ice pack over the cheek during the first 24 postoperative hours is essential to prevent edema, hematoma, and discomfort and should be obtained for the patient while he is still in the recovery room. The intrasinus and intranasal packing should be removed at the end of one or two postoperative days. If purulent secretions were encountered in the sinus, the postoperative administration of antibiotics is of value. The antibiotics may be altered according to culture and sensitivity tests.

FIGURE 6.3. *Caldwell-Luc operation—construction of nasoantral window.*

a. Diseased tissue is removed from the antrum with curettes and blunt cupped forceps. If the mucosal lining of the antrum is to be removed, it is first elevated with a blunt curved dissector. Dissection should be conducted with care in the region of the roof, for the infraorbital nerve may not have a bony covering. To construct the nasoantral window, a curved hemostat is passed into the nasal cavity along the floor and then directly lateralward beneath the inferior turbinate. The tip of the hemostat is moved from side to side in order to enlarge the opening sufficiently to admit a small Kerrison or Hajek forceps.

b. The nasoantral fenestration is enlarged in an anterior direction with Kerrison forceps and posteriorly with ring forceps.

The bony and membranous layers are removed simultaneously, exposing the inferior turbinate. There are a number of techniques for the construction of a flap from the medial wall of the antrum to be reflected laterally. These are somewhat difficult to fashion and have a tendency to resume their anatomic position, thus closing the fenestra.

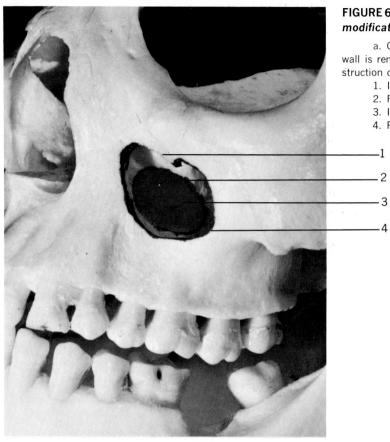

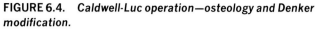

FIGURE 6.4. *Caldwell-Luc operation—osteology and Denker modification.*

a. Osteology of the Caldwell-Luc operation. Sufficient anterior wall is removed to facilitate removal of diseased tissue and construction of a nasomaxillary fenestra.

1. Infraorbital foramen
2. Rim of nasoantral window
3. Inferior turbinate
4. Rim of surgical defect of anterior wall of antrum

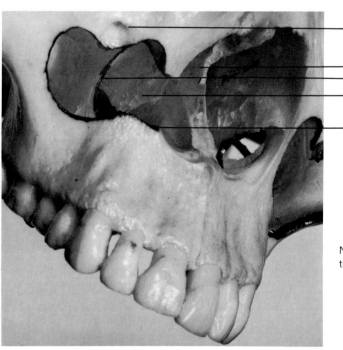

b. The Denker modification of the Caldwell-Luc operation. Note that a rim of bone remains intact below the infraorbital foramen to prevent fracture and injury to the nerve.

1. Infraorbital foramen
2. Nasal septum
3. Posterior rim of surgical defect of lateral nasal wall
4. Inferior turbinate
5. Inferior margin of surgical defect at junction of lateral wall and anterior wall of antrum

Oroantral Fistula

Diagnosis. The number of upper premolars and molars in intimate contact with the floor of the maxillary sinus is dependent upon the size of the sinus. The sinus may be separated from the roots of these teeth by a thin layer of bone, or there may be an absence of bone. On occasion the roots may extend into the maxillary sinus. An oroantral fistula may occur following the extraction of a non-diseased tooth. There are two predisposing factors to oroantral fistulas: the close proximity of premolar and molar roots to the sinus floor, and the presence of either an apical abscess or a maxillary sinusitis with poor drainage at the time of an upper molar or premolar extraction. An oroantral fistula may be secondary to a compound maxillary fracture, neoplasm of the antrum (especially after radiation therapy), or following a radical antrum operation.

The symptoms of an oroantral fistula, if of recent origin, are blood in the nasal cavity, and an escape of air from the fistulous tooth socket. Liquids taken into the mouth may escape through the nostril. If infection is present it usually is manifested within one or two days following the extraction of the tooth. Pain over the maxillary sinus and a profuse odoriferous nasal discharge are characteristic. The patient complains of foul taste. Purulent discharge can be seen exuding from the extraction site. This discharge may increase when the patient holds his nose and increases the intranasal pressure. The patient may have difficulty in developing a negative intraoral pressure such as when drinking through a straw.

The diagnosis is made from the history, signs and symptoms, x rays of the sinuses, and probing of the fistulous tract with a small-caliber lacrimal probe.

Indications for Surgical Procedure. The surgical procedure is determined by:

1. The size of the fistula
2. The presence or absence of adjacent teeth
3. Previous unsuccessful attempts for closure
4. Severity of the associated maxillary sinusitis
5. Epithelialization of the fistulous tract

On occasion an oromaxillary fistula may occur following the extraction of a non-diseased tooth. This usually heals rapidly after local repair, administration of antibiotics, and prohibiting the patient from nose-blowing. If a tooth root is broken off during extraction and found to lie within the antrum but submucosally, it is best left alone if there is no infection. If infection is present, antibiotic therapy plus local irrigation may result in resolution of the infection and healing. Otherwise a more radical procedure is necessary both to remove the foreign body and to close the oroantral fistula.

Repair of Fistula When Teeth Are Present. If the fistula is small and teeth are present it is closed by using a combination of gingival and palatal incisions adjacent to the teeth (Figs. 6.5a and 6.6). Antibiotic therapy is instituted several days before operation. The patient is prepared for operation as outlined for the Caldwell-Luc procedure. The incision is made near the gingival margin. The periosteum is elevated over the anterior wall of the maxillary sinus. The antrum is entered and a Caldwell-Luc operation is carried out, making certain that a large nasoantral window is fashioned. It is most important to obtain a culture so that sensitivity tests can be performed. All granulation tissue and diseased bone are curetted from both the sinus and oral orifices of the fistula. An incision is made on the palatal side of the alveolar ridge. A counter incision is made over the hard palate; this incision may extend beyond the junction of the hard and soft palate if necessary.

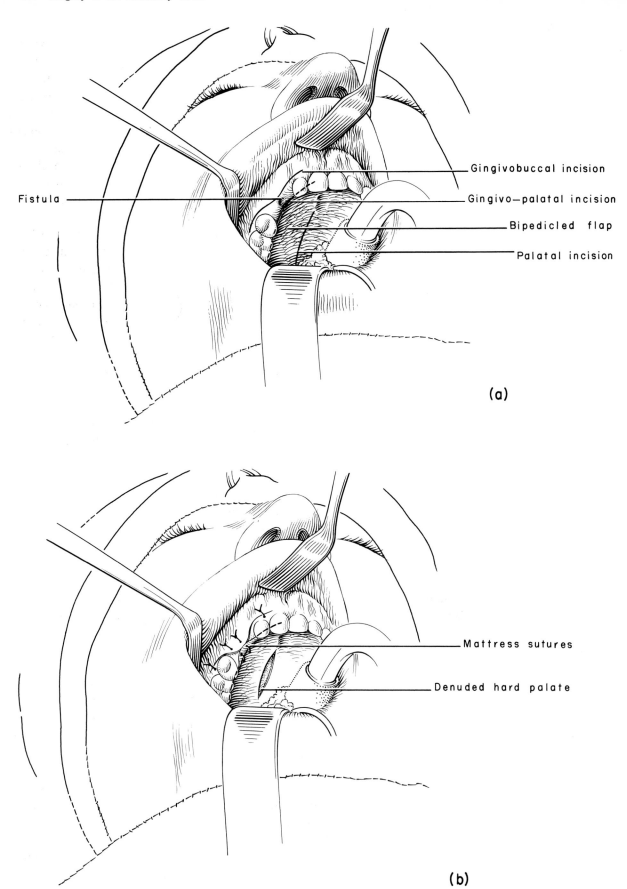

Fistula

Gingivobuccal incision

Gingivo—palatal incision

Bipedicled flap

Palatal incision

(a)

Mattress sutures

Denuded hard palate

(b)

FIGURE 6.5. *Repair of oroantral fistula when teeth are present.*

a. The gingivobuccal incision is made just above the gingival margin. The periosteum is elevated over the canine fossa and a Caldwell-Luc operation completed. A gingivo-palatal incision parallel to the above incision is made just medial to the gingival margin. A third incision begins behind the incisor teeth near the midline and extends posteriorly over the entire length of the hard palate. The mucosa between the latter two incisions is elevated from the hard palate, creating a bipedicled flap.

b. All diseased bone is removed from the bony fistulous tract. The two flaps are secured over this bony defect with mattress sutures. These flaps can be advanced into position by additional sutures if necessary. A defect over the hard palate is created as the bipedicled flap is advanced in the direction of the fistula.

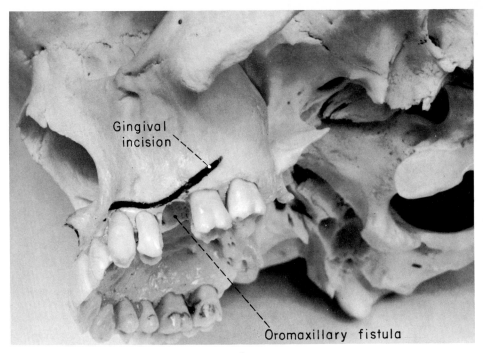

a

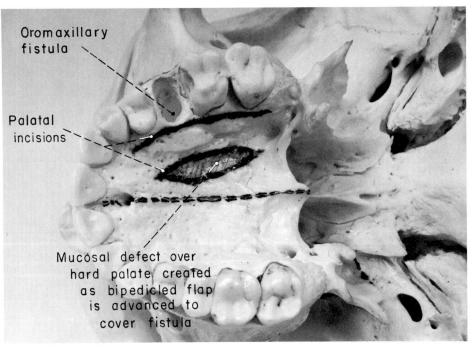

b

FIGURE 6.6. *Osteology of oroantral fistula repair when teeth are present.*

a. The gingivobuccal incision is extended to the margin of the fistula on the alveolar ridge.

b. The fistulous opening is viewed from below. The gingivo-palatal incision also extends to the margin of the fistula. The area of denuded palate that occurs as the bipedicled palatal flap is advanced and sutured to the gingivobuccal flap is indicated.

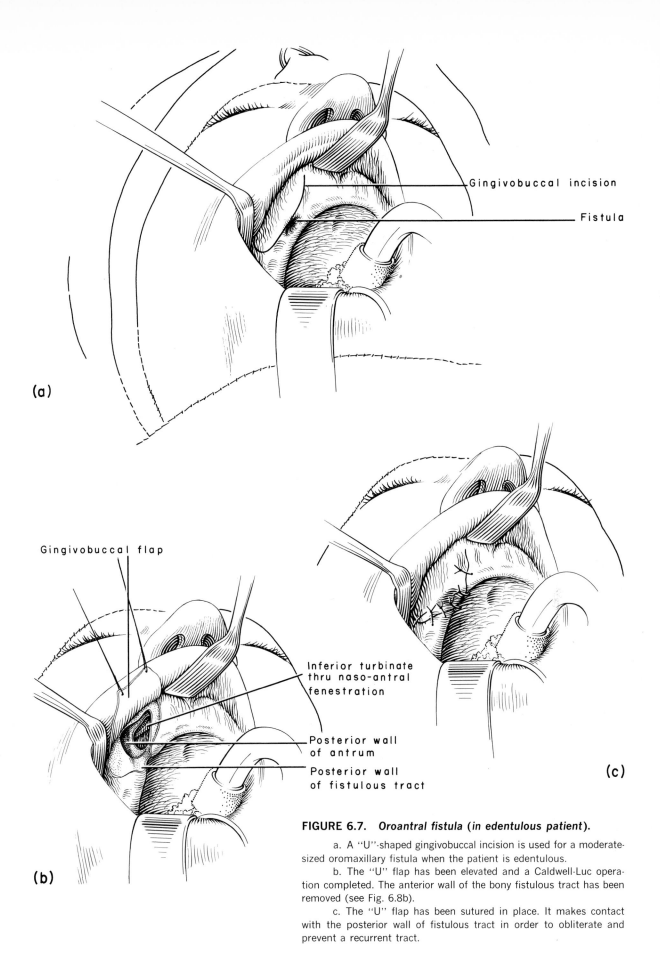

(a)

Gingivobuccal incision

Fistula

Gingivobuccal flap

Inferior turbinate
thru naso-antral
fenestration

Posterior wall
of antrum

Posterior wall
of fistulous tract

(b)

(c)

FIGURE 6.7. *Oroantral fistula (in edentulous patient).*

a. A "U"-shaped gingivobuccal incision is used for a moderate-sized oromaxillary fistula when the patient is edentulous.

b. The "U" flap has been elevated and a Caldwell-Luc operation completed. The anterior wall of the bony fistulous tract has been removed (see Fig. 6.8b).

c. The "U" flap has been sutured in place. It makes contact with the posterior wall of fistulous tract in order to obliterate and prevent a recurrent tract.

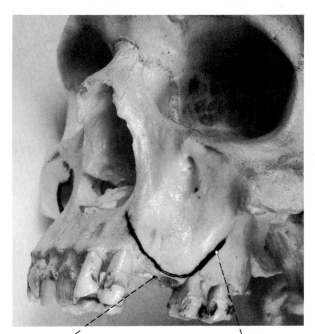

Oromaxillary
fistula

U-incision for
large oro-
maxillary
fistula

FIGURE 6.8. *Oroantral fistula (with teeth missing).*

a. The gingivobuccal flap is used for an oromaxillary fistula when the patient is edentulous or when several teeth are missing in the area of the fistula.

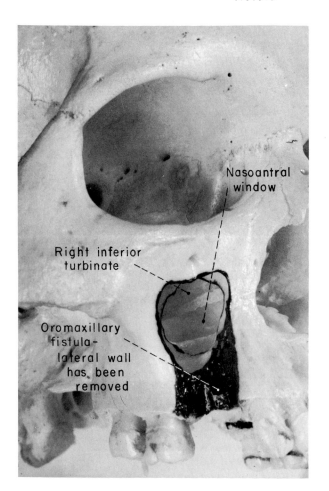

Nasoantral
window

Right inferior
turbinate

Oromaxillary
fistula-
lateral wall
has been
removed

b. The lateral wall of the fistula has been removed. The resulting defect is flattened so that when the "U" flap is replaced it makes contact with the entire surface of the bony trough.

A Caldwell-Luc operation has been completed. Note the lower margin of the inferior turbinate seen through the nasoantral fenestration.

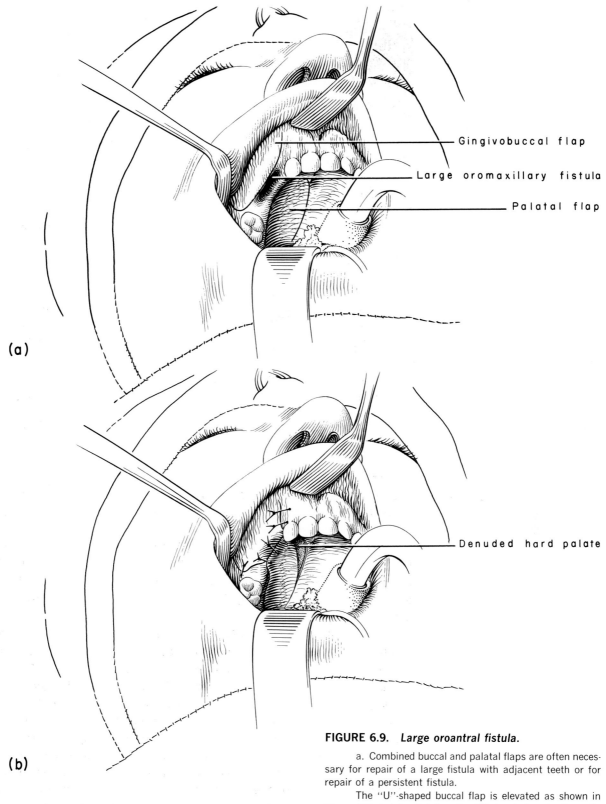

Gingivobuccal flap

Large oromaxillary fistula

Palatal flap

(a)

Denuded hard palate

(b)

FIGURE 6.9. *Large oroantral fistula.*

a. Combined buccal and palatal flaps are often necessary for repair of a large fistula with adjacent teeth or for repair of a persistent fistula.

The "U"-shaped buccal flap is elevated as shown in Figure 6.7 and the fistulous tract is treated as is shown in Figures 6.8b and 6.10.

b. The palatal flap, which is based posteriorly on the greater palatine vessels, is advanced towards the alveolar ridge where it is sutured to the buccal flap.

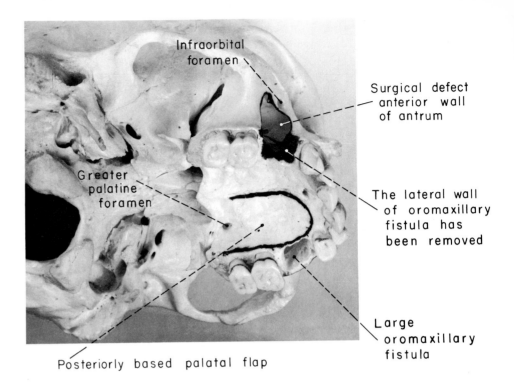

FIGURE 6.10. *Oroantral fistula (posteriorly based palatal flap).*

    The left greater palatine foramen is shown at the base of the posteriorly based palatal flap. A fistulous opening is shown on the left alveolar ridge. On the right side a similar fistula has been prepared by removing the lateral bony wall after a Caldwell-Luc operation has been completed.

The bipedicled flap thus created is elevated so that it may be advanced laterally in order to obtain tension-free approximation of the flaps. The flaps are securely sutured over the fistula with mattress sutures (Fig. 6.5b). The antrum is firmly packed with 1-inch Aureomycin-ointment impregnated iodoform gauze.

    Postoperatively the patient is maintained on antibiotics. The iodoform packing is removed on the fifth postoperative day by way of the nasoantral window. If the suture material used is #3-0 silk rather than chromic catgut it is removed on the tenth postoperative day. The patient is warned against nose-blowing until healing is complete.

    Procedure in Edentulous Patient. If the fistula is small or of moderate size, and there are no teeth present in the adjacent alveolar ridge, a gingivobuccal "U" flap is used to repair the defect (Figs. 6.7 and 6.8a). The "U" flap is elevated and a Caldwell-Luc operation is carried out. The lateral wall of the fistulous tract is completely removed from the alveolar ridge to the antrum. Adjacent bone is also removed laterally so that the "U" flap may be placed in contact with the entire surface of the trough thus created (Figs. 6.7b and 6.8b). The "U" flap is then secured in place with #3-0 chromic catgut or silk suture material (Fig. 6.7c).

    Procedure for Large or Persistent Oroantral Fistula. There are numerous surgical procedures for the correction of a persistent or large oroantral fistula. Probably the simplest and the most successful method is that of providing a posteriorly based palatal flap combined with a buccal flap (Fig. 6.9). It may be necessary to remove adjacent teeth if they are in close proximity to the fistula. In preparing the palatal flap it is important to be cognizant of the location of the greater palatal foramen and artery (Fig. 6.10). The location of the greater palatal foramen is approximately 0.5 cm medial to the last molar tooth. The lateral wall of the fistulous tract is removed in a manner similar to that previously described. A more extensive resection of the alveolar ridge may also be necessary. The palatal flap is then advanced laterally so that it may be sutured to the gingivobuccal flap without tension (Fig. 6.9b).

A connective tissue flap derived from the area above the gingivobuccal flap may be reflected inferiorly into a large oroantral fistula. This is sometimes necessary in conjunction with the palatal and buccal flap to close a very large oroantral fistula.

Vidian Nerve Section for Vasomotor Rhinitis

Indications. Patient has persistent discomfort from vasomotor rhinitis. The candidates complain of perennial bilateral nasal obstruction associated with constant or intermittent profuse watery discharge, which is aggravated by physical changes such as heat, cold, humidity, and chemical irritants including cigarette smoke, perfume, and strong odors. Emotional and endocrine changes are factors as well. Vasomotor rhinitis patients have negative or nonspecific responses to allergy skin tests, normal serum IgE levels, and should have no complicating bacterial infection. Surgical candidates are those who are unresponsive to intensive, conservative medical management.

On physical examination, these patients have engorged nasal mucosa which is pink to bluish in color obstructing most of the airway bilaterally and associated with watery secretions. In our experience vasomotor rhinitis is an uncommon disorder, occurring much less often than nasal allergy, but it is possible the two conditions occur simultaneously in a small minority of patients. In order to ensure good results, careful distinction must be made between the allergic patient and the vasomotor patient suffering primarily from the cholinergic effects of the parasympathetic fibers coursing the vidian nerve. The relationship of vasomotor rhinitis, nasal polypoid disease, and sinusitis is poorly understood.

Excision of the sphenopalatine ganglion may be indicated for atypical unilateral facial pain which is felt deep in the orbit, ethmoid, nose, cheek, and sometimes neck. This pain does not conform to the sensory distribution of any of the cranial nerves and does not have the paroxysmal characteristics of a true tic douloureux. The nose must be carefully examined for sharp septal spurs that may cause a similar pain syndrome that can be corrected by submucous resection of the spur-bearing portion of the septum. There should be no evidence of sinus or ophthalmologic disease.

Sphenopalatine ganglion neuralgia is often a tenuous diagnosis; however, one method of attempting to establish a relationship between the ganglion and the pain syndrome attributed to it is the injection of the ganglion with Xylocaine solution by way of the greater palatine foramen. The foramen is palpated as a shallow depression opposite the last molar tooth and just anterior to the posterior border of the hard palate. A $2\frac{1}{2}$-inch #22 hypodermic needle that is bent 90 degrees 2 cm from the point is inserted through the foramen for 2 cm into the pterygopalatine foramen up to the region of the sphenopalatine ganglion. After aspirating to ensure the needle tip is not within the lumen of a blood vessel, 1 cc of 2% Xylocaine solution without epinephrine is injected. Total relief of pain should occur within a few minutes and last from 3 to 4 hours. Temporary diplopia lasting 3 to 4 hours can

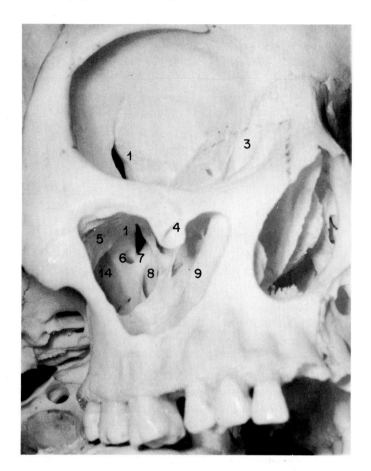

FIGURE 6.11. *Pterygomaxillary fossa.*

1. Superior orbital fissure
2. Optic foramen
3. Lacrimal fossa
4. Infraorbital foramen
5. Margin posterior wall of antrum
6. Foramen rotundum
7. Bony ridge between foramen rotundum and vidian canal
8. Vidian canal
9. Median wall of antrum
10. Nasoantral window
11. Fenestra into posterior ethmoid cell
12. Fenestra into sphenoid sinus
13. Sphenopalatine foramen
14. Pterygomaxillary fissure
15. Sphenoid sinuses
16. Attachment of middle turbinate (represented by a dotted line)
17. Hiatus semilunaris
18. Maxillary sinus
19. Inferior turbinate

a. A view of the pterygomaxillary fossa in relation to the orbit, maxillary sinus, and nasal cavity. In this specimen much of the anterior wall of the right maxillary sinus has been removed, preserving the infraorbital foramen. The posterior wall has also been removed, exposing the pterygomaxillary fossa. Note the close proximity of the foramen rotundum to the superior orbital fissure and the funnel-shaped vidian canal which is nearly in direct line with the medial wall of the antrum.

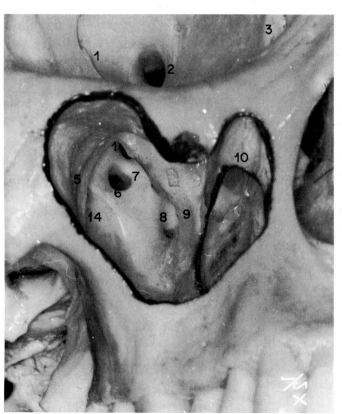

b. A closer view of the posterior wall of the pterygomaxillary fossa, to emphasize the close proximity of the foramen rotundum to the superior orbital fissure, the direction of the vidian canal from the foramen rotundum, the bony ridge between the foramen rotundum and the vidian canal, and the location of the vidian canal as related to the medial wall of the maxillary sinus.

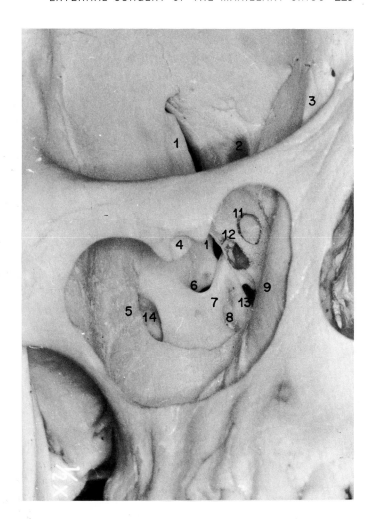

FIGURE 6.11. (Continued)

c. This specimen demonstrates the relationship among the vidian canal, sphenopalatine foramen, and medial wall of the antrum. A small fenestra has been fashioned into the posterior ethmoid and the sphenoid sinuses.

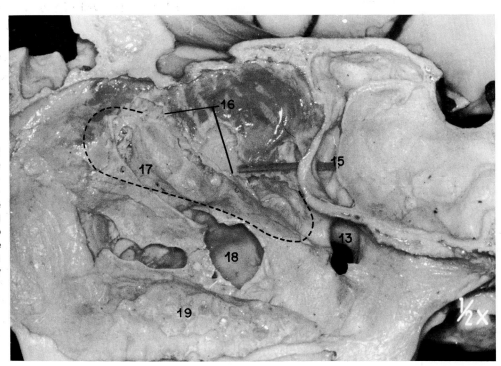

d. A close-up photograph of the right lateral nasal wall. The middle turbinate has been removed, exposing the hiatus semilunaris. The outline of the middle turbinate is indicated by a dotted line. Just behind the posterior tip of the middle turbinate is the sphenopalatine foramen and a view into the pterygomaxillary fossa.

also occur following this injection, and because of the possibility of permanent oculomotor nerve injury, alcohol injections in this region should never be used.

Anatomy of the Pterygomaxillary Fossa. The pterygomaxillary fossa is bound:
1. anteriorly, by the infratemporal surface of the maxilla (posterior wall of the maxillary sinus)
2. superiorly, by the undersurface of the sphenoid bone and the orbital process of the palatine bone
3. medially, by the perpendicular plate of the palatal bone
4. posteriorly, by the base of the pterygoid process and lower part of the anterior surface of the greater wing of the sphenoid bone (Fig. 6.11).

The pterygomaxillary fossa contains the third division of the internal maxillary artery, the accompanying veins, the vidian nerve, the sphenopalatine ganglion, and the second division of the trigeminal nerve. The spaces between these structures are filled with adipose tissue.

The openings into the pterygomaxillary fossa are as follows (Fig. 6.11):
1. The inferior orbital fissure is the communication between the pterygomaxillary fossa and the orbit.
2. The pterygomaxillary fissure is located laterally at the junction of the second and third division of the internal maxillary artery.
3. The sphenopalatine foramen is found close to the posterior tip of the middle turbinate. The sphenopalatine artery and nerves are distributed to the septum and the lateral wall of the nose through this foramen.
4. The foramen rotundum is readily identified in the posterior superior wall of the pterygomaxillary fossa. The second division of the trigeminal nerve enters the fossa by way of the foramen rotundum.
5. The vidian canal is a funnel-shaped opening on the posterior wall situated medial and slightly inferior to the foramen rotundum. A 7 to 10 mm wide vertical crest of bone separates the foramen rotundum from the vidian canal. The vidian canal is often difficult to view because of its close proximity to the medial wall of the antrum (lateral wall of the nasal cavity). The vidian nerve exits from this canal to join the overlying sphenopalatine ganglion.
6. The pharyngeal canal is an opening into the lateral aspect of the roof of the choanae. The pharyngeal branches of the sphenopalatine ganglion and the pharyngeal branches of the internal maxillary artery reach the nasopharynx by way of this canal.
7. The posterior palatine canal, found in the floor of the pterygomaxillary fossa, provides passage for the descending palatine nerves and the greater palatine artery.

Anatomy of the Vidian Nerve. The vidian nerve is made up of both sympathetic and parasympathetic fibers. The sympathetic innervation arises from the cervical ganglion of the carotid plexus. The parasympathetic innervation originates in the superior salivatory nucleus and accompanies the facial nerve to form the greater superficial petrosal nerve, which exits from the temporal bone through the hiatus facialis on the anterior surface of its petrous portion. Shortly thereafter the greater superficial petrosal nerve joins the sympathetic fibers from the carotid plexus to form the vidian nerve. The vidian nerve joins the overlying sphenopalatine ganglion shortly after its exit from the vidian canal. It proceeds to provide the parasympathetic and sympathetic nerve supply of the nasal cavities.

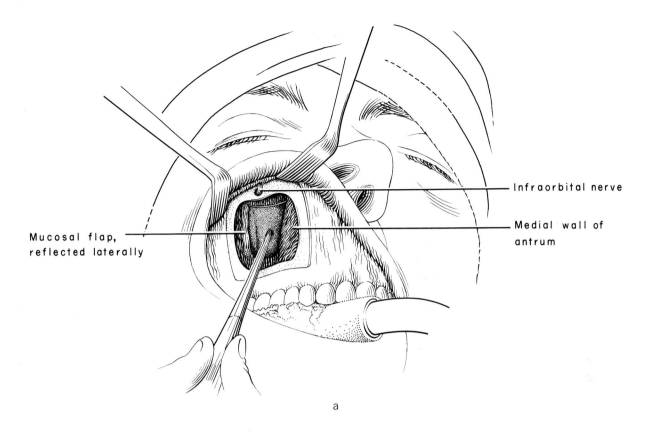

Mucosal flap,
reflected laterally

Infraorbital nerve

Medial wall of
antrum

a

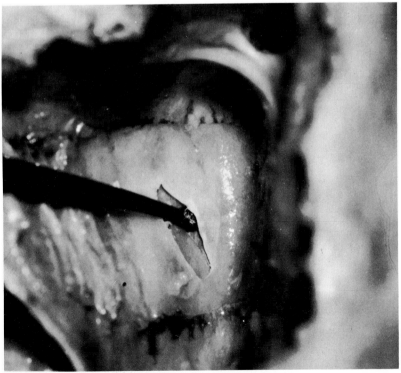

b

FIGURE 6.12. *Vidian nerve section.*

a. Most of the anterior wall of the right
maxillary sinus has been removed with preservation
of the infraorbital foramen and nerve. In this
dissection the mucosal flap of the posterior wall is
based and reflected laterally. A small opening is
made through the posterior wall of the maxillary
sinus with care being taken to preserve the underlying periosteum.

b. An opening through the posterior wall of
the maxillary sinus has been made with a sharp
curette. This is enlarged sufficiently to admit a Hajek
bone-cutting forceps. The entire posterior wall of
the sinus is removed with the Hajek forceps, care
being taken to preserve the underlying periosteum.

Technique of Vidian Nerve Section. The procedure may be performed with the patient under either general or local anesthesia. When local anesthesia is the choice, 2% Xylocaine with 1 : 100,000 epinephrine is injected into the gingivobuccal sulcus and around the infraorbital nerve. Following this injection, a curved needle is inserted 2 cm into the greater palatine foramen and 2 cc of the same local anesthetic agent previously used are slowly injected into the canal and pterygomaxillary fossa.

A Caldwell-Luc incision is employed. The periosteum is elevated from the anterior wall of the antrum in the region of the canine fossa. A curette, chisel, or rotating bur is used for entry into the antrum. As much of the anterior wall of the antrum is removed as is possible without damaging the infraorbital nerve (Fig. 6.12a). Removal can be accomplished with Kerrison forceps, but is best done with a rotating bur. A cocaine pack is placed in the antrum for a few minutes to further anesthetize the antral mucosa and decrease bleeding. A mucosal flap, based laterally or inferiorly, is elevated from the posterior wall of the antrum (Fig. 6.12a). A self-retaining retractor is applied to elevate the upper lip and periosteum.

The surgical microscope, with a 300 mm lens, should be used during the remaining dissection. The thin posterior wall is opened with a curette or small chisel (Fig. 6.12b). The underlying periosteum is easily separated and the posterior sinus wall can then be removed with Hajek or Citelli bone-cutting forceps. It is important to extend this bony dissection as far medially as is possible, for the vidian canal is often found directly posterior to the medial wall of the antrum.

Next the periosteum must be opened. Because there are many small blood vessels directly beneath the periosteum in the pterygomaxillary space, it is best to use electrocoagulation to make a cruciate incision. The four flaps that are formed are easily elevated to expose the underlying vessels and adipose tissue.

Pulsations of the internal maxillary artery can often be seen, giving the surgeon some indication as to the location of this artery. Adipose tissue is removed with dissectors, alligator and cup forceps, and suction tips, all especially designed for this purpose. Once the main artery is identified, it is elevated with an artery hook so that its branches may be more readily dissected free.

The sphenopalatine ganglion is often quite difficult to see because of the overlying internal maxillary artery. The artery may also interfere with the dissection in a medial and inferior direction to the vidian canal. In such cases it is ligated and sectioned medial to the origin of the infraorbital artery (Fig. 6.13). Once the sectioned artery is reflected medially, the rounded vertical bony ridge which separates the foramen rotundum from the vidian canal can be identified. The rather large, funnel-shaped vidian canal is found medial and slightly inferior to the foramen rotundum, nearly in a direct line with the medial wall of the antrum (Fig. 6.14b).

The sphenopalatine ganglion is held forward with a right-angle hook, and the emerging vidian nerve is seen. The vidian nerve is sectioned with a small sickle knife or a small curette. If the ganglion is to be removed, it is grasped in forceps and cut free with the nerve. A frozen section will confirm the presence of ganglion cells. Bone wax, Oxygauze, or bone chips can be packed into the vidian foramen; however, cautery deep in the vidian canal should be avoided. The posterior antral wall mucosal flap is placed over the pterygomaxillary fossa and covered with a layer of Gelfoam. A nasal antral window is made and the Caldwell-Luc operation is completed.

Postoperative Care. The postoperative care is similar to that after a Cald-

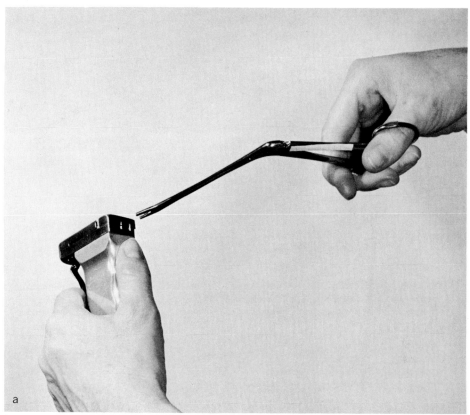

FIGURE 6.13. *Clip dispenser and self-locking clip.*

a. The clip dispenser is used to insert the self-locking clip into forceps especially designed for its application. The two jaws of the clip are inserted into their respective spots in the apparatus; as the knob is depressed, a clip is inserted into the forceps.

b. The upper loop is passed over and beyond the "artery."

c. As the forceps is compressed, the lower end of the clip bends so that it is extended into the loop.

d. As the clip is further compressed, it becomes locked and resembles a miniature safety-pin.

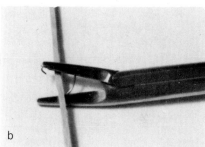

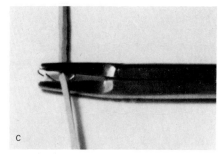

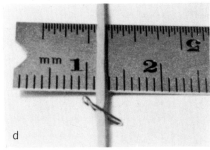

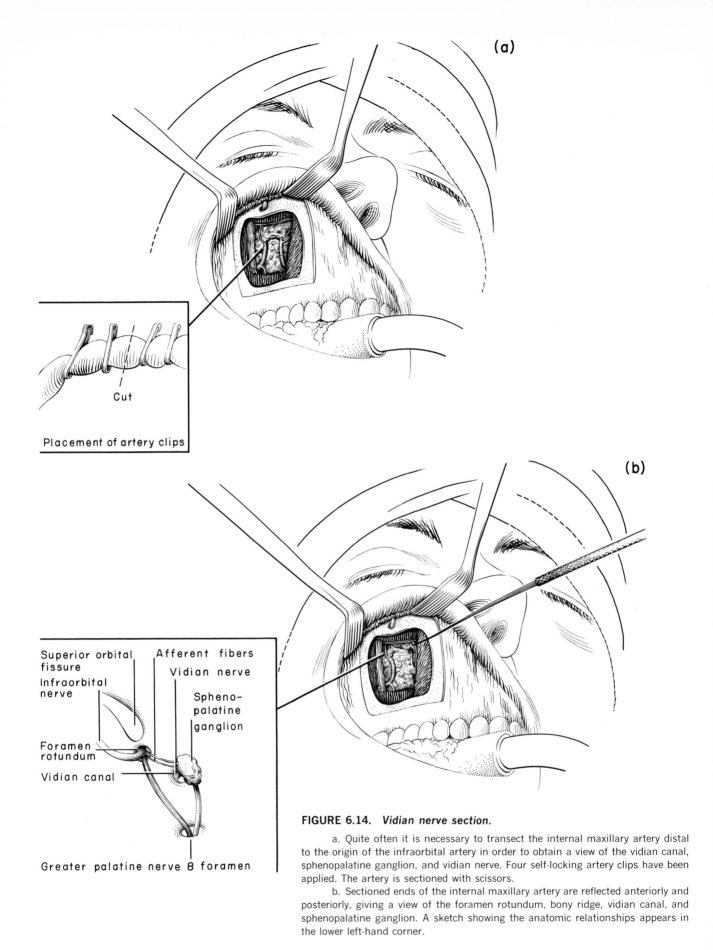

(a)

Cut

Placement of artery clips

(b)

Superior orbital
fissure

Afferent fibers

Infraorbital
nerve

Vidian nerve

Spheno-
palatine
ganglion

Foramen
rotundum

Vidian canal

Greater palatine nerve 8 foramen

FIGURE 6.14. *Vidian nerve section.*

    a. Quite often it is necessary to transect the internal maxillary artery distal to the origin of the infraorbital artery in order to obtain a view of the vidian canal, sphenopalatine ganglion, and vidian nerve. Four self-locking artery clips have been applied. The artery is sectioned with scissors.

    b. Sectioned ends of the internal maxillary artery are reflected anteriorly and posteriorly, giving a view of the foramen rotundum, bony ridge, vidian canal, and sphenopalatine ganglion. A sketch showing the anatomic relationships appears in the lower left-hand corner.

well-Luc procedure or ligation of the internal maxillary artery. Following the section of a vidian nerve, absence of lacrimation may give temporary discomfort. This is alleviated by methyl cellulose eye drops.

It should be noted that Gergely (1935) states that in one-third of the cases of vasomotor rhinitis unilateral sectioning of the vidian nerve shows bilateral improvement. This usually becomes apparent approximately 2 weeks after the operation, and thus a contralateral operation should be delayed for at least 1 month.

PARTIAL MAXILLECTOMY

During the past decade I have performed a gradually decreasing number of total maxillectomies along with an increasing number of subtotal maxillectomies combined with postoperative radiation therapy. At the present time my only indication for a total maxillectomy is extensive disease of the maxillary sinus with involvement of the alveolar ridge, palatal bone, or pterygoid region. A subtotal maxillectomy, performed by way of a lateral rhinotomy incision and/or an extended gingivobuccal incision, allows the surgeon to encompass the disease as well as a total maxillectomy in most cases. This, followed by a full course of postoperative radiation therapy, offers our patients an equal chance for cure as compared to those patients subjected to a total maxillectomy.

There are a number of reasons for a change from total maxillectomy to subtotal maxillectomy:

1. Our techniques for a partial maxillectomy have improved.
2. Preoperatively, the sites of extension of the disease can be accurately assessed by improved radiographic studies such as polytomography and CT body scanning.
3. As a result of these improved diagnostic procedures, the surgeon can plan his operation so as to encompass only the diseased segment and its surrounding tissue rather than a large block of tissue which is not diseased. Potential sites for recurrent disease can be accurately designated and reported so that the radiotherapist can concentrate on and include these in his field of radiation therapy.
4. In most cases, the disease can be encompassed as well by the subtotal maxillectomy as compared to the total maxillectomy.
5. During recent years, techniques for radiotherapy have improved sufficiently so that the sites for potential recurrence may be treated with a full course of radiation therapy without injury to surrounding structures.
6. The subtotal maxillectomy results in excellent cosmesis as compared to the unsightly appearance and facial asymmetry that results from a total maxillectomy.

The obvious disadvantage for this conservative therapy is the difficulty in observing the cavity for recurrent disease and the problem of keeping the cavity free from crusting. These problems have been overcome with the use of straight and angulated fiberoptic scopes for visualization of the cavity along with periodic polytomography. The crusting can be controlled by a lubricating spray such as Spray B (200 mg camphor, 200 mg menthol, 0.2 ml eucalyptol, petrolatum liquid q.s. ad 100 ml). Crusting is also controlled by irrigating the cavity with warm saline solution (1 tsp salt/glass warm water) or Alkalol solution to which has been added an equal part of hot tap water. The patient thus irrigates with warm, half-strength Alkalol solution.

Nasal irrigations are accomplished by inserting the end of an ulcer or baby enema syringe into the nostril while the patient leans forward, face down over a sink with the mouth open.

Irrigations are usually commenced 10 days to 2 weeks following surgery when the patient is completely healed. They are continued two or three times a day until crusting becomes minimal. After this, irrigations are carried out several times a week as indicated.

Crusting in a subtotal or total maxillectomy can lead to serious consequences. The accumulation of crusts is a formal invitation for bacterial growth, which, in turn, produces an offensive odor, loss of underlying mucous membrane, and localized osteomyelitis. We have seen a case of metastatic osteomyelitis of the cervical spine resulting from untreated subtotal maxillectomy cavity crusting. Thus, when a patient appears with a much crusted cavity, a culture is taken, the patient is placed on high dose antibiotic therapy (erythromycin), and irrigations are carried out with sufficient frequency so as to eliminate crusting.

On occasion, a small fistula will develop weeks or months after the completion of radiation therapy in the upper end of the lateral rhinotomy incision. This complication occurs frequently enough in my series of patients so that it is referred to as the circular bandaid syndrome.

For some reason, this complication is of little concern to the patient, which is indeed fortunate, for our attempts to close this small defect in radiated tissue have been completely unsuccessful.

TOTAL MAXILLECTOMY

Maxillectomy is the treatment of choice for a carcinoma confined to the antrum. Unfortunately, these cases are few and far between, for carcinoma in the maxillary sinus usually extends beyond the confines of the sinus to produce signs and symptoms which bring the disease to the attention of the patient.

As a general rule, inferiorly located carcinoma of the maxillary sinus has the best chance for cure. If the lesion has broken through the anterior wall of the sinus, everything under the cutaneous cheek must be removed, and, on occasion, the skin of the cheek must be included with the resected specimen. If the carcinoma has broken through the roof of the antrum, the orbital contents must be resected with the maxilla. If the tumor invades the anterior ethmoid cells, the nasal septum and entire ethmoid labyrinth, including the roof of the labyrinth and the cribriform plate, must be removed. Tumors which extend through the posterior wall of the antrum into the posterior ethmoid cells, sphenoid sinus, or apex of the orbit have a poor prognosis even with preoperative or postoperative radiation therapy. If the carcinoma extends into the frontal sinus, the frontal bone in this area should be resected.

If the disease extends beyond the confines of the antrum and the site of extension can be accurately outlined, preoperative radiation therapy should be instituted. The advantage here is that a larger dose of radiation can be given with less chance of tumor spread by the surgical procedure, and there will be fewer postoperative complications. Postoperative radiation therapy is given when the site of extension is discovered at the time of the operation. In such cases, a radiotherapist can administer the radiation more accurately than would have been possible prior to the operation, but the amount must be limited because of almost certain injury and breakdown of surrounding normal tissues.

Is a maxillectomy ever done when there is no chance for cure? Yes, it is undertaken to remove diseased tissue and the products of palliative radiation therapy when such complications as bone sequestration, severe odor, uncontrollable pain, and trismus result from this therapy.

Preoperative Management. Permission for removal of the orbit must be obtained preoperatively in all cases, for an unsuspected extension of disease is not uncommon. The surgeon may choose to begin antibiotic therapy before the operation, especially if the carcinoma is accompanied by secondary infection. Anteroposterior and lateral planograms of the maxillary sinus are often most helpful in determining the extent of the disease. It is preferable to obtain upper and lower dental impressions before the maxillectomy rather than during the immediate postoperative period. If this is not possible, the impression can be taken either immediately after the operation or following removal of the packing. The patient's blood is cross-matched with at least 1500 cc of whole blood, which should be in readiness at the time of the operation. In the past, ligation of one or both external carotid arteries has been a prelude to maxillectomy. For the most part, this has been abandoned, and hemorrhage is controlled and blood replaced as the problem is encountered.

Since the incidence of carcinoma of the maxillary sinus is high among persons of the older age group, a careful preoperative evaluation of the patient's general health is essential.

Anesthesia. Hypotensive anesthesia facilitates this extensive and bloody surgical procedure; however, only about 50% of patients with carcinoma of the maxillary sinus can fulfill the necessary qualifications for hypotensive anesthesia, which requires that the systolic blood pressure be maintained at 60 mm and even slightly lower if the patient is young and healthy. A cuffed endotracheal tube should be inserted through the nasal cavity opposite to the side being operated upon. Pharyngeal packing is inserted to prevent blood from entering the esophagus or trachea. The anesthetic agent of choice is one which allows the surgeon to use cautery and epinephrine solution simultaneously.

Maxillectomy with Orbital Exenteration

The patient is placed on the operating table in the supine position. His head is elevated above the level of the thorax in order to reduce the venous pressure. Maxillectomy is a difficult, bloody, and high-risk operation. Heavy equipment is necessary.

The anatomic parts to be removed are: the orbital contents, the floor and medial wall of the orbit, the malar bone, a portion of the zygomatic arch, the antrum, the ethmoid sinuses, the anterior wall of the sphenoid sinus, the pterygoid plate, the hard palate, and the nasal septum if the ethmoid or nasal cavity is involved with the tumor (Figs. 6.15a and b).

Incisions. The eyelids are sewed together with #5-0 silk or polyethylene suture material. The incision begins over the lateral aspect of the nasal dorsum, just above the level of the inner canthus. It is made directly to the bone (Fig. 6.16a). It is extended down over the nasal bone midway between the lateral nasal crease

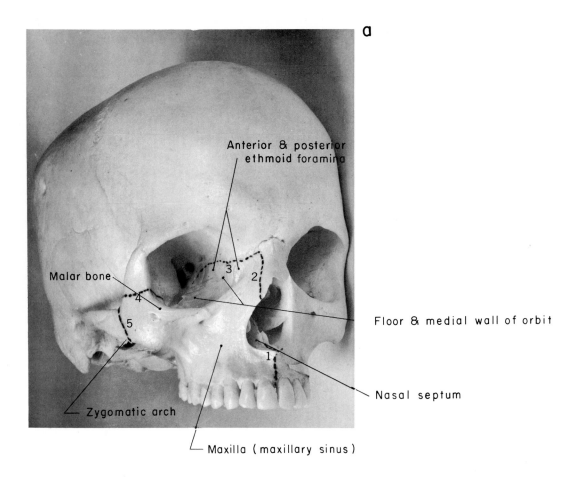

a

Anterior & posterior
ethmoid foramina

Malar bone

3

2

4

Floor & medial wall of orbit

5

1

Nasal septum

Zygomatic arch

Maxilla (maxillary sinus)

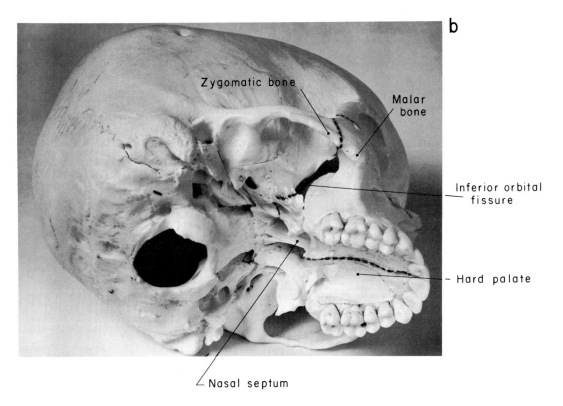

b

Zygomatic bone

Malar
bone

Inferior orbital
fissure

Hard palate

Nasal septum

and the dorsum of the nose, around the ala and the nasal labial crease, to the midline under the columella. Cross hatching of the incision is carried out in order to ensure a more accurate closure. A vertical midline incision is used to split the upper lip. The upper lip is compressed with a finger and thumb on each side while the lip-splitting incision is made. As pressure is released the superior labial and lateral nasal branches of the external maxillary artery are easily identified and ligated.

The incisions above and below the eyelid margin are made approximately 2 mm away from the tarsal plates. They rejoin lateral to the external canthus and extend laterally an additional 2 cm. Some surgeons advocate preservation of the lids so that a prosthesis may be worn. The cosmesis attending this operation is not entirely satisfactory and preservation of the lids is often not advisable, because the orbital defect is needed for long-term inspection and the detection of recurrent disease.

An incision is made along the entire length of the gingivobuccal sulcus and posteriorly around the maxillary tuberosity (Fig. 6.16b). If teeth are present, the median incisor on the side of the maxillectomy is removed.

Either of two methods is used to approach the hard palate. If the lesion extends to, or involves, the hard palate, then the mucous membrane over the hard palate must be removed with the specimen. In such cases a midline incision is made from the anterior midline alveolar ridge to the junction of the hard and soft palates. An incision is then made along the posterior rim of the hard palate. This connects with the gingivobuccal incision which has been extended around the maxillary tuberosity.

If the hard palate is not involved, the mucosal incision is made along the palatal side of the alveolar ridge parallel to the gingivobuccal incision (Fig. 6.16b). This connects with the gingivobuccal incision around the posterior aspect of the maxillary tuberosity. A mucous membrane flap is elevated, exposing the hard palate on the side upon which the maxillectomy is being performed (Fig. 6.16c).

Elevation of the Facial Flap. The nasal cavity is entered interiorly after the upper lip has been reflected laterally (Fig. 6.17a). An electrocautery knife is useful here. This incision is extended laterally and then superiorly in the pyriform aperture to a point on the inferior margin of the nasal skeleton at the junction between the nasal bone and the ascending process of the maxilla (Fig. 6.17b). The periosteum is elevated over the nasal bone and ascending process of the maxilla to the level of the nasal process of the frontal bone, while the nose is retracted to the opposite side.

FIGURE 6.15. *Maxillectomy—anatomic parts to be removed and bone incisions.*

a. The parts to be removed are: (1) floor of orbit; (2) malar bone; (3) zygomatic arch (medial aspect); (4) ethmoid sinuses and anterior wall of sphenoid; (5) lateral wall of nose with the turbinates; (6) hard palate; (7) entire maxillary sinus; and (8) pterygoid plates.

Bone incisions from left to right: (1) anterior alveolar ridge and premaxilla, just to the right of the nasal septum; (2) between the nasal bone and ascending process of the maxilla to the level of the nasal process of the frontal bone; (3) along the superior aspect of the medial orbital wall, just inferior to the ethmoid foramina and the suture line between the orbital plate of the frontal bone and the lamina papyracea; (4) across the malar bone, connecting with the lateral aspect of the inferior orbital fissure; (5) transecting the zygomatic arch, medially.

b. The parts to be removed are: (1) malar bone; (2) maxillary sinus; (3) right alveolar ridge; (4) hard palate; (5) nasal septum (if disease is present in the nasal cavity); and (6) pterygoid plates.

Bone incisions: (1) malar bone; (2) zygomatic arch; (3) across the base of the pterygoid process (this incision may be made between the posterior wall of the maxilla and the pterygoid plates if the former remains intact and free of tumor invasion); and (4) the hard palate, split in the midline.

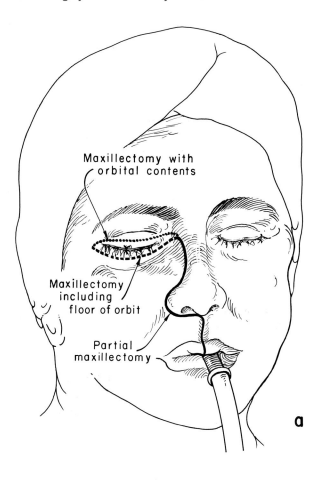

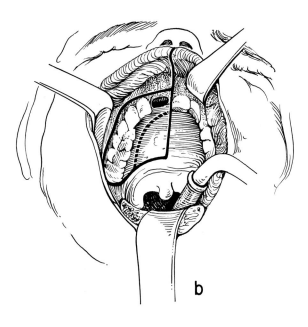

FIGURE 6.16.   *Maxillectomy—incisions.*

Incisions: ———— indicates partial maxillectomy; ——————— indicates maxillectomy including floor of orbit; ·········· indicates maxillectomy with orbital contents.

a. The incision begins at a point midway between the inner canthus and the nasal dorsum. It extends inferiorly, anterior to the nasofacial crease, until the alar sulcus is reached. It follows the alar sulcus and continues on just below the nasal orifice to the midline. The upper lip is split in the midline.

If the floor of the orbit is to be included, the incision must be extended laterally within 4 mm of the tarsal plate inferiorly.

An incision just above the tarsal plate in the upper lid is added if the orbital contents are to be included in the resection. The horizontal incisions above and below the lids are connected just lateral to the external canthus and extended lateralward about a centimeter.

b. The buccal side of the upper lip is split vertically in the midline. The mucosal incision is continued across the space previously occupied by the right median incisor. The mucous membrane over the hard palate is incised in the midline.

At the junction of the soft and hard palate the incision is directed laterally toward the posterior margin of the alveolar ridge.

The mucous membrane in the gingivobuccal sulcus is incised along the entire length of the alveolar ridge and connected to the palatal incision.

The interrupted line indicates an alternate incision which is used when preserving the mucous membrane over the hard palate. This incision can be made along the alveolar ridge rather than in the gingivo-palatal sulcus.

c. The mucous membrane is being elevated away from the hard palate. It is unwise to preserve this tissue when the floor of the antrum is invaded by tumor.

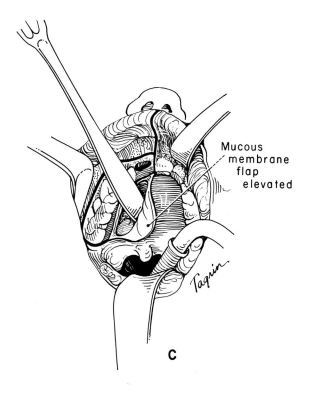

Mucous membrane flap elevated

Elevation of the facial flap is continued in a subcutaneous plane. The skin of the lids is elevated superficial to the orbicularis oculi muscle. (On the other hand, if the tumor does not extend to this region, the orbicularis oculi muscle may be preserved with the facial flap to give a better cosmetic result.) The buccinator muscle is preserved with the facial flap. All other facial muscles attached to the anterior wall of the antrum must be transected. The buccinator can be followed easily, for its fibers are continuous with those of the orbicularis oris muscle and run in a posterior direction. That portion of the buccinator muscle which attaches to the maxilla is transected. Elevation of the flap is continued posteriorly to the anterior aspect of the zygomatic arch and to the lateral aspect of the malar bone.

Orbit. As has been mentioned, the skin of the upper lid is usually elevated to include the orbicularis oculi muscle unless there is extension of disease into the orbit. The superior orbital rim is identified. The periosteum is incised along the superior orbital rim and also on the medial and lateral orbital rims, to the level of the inner and external canthi (Fig. 6.18). Elevation of the periosteum is begun superiorly, and the contents of the orbit are dissected inferiorly (Fig. 6.18b). The optic nerve and vessels are transected with curved scissors. Troublesome bleeding can be controlled with packing left in place for a short time.

Malar Bone. The inferior orbital fissure is identified. A long, curved hemostat is inserted under the malar bone and up and out through the inferior orbital fissure (Fig. 6.19a). This hemostat is used to grasp one end of a Gigli saw, which is pulled through and used to transect the malar bone (Fig. 6.19b). The malar bone can also be incised with a Stryker saw (Fig. 6.19c). On occasion it may be necessary to remove the superior and lateral bony walls of the orbit, thus exposing the dura.

Zygomatic Arch. After detaching the anterior attachment of the masseter muscle, the zygomatic arch is transected (Fig. 6.20a and b) with either a Gigli or a Stryker saw (Fig. 6.20c).

Hard Palate. The simplest way to transect the hard palate is with a 2-cm osteotome (Fig. 6.21a). The transection may be accomplished by inserting a Gigli saw into the nasal cavity and out at the junction of the hard and soft palates. The saw is grasped by a curved hemostat inserted through the incision at the junction of the hard and soft palates (Fig. 6.21b). When sawing, it is necessary to pull slightly toward the opposite side so that the saw will approximate the midline (Fig. 6.21c). Troublesome bleeding may occur from the greater palatine artery, but this can be controlled by packing or by inserting a cautery tip into the greater palatine foramen. In order to decrease the amount of bleeding, the electrocautery knife can be employed on the buccal and nasal sides of the hard palate prior to using the osteotome or Gigli saw.

Ethmoid. The upper nasal cavity is entered by one of two methods. A 1-cm osteotome is placed between the nasal bone and the ascending process of the maxilla. The osteotome is inserted to the level of the nasal process of the frontal bone (Fig. 6.22a). This is approximately at the level of the inner canthus, cribriform plate, roof of the ethmoid labyrinth, anterior and posterior ethmoid arteries, and the suture line between the orbital process of the frontal bone and the lamina papyracea. The exposure also can be accomplished by removing the ascending process of the maxilla with a rongeur (Fig. 6.22b).

The periosteum is elevated laterally, exposing the lacrimal sac and lamina papyracea. The anterior and posterior ethmoid arteries are identified and cauterized. The anterior and posterior ethmoid foramina accurately identify the level of

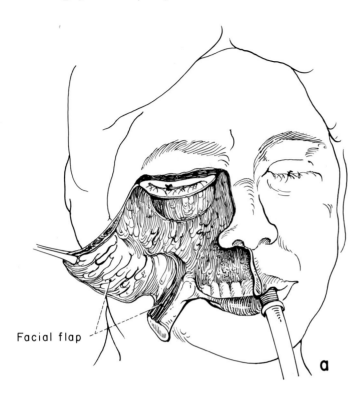

Facial flap

FIGURE 6.17. *Maxillectomy—elevation of the facial flap.*

a. The eyelids are sutured and the facial flap is dissected laterally exposing the masseter muscle, zygomatic arch, and malar bone.

b. The nasal cavity is entered laterally. This incision is carried superiorly to the junction of the nasal bone and the ascending process of the maxilla.

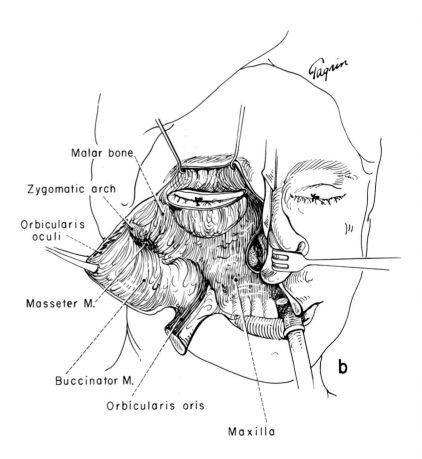

Malar bone

Zygomatic arch

Orbicularis oculi

Masseter M.

Buccinator M.

Orbicularis oris

Maxilla

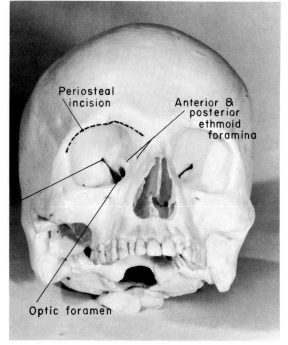

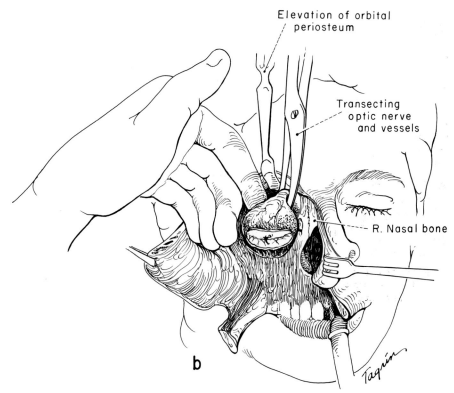

FIGURE 6.18. *Maxillectomy—the orbit.*

a. The upper lid is dissected and retracted superiorly. The periosteum over the supraorbital rim is incised, as indicated.

b. The periosteum is elevated from the superior, medial, and lateral walls of the orbit. As the orbital contents are retracted inferiorly with the index finger, a pair of long, curved scissors is inserted, cutting the optic nerve and vessels. The superior orbit is packed tightly with a moist gauze strip to control the bleeding.

FIGURE 6.19. *Maxillectomy—the malar bone.*

a. The orbital contents are retracted medially, exposing the lateral aspect of the inferior orbital fissure. A curved hemostat is inserted under the malar bone and out the inferior orbital fissure in order to grasp one end of a Gigli saw.

b. The malar bone is transected as far superiorly as is possible with the Gigli saw.

c. A tangential Stryker saw with a sinus blade can be used for this bone incision.

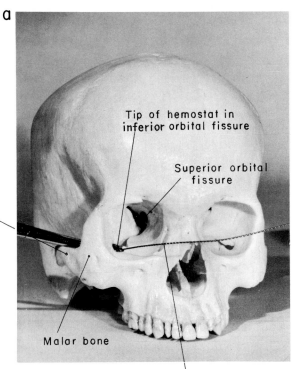

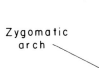

a

Tip of hemostat in inferior orbital fissure

Superior orbital fissure

Zygomatic arch

Malar bone

Gigli saw

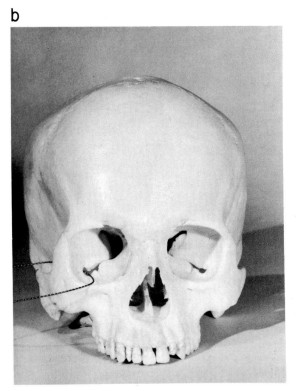

b

Gigli saw extending from infratemporal fossa – through inferior orbital fissure and around malar bone

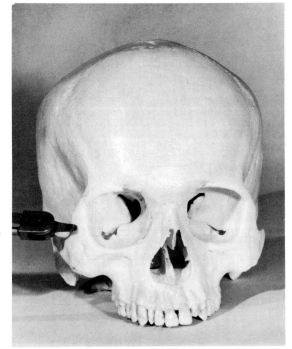

c

Stryker saw in readiness to transect the malar bone

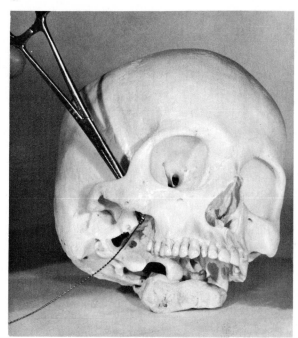

a

Hemostat inserted
behind zygomatic
process of
malar bone

Tip of hemostat grasping
Gigli saw

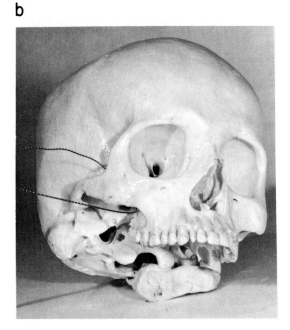

b

Gigli saw in position to
transect the zygomatic
process of the
malar bone

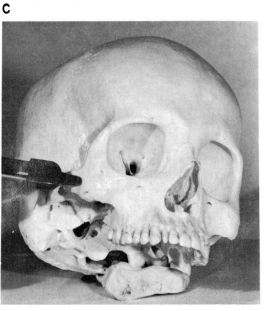

c

Stryker saw used
to transect
zygomatic
process of
malar
bone

FIGURE 6.20. *Maxillectomy—
zygomatic arch.*

a. A curved hemostat is inserted
under the zygomatic arch to grasp one end
of a Gigli saw.

b. The zygomatic arch is transected
just lateral to the malar eminence.

c. A tangential saw can be used to
section the zygomatic arch.

FIGURE 6.21. *Maxillectomy—sectioning the hard palate.*

a. The simplest method of sectioning the hard palate is with the use of a wide osteotome. The blade is placed in the midline on the alveolar ridge and just to the right (maxillectomy side) of the nasal septum in the nasal cavity.

b. The Gigli saw can be used to section the hard palate. A hemostat is inserted into the right nasal cavity for grasping one end of the Gigli saw which has been inserted in the midline at the posterior margin of the hard palate.

c. As the hard palate is being sectioned, the Gigli saw is pulled slightly to the left (opposite maxillectomy side).

An osteotome used to split the hard palate

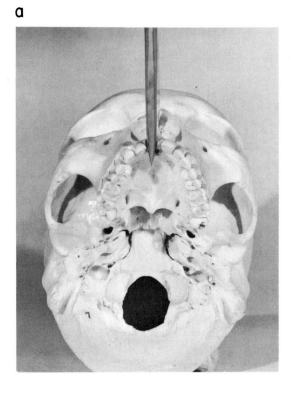

a

Hemostat in right nasal cavity grasping tip of Gigli saw which has been inserted through incision at junction of hard and soft palate

b

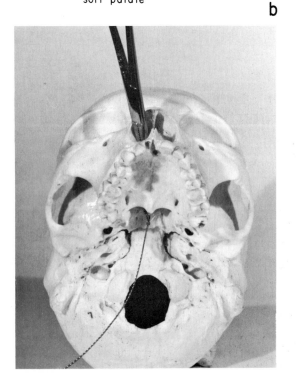

Gigli saw in position to transect the hard palate

c

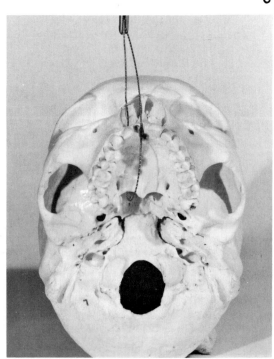

a

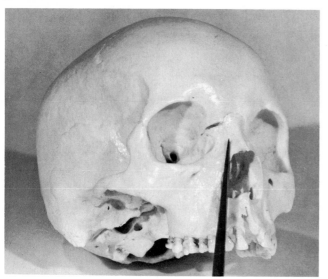

Chisel used to separate
nasal bone from the ascending
process of the maxilla

b

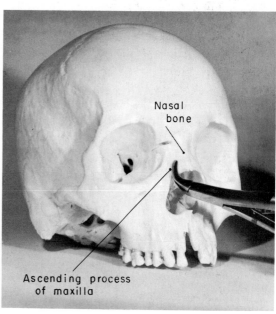

Nasal
bone

Ascending process
of maxilla

FIGURE 6.22. *Maxillectomy—nasal bone.*

a. The nasal bone is separated from the ascending process of the maxilla by inserting an osteotome between the two. The osteotome is introduced to the level of the nasal process of the frontal bone.

b. This dissection can also be accomplished by removing a portion of the ascending process of the maxilla adjacent to the nasal bone with a rongeur.

the cribriform plate and roof of the ethmoid sinuses. An osteotome is used to transect the specimen just below the roof of the ethmoid sinuses (Fig. 6.23a). This osteotome is extended posteriorly to the depth of the posterior ethmoid artery (Fig. 6.23b). If the disease involves the ethmoid sinuses, their bony roof and cribriform plate should be removed, thus exposing the dura. In such cases, cerebrospinal fluid leakage usually occurs. Repair is made with a split-thickness skin graft or a mucosal flap from the septum (p. 208). When the ethmoid sinuses are grossly involved, it is also advisable to resect the nasal septum.

Posterior Dissection (Fig. 6.24). The masseter muscle is detached from the maxilla. There are two methods to handle the posterior dissection. If the posterior wall of the antrum remains intact, an osteotome is inserted between the maxilla and the pterygoid process (Fig. 6.24a). Most often it is impossible to determine whether or not the posterior wall of the antrum is involved with the tumor and thus an alternate method must be used. The pterygoid muscles are detached from the medial and lateral pterygoid plates. A large curved osteotome is placed behind the pterygoid plates, and the pterygoid process is transected near its origin from the remainder of the sphenoid bone (Fig. 6.24b). Brisk bleeding from the internal maxillary artery may be encountered in this area.

Specimen Removal (Fig. 6.25a and b). After the pterygoid processes have been freed the specimen is attached only by the posterior and medial aspect of the bony orbit and the pterygomaxillary fossa. A heavy pair of scissors is placed

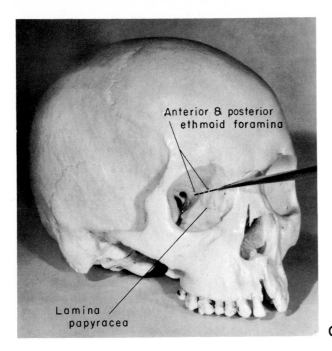

Anterior & posterior
ethmoid foramina

An osteotome transecting the
ethmoid labyrinth just below
the ethmoid foramina

Lamina
papyracea

a

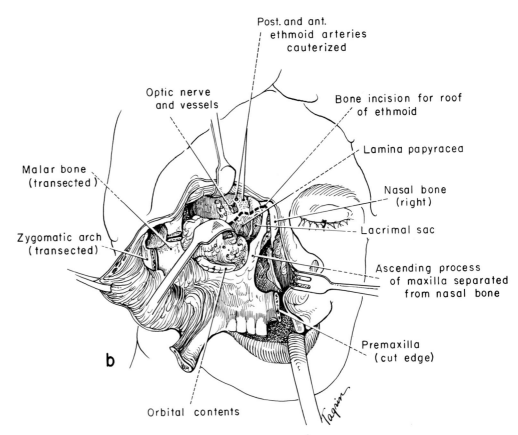

Post. and ant.
ethmoid arteries
cauterized

Optic nerve
and vessels

Bone incision for roof
of ethmoid

Lamina papyracea

Malar bone
(transected)

Nasal bone
(right)

Zygomatic arch
(transected)

Lacrimal sac

Ascending process
of maxilla separated
from nasal bone

Premaxilla
(cut edge)

b

Orbital contents

FIGURE 6.23. *Maxillectomy—roof of ethmoid sinus.*

The medial wall of the orbit is exposed by retracting the orbital contents downward and laterally. The anterior and posterior ethmoid arteries are cauterized and sectioned. An osteotome is placed just below the suture line between the orbital process of the frontal bone and the lamina papyracea, using the ethmoid foramina as guides.

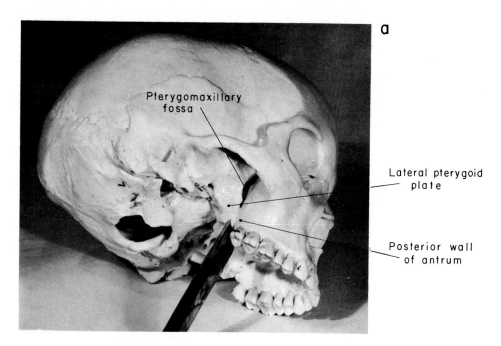

Osteotome placed between
the maxilla and the
pterygoid plates

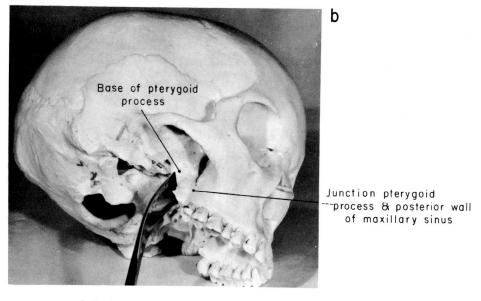

Osteotome transecting the
pterygoid processes at
their base

FIGURE 6.24. *Maxillectomy—pterygoid process.*

a. If it can be determined preoperatively that the posterior wall of the antrum is intact, the dissection is accomplished between the pterygoid plates and the maxilla.

b. Usually it is necessary to remove the pterygoid plates with the specimen. The external and internal pterygoid muscles are sectioned at their origin. A curved osteotome is inserted behind the pterygoid plates, and the pterygoid process is sectioned at its base.

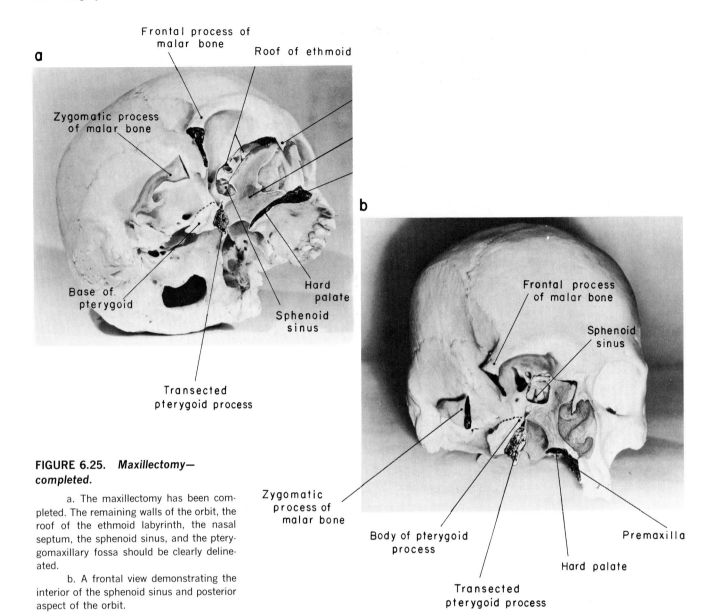

FIGURE 6.25. *Maxillectomy— completed.*

a. The maxillectomy has been completed. The remaining walls of the orbit, the roof of the ethmoid labyrinth, the nasal septum, the sphenoid sinus, and the pterygomaxillary fossa should be clearly delineated.

b. A frontal view demonstrating the interior of the sphenoid sinus and posterior aspect of the orbit.

behind the pterygoid plates and then wherever the specimen remains intact. As soon as the specimen is removed, a large hot-pack is inserted into the cavity. Time can now be taken for examination of the specimen to determine the extent of the disease. The packing is removed and the internal maxillary artery is ligated. The remaining portions of the ethmoid labyrinth, the anterior wall of the sphenoid sinus, and other areas where there could be possible extension of the disease are resected (Fig. 6.26a).

Skin Grafting. A .0015- to .0018-inch thickness skin graft is obtained from the medial aspect of the thigh, a nonhair-bearing area. All areas void of mucous membrane are grafted. One graft is used to line the orbit, roof of the ethmoid sinuses, and the cribriform area. A second graft extends from the anterior wall of the sphenoid sinus to the anterior skin incision, thus lining the skin flap. This graft is sutured to the gingivobuccal incision inferiorly and subcutaneously anteriorly. Chromic catgut (#4-0) is used for suturing the skin graft (Fig. 6.26b). Over-

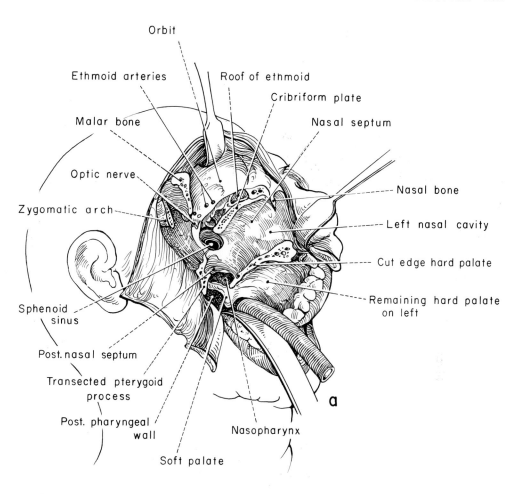

FIGURE 6.26. *Maxillectomy—skin grafting and packing.*

a. A sketch showing the parts mentioned in Figure 6.25 in relation to the surrounding soft tissues.

b. All areas void of mucous membrane are grafted with a split-thickness skin graft obtained from the inner aspect of the thigh. Usually two pieces of graft are used. A smaller piece is used to cover the cribriform area, roof of the ethmoid sinuses, and the orbit. A second piece extends from the front face of the sphenoid sinus, covering the inner aspect of the facial flap.

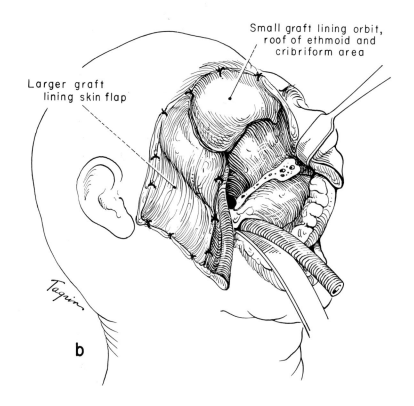

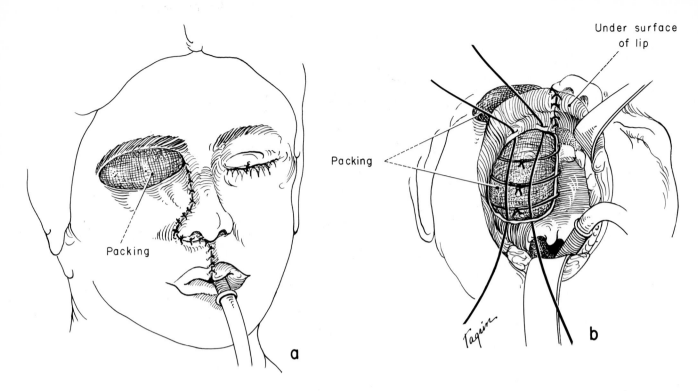

Under surface
of lip

Packing

Packing

a

b

FIGURE 6.27. *Maxillectomy—skin closure.*

a. The skin graft is covered with a layer of Gelfoam to prevent the graft from being pulled away when the packing is removed.

The maxillectomy cavity is packed with 1-inch Aureomycin-impregnated iodoform gauze prior to replacement of the facial flap.

The incisions are closed subcutaneously with interrupted #3-0 chromic catgut and the skin edges are approximated with #5-0 dermal suture material.

b. Chromic catgut sutures (#00) are bridged across the palatal defect in lateral and antero-posterior directions to prevent downward displacement of the packing.

lapping portions of the graft can be trimmed, postoperatively, after the packing has been removed. As a general rule these grafts take very well and it is not necessary to suture them carefully in place. The entire skin-grafted cavity is lined with a layer of absorbable gelatin material, so that when the gauze packing is removed the skin graft will not be pulled away. The defect (cavity) is packed with Aureomycin ointment-impregnated iodoform gauze. This packing is held in place with a temporary prosthesis or by bridging #00 chromic catgut or #3-0 Dermalene sutures from the midline to the gingivobuccal incision (Fig. 6.27b).

Skin Closure (Fig. 6.27a). Using the cross-hatchings as a guide, the flap is replaced subcutaneously with #3-0 chromic catgut sutures. The mucous membrane is sutured with #4-0 chromic catgut. Dermal suture material (#5-0) is used for the skin closure. A light dressing is placed over the orbit, face, and side of the nose. A nasogastric feeding tube is inserted by way of the nasal cavity opposite the operated side. This remains in place for approximately 4 days or until the patient is able to feed himself properly. If there is any sign of impending respiratory obstruction, or a radical neck dissection has been carried out with the maxillectomy, a tracheotomy should be performed.

Postoperative Care. The packing is removed between the seventh and tenth postoperative day. An impression for a temporary prosthesis is made at this time,

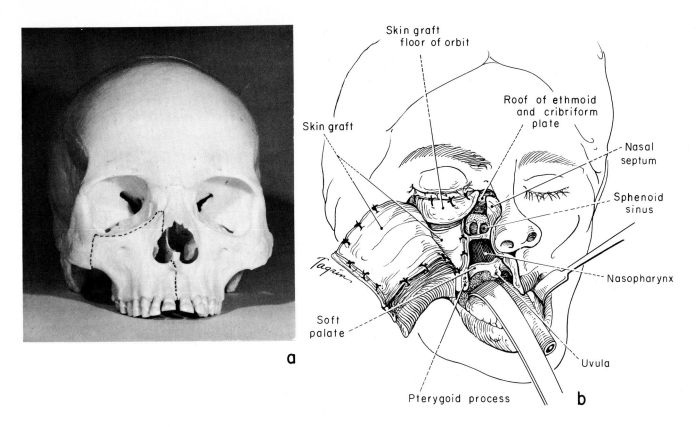

a

b

FIGURE 6.28. *Maxillectomy without orbital resection.*

a. The periosteal and bone incisions to be used when the bony floor of the orbit is to be preserved. Other bone incisions are similar to those shown in Figure 6.15.

b. Skin grafting is employed to cover either the bony floor of the orbit or the orbital periosteum. In the latter instance, the skin graft, as it contracts, provides support for the orbital contents. A second graft extends from the lateral margin of the front face of the sphenoid sinus laterally, lining the inner aspect of the facial flap.

if this was not done immediately after the operation. Moist cotton packing can be used temporarily to fill the defect. This is changed several times a day, especially after each meal. The cavity should be carefully cleaned each day with hydrogen peroxide solution and irrigated with warm saline solution. Excessive skin that has been grafted is trimmed. A permanent dental prosthesis is made four to six weeks postoperatively when all healing has taken place.

As a general rule a dental prosthesis is preferable to a reconstructed palate because this provides for easier inspection of the cavity, and recurrent disease can be identified at an early date. If the mucous membrane and periosteum of the hard palate have been preserved (Fig. 6.16b and c), the defect in the palate may be eliminated. When the hard palate is reconstructed, the resultant skin-lined cavity, which produces much debris, may result in a crusting and an odor problem. There are three methods for constructing the palate: (1) by using a pedicled flap consisting of the entire forehead based on one temporal artery (this is tunneled in through the cheek); (2) by using a cervical pedicled skin flap which is pulled up and through the cheek; or (3) by swinging the nasal septum, which has been incised anteriorly, superiorly, and posteriorly and hinged inferiorly, laterally to cover the palatal defect.

Maxillectomy with Preservation of the Orbit

A medial and lateral tarsorrhaphy (see Vol. II, pp. 252 to 254) should be performed prior to making the maxillectomy incision. This is done to prevent edema and ectropion of the lower lid postoperatively. The rhinotomy and the upper lip, gingivobuccal, and palatal incisions are made as described on pages 237 to 238. The horizontal incision under the eye extends across the lower lid within 2 to 3 cm from the tarsal plates (Fig. 6.16). The lower lid is elevated in a plane above the orbicularis oculi muscle. The flap is elevated, preserving the orbicularis oculi and buccinator muscles. The entire front face of the maxilla, ascending process, inferior orbital rim, zygomatic arch, and malar bone are exposed.

A periosteal incision is made along the inferior orbital rim (Fig. 6.28a). The periosteum is elevated from the floor and lower medial and lateral walls of the orbit. A curved hemostat is inserted under the malar bone, the tip presenting in the inferior orbital fissure (Fig. 6.20) in order to grasp one end of a Gigli saw, which is used to transect the malar bone. If the floor of the orbit is to be preserved, the orbital periosteum is not elevated from it.

The remainder of the operation is as has been described for maxillectomy with orbital exenteration. The ethmoid is usually transected at slightly lower level than is shown in Figure 6.23. The remainder of the ethmoid cells are carefully removed after the specimen has been resected.

There are two methods to obtain support for the orbit if the bony floor has been removed.

1. The temporalis muscle is detached from the coronoid process of the mandible. It is slung under the orbital periosteum and sutured in the region of the inner canthus. The temporalis muscle, as well as the remainder of the maxillectomy defect, is covered with a split-thickness skin graft.

2. An alternate, but not quite as effective, method to support the orbit is that of suturing a sling of skin graft under the orbital periosteum. As the graft becomes attached to the periosteum and contracts, it supplies a good support to the orbit.

It is best not to disturb the tarsorrhaphy incision for several weeks in order to prevent edema and ectropion of the lower lid. The remainder of the postoperative care is as has been outlined for maxillectomy with orbital exenteration.

REFERENCES

Adisman, I. K.: Removable Partial Dentures for Jaw Defects of the Maxilla and Mandible. Dent. Clin. N. Amer. 849–870 (Nov.) 1962.

Ashley, R. F.: A Method of Closing Antroalveolar Fistulae. Ann. Otol. 48:632–642 (Sept.) 1939.

Bakamjian, V.: A Technique for Primary Reconstruction of the Palate after Radical Maxillectomy for Cancer. Plast. Reconstr. Surg. 31:2:103–116 (Feb.) 1963.

Baker, R., Cherry, J., Lott, S., and Bischofberger, W. B.: Carcinoma of the Maxillary Sinus. Arch. Otolaryng. 84:201–204 (Aug.) 1966.

Bosley, R. J.: The Surgical Treatment of Persistent Antroalveolar Fistulas. Laryngoscope 73:1:60–70 (Jan.) 1963.

Chasin, W. D., and Lofgren, R. H.: Vidian Nerve Section for Vasomotor Rhinitis. Arch. Otolaryng. 86:129–135 (July) 1967.

Cocke, E. W., Jr., and Braund, R. R.: Superior Maxillary Resection. In: P. Cooper (Ed.): *The Craft of Surgery.* Boston, Little, Brown & Co., 1964, pp. 82–91.

Dunning, H. S.: Maxillary Sinusitis of Oral Origin. Laryngoscope 35:766–771, 1925.

Edgerton, M. T., and Devito, R. V.: Reconstruction of Palatal Defects Resulting from Treatment of Carcinoma of the Palate, Antrum, or Gingiva. Plast. Reconstr. Surg. *28*:3:306–319 (Sept.) 1961.

Gergely, Z.: Transmaxillary Ligature of the Arteria Maxillaris Interna (Seiffert's Method). Acta Otol. *22*:142–146, 1935.

Golding-Wood, P. H.: Observations on Petrosal and Vidian Neurectomy in Chronic Vasomotor Rhinitis. J. Laryng. *75*:232–247, 1961.

Golding-Wood, P. H.: Pathology and Surgery of Chronic Vasomotor Rhinitis. J. Laryng. *76*:969–977 (Dec.) 1962.

Ketcham, A. S., Wilkins, R. H., Van Buren, J. M., and Smith, R. R.: A Combined Intracranial Facial Approach to the Paranasal Sinuses. Amer. J. Surg. *106*:5:698–703 (Nov.) 1963.

Lingeman, R. E.: Management of Malignant Disease of the Accessory Nasal Sinuses. Personal communication.

McCoy, G., and Johnson T.: Malignancy of the Maxillary Sinus: Selection of Therapy. Laryngoscope *72*:5:586–596 (Feb.) 1962.

Montgomery, W. W., Lofgren, R. H., and Chasin, W. D.: Analysis of Pterygopalatine Space Surgery. Laryngoscope, *LXXX* (8):1190–1200 (Aug.) 1970.

Schuknecht, H. F.: The Surgical Management of Carcinoma of the Paranasal Sinuses. Laryngoscope *61*:9:874–890 (Sept.) 1951.

Sisson, G. A.: Cancer of the Maxillary Sinus. Pacif. Med. Surg. *73*:251–257 (July–Aug.) 1965.

Stemmer, A. L.: Planning and Management of the Bilateral Subtotal Maxillectomy. Plast. Reconst. Surg. *34*:4:390–402 (Oct.) 1964.

Turnbull, F. M., Jr., and Hara, H. J.: Carcinoma of the Paranasal Sinuses and the Nasal Cavities. Trans. Pacif. Coast Otoophthal. Soc. 1955.

Weaver, D. F.: Tumors of the Maxillary Antrum. Laryngoscope *62*:2:139–159 (Feb.) 1952.

7

Facial Fractures

Of first concern when confronting a patient with facial trauma is his general medical status, with particular attention to possible airway obstruction, hemorrhagic shock, and existent or potential central nervous system damage. Specialized treatment of the facial injury may be immediate or delayed, depending upon such factors as the condition of the involved tissues, the time lapse since the traumatic insult, or—of most importance—the presence of other medical problems demanding more urgent attention. In all cases, the soft-tissue wounds should be cleansed, debrided of devitalized tissue, and protected from further injury while awaiting definitive therapy.

Facial lacerations should be sutured as soon as the patient's condition permits, preferably within 24 hours, but primary closure may, on occasion, be delayed as long as several days. When possible, open wounds of the face should be used to gain access to underlying fractures for inspection, reduction, and internal fixation. The surgeon should search these wounds carefully for foreign particles such as soil, stone, glass, cloth fragments, pieces of wood or metal, vegetative matter, and other debris that may be hidden within the traumatized tissues. All abraded epithelium must be diligently examined for impregnated bits of asphalt and other particulate matter that may require removal by scrubbing or dermabrasion if the "debris tattooing" mentioned by Shumrick and by Dickinson is to be avoided. Segments of bone are potential centers for osteogenesis, so none that have a chance for survival are removed; small fragments that are completely detached usually do not survive and should be removed. If reduction and fixation of facial fractures must be delayed, the time interval should not exceed 2 or 3 weeks, depending upon the site of the fracture. Early application of a barrel bandage or simple wire ligature of the teeth may stabilize fracture fragments enough to minimize pain and reduce blood loss in patients with maxillary or mandibular fractures. Prophylactic treatment for tetanus is administered, and the systemic use of broad-spectrum antibiotics, such as penicillin, is advisable. Corticosteroids and anti-inflammatory enzymes are of questionable value in these patients.

It may be necessary to seek consultation from a neurosurgical, ophthalmologic, and/or dental colleague.

A tracheotomy is performed if there is any indication of impending airway obstruction.

The objectives of the treatment of facial fractures are based on prevention of the following:

1. Abnormalities in the position and motility of the ocular globe
2. Dental malocclusion
3. Facial disfigurement
4. Nasal obstruction
5. Interference with sinus drainage
6. Sensory and motor nerve dysfunction
7. Temporomandibular joint ankylosis
8. Osseous nonunion with chronic pain or tenderness
9. Osteomyelitis or sequestration of bone fragments

The examination should include a search for the following signs and symptoms:

1. Soft tissue injury: edema, contusions, abrasions, and lacerations (including gingival tears)
2. Ecchymosis: subconjunctival, periorbital, and intraoral
3. Epistaxis: anterior and posterior
4. Deformities: obvious by inspection and/or palpation
5. Ophthalmic problems: loss of visual acuity, decreased visual field, abnormal ocular motility, diplopia, displacement of globe, corneal abrasion or laceration, hyphema, pupillary dysfunction, abnormal funduscopic exam, telecanthus, epiphora
6. Sensory nerve dysfunction: anesthesia or hypesthesia of any of the three divisions of the fifth cranial nerve, with particular attention to the areas of distribution of the infraorbital and mental nerves
7. Motor nerve dysfunction: paresis or paralysis of any or all divisions of the seventh cranial nerve
8. Trismus
9. Malocclusion
10. Subcutaneous emphysema
11. Bony crepitus with pathologic mobility of mandible, maxilla, or nasal bones
12. Cerebrospinal fluid rhinorrhea
13. Pain and tenderness
14. Evidence of infection: soft tissue wound infection; sinus infection (suppurating antral hematoma)
15. Dental fractures and avulsions
16. Nasal obstruction: septal hematoma or septal fracture and dislocation

NASAL FRACTURES

This group of facial fractures occurs most frequently. An accurate history of previous nasal trauma or operations, as well as an account of the current injuring force, is important. Radiographs are taken and should include the Waters' projec-

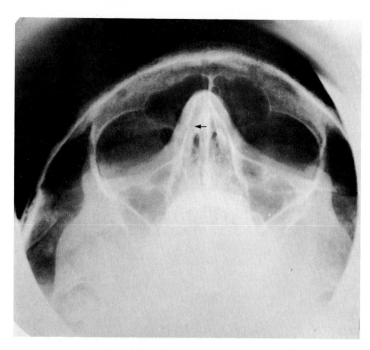

FIGURE 7.1. *Fracture of the nasal bones with minimal displacement.*

a. An end-on view of the nasal bones. The arrow points to a fracture line. The slight displacement of the nasal bones to the right is apparent.

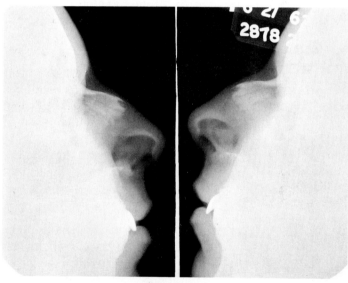

b. Lateral views (same patient as 7.1a). The fracture line is not clearly demonstrated by these views. The longitudinal grooves are often mistaken for fracture lines.

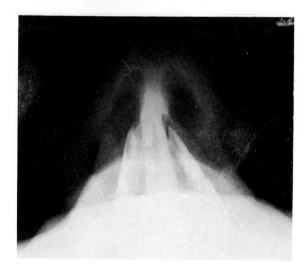

c. The sublabial view is useful to show the degree of displacement of the bony nasal pyramid, as compared with view in 7.1a.

tion, soft tissue lateral view, and a projection of the nasal bones from above, obtained by placing an occlusal x-ray film in the mouth, just under the hard palate (Fig. 7.1).

Simple Nasal Fracture

Anesthesia. The key to acceptable reduction of nasal fractures is adequate anesthesia. Young children, uncooperative adults, and patients with complex nasal fractures require a general anesthetic; all others may have their nasal fractures treated under local anesthesia. A solution of 1% lidocaine with 1:100,000 parts epinephrine has proven to be an effective and safe agent when used within the limits of safe pharmacologic dosage.

The technique for anesthesia following nasal fracture is identical to that used for rhinoplasty. Subcutaneous deposition of anesthetic solution midway between the nasion and medial canthus effectively anesthetizes branches of the infra-trochlear nerve. A bilateral infraorbital nerve block anesthetizes the lower lateral portions of the nose as well as the entire upper lip. The nasal tip is anesthetized by subcutaneous infiltration of the line of junction between the anteroinferior margin of the nasal bones and the attached upper lateral cartilages, where the external nasal branches of the anterior ethmoid nerve assume a subcutaneous course. Finally, a small amount of lidocaine injected into the base of the columella, in the vicinity of the anterior nasal spine, will anesthetize the branches of the nasopalatine nerve contributing sensation to that area.

The mucous membrane of the nasal interior is innervated by branches from the pterygopalatine ganglion with the exception of the olfactory area that occupies a small region near the roof of the nasal cavity. The pterygopalatine ganglion itself can be blocked directly either via the greater palatine foramen or from an external approach across the mandibular notch and into the pterygopalatine fossa. Techniques for these particular nerve blocks are well described elsewhere, e.g., by Adriani. More commonly, the nasal mucous membrane is anesthetized by topical application of cocaine solution (not to exceed 200 mg of cocaine in the average adult). In addition to producing adequate anesthesia, topical cocaine is a very effective vasoconstrictor, decongesting engorged mucosa and minimizing bleeding from mucosal tears incurred during fracture reduction. Six cotton pledgets, moistened with 5% cocaine solution, are prepared, and three are placed in each nostril.

FIGURE 7.2. *Reduction of nasal fractures.*

a. The instruments used for reduction of nasal fractures are Asch forceps, straight nasal fracture elevator, and Walsham forceps.

b. A fracture of the nasal bone with lateral displacement is reduced by using firm, gradually increasing pressure.

c. For elevation of a depressed nasal tip, the straight elevator is inserted into the nasal cavity. Reduction of the nasal fracture is guided by external palpation.

d. For reduction of a medially displaced nasal bone, a straight elevator, placed within the ipsilateral nostril, elevates the nasal bone under the guidance of external palpation.

e. The Walsham forceps is especially useful in reducing a fracture of the nasal bones when there is severe impaction or when reduction is delayed more than a few days following injury. It is used to grasp the nasal bone or fragments firmly and then to manipulate them into proper position.

f. For a fracture-dislocation of the entire nasal pyramid, one blade of the Asch forceps is inserted into each nasal cavity. The nasal pyramid is elevated in an anterosuperior direction and then replaced in the midline. This technique is also used for replacing the nasal septum to its midline position.

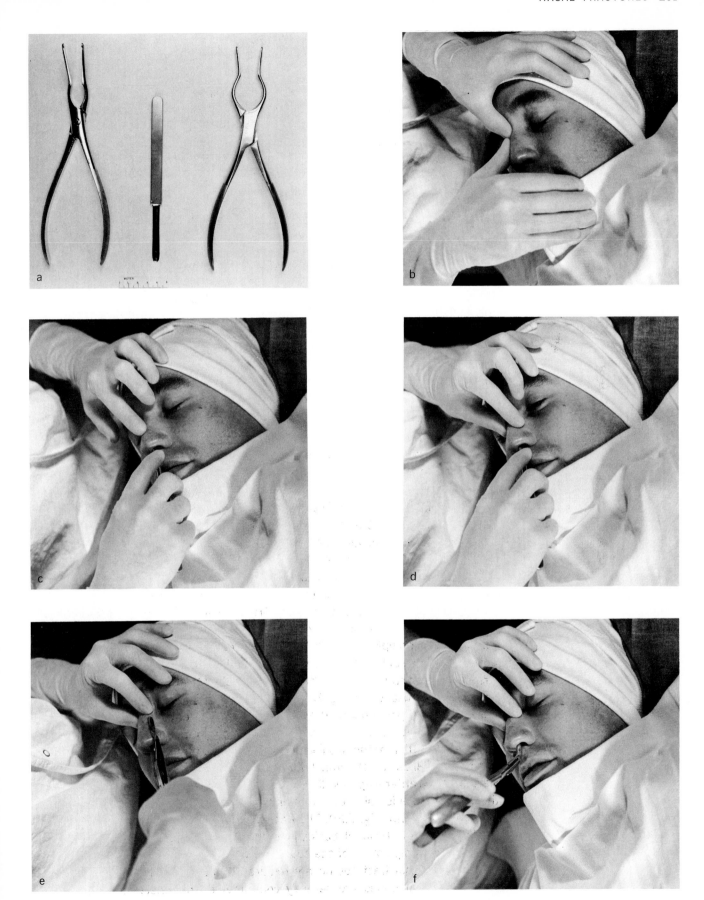

The first pledget is placed beneath the nasal bones and into the superior meatus. The second is positioned between the middle turbinate and the nasal septum, with the leading end of the pledget passing beyond the posterior attachment of the middle turbinate to the vicinity of the sphenopalatine foramen (through which most of the nasal branches of the pterygopalatine ganglion pass). The final pledget is placed between the inferior turbinate and the adjacent nasal septum. The preceding steps having been taken, at least 10 minutes should elapse before manipulation of the nasal bones is attempted. This time interval will permit maximum anesthesia and vasoconstriction.

Technique of Reduction

Primary treatment affords the best opportunity to achieve a satisfactory correction of a nasal fracture. If reduction can be performed within the first hour or two following trauma, edema will be slight and the task, therefore, will be easier. If this initial opportunity is lost, edema will usually prevail. Nevertheless, primary reduction of nasal fractures may be attempted as late as 7 to 10 days following trauma if necessary. Beyond that period of time, however, early healing and malunion may prevent closed reduction and make secondary rhinoplasty the procedure of choice.

The instruments used for primary reduction of a nasal fracture consist of a straight blunt-end elevator (e.g., Boies nasal fracture elevator), Asch forceps, and Walsham forceps (Fig. 7.2a). If these instruments are unavailable, a No. 3 scalpel handle and a large Kelly forceps, with protective rubber tubing placed over the tips, may be substituted. Nondisplaced nasal fractures require no specific therapy.

A laterally displaced fracture of the nasal bones may occasionally be reduced by simple digital manipulation using firm, gradually increasing pressure toward the midline (Fig. 7.2b). More often, however, the nasal bones sustaining the force of injury are displaced medially and become depressed as well. These depressed nasal bones can usually be reduced only by elevating them into place with a straight elevator, while the operator uses the index finger and thumb of his nondominant hand for palpating and molding the bones into position (Fig. 7.2c and d).

Fractures of the nasal bones that are impacted or angulated and fail to be placed in acceptable reduction by the preceding techniques may often be reduced with Walsham forceps. One blade of the instrument is placed in the nasal cavity on the undersurface of the depressed nasal bone while the other blade (protected with a short sleeve of soft rubber tubing) remains against the nasal skin on the external surface of the nasal bone (Fig. 7.2e). Manipulation, controlled by digital palpation, will result in proper placement of the fractured segment.

If there is deviation of the entire nasal pyramid to one side and buckling or fracture-dislocation of the nasal septum, one blade of the Asch forceps is inserted into each nasal cavity. The initial manipulation with the forceps in this position is elevation in an anterosuperior direction to disimpact the depressed segments while the external nose is palpated and manipulated with the fingers of the surgeon's nondominant hand (Fig. 7.2f). The nasal pyramid is then returned to its midline position, and any residual buckling of the nasal septum is then corrected by appropriate manipulation of the septum itself with the Asch forceps.

Simple nasal fractures do not require intranasal packing. If, on the other hand, the nasal bones are severely comminuted and unstable, careful nasal packing with either antibiotic-impregnated iodoform gauze or a finger-cot pack will support the fragments until they are fixed in place. Occasionally brisk epistaxis will in itself necessitate packing after reduction of a nasal fracture. It is in most cases advisable to apply an external splint, such as that employed following a rhinoplasty, if for no other reason than to forewarn others of the patient's healing injury.

Certain nasal fractures, especially those associated with fracture-dislocation or buckling of the nasal septum, cannot be reduced by the closed techniques. Treatment should consist of open reduction and one of the various septorhinoplasty techniques. Associated septal hematoma or abscess warrants emergency surgical intervention as discussed in Chapter 8.

Open Nasal Fractures

All displaced nasal fractures are open fractures on the basis of the laceration that occurs in the delicate mucoperiosteum of the involved nasal bone. Many nasal fractures are open externally as well. In these cases, the soft tissue wound should be cleansed, debrided as necessary, and sutured with good soft tissue technique. The fractures are otherwise handled as mentioned previously. If there is actual loss of nasal skin precluding primary closure, a local flap may be required for osseous coverage (see Chapter 8).

Nasomaxillary Fractures

When subjected to a severe force from an anterior direction, the nasal pyramid (nasal bones, ascending processes of the maxillae, and nasal processes of the frontal bone) is fractured from its attachments and becomes a projectile body, driven into the interorbital space and tearing through the delicate bone and soft tissue structures until it comes to rest in a posterior position. The resultant deformity has been variously termed the nasomaxillary fracture, naso-orbital fracture, or the nasoethmoidal fracture. Its significance lies in the vast variety of immediate complications and late sequelae with which it may be associated. The following is only a partial list of these problems:

A. Neurologic
1. Dural tear
2. Cerebrospinal fluid leak and possible meningitis
3. Aerocele
4. Brain laceration
5. Avulsion of olfactory nerve perforating cribriform plate
6. Epidural or subdural hematoma
7. Brain contusion and necrosis of brain tissue
B. Ophthalmic
1. Traumatic telecanthus (pseudohypertelorism)
2. Traumatic orbital hypertelorism
3. Orbital hematoma (lacerated anterior ethmoidal artery)
4. Optic nerve injury with potential blindness
5. Epiphora secondary to disrupted lacrimal excretory system
6. Ptosis secondary to injury of the levator palpebrae superioris
7. Disruption of trochlea

    8. Injury to or entrapment of medial rectus muscle

    9. Ocular globe injury (e.g., perforations, hyphemas, retinal edema, retinal tears or detachments, and choroidal ruptures)

C. Rhinologic

    1. External nasal deformity

    2. Nasal obstruction secondary to septal fracture-dislocation and/or hematoma

    3. Anosmia

    4. Severe posterior epistaxis

    5. Nasofrontal duct disruption with secondary chronic frontal sinusitis or mucocele

Although most "smashed noses" are accompanied by few, if any, of the preceding complications, a diligent effort should be made to rule out all of these possibilities prior to dismissing the injury as a simple nasal fracture. If there has been a history of unconsciousness subsequent to the injury or if there are any signs suggestive of central nervous system damage, a neurosurgeon must be immediately consulted. Likewise, an ophthalmologist should be called to evaluate the ocular globes in all of these patients to detect occult damage or to establish a baseline if the examination proves normal. These fractures are frequently overlooked or neglected during the initial days following injury when the best opportunity for good surgical correction presents itself. The maxillofacial surgeon must have full familiarity with the complex anatomy of the area, be prepared to utilize microsurgical techniques, and be capable of restoring osseous continuity and soft tissue integrity if a satisfactory end result is to be expected.

Discussion of the surgical repair of many of these problems is far beyond the intended scope of this book. Other areas are treated in depth in other chapters. Of particular relevance here, however, is the proper management of three of the more consistent findings associated with these fractures: the osseous deformity, medial canthus disruption, and the acutely damaged lacrimal execretory system.

The Osseous Deformity. Nasomaxillary fractures frequently cannot be managed by simple closed reduction, internal packing, and external splinting, even in the absence of nasolacrimal or other soft tissue injury that would mandate surgical exploration and repair. An excellent way of treating these fractures is by the use of two pieces of #26-gauge stainless steel wire and lead or plastic plates (Fig. 7.3). The nasal bones are elevated and held in position by an assistant while the wire, on a heavy straight needle, is passed through the skin, a posterior fracture line in the ascending process of the maxilla, the nasal septum, and out, again, by way of a posterior fracture line of the opposite ascending process and its overlying skin. Two such wires are passed, one located superiorly near the frontomaxillary suture and the other anteroinferiorly near the maxillary contribution to the pyriform aperture. The free ends of the two wires on each side are then passed through a piece of thin Silastic* sheeting (to help protect the skin surface) followed by a lead or plastic plate trimmed to the appropriate size and shape. The two adjacent wires are then twisted down bilaterally to fix the fracture fragments in a sandwiched position between the two plates. To help obtain the proper convergence of the nasal bones and ascending processes, the anterior borders of the plates can be manually approximated to the desired extent and held with a piece of adhesive tape between

---

*Dow Corning Corporation, Midland, Michigan

Silicone sheeting

Lead sheeting

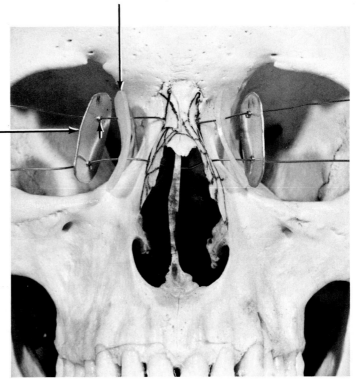

FIGURE 7.3. *Splinting a severely comminuted and depressed fracture of the nasal bones.*

   a. Two pieces of lead and silicone rubber sheeting are cut to size and sterilized. Number 26-gauge stainless steel wire is placed on a heavy, curved cutting needle. The needle is passed through one end of the lead and silicone rubber sheeting. As the fragments are elevated, the needle is passed directly through both nasal bones and the nasal septum. The wire continues on through the silicone rubber and lead sheeting on the opposite side of the nose. A second wire is passed in a similar fashion.

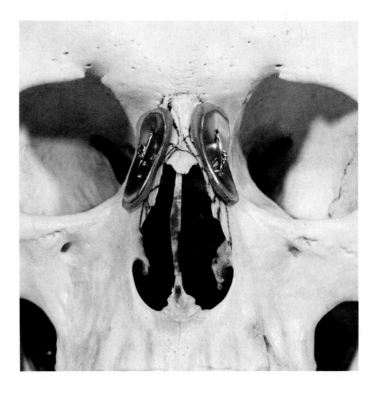

   b. The final result of external nasal splinting. The wires are twisted on each surface of the lead sheeting. The silicone rubber sheeting is used as a cushion to prevent pressure necrosis.

the plates, across the nasal dorsum. If passing the wires through existent fracture lines proves to be unsatisfactory or impossible, the surgeon can use a hand drill to establish a better path. The reduction may be given additional support by suturing Silastic plates to each side of the nasal septum. Intranasal packing may also be required. Since contamination is likely in this location, it is important to use antibiotic-impregnated iodoform gauze for this purpose. The packing can be removed at the end of 5 days; the external splints should remain in place approximately 10 days. This same method of splinting is often useful in conjunction with surgical exploration of the traumatized area and open reduction of the larger fracture fragments.

Medial Canthal Disruption. Understanding the pathophysiology of medial canthal deformity associated with nasomaxillary fracture is dependent upon a fundamental knowledge of the anatomy of this area of the medial orbital wall. In 1966, Converse and Smith discussed this problem in detail, and in 1976, Jones provided exacting anatomic information lending strong support to the earlier publications.

The pretarsal portions of the orbicularis oculi muscle, of the upper and lower eyelids, pass from the medial margins of the upper and lower tarsi, respectively, toward their insertion into the medial orbital wall. In doing so, they each split into a larger superficial head and smaller deep head. The two superficial heads join one another prior to their insertion in front of the anterior lacrimal crest of the ascending process of the maxilla and thereby form the medial canthal tendon. Likewise, the two deep heads join one another prior to their insertion behind the posterior lacrimal crest and are referred to as the tensor tarsi muscle (Horner's muscle). The lacrimal sac, lying in the lacrimal fossa, is thus straddled by the medial canthal ligament anteriorly and the tensor tarsi muscle posteriorly. The normal angular shape of the medial canthus and the normal exposure of the lacrimal caruncle are dependent upon the integrity of this ligament and muscle which anchor the orbicularis oculi muscle to the medial orbital wall. Disruption of this system, either by severance of these anchoring structures or, more commonly, by lateral fracture-dislocation of small fragments of bone into which they insert, will lead to lateral displacement of the soft tissue structures of the medial canthus. This displacement is caused by the unopposed pull of the orbicularis muscle, in a lateral direction, resulting in a rounding off of the normally angular medial canthus and an associated disappearance from view of the lacrimal caruncle. The interpupillary distance is unaffected by this form of injury and the widened intercanthal distance has been termed traumatic telecanthus. Epiphora may ensue secondary to altered lacrimal excretory physiology or actual transection of the lacrimal excretory apparatus.

Converse and Smith describe two mechanisms of occurrence of this medial canthal injury. In one, the nasal pyramid becomes abruptly displaced posteriorly but, traveling medial to the medial orbital rim and wall, it fragments the latter structures in a lateral direction and leaves the medial canthal tendon inserted into its bony fragment. In the second mechanism of injury, the nasal pyramid telescopes upon the lateral surface of the medial orbital rim and wall and, in so doing, severs the medial canthal tendon, leaving it unattached to an osseous fragment. The resultant clinical findings differ in these two injuries in that the lacrimal excretory system has a higher likelihood of damage with the second mechanism.

Whenever medial canthal deformity is present following severe nasomaxillary trauma, surgical exploration is indicated as soon as the patient's general condition permits. An external ethmoidectomy-type skin incision is made midway between the medial canthus and the midline of the nasal dorsum. Soft tissue dissection proceeds posteriorly staying lateral to the periosteum until the level of the lacrimal fossa is encountered. In this vicinity, if the ruptured medial canthal ligament is not immediately encountered (it is most easily identified by its firm attachment to a fragment of bone avulsed from the medial orbital margin), gingerly dissecting laterally toward the medial ends of the tarsal plates should allow its identification. The intimate association of the lacrimal canaliculi with the medial canthal tendon warrants cannulation of the canaliculi with a size 00 lacrimal probe and their positive identification (preferably with the use of a microscope or loupes with 4X magnification) prior to dissecting out the tendon. Once isolated, the medial canthal tendon of one or both sides is wired with #30-gauge stainless steel wire to the medial orbital wall in the vicinity of the normal location of the posterior lacrimal crest, utilizing a transnasal wiring technique if no rigid support can be found at the ipsilateral posterior lacrimal crest. Various medial canthoplasty techniques have been proposed in the literature, the one described by Beyer and Smith being dependable when sufficient medial orbital wall persists. Primary medial cantho-plasty provides a much greater chance of satisfactory repair than does a second-ary effort at a later date. It is, therefore, the obligation of the maxillofacial surgeon to be suspicious of this injury whenever confronted with injury to the nasomaxillary area.

The Acutely Traumatized Lacrimal Excretory System

As mentioned previously, the lacrimal excretory system is susceptible to disruption of its anatomic and functional integrity as a consequence of naso-maxillary fractures. If untreated, these injuries may result in epiphora, repeated dacryocystitis, mucocele, or a lacrimal sac fistula. Surgical repair, once one of these problems has become established, requires a dacryocystorhinostomy if the site of lacrimal obstruction is distal to the internal common punctum (Chapter 3) or, as described by Jones in 1976, a conjunctivodacryocystorhinostomy should the canaliculi themselves become obliterated. Provided with a knowledge of the anat-omy of the lacrimal system (Chapter 3) and skill in the use of microsurgical techniques, the maxillofacial surgeon should be capable of cannulating the entire lacrimal apparatus, identifying the site and nature of the defect, and, if necessary, performing a reanastomosis of lacerated segments using #8-0 or #9-0 monofila-ment nylon sutures. This procedure will, by no means, guarantee normal lacrimal function, but it will maximize the chance of achieving that end result with avoid-ance of revision surgery at a later time.

FRACTURE OF THE ZYGOMATIC BONE (ZYGOMA OR MALAR BONE)

The zygomatic bone articulates with the temporal bone, frontal bone, greater wing of the sphenoid bone, and the maxillary bone. It forms the prominence of the cheek, contributing as well to the lateral and infraorbital margins, the lateral orbital wall, and the zygomatic arch. Fractures of the zygoma are often erroneously referred to as "tripod" or "tri-malar" fractures. These terms should be avoided since they are nondescriptive and misleading. A classification of zygomatic fractures proposed by Knight and North is of academic interest, but has not proven to be of major importance in the selection of appropriate therapy for individual cases:

CLASSIFICATION OF ZYGOMATIC FRACTURES

GROUP I	(6%)	No significant displacement
GROUP II	(10%)	Zygomatic arch fractures
GROUP III	(33%)	Unrotated body fractures
GROUP IV	(11%)	Medially rotated body fractures (counterclockwise on L; clockwise on R)
		Type A: Down at infraorbital margin and outward at zygomatic prominence
		Type B: Down at infraorbital margin and inward at zygomaticofrontal suture
GROUP V	(22%)	Laterally rotated body fractures (clockwise on L; counterclockwise on R)
		Type A: Inward at zygomatic prominence and upward at infraorbital margin
		Type B: Inward at zygomatic prominence and outward at zygomaticofrontal suture
GROUP VI	(18%)	Complex fractures

Signs and Symptoms

The signs and symptoms of fracture of the zygomatic bone can be summarized as follows:

1. Flattening of the upper cheek
2. Diplopia
3. Limited ocular motility (positive forced duction test)
4. Periorbital edema and/or ecchymosis
5. Subconjunctival hemorrhage
6. Enophthalmos
7. Ptosis (secondary to inferior displacement of the lateral canthus)
8. Palpable bony "step" deformity of the infraorbital margin or, occasionally, a palpable bony defect at the zygomaticofrontal suture
9. Anesthesia or hypesthesia of the infraorbital nerve
10. Decreased mandibular excursion
11. Ecchymosis of the gingivobuccal sulcus on the involved side with palpable submucosal osseous fragmentation in the sulcus
12. Subcutaneous emphysema
13. Epistaxis (bleeding from the antrum)

Diagnosis

Flatness of the cheek may be quite obvious unless obscured by edema and hematoma. The infraorbital margins are carefully bimanually palpated. The "step" deformity or notching of the rim is characteristic of this fracture (Fig. 7.4b). Sensation is tested over the nose, cheek, and upper lip and compared with that on

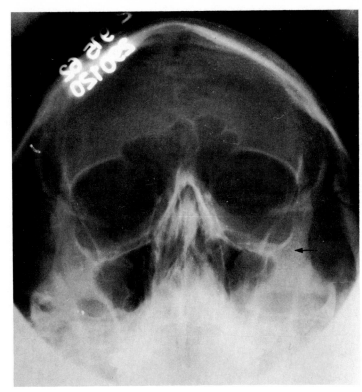

a

FIGURE 7.4. *Fracture of the zygomatic bone.*

a. The left zygoma is fractured with displacement in a posteroinferior and medial direction (arrow). This fracture gives a depressed cheek bone appearance. Note the narrowed width of the orbit and density in the lateral aspect of the left maxillary sinus. This type of fracture usually requires open reduction and wiring in the zygomaticofrontal and infraorbital rim regions.

b. The left zygoma is depressed and rotated laterally (arrow). Note the step deformity of the infraorbital rim.

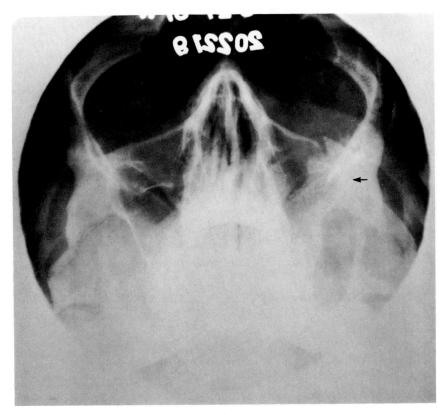

b

the uninjured side. Since the thinnest bone is in the region of the infraorbital groove and foramen, the infraorbital nerve is quite often involved (Figs. 7.4a and 7.5a). The zygomatic arch is carefully palpated since it may be depressed (Fig. 7.11). Painful or limited excursion of the mandible is indicative of a depressed zygomatic bone impinging on the underlying coronoid process. Escape of air into the soft tissues may produce periorbital emphysema. Bony crepitus, if present, is pathognomonic of zygomatic bone fracture. Palpation of the maxilla through the buccal sulcus will often reveal osseous disruption.

The patient is tested for diplopia and ocular motility. Diplopia is present in approximately 10% of cases according to Knight and North, Barclay, and Tempest. It may be due to orbital edema, entrapment or paralysis of an extraocular muscle, or displacement of the ocular globe. The forced duction (traction) test should be performed to rule out muscle entrapment (Fig. 7.16). Asymmetric palpebral fissures are due to displacement of the lateral canthal ligament with the fractured lateral orbital wall. Transillumination of the sinuses will usually disclose decreased translucency of the fractured antrum. This lowered translucency is caused by mucosal edema and the presence of blood within the antrum. Conventional radiographs (Caldwell, Waters', lateral, and basal projections) will also demonstrate opacification of the maxillary sinus and, possibly, air in the orbital or periorbital tissues. They will reveal the amount of fragmentation and nature of displacement. Modern techniques of polytomography permit even more sophisticated analysis of the osseous injury, elucidating otherwise occult disease.

Treatment

In approximately 6% of these fractures, according to the figure of Knight and North, there is no significant displacement and no therapy is required (Fig. 7.5). Most fractures of the zygomatic bone are the result of a direct blow over the malar prominence, which produces posterior and medial displacement of the bone (directly into the antrum). Other zygomatic fractures are characterized by lateral (Fig. 7.9a) or medial (Fig. 7.9b) rotation. With lateral rotation (i.e., clockwise on the left and counterclockwise on the right), the infraorbital rim is displaced upward; with medial rotation (i.e., counterclockwise on the left and clockwise on the right), the infraorbital rim is displaced downward.

If, upon initial evaluation, severe edema and ecchymosis are present, it probably does no harm to wait until these conditions have subsided, at which time reduction will be more easily accomplished. As a rule, however, it is not possible to reduce these fractures later than 3 weeks following their occurrence.

Indirect Reduction (described by Keen and by Goldthwaite; Fig. 7.7a). In this method, reduction is performed via the gingivobuccal sulcus. A small incision is made in the buccal mucosa behind the maxillary tuberosity. A curved elevator (Fig. 7.6a) is inserted behind the tuberosity, and sufficient force is applied to manipulate the displaced malar bone into its normal anatomic position. The maneuver can be guided externally by the operator's hand that is not holding the elevator. Often reduction of the fracture is accomplished easily and effectively by this method. Some object to this approach because oral contamination of the field of the fracture may occur and because, when used alone, it does not provide a method for fixation of the reduced fracture, which may subsequently redisplace.

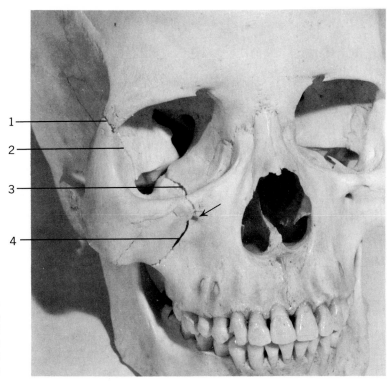

a

FIGURE 7.5. *Malar fracture.*

a. A front view of a malar fracture with no significant displacement. The fracture lines include the front face of the maxillary sinus in the region of the infraorbital foramen, the infraorbital groove, the greater wing of the sphenoid bone, the zygomaticofrontal suture line, the zygomaticotemporal suture line, and the lateral wall of the maxillary sinus.

Fractures across:
1. Zygomaticofrontal suture
2. Greater wing of sphenoid
3. Infraorbital groove
4. Anterior wall of maxillary sinus

b. A lateral view of the malar fracture showing the fracture lines through the zygomaticofrontal and zygomaticotemporal suture lines, the greater wing of the sphenoid bone, and the lateral wall of the maxillary sinus.

Fractures of:
1. Zygomaticofrontal suture
2. Greater wing of sphenoid
3. Zygomaticotemporal suture
4. Lateral wall of antrum

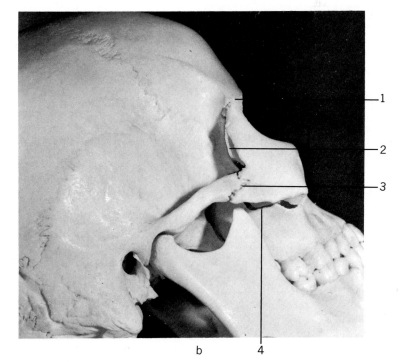

b   4

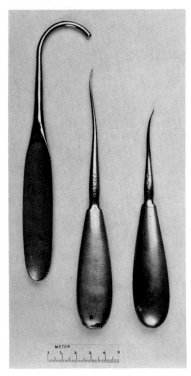

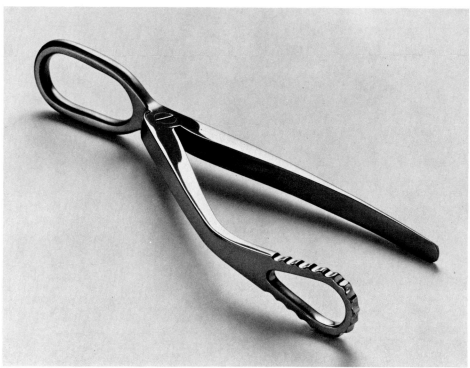

a   b

FIGURE 7.6. *Instruments for reduction of malar fracture.*

    a. Malar fracture hook, Cushing periosteal elevator, and a small periosteal elevator (shown left to right).

    b. Rowe's pattern zygomatic elevator.

Percutaneous Route (described by Matas, by Codman, by Manwaring, and by W. D. Gill; Fig. 7.7c). Since the description by Matas of looping a copper wire around the zygomatic arch and applying manual traction to achieve reduction, various instruments have been used to grasp the fractured zygoma percutaneously and to reduce such fractures. Gill's 1928 technique, employing a towel clip to engage the zygomatic arch, lateral orbital rim, or infraorbital margin, is simple and still of value in selected instances as a primary or ancillary procedure for these reductions. Fixation is not possible, however, with this method.

Temporal Route (described by Gillies, Kilner, and Stone; Fig. 7.7b). Strong and effective force can be applied through this approach. An incision is made within the hairline over the temporal fossa. The elevator must be passed deep to the temporal fascia but not through the temporal muscle. The fascia attaches to the zygomatic arch and thus guides the instrument deep to that structure, where it can be effectively used to reduce the fracture. While mobilizing the fragments into proper position with one hand on the elevator, the surgeon uses his other hand to assist with the manipulation. Care must be taken to avoid using the patient's temporal fossa as a fulcrum for the leverage required; the skull here is thin and an iatrogenic fracture may be incurred. A safer method is to pad the temporal area with a folded towel, which will disperse the pressure should leverage prove necessary. Otherwise, direct pull on the elevator in the direction necessary for reduction is the preferred technique. This procedure is facilitated by the use of a Rowe's pattern zygomatic

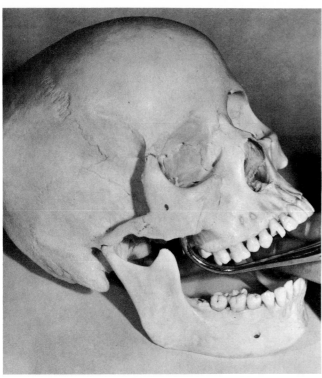

a

FIGURE 7.7. *Reduction of malar fractures.*

a. Keen technique for reduction. A curved elevator is inserted behind the tuberosity of the maxilla, and the necessary force is applied to manipulate the displaced malar bone into its proper position.

b. The Gillies technique of reduction. The elevator is passed through the temporal fascia, but not through the temporalis muscle. Strong and effective force can be implemented through this approach.

c. Gill method. A large sharp towel clip is used percutaneously to grasp the mobile zygomatic fragment and to manipulate it into position.

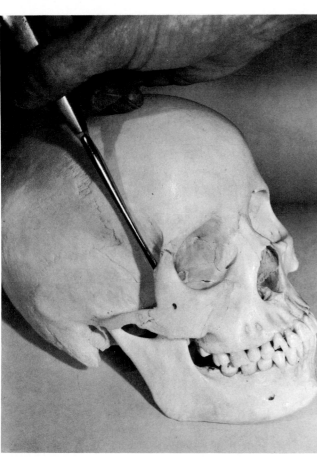

b

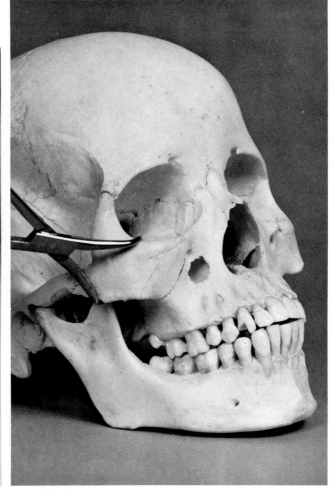

c

elevator* (Fig. 7.6b), which enables the operator to apply a great amount of force to the fracture fragment without levering against the patient. As with the indirect method, there is no way to provide fixation of the fracture fragments.

Intranasal Technique (described by Shea; Fig. 7.8a). A nasoantral window is made in the inferior meatus in the usual fashion. A large curved trochar or sound is inserted into the antrum. With leverage via this route and external palpation, the fractured bone can be manipulated into place. The objections to this method are the same as those to the indirect reduction.

Transantral Route (described by Weir and by Lothrop; Fig. 7.8b). A Caldwell-Luc incision is made on the fractured side. A heavy, curved elevator or urethral sound is introduced into the antrostomy opening in the canine fossa and used to realign the bones. If the fragment(s) is not stable, the maxillary sinus can be packed with $\frac{1}{2}$-inch iodoform gauze stripping, impregnated with antibiotic ointment. The end of the gauze is introduced into the nasal cavity through a nasoantral window, allowing easy removal after 7 to 10 days. The packing is very effective in stabilizing the fractured bone, thus making this route more practical than the transnasal approach. Care must be taken to inspect the roof of the antrum for vertically oriented comminuted fragments, which could be unintentionally driven into the orbit during placement of the gauze. Likewise, a layer of Gelfoam† above the gauze will ensure that a sharp bony fragment will not become attached to the packing.

Open Reduction (Fig. 7.9c). All displaced fractures in which it is impossible to manipulate the fragments into position or in which the fragments are unstable after reduction must be treated by open technique with internal wire fixation. The most practical places for interosseous wiring are in the region of the zygomatico-frontal suture line and the infraorbital margin. These areas are approached, respectively, by incisions in the lateral aspect of the eyebrow and in the wrinkle line of the lower eyelid just above the infraorbital rim. The latter incision (rim incision) is carried through the orbicularis oculi muscle and then follows a plane superficial to the septum orbitale down onto the infraorbital margin. Holes are drilled with a small perforating drill bit after the fracture has been reduced and stabilized. Instruments such as the Kocher forceps, the Lahy thyroid clamp, towel clips, bone hooks, and the Dingman bone-holding forceps are useful for this manipulation. Usually #26-gauge or #28-gauge wire is suitable for fixing the fragments. The wire is tightened by twisting. After cutting the wires, it is important to bend the ends into drill holes or fracture lines to prevent them from eroding overlying skin. Should a laceration overlie a fracture site on the zygomatic arch, this fracture may be wired as well, although wire fixation of this fracture site is usually unnecessary.

If all methods of reducing an old fracture are unsuccessful, the malar deformity and floor of the orbit are repaired by using autogenous bone grafts. The bone can be obtained from the iliac crest; on occasion, however, the nasoseptal cartilage and bone of the anterior wall of the antrum will provide sufficient material for the graft.

Kirschner Wire Technique (described by Brown, Fryer, and McDowell; Fig. 7.10). Kirschner wires, which come in three diameters (.062, .045, and .035 inch), can be drilled into bone without making a dermal incision. The wire must not

---

*Chas. F. Thackeray, Ltd., Leeds, England
†The Upjohn Co., Kalamazoo, Michigan

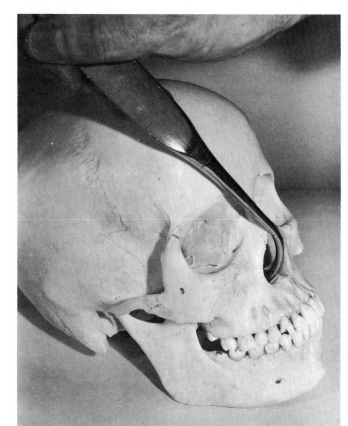

FIGURE 7.8. *Reduction of malar fractures.*

  a. Shea method. A large, curved trocar is inserted, through a nasoantral window, into the antrum. With this leverage and with external palpation, the fracture can be manipulated into place.

  b. Lothrop method. A heavy, curved elevator is introduced into the antrostomy opening made by a Caldwell-Luc incision. The maxillary sinus can then be packed.

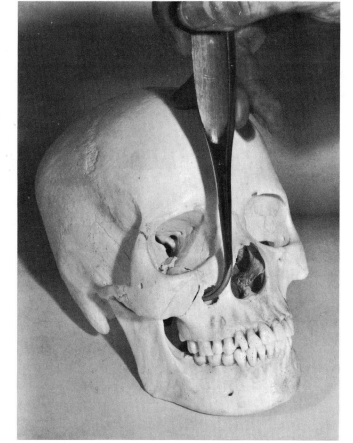

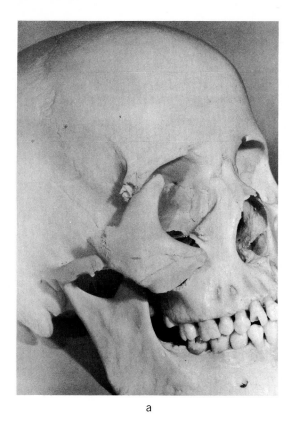

a

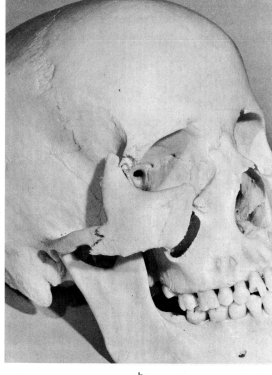

b

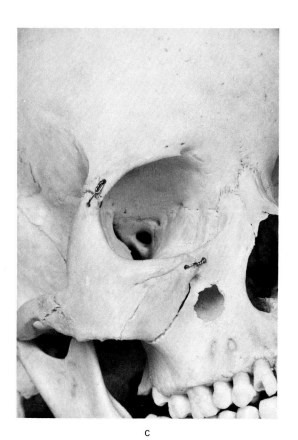

c

FIGURE 7.9. *Open reduction of malar fractures.*

a. A fracture of the malar bone with medial rotation. The lateral aspect of the infraorbital rim is depressed.

b. A fracture of the malar bone with lateral rotation. The lateral aspect of the infraorbital rim is displaced superiorly.

c. The usual sites for wire fixation of the malar fracture:

1. A skin incision along the inferior margin of the lateral aspect of the eyebrow is made to expose the zygomaticofrontal fracture line.

2. The infraorbital rim fracture is approached through an incision along a natural crease in the overlying skin or through a lower lid blepharoplasty type of skin incision. A transconjunctival approach has been advocated by Tessier.

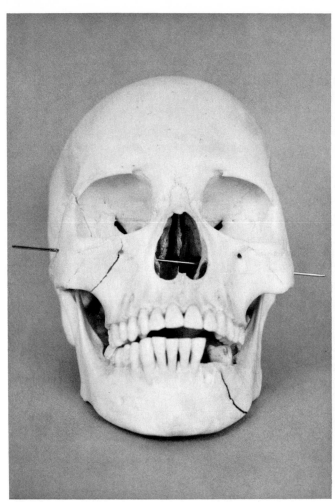
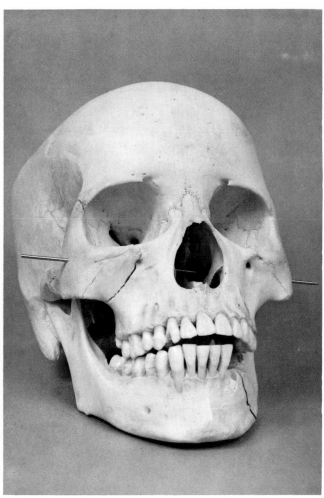

a   b

FIGURE 7.10. *Kirschner wire technique for reduction and fixation of the malar fracture.*

a. The Kirschner wire is placed in the drill chuck. After piercing the skin and subcutaneous tissues, the wire is drilled into the fractured malar bone. The malar bone is placed into its normal position by manipulation with the Kirschner wire or by any of the other methods of reduction (Figs. 7.7 and 7.8). The Kirschner wire is then drilled through the nasal cavity and through the opposite zygoma.

b. An oblique view showing the Kirschner wire in place. The end(s) of the wire is cut ½ inch from the skin and covered with a sterile cork.

extend more than 2 inches beyond the chuck of the drill in order to prevent bending and misdirection. An unstable zygoma, after simple reduction by the previously described methods, can be fixed by drilling a Kirschner wire through its body, across the nose, and into the opposite malar bone, while the fragment is held in the proper position. The wire is cut off ½-inch external to the skin surface and then either bent to lie tangent to the skin surface or covered with a sterile cork.

FRACTURES OF THE ZYGOMATIC ARCH

The diagnosis of a zygomatic arch fracture is usually not difficult, for the pain in this region is aggravated by talking and chewing. Trismus may be present, with impaired excursion of the jaw. The symptoms are caused by the contact of the medially displaced zygomatic arch with the coronoid process and the temporal muscle. The depressed fracture can be seen as a loss of normal projection in this area and is easily palpated (Fig. 7.11). Nondisplaced fractures require no specific treatment.

Method of Reduction

A fracture of the zygomatic arch, without severe displacement or comminution can be treated percutaneously by elevation with a heavy bone hook, according to Patterson, or with a towel clip, according to W. D. Gill. The hook is inserted beneath the arch from below, and the fracture is reduced by lateral traction. Use of the towel clip has been discussed in the section on zygomatic (malar) fracture.

The Gillies technique may likewise be used to reduce a fracture of the zygomatic arch (Fig. 7.7b), especially when it is combined with a malar fracture.

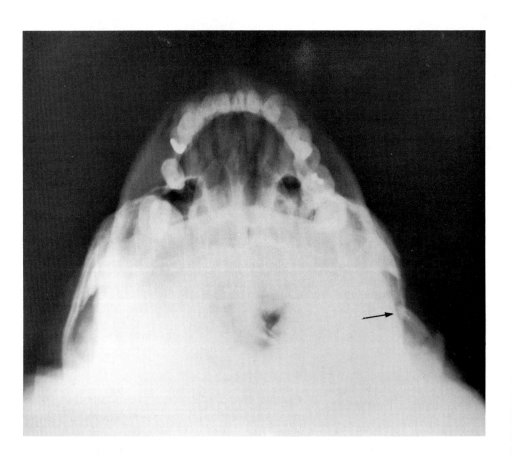

FIGURE 7.11. *Fracture of zygomatic arch.*

The arrow indicates a depressed fracture of the zygomatic arch. A central fragment was markedly displaced.

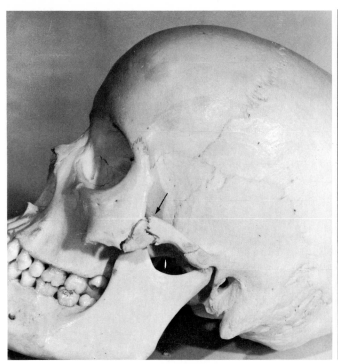
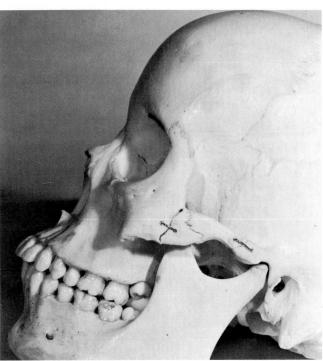

a   b

FIGURE 7.12. *Fracture of the zygomatic arch.*

a. The arrow points to a fracture of the zygomatic arch with medial displacement. The fracture lines are located both anterior and posterior to the zygomaticotemporal suture.

b. If this fracture cannot be satisfactorily reduced by other techniques, open reduction and wiring are required; both fractures are wired using drill holes and #26-gauge stainless steel wire.

From this approach, the fracture, if unstable, can be packed out in a reduced position with rubber dam packing or finger-cot packs. These packings are removed in 1 week.

Open reduction and wiring of zygomatic arch fractures is rarely indicated and should be routinely utilized only when a laceration overlies an unstable fracture site. The reduced fragment ends are then drilled and wired with #26-gauge stainless steel wire (Fig. 7.12b). If there is no laceration and the fragments cannot be reduced via other routes, a direct approach is necessary. An auriculotemporal incision is cosmetically acceptable and consists of an oblique limb in the temporal hairline running from an anterosuperior point to a posteroinferior one at the superior pole of the preauricular crease. It then drops into a vertical limb following the preauricular crease to the level of the tragus or just below. A skin flap is then raised anteriorly, in a superficial plane immediately deep to the hair follicles. Care must be taken to avoid injury to the frontal branch(es) of the facial nerve, which courses across the zygomatic arch near its midpoint; this preventive measure is facilitated by positive identification utilizing a nerve stimulator and magnification. Ginger dissection down to the arch will then allow the necessary exposure for the previously described wire fixation.

MIDFACIAL (MAXILLARY) FRACTURES

Midfacial fractures should be treated as early as possible in order to restore normal function and effect a good cosmesis. The objectives of therapy are to obtain normal dental occlusion and facial contour and to prevent infection.

During the immediate post-injury period, attention should be directed toward maintenance of an adequate airway and prophylaxis against infection. If the airway is compromised by pharyngeal edema or by displaced bony support, a tracheotomy should be performed. Severe hemorrhage from the internal maxillary artery, one of its branches, or the anterior ethmoidal artery is not uncommon in association with a midfacial fracture. This hemorrhage is controlled by local packing. If this procedure is not successful, ligation of the internal maxillary artery, the external carotid artery, or the anterior ethmoidal artery should be considered.

If the patient's condition is satisfactory shortly after the accident, the reduction of the midfacial fracture is usually not difficult unless the bone is severely comminuted or infection is present. On occasion, reduction of a fracture is delayed either because of the patient's neglect or because of an associated severe injury, such as a cervical spine fracture or closed head injury. In these instances, granulation tissue and fibrosis interfere with reduction. It may be necessary to expose the fracture line and separate the malfixation with an osteotome. Various methods are available to accomplish fixation of midfacial fractures:

1. External support with a barrel bandage, when the midfacial fracture is stable and not displaced.
2. Intermaxillary fixation, using arch bars or wiring artificial dentures in place (Figs. 7.24, 7.25, and 7.26), combined with some form of internal wire suspension (Fig. 7.14)
3. Open reduction and interosseous wiring of fracture segments
4. Internal pin fixation (Fig. 7.10)

Classification of Midfacial Fractures (Fig. 7.13)

Although preceded 35 years by Guerin's description of the transverse fracture of the maxilla, Le Fort is responsible for the classification of maxillary fractures into three general categories, which bear his name and are still utilized for descriptive purposes.

The Le Fort I fracture (Guerin fracture) involves the lower midface. It may be unilateral or bilateral. The fracture line is transverse through the lower maxilla and into the lower nasal cavity. The resulting segment of the maxilla includes the alveolar process, a portion of the maxillary sinus, the hard palate, and, on occasion, the lower aspect of the pterygoid plates. Abnormal mobility of the fracture fragment may be easily demonstrated by digital manipulation. An associated vertical fracture may occur, usually in the midline, dividing the lower midface into two segments.

The Le Fort II fracture (pyramidal fracture) passes through the nasal bone, lacrimal bone, floor of the orbit, infraorbital margin and across the upper portion of the maxillary sinus and pterygoid plates to the pterygopalatine fossa. Fractures of the cribriform plate and roof of the ethmoid cells (with spinal fluid rhinorrhea) and damage to the lacrimal system may occur with this fracture. Because the fracture segment is mobile, it has been termed a "floating maxilla."

FIGURE 7.13. *Le Fort classification of midfacial fractures.*

On each skull the numeral 1 indicates Le Fort I fracture; the numeral 2, Le Fort II; the numeral 3, Le Fort III.

a. Anterior ethmoid foramen
b. Posterior ethmoid foramen
c. Optic canal
d. Superior orbital fissure
e. Inferior orbital fissure
f. Lacrimal fossa
g. Nasal septum
h. Nasal bone
i. Infraorbital foramen
j. Nasal spine

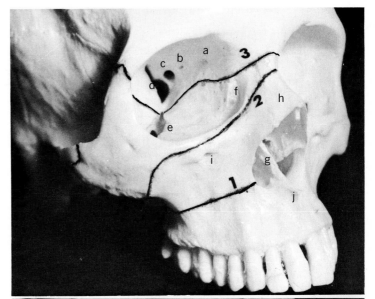

a. External auditory canal
b. Glenoid fossa
c. Lateral pterygoid plate
d. Lacrimal fossa
e. Nasal spine
f. Infraorbital foramen

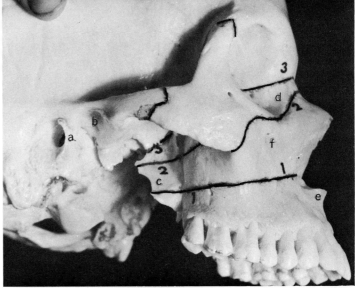

a. Foramen magnum
b. Middle turbinate
c. Inferior turbinate
d. Nasal septum
e. Base of pterygoid process
f. Medial pterygoid plate
g. Lateral pterygoid plate
h. Zygomatic process of temporal bone
i. Malar bone

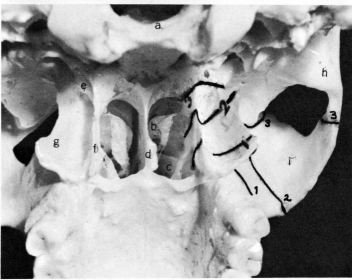

The Le Fort III fracture (craniofacial disjunction) is a complete separation of the facial bones from their cranial attachments. The fracture line extends across the nasofrontal suture, along the ethmoid junction with the frontal bone, through the superior orbital fissure, and across the lateral wall of the orbit, the zygomaticofrontal suture, and the temporozygomatic suture. A high fracture of the pterygoid plates is usually present. The Le Fort III fracture is most often comminuted producing the "dish-face" deformity. It is commonly associated with intracranial complications such as spinal fluid leaks via the roof of the ethmoid cells and the cribriform plate.

Specific Treatment

Le Fort I (Fig. 7.13). Stable fractures of the lower midface which are not displaced can be treated by using a snug barrel-type dressing. This treatment is effective even when the patient is edentulous and wears dentures. In such cases the maxillary dental plate is applied and adjusted so that it is in occlusion with either the mandibular teeth or the lower denture. Stabilization is carried out for 2 days by using a barrel-type dressing. The patient is placed on a liquid diet for 2 weeks. At the end of this period the fracture is usually well healed.

When occlusion is perfect and the fracture segment does not move with palpation, the barrel-type bandage may be omitted. The patient, however, should be placed on a liquid diet for a period of 2 weeks.

Intermaxillary fixation must be employed when dental occlusion is not perfect. The technique of establishing this arch bar fixation is discussed under the section on mandibular fracture (Figs. 7.24, 7.25, and 7.26). After satisfactory occlusion is thus obtained, the inevitable downward drift of the maxillary fracture segment, which has been ligated to the mobile mandibular arch, is prevented by internal wire suspension of the fragment to the first available stable osseous structure superiorly. A #24- or #25-gauge stainless steel wire passed from arch bar to pyriform margin anteriorly and from arch bar to zygomatic arch posteriorly will usually provide the necessary support. The pyriform margin is approached through an incision anteriorly in the gingivolabial sulcus, and the wire, having been passed through a drill hole in the stable osseous margin of the pyriform aperture, is ligated to the anterior aspect of the maxillary arch bar. To pass the wire around the zygomatic arch, a percutaneous technique, using a spinal needle or Dingman wire passer in a manner similar to that utilized for circumferential wiring of the mandible (Fig. 7.30), is employed. As an alternative to suspension from the preceding sites, internal wires may be passed through the infraorbital rims or zygomaticofrontal sutures and ligated inferiorly to the maxillary arch bar. For anterior suspension, a small skin incision is made over the infraorbital rim, and a long segment of #24- or #25-gauge stainless steel wire is inserted through a drill hole in the rim. Both ends of this wire are inserted into a Dingman wire passer, which has been passed from the rim incision to the ipsilateral labial sulcus, coursing along the front face of the maxilla. As the wire passer is withdrawn, the ends of the wire are delivered into the oral cavity through the labial sulcus puncture site. One end is passed on each side of the maxillary arch bar, and, with the maxillary fracture segment held in reduction, the ends are twisted together until tight. For posterior support the wire passer is passed from the zygomaticofrontal suture, medial to the zygomatic arch, and into the posterior aspect of the ipsilateral buccal sulcus. A long wire placed through a drill hole at the suture is then led through the wire passer into the mouth as described previously. It is ligated to the posterior aspect of the arch bar after reduction of the maxillary fragment (Fig. 7.14). Although the Dingman wire passer is utilized in the preceding examples, a #18-gauge spinal needle can also be used. In the latter case, however, care must be given to properly direct

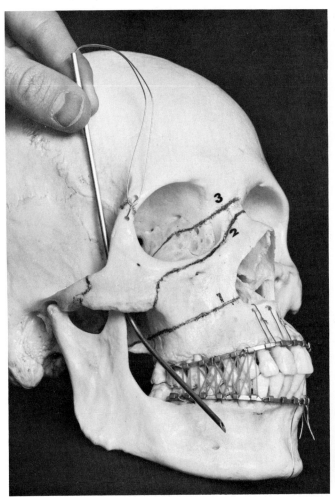

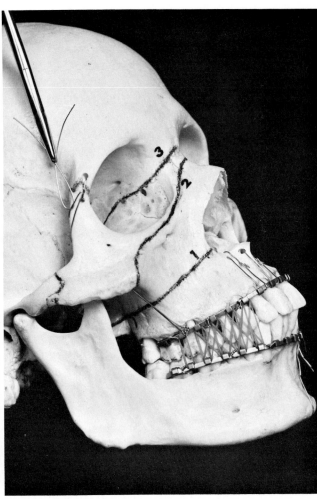

a   b

FIGURE 7.14. *Midface fracture—internal wire suspension.*

As in Figure 7.13, the numeral 1 indicates Le Fort I; 2, Le Fort II; 3, Le Fort III.

a. Both ends of a long segment of #25-gauge stainless steel wire are inserted through a drill hole or wire in the zygomaticofrontal region and into a Dingman wire passer. The latter instrument has been inserted through the temporal fascia, at the operative site, and directed into the ipsilateral buccal sulcus, coursing medial to the zygomatic arch. The wire passer, having no handle or hub, is then removed via the oral cavity, leaving the ends of the wire protruding through the puncture site of the buccal sulcus.

b. One end of the wire is placed medial to the maxillary arch bar and the other lateral to it. After reduction of the fracture, the ends of the wire are twisted until tight against the arch bar.

A second segment of wire may be passed through the loop of the suspension wire (at the zygomaticofrontal suture) and left in place, just deep to the skin incision. At the end of the period required for fixation of the fracture, the suspension wire is disconnected from the arch bar. Under local anesthesia of the zygomaticofrontal site, the suspension wire is removed by making a small incision and grasping the pull-out wire which has been placed through its upper loop.

the instrument so as to allow removal of the needle "hub first" and yet deliver the wire end(s) to the desired location. The spinal needle must be passed from an intra- to an extraoral direction, while the Dingman wire passer can be inserted in a similar or opposite direction and, lacking a hub, still be withdrawn from the intraoral site.

Loose teeth should be considered. Most often a loose tooth, unless very unstable, will become fixed in place without treatment. If a tooth is very loose, it is wired to adjacent teeth with a #26-gauge stainless steel wire. A dental arch bar is applied and wired in place to stabilize a number of loose teeth when fractured segments of alveolus occur. In the latter instance it is necessary also to apply a mandibular arch bar and elastics for intermaxillary fixation to assure proper dental occlusion.

On occasion there is loss of a portion of the maxillary alveolus with exposure of the maxillary sinus. This condition must be treated as an oroantral fistula (Chapter 6). A packing in the maxillary sinus with its end protruding into the nasal cavity through a nasoantral window is essential in these cases.

A fractured alveolar segment in an edentulous patient may be handled in one of the following ways:

1. A good reduction and positioning of the segment may be accomplished by inserting the dentures and securing immobilization with a barrel-type bandage.
2. The fracture line is exposed and the segment is fixed in place by direct wiring.
3. The alveolar segment may be fixed by inserting a Kirschner wire after proper repositioning of the fractured segment.

Vertical Fractures with Le Fort I. In a vertical fracture associated with a lower midfacial fracture, if no displacement is present, no specific therapy is necessary. When the vertical fracture line is either separated or displaced and the patient has upper teeth, one side of the arch bar is applied and wired in place, and the vertical fracture is reduced. The opposite side of the arch bar is then wired in place. If the teeth are widely separated in the anterior midline, they should be wired together before the dental arch bars are applied. The application of a mandibular arch bar and intermaxillary fixation are necessary to ensure normal dental occlusion.

Direct exposure of the fracture line and wiring of the fragments is the treatment of choice when confronted with a vertical fracture in which there is displacement and the patient's upper jaw is edentulous. A Kirschner wire may be used to pin a unilateral segment (produced by a unilateral Le Fort I terminating near the midline, in a vertical fracture) to the stable opposite side. If bilateral segments are present, each may be pinned to the opposite zygoma.

Le Fort II Fracture (Fig. 7.13). In the Le Fort II fracture, undisplaced and stable fragments are treated conservatively as has been described for Le Fort I fractures. A superiorly displaced segment is rocked loose and pulled inferiorly. Downward traction and restoration of normal dental occlusion can be accomplished by intermaxillary fixation with arch bars and elastics. Internal wire suspension is required as described previously.

In a unilateral Le Fort II fracture, immobilization can be secured with a Kirschner wire directed through the unstable fragment and into the stable opposite side.

A Le Fort II fracture in which the segments are displaced downward is much less stable and much more difficult to manage. It is approached by direct wiring of the infraorbital margin fracture and the application of dental arch bars and internal suspension wires (Fig. 7.14).

Le Fort III Fracture (Fig. 7.13). It is difficult to outline specific methods for reduction and fixation of the Le Fort III fracture, for they are usually comminuted and associated with other facial fractures. The general principles are to secure good occlusion by intermaxillary fixation and to immobilize the fracture by internal wire suspension and direct wiring of component displaced fractures. Careful assessment of these patients and appropriate application of the various techniques mentioned previously usually assure satisfactory healing.

FRACTURES OF THE ORBIT

As with midfacial fractures, the incidence of orbital fractures tends to vary directly with the incidence of motor vehicle accidents. This incidence has generally increased yearly, with the exception of 1973 and 1974 when a gasoline shortage resulted in a slower maximum speed limit. The advent of seat belts has contributed to more frequent preservation of life in severe collisions but, in so doing, has presented the maxillofacial surgeon with an increased number of severe facial fractures in patients who otherwise would have become mortality statistics. Vehicular accidents cause approximately 50% of orbital fractures. The human fist accounts for about 20%, while a ball, elbow, or fall combine to account for about 25%. The remaining 5% are due to various unusual accidents.

Anatomy

In order to understand the pathophysiology of the orbital fracture, certain anatomic relationships must be studied. The lateral wall of the orbit is formed by the frontal process of the zygomatic bone and the greater wing of the sphenoid bone. This wall is relatively thick and quite sturdy. The orbital process of the frontal bone forms the roof of the orbit, also a durable structure. The medial wall is formed by the lacrimal bone and the lamina papyracea of the ethmoid bone. As its name implies, the lamina papyracea is quite thin, but it is well supported by the many osseous ethmoid cell partitions. The floor of the orbit is formed by the orbital processes of the maxillary and zygomatic bones and extends posterosuperiorly on an inclined plane. A very thin area of bone is located immediately anterior to the inferior orbital fissure. The orbital floor is further weakened by the canal through which the infraorbital nerve passes.

Due to the conical shape of the orbit, a blow from an anterior position will displace the orbit's contents posteriorly, resulting in the blowout type of fracture. According to Jones and Evans, this type usually occurs in the thin area just anterior to the inferior orbital fissure and medial to the infraorbital canal or groove, although it may occur in other areas of the floor as well.

Blowout fractures must occur by the preceding mechanism and are to be distinguished from the orbital floor fractures which occur as the posterior components of orbital margin fractures. Rarely, the medial orbital wall or orbital roof may be the site of fracture (see reports by Edwards and Riley and by McClurg and Swanson).

Signs and Symptoms of Orbital Fracture

Enophthalmos. Fracture of the orbit may result in varying degrees of enoph-thalmos, which is disfiguring when in excess of 5 mm. It may not be apparent immediately after the injury because of edema or hemorrhage. As would be suspected from knowledge of the anatomy of the orbit, numerous mechanisms or combinations thereof are responsible for the finding:

1. There may be an escape of orbital fat into the maxillary sinus accompany-ing the fracture of the floor of the orbit. This situation may occur with the comminuted fracture or the hinged, or so-called "trapdoor," fracture. In some instances the maxillary sinus has been found to be filled with this orbital fat.
2. The inferior rectus or inferior oblique muscles may herniate into the antrum and be entrapped by bony fragments in a blowout fracture. This occurrence may tether the ocular globe in a retrodisplaced position.
3. Atrophy of orbital fat may occur subsequent to contusion or infection. This condition decreases the volume of soft tissue within the fixed volume of the bony orbit, allowing retrocession of the globe.
4. Enophthalmos may also occur as a result of fracture and downward displacement of a large segment of the orbital floor. This complication expands the volume of the bony orbit, with a fixed quantity of soft tissue within, allowing the globe to recede posteroinferiorly. When this fracture accompanies a fracture-dislocation of the infraorbital margin, it is usually associated with more complex fractures of the maxilla and/or zygoma.

Exophthalmos. Occasionally, the orbital floor is fractured and displaced upward, causing exophthalmos. In such fractures, the infraorbital rim is usually involved. The force causing this type of fracture has been applied over the anterior wall of the maxillary sinus, just inferior to the infraorbital margin. The margin with its attached orbital plate is thus shifted so as to displace the latter upward, reduce the volume of the osseous orbit, and consequently force the soft tissues and globe anteriorly.

Diplopia. Disturbance in ocular motility is a relatively common finding in patients with fracture of the floor of the orbit, because the most common site of the blowout type fracture is in that portion of the floor which is weakened by the infraorbital canal or groove. The inferior oblique muscle arises from the orbital floor near the lateral margin of the upper aperture of the nasolacrimal canal, and the inferior rectus muscle is located, in direct relation with the infraorbital canal, on the inferior aspect of the orbital contents.

The inferior oblique and inferior rectus muscles are those involved with disturbances in oculomotor function associated with fractures of the orbital floor. The site of fracture and entrapment of these muscles has much to do with the clinical picture. If the muscle is entrapped anterior to the equator of the globe (Fig. 7.15a), the involved eye will be fixed in a downward position. The oculomotor imbalance will not be obvious with downward gaze but becomes much exaggerated with upward gaze. If the muscle is entrapped posterior to the equator of the globe, the involved eye will be fixed in the elevated position. In this case, the oculomotor imbalance may be unapparent with upward gaze and exaggerated with downward gaze (Fig. 7.15b). If the inferior rectus muscle is entrapped at the level of the

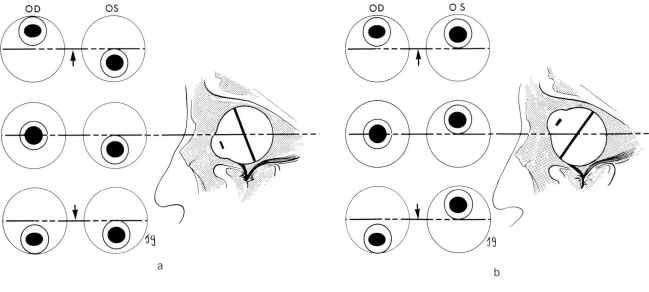

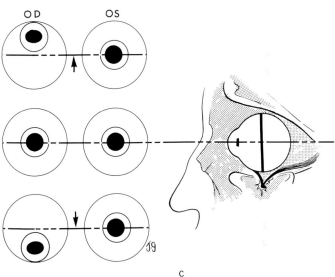

FIGURE 7.15. *Disturbance of oculomotor function due to fracture of orbital floor. (From Aiello, L. M., and Myers, E. N.: Blow-out Fracture of the Orbital Floor. Arch. Otolaryng. 82:638–648 [Dec.] 1965.)*

a. Vertical gaze imbalance with the left inferior rectus muscle entrapped anterior to the equator of the globe.

b. Vertical gaze imbalance with the left inferior rectus muscle entrapped posterior to the equator of the globe.

c. Vertical gaze imbalance with the left inferior rectus muscle entrapped at the equator of the globe.

equator of the globe, the involved eye will appear normal in the primary position but will remain fixed when downward or upward gaze is attempted (Fig. 7.15c). In fractures of the orbital floor lateral to the infraorbital canal, oculomotor function is rarely affected.

The branch of the oculomotor nerve supplying the inferior rectus muscle courses along the upper surface of this muscle before entering it at the junction of its posterior and middle thirds. The branch to the inferior oblique muscle follows the lateral border of the inferior rectus muscle to the point where the two muscles cross and then penetrates the ocular surface of the former muscle. Injury to these branches of the third cranial nerve, especially the inferior oblique branch, can be associated with orbital floor fractures, and the manifestations of such injury must be differentiated from those due to muscle entrapment. This discrimination is most easily accomplished with the forced duction test (traction test) discussed later. Dysfunction of an extraocular muscle due to laceration, avulsion from its origin or insertion, or muscle contusion and hemorrhage must also be considered as possible causes for diplopia.

Transient diplopia may be associated with fracture and dislocation of the zygoma. It is most commonly seen when the bone has been displaced as a single fragment. The causes are hemorrhage and edema which produce superior displacement of the globe.

Facial Asymmetry. This finding is not usual in patients with a blowout fracture of the orbital floor. It is typical, however, when the fracture involves the infraorbital margin or when fracture-dislocation of the zygoma occurs.

Sensory Nerve Injury. Hypesthesia or anesthesia of the sensory area of distribution of the infraorbital nerve may be associated with fracture of the floor of the orbit. When present, this sign implies fracture involvement of the infraorbital canal. Furthermore, disturbance in the function of the infraorbital nerve associated with an intact orbital rim is strongly suggestive of a blowout type of orbital floor fracture, again with involvement of the infraorbital groove or canal. Prolonged anesthesia of the infraorbital nerve is a positive indication for exploration and decompression of the nerve.

Ocular Complications. Many ocular complications can occur in association with orbital fracture:

1. Subconjunctival hemorrhage and periorbital ecchymosis are the usual findings following blunt trauma to the orbit. They are transient and only rarely complicated by cicatricial entropion.
2. Corneal abrasion may occur, but is not common because of reflex closure of the lids at the time of injury.
3. Injury to the pupil and iris may produce mydriasis or iridodialysis.
4. The lens may be dislocated anteriorly or posteriorly; this situation can be further complicated by anterior uveitis, secondary glaucoma, or corneal edema.
5. Hyphema (hemorrhage into the anterior chamber of the eye) is not uncommon in this type of injury. It usually clears spontaneously but may be complicated by secondary glaucoma, corneal pigmentation, or heterochromia of the iris.
6. Glaucoma may well be the most common chronic sequela to orbital injury producing a fracture. The increased intraocular pressure may not occur for weeks or even years after the injury.
7. Injury to the retina may be associated with fracture of the floor of the orbit. Edema of the retina is common and usually transient.

Diagnosis

In a fracture of the floor of the orbit with a resultant disturbance in ocular motility, infraorbital nerve injury, enophthalmos, facial asymmetry, or other complication, diagnosis is not difficult. On the other hand, this fracture can be overlooked when it is associated with devastating bodily injuries that require immediate lifesaving measures. Also, the symptoms can be masked by edema, ecchymosis, or hematoma. On occasion, the defect may not become apparent for a number of weeks after the initial injury.

Certainly a patient with a history of injury to the orbit, a unilateral enophthalmos, disturbance of eye muscle function, and anesthesia or hypesthesia of the infraorbital nerve, associated with an intact orbital rim, should be considered to have a blowout fracture of the orbit. A break in the continuity of the orbital margin further elucidates the pathology.

Entrapment of the inferior oblique or inferior rectus muscle (Fig. 7.15) is suggested by an abnormal version test in the vertical plane. The diagnosis is confirmed by the forced duction test (traction test), which is carried out as follows:

The conjunctiva is anesthetized with a drop of topical anesthetic solution.

The conjunctiva and the tendon of the inferior rectus are then grasped with fine-toothed Bishop-Harmon forceps, and gentle superior rotation is attempted. Entrapment of the muscle is demonstrated by a restriction of ocular excursion. The test is repeated for all the cardinal positions of gaze to rule out entrapment of the other extraocular muscles as well (Fig. 7.16).

Radiographs are of extreme value in diagnosing fractures of the floor of the orbit (Fig. 7.17). The Waters' view gives a good picture of the contour of the floor of the orbit and rim in relation to the maxillary sinus. The Caldwell view also demonstrates the floor of the orbit. The typical finding is that of depression and fragmentation of the floor of the orbit with prolapse of orbital contents into the antrum. A maxillary sinus completely opacified by blood may mask these findings. A fracture may also occur in the lamina papyracea of the ethmoid bone, producing radiographic findings of subcutaneous emphysema or air in the orbit. Anteroposterior laminograms of the orbit provide the ultimate radiographic information in diagnosing orbital floor fractures.

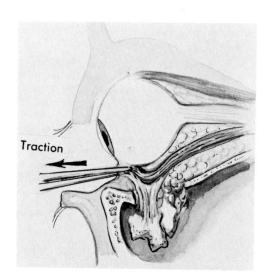

FIGURE 7.16. *Traction tests. (From Converse, J. M., Smith, B., Obear, M. F., and Wood-Smith, D.: Orbital Blowout Fractures: A Ten-Year Survey. Plast. Reconstr. Surg. 39:20–36, 1967.)*

a. The forced duction test. The tendon of the inferior rectus muscle is grasped with a tooth forceps. Entrapment is demonstrated by reduction of upward ocular excursion.

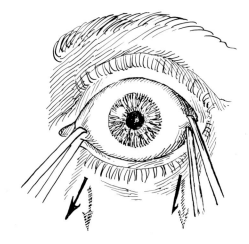

b. The forward traction test. Two forceps grasp the medial and lateral recti muscles and exert a forward traction on the eyeball. Freedom of forward displacement of the orbital contents is a favorable prognostic sign for the correction of enophthalmos by orbital implants; resistance to forward traction is a poor prognostic sign.

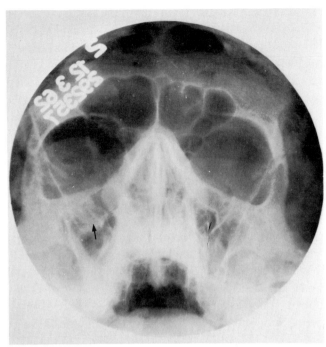
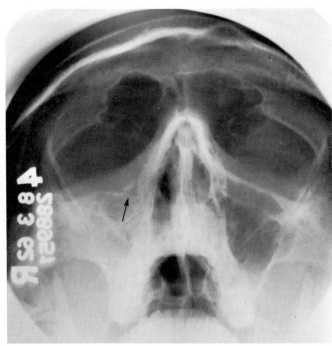

a   b

FIGURE 7.17. *Fracture of floor of orbit.*

a. There is evidence of a blow-out fracture on the right side as well as evidence of soft-tissue herniation into the right maxillary sinus from the orbit. Air is present in the soft tissues of the right orbit.

b. This x ray demonstrates a fracture of the medial aspect of the infraorbital rim associated with a blow-out fracture. Medial displacement of the paper plate of the right ethmoid was also present in this patient.

Treatment

Indications for surgical treatment of orbital floor fracture are (1) the presence of enophthalmos; (2) a disturbance in the eye muscle function manifested by diplopia; (3) facial deformity; and/or (4) a persistent anesthesia in the distribution of the infraorbital nerve.

Surgery is performed with the patient under general anesthesia. The patient's entire face is prepared so the surgeon may have access to the floor of the orbit by way of the antrum as well as through an infraorbital incision. The face is draped, leaving both sides exposed so the normal side can be used for comparison.

The degree of enophthalmos is determined by comparison with the unaffected orbit. The ocular motility is tested by forced duction for each of the extraocular muscles, and these findings are compared with the freedom of motion of the opposite normal side.

Fracture of the floor of the orbit, especially when the patient is treated within 2 or 3 weeks of injury, can quite often be satisfactorily reduced by way of the maxillary sinus. The anterior wall of the maxillary sinus is exposed by using a Caldwell-Luc incision. The periosteum is elevated from the entire front face of the maxillary sinus, so the infraorbital nerve and foramen may be examined. The size and contour of the maxillary antrum are determined by viewing the radiographs.

The intact anterior wall is carefully removed with a small cutting bur so it can be used, if necessary, as an autogenous bone graft to the floor of the orbit. Sufficient exposure is necessary for viewing the orbital floor from below and, also, for the insertion of a finger for palpation of the fracture.

Prior to reduction of the fracture with a finger in the maxillary sinus, it is useful to reduce the enophthalmos from above by using traction sutures of #4-0 silk passed around the tendons (Fig. 7.18) of the superior and inferior rectus muscles. This technique has two results: (1) it will usually free an entrapped muscle, and (2) it provides additional space for replacement of the orbital contents and elevation of the floor of the orbit. In most instances, when the orbital contents are replaced and the fracture reduced, the orbital contents and floor remain in place. Whether or not the orbital floor remains in good position, the antrum should be packed. This procedure is a requisite especially when the fracture is associated with discontinuity of the orbital rim or a depressed malar fracture. If the presence of vertically aligned bone fragments is likely, it is preferable to expose the orbital floor from above and provide ocular protection during reduction and packing. A layer of Gelfoam is placed against the roof of the antrum so that the packing will not become adhered to or involved with bone spicules. The entire antrum is packed with antibiotic-impregnated gauze, the end of which projects into the nasal cavity through a nasoantral window. The Caldwell-Luc incision is sutured in the usual fashion.

The infraorbital approach to the floor of the orbit is used in those cases in which reduction is not readily attained by the inferior approach and when an associated orbital rim fracture necessitates open reduction and wire fixation. The incision for this approach is made in the natural skin fold of the lower lid, approximately 3 mm below the margin of the tarsal plate. It is extended obliquely down-

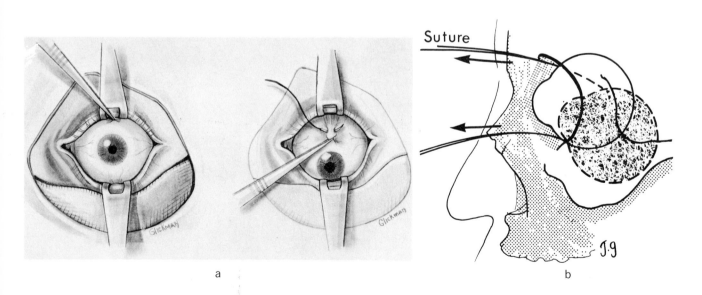

a   b

FIGURE 7.18. *Reduction of enophthalmos. (From Aiello, L. M., and Myers, E. N.: Blowout Fracture of the Orbital Floor. Arch. Octolaryng. 82:638–648 [Dec.] 1965.)*

a. Technique of forced duction of the extraocular muscles (left). Technique for inserting traction sutures (right).

b. Traction moves the globe anteriorly out of the orbit, providing space for reduction of orbital contents.

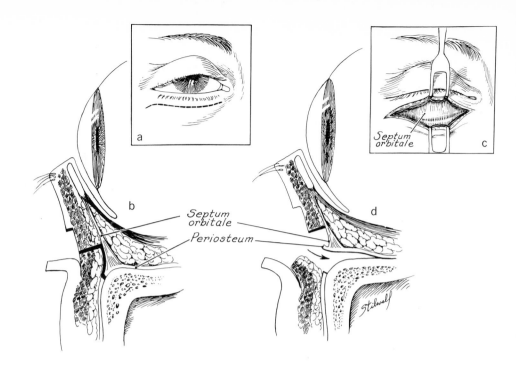

FIGURE 7.19. *Technique of exposure of the floor of the orbit. (From Converse, J. M., Cole, G., and Smith, B.: Late Treatment of Blow-out Fracture of the Floor of the Orbit. A Case Report. Plast. Reconstr. Surg. 28:2:183–191 [Aug.] 1961.)*

a. Outline of skin incision.

b. The skin is raised from the orbicularis oculi muscle, the muscle fibers are separated at a lower level, and the septum orbitale is followed down to the orbital rim.

c. The septum orbitale has been exposed; this structure is the guide to the orbital rim.

d. The periosteum is incised along the inferior orbital rim and elevated from the floor of the orbit.

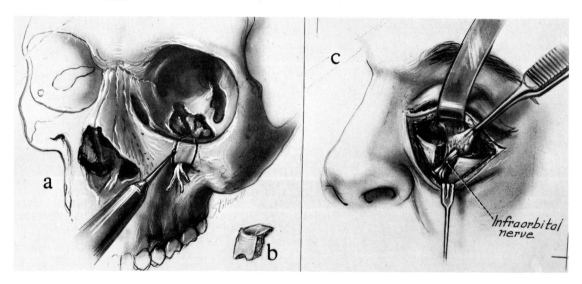

FIGURE 7.20. *Decompression and identification of the infraorbital nerve. (From Converse, J. M., Smith, B., Obear, M. F., and Wood-Smith, D.: Orbital Blowout Fractures: A Ten-Year Survey. Plast. Reconstr. Surg. 39:1:20–36 [Jan.] 1967.)*

a. When difficulty is encountered in dissecting the infraorbital nerve in the orbital fracture area, the nerve is exposed at the infraorbital foramen, and a section of bone is outlined for removal in order to uncover the infraorbital canal.

b. Block of bone removed and set aside for later replacement.

c. The infraorbital nerve is traced back to the blow-out fracture and dissected from the orbital contents. The block of bone illustrated in b is then replaced.

ward in its lateral portion (Fig. 7.19a) to avoid a "trap door" scar deformity. The skin is elevated from the orbicularis oculi muscle for a short distance inferior to the incision (Fig. 7.19b). At this point the orbicularis oculi muscle is split longitudinally. The orbital septum is encountered and followed downward to the point where it is inserted into the infraorbital margin. The periosteum is incised along the margin and elevated from the floor of the orbit. The floor of the orbit can be gradually exposed by progressive insertion of an orbital retractor. During this procedure, a finger in the antrum often facilitates the maneuver; it aids in reducing the herniated orbital contents and replacing bony fragments. Traction on the sutures around the inferior and superior rectus muscle insertions is also helpful at this time. Any of several autogenous and alloplastic materials can be utilized to reconstitute a severely comminuted orbital floor. Among these materials are iliac bone, anterior antral wall, nasal septum, fascia lata, Teflon* and Silastic sheeting. As with any similar procedure, use of autogenous material offers the best chance for success and for avoiding complications. The iliac bone is taken from the inner aspect of the ilium. The cortical surface of the bone should face upward.

If an additional space-occupying substance is needed, especially in an old fracture with marked increase in the overall orbital volume, fascia lata may be placed superior to the bone graft in order to further support the orbital contents and eliminate the enophthalmos.

Regardless of the material selected, care must be taken to trim the implant to a size sufficient to provide the necessary support without encroaching upon the optic nerve posteriorly. When using alloplastic sheeting, a small tab cut into its anterior edge can be placed beneath the anterior edge of the orbital floor defect and thereby prevent anterior migration of the implant with eventual extrusion.

Anesthesia of the Infraorbital Nerve. If complete anesthesia occurs in the area of the infraorbital nerve distribution, and the fracture is found to involve the infraorbital canal and foramen (Fig. 7.5a), a decompression procedure (Fig. 7.20) is accomplished via the infraorbital incision. A block of bone which includes the infraorbital canal is removed. The nerve is carefully dissected and decompressed and the block of bone replaced.

FRACTURES OF THE MANDIBLE

This type of facial fracture is the most common when simple nasal fractures are excluded. This frequency is to be expected, taking into consideration the position of the jaw in relation to the remainder of the skull. Management of these fractures is most important not only for satisfactory cosmesis, but also for good dental occlusion and mastication.

Anatomy

In order to evaluate and treat a fracture of the mandible properly, knowledge of the anatomy of this bone and its surrounding structures is essential. Familiarity with the origin, insertion, and direction of pull of the various muscles of the mandible simplifies evaluation of any particular fracture with reference to its

* E. I. DuPont de Nemours & Co., Inc., Wilmington, Delaware

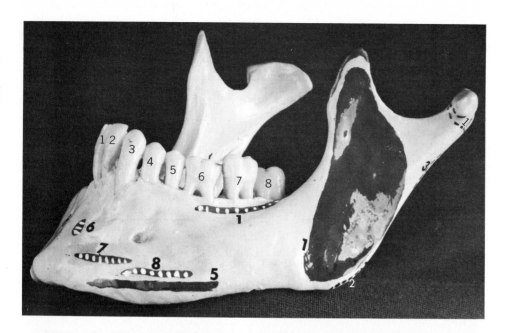

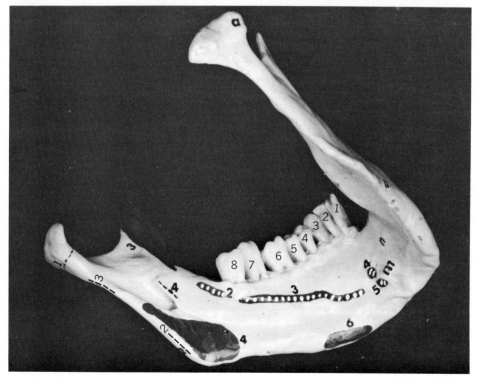

FIGURE 7.21. *The mandible.*

Ligaments (interrupted lines)
1. Temporomandibular joint capsule
2. Stylomandibular ligament
3. Temporomandibular ligament

Teeth

	1	2	3	4	5	6	7	8
erupted	½	1	2	1½	3	6	12	adult
replaced	7	8	11	9	10			

Muscles
  Origins (stippled)
1. Buccinator   7
2. Superior constrictor   10
3. Mylohyoid 5^{III}
4. Genioglossus   12
5. Geniohyoid   12
6. Mentalis   7
7. Depressor labii inferioris   7
8. Depressor anguli oris   7

Muscles
  Insertions (plain)
1. Masseter 5^{II}
2. Lateral pterygoid 5^{III}*
3. Temporalis 5^{III}*
4. Medial pterygoid 5^{III}
5. Platysma   7
6. Digastric 5^{III}

  *Insertions 2 and 3 are
shown in Fig. 7.22a).

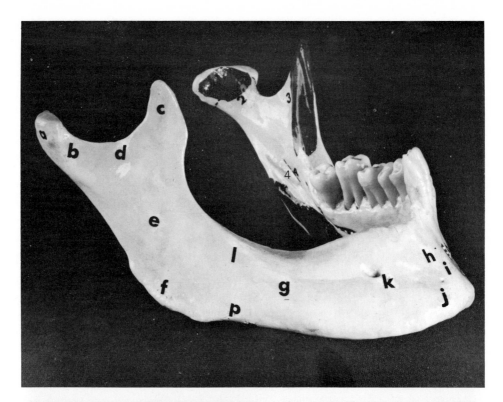

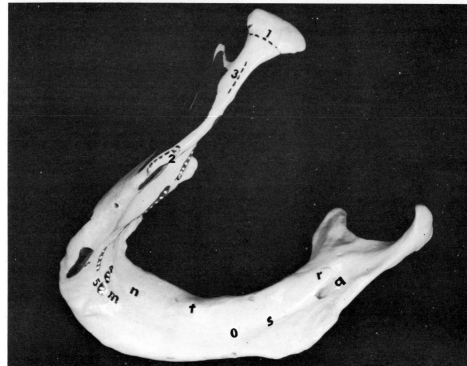

FIGURE 7.22. *The mandible.*

Ligaments
1. Temporomandibular joint capsule
2. Stylomandibular ligament
3. Temporomandibular ligament
4. Sphenomandibular ligament

Muscles

　Origins (stippled)
　　1. Buccinator　7*
　　2. Superior constrictor　10*
　　3. Mylohyoid　5^{III}*
　　4. Genioglossus　12
　　5. Geniohyoid　12
　　6. Mentalis　7*
　　7. Depressor labii inferioris　7*
　　8. Depressor anguli oris　7*

　*Origins 1 through 3, and 6
through 8 are shown in Fig. 7.21.

Landmarks
　a. Head ⎫Condyloid process
　b. Neck ⎭
　c. Coronoid process
　d. Mandibular notch
　e. Ramus
　f. Angle
　g. Body
　h. Symphysis
　i. Mental protuberance
　j. Mental tubercle
　k. Mental foramen
　l. Oblique line
　m. Sublingual fossa
　n. Genial tubercle
　o. Submandibular fossa
　p. Groove for facial artery
　q. Mandibular foramen
　r. Lingula
　s. Mylohyoid groove
　t. Mylohyoid line

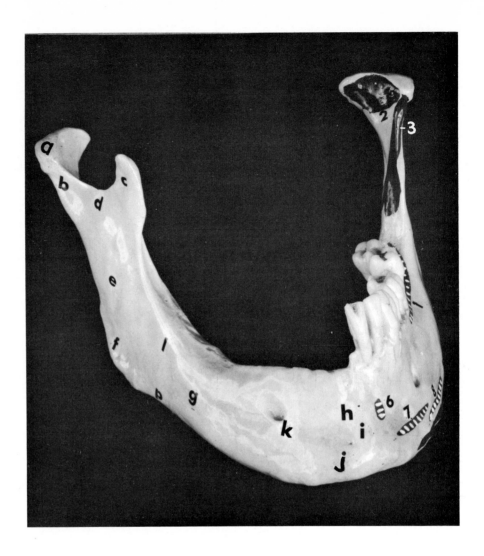

FIGURE 7.23. *The mandible.*

a. Landmarks
a. Head ⎫ Condyloid process
b. Neck ⎭
c. Coronoid process
d. Mandibular notch
e. Ramus
f. Angle
g. Body

h. Symphysis
i. Mental protuberance
j. Mental tubercle
k. Mental foramen
l. Oblique line
m. Sublingual fossa*
n. Genial tubercle*
o. Submandibular fossa*

p. Groove for facial artery*
q. Mandibular foramen*
r. Lingula*
s. Mylohyoid groove*
t. Mylohyoid line*

*Landmarks (m) through (t) are shown in Figure 7.21.

displacement, and it helps in determining the best method for reduction and immobilization.

Muscles of the Mandible (Figs. 7.21 through 7.23). Three groups of muscles provide the variety and versatility of mandibular function—the elevators, the depressors, and the protrusors. The origins and insertions of these muscles on the mandible and the various ligaments of the mandible are shown in Figures 7.21, 7.22, and 7.23.

Elevators of the Mandible. The *masseter* muscle extends from the zygomatic arch to the lateral surface of the mandible. Its insertion covers most of the lateral

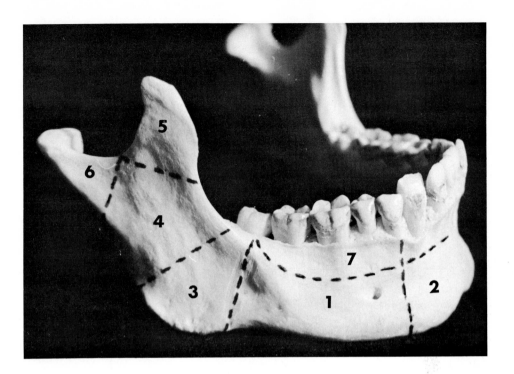

FIGURE 7.23. (Continued)

b. Dingman classification of mandibular fractures:

1. The region of the *body* is that portion of the mandible between an anterior vertical line, drawn at the interproximal plane of the cuspid and first bicuspid teeth, and a posterior line, following the anterior border of attachment of the masseter muscle (21% of mandibular fractures).

2. The *symphysis* area is that portion of the mandible between the anterior boundaries of the region of the body of each side (15% of mandibular fractures).

3. The region of the *angle* is defined as that portion of the mandible lying deep to the area of attachment of the masseter (20% of mandibular fractures).

4. The *ramus* of the mandible is that portion located below a right angle, the vertex of which is at the mandibular notch, and above the posterior border of insertion of the masseter muscle (3% of mandibular fractures).

5. The *coronoid process* is that portion above the anterior limb of the right angle which forms the anterosuperior border of the ramus (2% of mandibular fractures).

6. The *condylar process* is that portion of the mandible above the posterior limb of the right angle which is the posterosuperior border of the ramus (36% of mandibular fractures).

7. Fractures of the *alveolar process* involve the teeth and the alveolar process immediately inferior (3% of mandibular fractures).

surface of the coronoid process, ramus, and angle of the mandible. The masseter muscle elevates the mandible.

The *temporal* muscle arises in the temporal fossa, descends medial to the zygomatic arch, and inserts on the medial surface and anterior margin of the coronoid process. It both elevates and retracts the mandible.

The *medial pterygoid* muscle arises from the medial surface of the lateral pterygoid plate, the pyramidal process of the palatal bone, and a small slip from the maxillary tuberosity. It inserts on the medial and inferior surface of the ramus of the angle, below the mylohyoid groove. By exerting a force directed upward, forward, and inward, it elevates the mandible.

Depressors of the Mandible. The *geniohyoid* muscles originate from the body of the hyoid and insert, on each side of the midline, into the posteroinferior aspect of the mandible (Fig. 7.21). They pull the anterior mandible inferiorly.

The tendon joining the anterior and posterior bellies of the *diagastric* muscle is attached, but not fixed, to the hyoid bone by a pulley made of deep cervical fascia. The anterior belly inserts into the digastric fossa (Fig. 7.21) on the inner surface of the anterior mandible. The digastric muscle depresses and pulls back the anterior mandible.

Protrusors of the Mandible. The *lateral pyerygoid* muscle originates with two heads, the superior from the infratemporal surface of the greater wing of the sphenoid and the inferior from the lateral surface of the lateral pterygoid plate. It inserts into the articular capsule and disk of the temporomandibular joint (primarily the superior head) and into the pterygoid fovea on the condylar neck (primarily the inferior head). It pulls the condyle forward and medially, the lowermost fibers exerting a downward component as well. This action slides the head of the condyle forward onto the articular tubercle. Protrusion, therefore, tightens the stylomandibular and sphenomandibular ligaments so as to cause the mandible to rotate on these as a pivot point and thereby open the mouth wider.

The *mylohyoid* muscle extends from the mylohyoid line (Fig. 7.21) in a medial, inferior, and posterior direction to meet its contralateral half along the median raphe. The latter extends from the chin to the hyoid bone. This muscle does not influence mandibular function except when a fracture of the symphysis or anterior body regions occurs. Under these circumstances, it either pulls the fragments together or causes overriding of the fracture.

Diagnosis of Mandibular Fracture

The diagnosis of a fracture of the mandible is not difficult to make when there is a history of injury to the jaw, and the following signs and symptoms are present:

1. Swelling, ecchymosis, or laceration of the skin overlying the mandible or laceration of the intraoral mucous membranes.
2. Pain. Following fracture of the mandible, pain due to injury of the inferior alveolar nerve, mandibular periosteum, and soft tissues can be quite severe. Pain may also be the result of entrapment of muscle between the fragments and/or muscle spasm.
3. Anesthesia. It may occur on one side of the lower lip, the alveolar ridge, and teeth where the inferior alveolar nerve is injured or sectioned. This condition indicates a fracture of the mandibular body.
4. Tenderness elicited by either external or intraoral palpation.
5. Malocclusion. Any displacement associated with fracture of the mandible will produce at least a degree of malocclusion which is noted by the patient. The patient will not only complain that his teeth do not meet properly but also be able to indicate the site of displacement. The edentulous patient will complain that he is unable to insert his dentures and that any attempts to do so are painful.
6. Mobility and crepitation. Manipulation of the mandible will elicit mobility at the fracture site. This motion often produces crepitation. In the edentulous patient, on intraoral palpation, a ridge may be detected at the site of the fracture.
7. Malfunction. Trismus or complaints of abnormal and painful mastication are not uncommon. Interference with verbal articulation may also occur. Mandibular excursion may follow a path deviating from midline.

8. Impairment of airway. Severe fracture of the mandible with displacement, trismus, hematoma, and edema of the soft tissues renders the patient unable to cope with his salivary secretions and bleeding. This problem can lead to complete upper airway obstruction, necessitating an emergency tracheotomy.

9. Drooling. This condition results from reflex hypersecretion by the salivary glands coupled with the patient's inability to swallow effectively.

10. Distortion of normal facial symmetry. Other than the soft tissue edema, disruption and displacement of the mandibular arch produce an altered facial appearance. This change may be more noticeable to the patient and his family than to the physician examining the patient for the first time.

Classification of Mandibular Fractures

The Dingman classification of mandibular fractures is both practical and simple (Fig. 7.23b). The mandible is divided into seven regions: body, symphysis, angle, ramus, coronoid process, condylar process, and alveolar process. The management of fractures of each of these areas will be discussed separately.

General Treatment of Mandibular Fractures

For the proper management of the mandibular fracture, certain factors and principles must be observed. Usually the patient can describe the severity, direction, and force of the blow that caused the fracture. This information is of value in determining the site and severity of the bone injury.

Whether or not there is displacement of the fractured bone must be determined. The site of the fracture can be ascertained roughly by palpation but more accurately with appropriate radiographs. With regard to mandibular injury the following x-ray projections should be obtained: posteroanterior, lateral, modified Towne's, right and left lateral oblique, inferosuperior intraoral occlusal of parasymphysial area, and tomography of the temporomandibular joints (if indicated).

The direction of the fracture line is often important. For example, in a fracture in the region of the body and extending downward and forward from the posterior alveolus, the segments are relatively stable and are not likely to be displaced because of muscular action. This is termed a favorable fracture. On the other hand, a fracture in the same region extending downward and posteriorly from the posterior alveolus is unstable and quite apt to be displaced by muscular action; hence, it is an unfavorable fracture.

The bevel of a fracture is also a determinant of favorability. If the edges of the bone in a fracture are beveled in an anteromedial direction, the posterior segment will be displaced medially and the fracture is unfavorable. If they are beveled in the opposite direction, the mandible will be rendered stable by muscle pull and the fracture is a favorable one.

In general, with a knowledge of the origins and insertions of the muscles and ligaments attached to the mandible, along with knowledge of the location and direction of the fracture, the surgeon should be able to predict the likelihood and direction of displacement.

Less than 50% of mandibular fractures are single isolated entities; the majority occur as multiple mandibular fractures, according to Rowe and Killey. For this reason, all such patients should be thoroughly scrutinized for multiplicity of fractures, and each fracture thus found should be considered separately.

It is important to determine whether a tooth is involved in the fracture line. As a rule, the presence of teeth renders the fracture segments more stable than they would be in an edentulous mouth, particularly if teeth are present on both sides of the fracture line. On occasion a tooth may become displaced and interposed between fracture segments, making reduction difficult and necessitating the tooth's extraction.

If the patient is edentulous or partially so, it is important to learn whether he has a denture. If the denture has been broken at the time of injury, it should be repaired immediately so it can be utilized for both splinting and immobilization of the mandible.

Mandibular fractures do not necessarily require immediate reduction. It is often wise to delay several days so that other injuries may be evaluated, radiographs may be obtained as indicated, and measures may be instituted for resolving the edema and preventing infection.

Since all mandibular fractures through tooth-bearing alveolus must be considered compound, broad-spectrum antibiotic therapy is instituted along with vigorous oral hygiene. The use of a Water Pik* is of tremendous value for this purpose. Frequent oral irrigations with 1.5% hydrogen peroxide solution are also beneficial. Elevation of the patient's head by placing him in a semi-sitting position, and the application of cold compresses as soon as possible should assist in limiting the edema. Immobilization, with a barrel bandage or eyelet wires, will stabilize fragments temporarily, prevent further displacement and bleeding, and help to control muscle spasms and pain. The administration of steroids or enzymes is of unproven value.

Fractures of the Body of the Mandible (21%)

The body of the mandible is that portion delineated anteriorly by a vertical line drawn between the canine tooth and first premolar and delineated posteriorly by the anterior border of the attachment of the masseter muscle (Fig. 7.23b).

Treatment. In fractures of the body of the mandible, the segments are either stable (favorable fracture) or unstable (unfavorable fracture). In a fracture extending inferiorly and anteriorly from the molar region, the segments are relatively *stable,* and, because of muscle action, they are unlikely to be displaced. In a fracture of the body extending inferiorly and posteriorly from the molar region, the segments are likely to be *unstable* and to become displaced. Most fractures through the body of the mandible occur in patients with teeth and can be managed by closed reduction and intermaxillary fixation with arch bars and elastic traction (Figs. 7.24 through 7.26). The usual period of fixation is about 5 or 6 weeks, followed by a trial without traction, but with the bars in place, for several days. If the patient experiences no pain at the fracture site with mastication during the trial period, the bars can then be safely removed. If pain is elicited during this period,

---

* Teledyne Water Pik, Ft. Collins, Colorado

FIGURE 7.24. *Application of dental arch bars.*

a. A piece of #25-gauge stainless steel wire, approximately 6 inches long, is used to ligate each tooth to the arch bar. The wire is first inserted below the arch bar, between two teeth, in an intraoral direction (white arrow). One loop of wire is made around the neck of the tooth (a). Finally the end of the wire passes through the interdental space of the opposite side of the tooth, from an intraoral direction, exiting above the arch bar (black arrow). An alternate technique, which is simpler and faster, omits the complete loop around the neck of the tooth, allowing passage of the wire as a single loop around tooth and bar combined. The former method provides more secure fixation and is preferred for teeth with ill-defined neck regions (e.g., the cuspid teeth). The ends of the wire are crossed, grasped by a needle holder and twisted clockwise (by convention) until they are snug (tooth b). The twisted ends of the wire are cut approximately 5 mm from the arch bar and bent snugly against the arch bar so as to avoid soft tissue irritation (tooth c).

b. Prior to its application, the arch bar can be cut to a proper length so the ends can be tucked into an interdental space (black arrow) or contoured to the surface of the most distal tooth. The white arrow points to the twisted ends of the wire, which have been bent and placed securely against the arch bar.

c. A side view of the three steps (1, 2, 3) used to secure the arch bar in place.

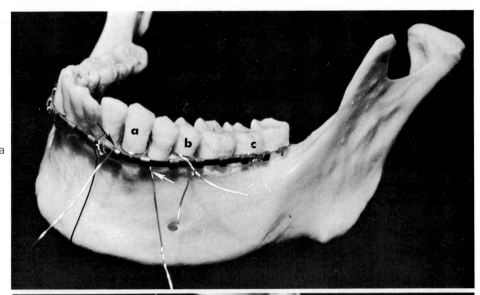

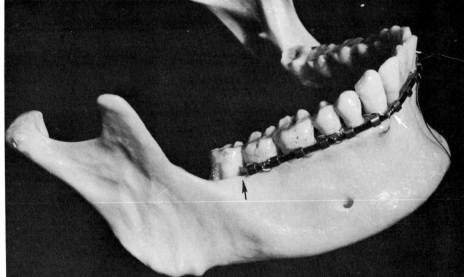

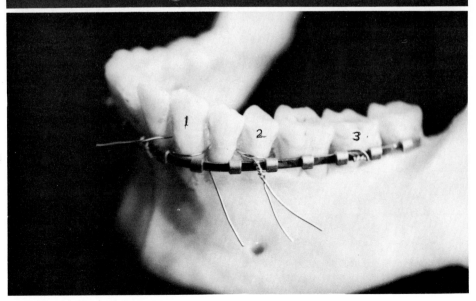

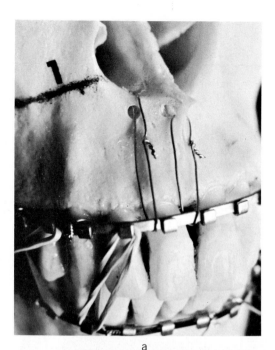

a

FIGURE 7.25. *Application of dental arch bars.*

a. If the upper incisors are missing, the anterior portion of the arch bar may be secured in place by wiring it to either the nasal spine or the rim of the piriform aperture.

b. If the lower incisors are missing, the arch bar can be secured in place by circumferential wiring to the symphysis (arrow). This technique is described in Figure 7.30.

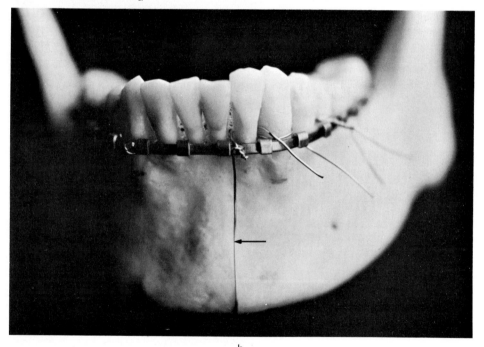

b

traction is reapplied for another couple of weeks after which another trial is made. In a stable fracture of the body of the mandible the segments can be immobilized by wiring together two teeth on each side of the fracture line (Fig. 7.27), or a single arch bar may be ligated to the mandibular teeth (monomaxillary fixation). If the fragments cannot be reduced or satisfactorily immobilized by application of an arch bar or if a large fragment of a comminuted fracture is displaced inferiorly, open reduction and inferior interosseous wiring is the treatment of choice (Fig. 7.28). If the mandible is edentulous, open reduction and superior interosseous wiring is

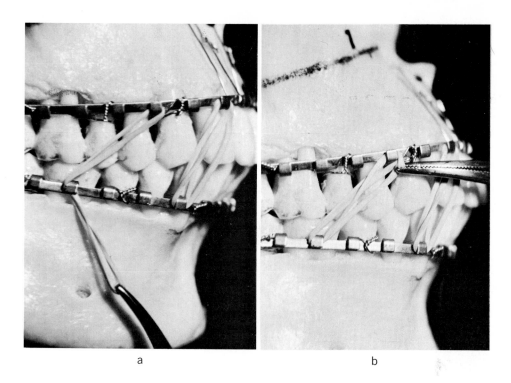

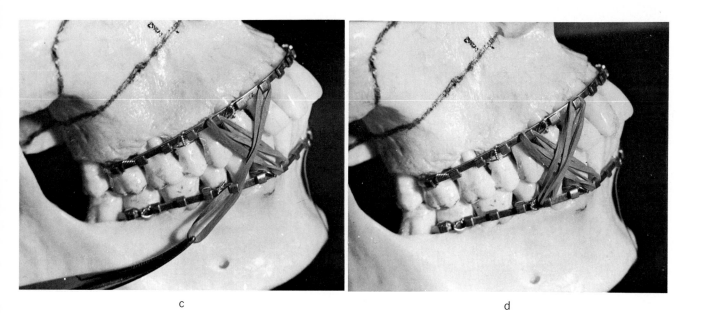

FIGURE 7.26.   *Method of applying rubber bands to the arch bars.*

a. One end of the rubber band is inserted over a hook of the upper arch bar while the other end is grasped by a mosquito hemostat. Both strands of the rubber band are looped around a hook on the opposite arch bar.

b. The end of the rubber band grasped by the hemostat is looped around the original hook in the upper arch bar.

c and d. Crisscrossing the rubber bands between the arch bars adds stability to the inter-maxillary fixation.

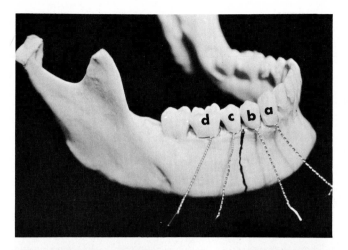

FIGURE 7.27. *Method of immobilization of a stable fracture of the mandibular body.*

a. A #25-gauge stainless steel wire is placed around two teeth on each side of the fracture line and twisted into place.

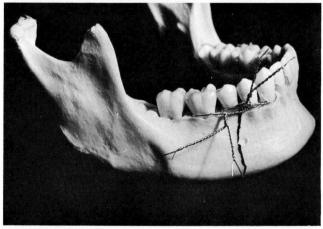

b. The wires attached to teeth (a) and (c), and the wires attached to (b) and (d) are twisted together.

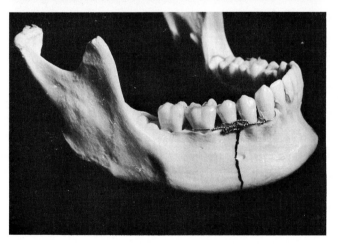

c. The resultant two twisted ends are cut at 5 mm lengths and bent inward so there is no irritation to the surrounding soft tissues.

required, with placement of the wire about 5 mm inferior to the alveolar crest, by the intraoral route (Fig. 7.29).

Considerable displacement occurs with bilateral fractures through the body of the mandible. The anterior fragments are depressed and the posterior fragments are displaced upward and medially. Bilateral open reduction, interosseous wiring (Fig. 7.30), and intermaxillary fixation are required in severe cases (Fig. 7.31). It may occasionally be necessary to use intramedullary pinning or external skeletal pin fixation to stabilize a severely comminuted fracture of the mandibular body.

FIGURE 7.28. *Interosseous wiring.*

a. A drill hole is made on each side of the fracture. A #25-gauge stainless steel wire is inserted into one drill hole, and the end is grasped on the medial aspect of the mandible and directed out through the opposite drill hole. The wires are crossed, grasped by a needle holder, and twisted tightly into place (arrow).

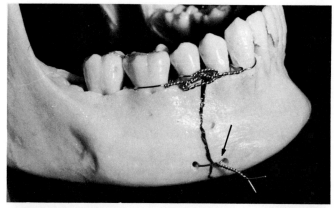

b. The twisted ends of the wire are cut at 4-mm lengths, and bent so that the ends can be inserted into one drill hole (arrow).

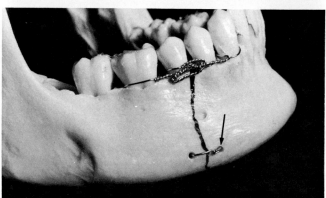

c. If the fracture of the mandibular body is unstable, then four drill holes are made. The wire is inserted into one lower drill hole and out the opposite lower drill hole. The same end of the wire is then inserted into the opposite upper drill hole and finally out through the fourth. The twisted ends of the wire are cut at 4 mm and tucked into one of the drill holes.

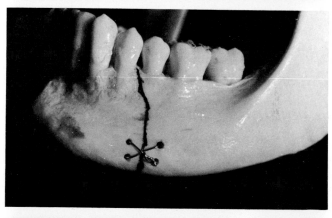

d. A fracture running from the outer to the inner aspect of the mandible, in an oblique direction, is best wired around the inferior border of the mandible through a single drill hole which includes both fragments.

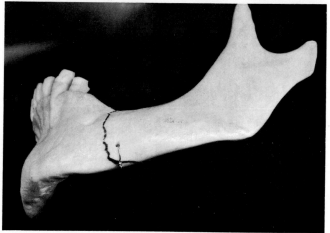

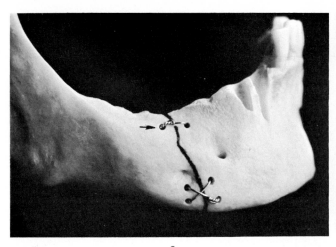

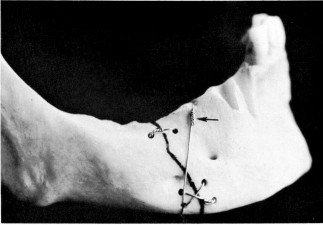

a   b

FIGURE 7.29. *Interosseous wiring in edentulous mandible.*

a. In an edentulous mandible, a fracture of the mandibular body with the fragments superiorly separated is best treated by intraoral interosseous wiring (arrow). The incision for exposure begins along the superior aspect of the lateral alveolar ridge posterior to the fracture line and continues anteroinferiorly over the body of the mandible. This provides a flap, which includes all layers over the bone, that can be reflected inferiorly and superiorly. The periosteum is elevated over the inner and outer aspect of the alveolar ridge on the side of the fracture. Drill holes are made 0.5 cm below the crest of the alveolar ridge. An elevator is placed on the inner aspect of the alveolar ridge when making the drill holes in order to avoid injury to the soft tissues. A #25-gauge stainless steel wire is inserted into one drill hole and out the other, care being taken not to injure the soft tissues. The wires are crossed, grasped with a needle holder, and twisted snugly, care being taken to avoid a loop of wire on the inner aspect of the mandible.

b. Circumferential wiring (arrow) of the mandible can be used for immobilizing and stabilizing an oblique fracture of the mandibular body (see Fig. 7.30).

Open Reduction. A 4-cm incision is made at least 1 cm below the inferior border of the mandible. The center of the incision is placed over the fracture line, and the dissection is carried through the platysma to underlying fascia. The mandibular branch of the facial nerve is superficial to this fascia and must be avoided. Usually, the facial artery and vein can be identified. These are ligated, transected, and reflected upward along with the fascia, thus preventing injury to the marginal mandibular branch of the facial nerve. The dissection is carried directly to, and through, the periosteum on the inferior border of the mandible. The periosteum is elevated medially and laterally on both sides of the fracture line. Granulation tissue, small bone fragments, and entrapped muscle must be removed from the site of the fracture.

In a fracture that follows an oblique course as it passes from the outer to the inner surface of the mandibular body, it is best to place a wire around the inferior margin of the mandible and through a single drill hole which includes both fragments (Fig. 7.28d).

In fractures without extreme obliquity from outer to inner surface, the fracture is reduced and the segments held in place by wiring through either two or four drill holes. These holes are made from 5 to 7 mm superior to the inferior border of the mandible in order to avoid the mandibular canal and inferior alveolar nerve and artery (Fig. 7.28). After twisting the wire, it is cut to a length of approximately 5 mm, bent at right angles, and tucked into one of the drill holes (Fig. 7.28b).

Interosseous wiring through four drill holes (Fig. 7.28c), in a figure-of-eight technique, is employed when the fracture segments are quite unstable.

The periosteum is carefully approximated, the subcutaneous layers are closed with #4-0 chromic catgut suture material, and the skin is closed with #5-0 monofilament synthetic suture material. A Penrose drain may be inserted if gross contamination has occurred or continued bleeding and hematoma formation are possible. In either case, postoperative antibiotic therapy is essential.

In order to accomplish a restoration of exact occlusion, intermaxillary fixation with arch bars and elastic traction is usually necessary in a patient with teeth.

In a fracture through the body of the mandible in an edentulous patient, with artificial dentures, stabilization may be attained by circumferential wiring (Figs. 7.29 and 7.30), which includes both the body of the mandible and the denture. Postoperative oral hygiene is extremely important with this type of fixation.

Intraoral Reduction of Any Edentulous Fracture. The superior aspect of the fracture site can be readily identified by the step deformity at the fracture line, which is easily palpated on the alveolar ridge. An incision is made along the superolateral aspect of the crest of the alveolar ridge posterior to the fracture line. It is continued anteriorly across the fracture and then slopes inferiorly over the lateral surface of the body of the mandible, so a flap of mucoperiosteum can be reflected inferiorly and superiorly. The periosteum is thereby elevated over the inner and outer aspect of the alveolar process on each side of the fracture. Drill holes are made 5 mm below the crest of the alveolar ridge. It is best to place an elevator medial to the mandible when making the drill holes so that the soft tissues will not be injured. A #25-gauge stainless steel wire is passed into one drill hole and out the opposite one so it can be twisted on the lateral surface of the mandible. The medial surface of the mandible must be inspected to make certain that a loop of wire does not remain there. The twisted end of the wire is cut and tucked into one of the drill holes (Fig. 7.29a). It is important to place this wire 5 mm below the alveolar crest so it will not interfere with the proper fitting of an artificial denture.

In a fracture that is extremely oblique as it runs from superior to inferior in an edentulous mandible, the fragments can be immobilized by circumferential wiring (Figs. 7.29b and 7.30).

Fractures of the Mandibular Symphysis (14%)

The portion of the mandible designated as the symphysis is the anterior region between vertical lines drawn bilaterally between the cuspids and first bicuspids. Approximately 14% of mandibular fractures occur in this area.

Treatment. Only a small percentage of these fractures occur in the exact midline because of the strength added to this area by the mental protuberance. These fractures are handled easily, for usually no displacement of the segments occurs and the fracture surfaces are held in apposition by the medially directed force of the mylohyoid muscles. A mandibular arch bar may be sufficient for immobilization, but intermaxillary fixation helps assure healing in an exact occlusal relationship.

A fracture of the region of the symphysis is usually oblique, is often accompanied by a condylar fracture, and is generally displaced (Fig. 7.32a). If the fracture is easily reduced by manipulation, intermaxillary fixation with arch bars for 5 or 6 weeks is employed. Frequently, the inferior aspect of the fracture does not respond

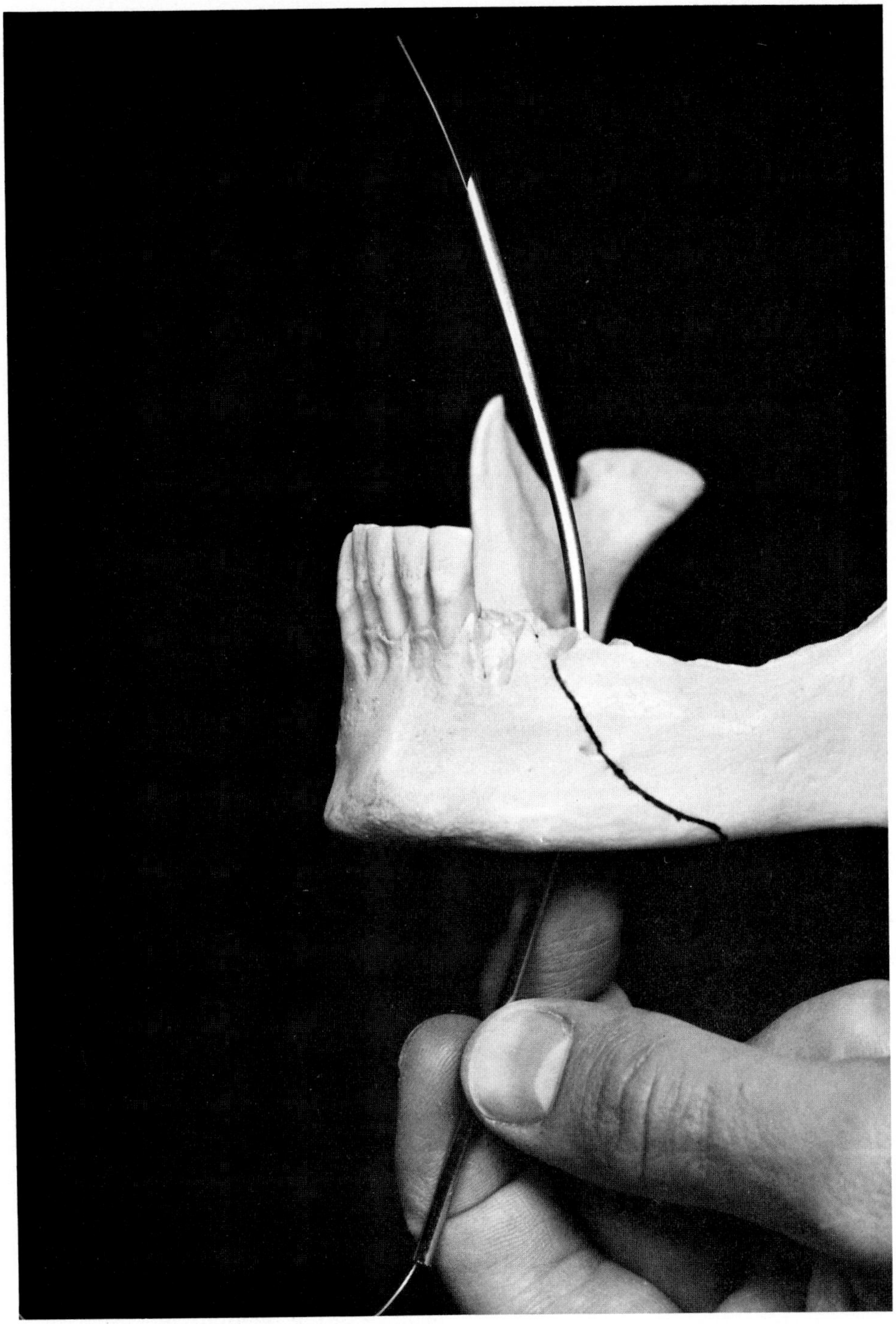

FIGURE 7.30. *Circumferential wiring of body of mandible.*

a. Circumferential wiring of the body of the mandible is accomplished by making a small stab incision just posterior to the inferior aspect of the mandibular body with a #11 scalpel blade. The incision is placed in a vertical line between the superior and inferior ends of the fracture line, which may be determined by palpation. A Dingman wire passer is inserted through the incision and along the lingual cortex of the mandible, entering the floor of the mouth adjacent to the alveolar ridge. A #25-gauge wire is threaded through the wire passer, the latter then being removed to leave the wire in place.

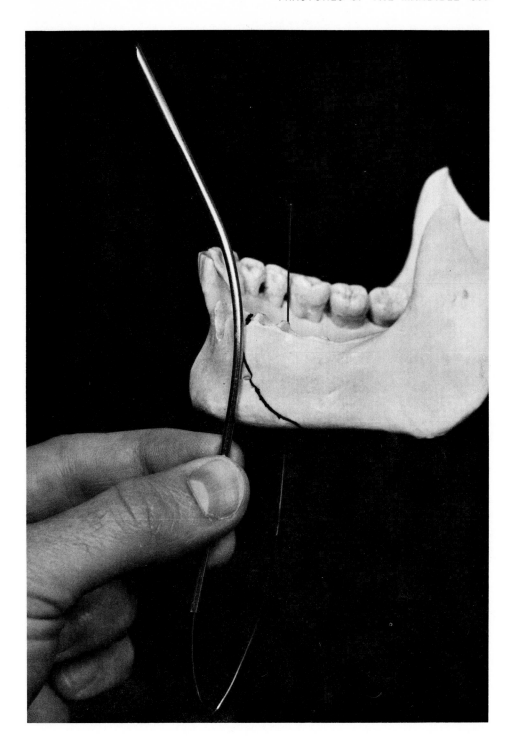

b. The wire passer is then reinserted into the same incision and directed into the buccal sulcus, coursing along the buccal cortex of the mandible. The inferior end of the #25-gauge wire is threaded through the wire passer, and the wire passer is then removed from its intraoral location, leaving this end of the wire protruding through the buccal sulcus puncture site. A small intraoral incision is made on the outer aspect of the mandible, just where the wire is to be twisted. The twisted end of the wire is bent inferiorly and tucked against the body of the mandible so that it will be covered by soft tissues (Fig. 7.29b).

If a #16-gauge spinal needle is to be substituted for the Dingman wire passer, the second pass of the needle must be from an intra- to an extraoral direction so it can be extracted via the oral cavity. The hub of the needle makes observance of this point essential.

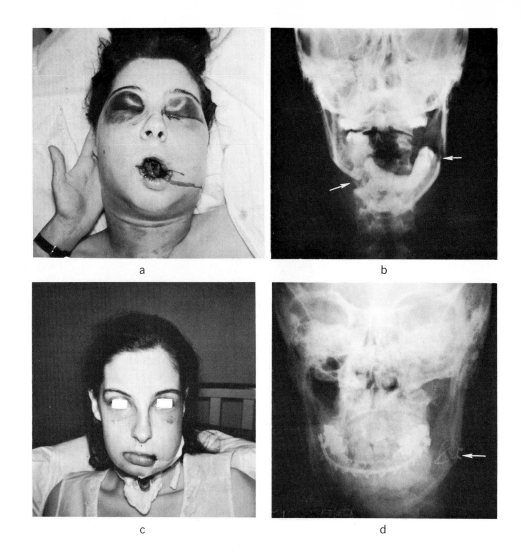

FIGURE 7.31. *Bilateral mandibular fracture.*

    a. The chin is displaced downward and inward.
    b. The two fracture lines are indicated by white arrows. Note the degree of displacement.
    c. Post-reduction photograph. The chin is again in the normal position.
    d. The fracture was reduced and the fragments stabilized by interosseous wiring and inter-maxillary fixation with a dental arch bar.

well to closed treatment and must be reduced by open technique and immobilized by interosseous wiring.

    The incision for open reduction is made 1.5 cm behind the inferior border of the mandible. This site is important, for a scar anterior to it will be quite noticeable. If there is edema and ecchymosis at the time of operation, the exact placement of this incision is difficult. Some surgeons find it easier to mark the line of incision preoperatively with the patient in the erect position.

    The incision should be about 4 cm in length and gently curved to run parallel to the mandibular contour. Dissection is carried through the platysma, directly to the inferior border of the mandible. A slight anterior retraction of the incision may be necessary for the dissection. All bleeding is controlled with electrocoagulation.

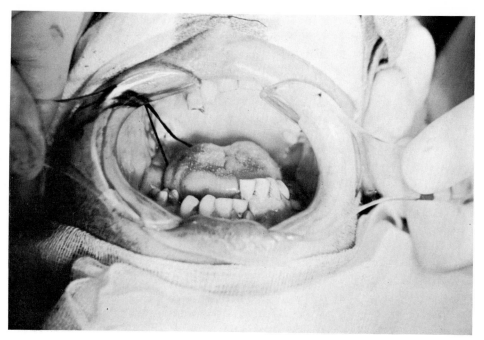

a

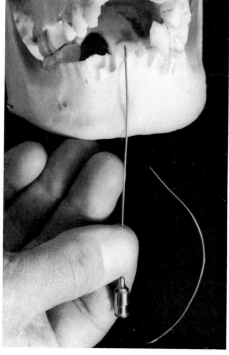

b

FIGURE 7.32. *Fracture of the mandibular symphysis with displacement.*

a. This fracture required open reduction, inferior interosseous wiring, and dental arch bar intermaxillary fixation.

b. Technique for circumferential wiring of the symphysis in the edentulous patient. Refer to Figure 7.30 for details.

As soon as the inferior border of the mandible is approached, the fracture line should be easily palpable. The periosteum of the inferior border of the mandible is incised on each side of the fracture line and then elevated anteriorly and posteriorly. In so doing, the attachment of the anterior belly of the digastric muscle is detached. The dissection is continued until both segments of the fracture are clearly viewed. Bone chips and granulation tissue are removed. Muscle that has become trapped in the fracture must be dissected free.

The fracture is reduced with bimanual manipulation and also with the aid of bone forceps. If the reduction is simple and the segments do not tend to be unstable after the reduction, a hole is drilled through the mandible on each side of the fracture line. The mandible is then wired with a #24- or #25-gauge stainless steel wire (Fig. 7.28a). The twisted end is buried in one of the drill holes (Fig. 7.28b). The wound is closed without drainage by carefully approximating all layers. Hemostasis is imperative. A course of prophylactic antibiotics is given.

If the plane of the fracture is oblique to the outer surface of the mandible, it may be best to drill a hole directly through both fragments and twist the wire below the inferior mandibular margin (Fig. 7.28d), rather than place a drill hole on each side of the fracture line. Once the open reduction and interosseous wiring have been completed, the upper and lower arch bars are applied for intermaxillary fixation.

A *fracture of the symphysis in an edentulous patient* is somewhat more difficult to stabilize, especially when the fracture line runs obliquely from superior to inferior. Four holes are drilled for a figure-of-eight wiring (Fig. 7.28c). It also may be necessary to place a wire around the entire symphysis (Fig. 7.30 and 7.32). This wiring can be accomplished by inserting the wire into a Dingman wire passer and passing the latter around one surface of the symphysis. Then, after removing the wire passer and passing it around the opposite surface of the symphysis, the inferior end of the wire is threaded into the lumen of the wire passer, which is once again extracted. The wire is twisted intraorally, anterior to the superior portion of the mandible. If a spinal needle is used in place of the Dingman wire passer (Fig. 7.32b), the same precaution, discussed under the section on midfacial fractures, should be observed for successful placement of the wire.

Mandibular Fracture in the Region of the Angle (20%)

The region of the angle is defined as that portion of the mandible lying deep to the attachment of the masseter muscle. It is not uncommon for a fracture in this region to be accompanied by a fracture of the body of the mandible on the opposite side.

If little or no displacement of the fragments occurs, intermaxillary fixation with arch bars and elastic traction is the preferred treatment. This traction remains for 5 or 6 weeks and is then tested as with body fractures. If displacement is significant, open reduction and interosseous wiring must be utilized. As a general rule, the intraoral approach is used for open reduction in the edentulous mandible and is carried out as has been described for fractures of the mandibular body.

The extraoral open reduction should be employed in patients with teeth. A 4-cm incision is made 1.5 cm below the angle of the mandible. Dissection is carried through the platysma and then superiorly, to the inferior border of the mandible. The masseter muscle is identified and incised along the inferior margin of the mandible. The underlying periosteum is likewise identified and incised, along the margin, anterior and posterior to the fracture site, and elevated from the lateral and medial surfaces of the mandibular angle for the full length of the periosteal incision. When making the drill holes, it is important to protect the soft tissues medially with a retractor or elevator. The wiring technique has already been described. Figure-of-eight wiring may be necessary when the fragments are unstable. If a molar tooth interferes with proper reduction of the fracture, it must be extracted. Intermaxillary fixation with arch bars and elastic traction may or may not be necessary following open reduction.

Mandibular Fractures in the Region of the Ramus (3%)

The ramus of the mandible is that portion above the posterior border of the insertion of the masseter muscle and below the coronoid process and neck of the mandible.

Fractures in this region are uncommon because of the thickness of this structure and the protection afforded it by the masseter, temporal, and medial pterygoid muscles. They represent only 3% of all mandibular fractures. The fragments are usually adequately treated by intermaxillary fixation for 5 or 6 weeks, much natural splinting being afforded by the attached muscles just mentioned.

Mandibular Fractures of the Coronoid Region (2%)

The coronoid process is divided from the ramus by a line extending downward and forward from the most inferior point of the mandibular notch to intersect the anterior border of the ascending portion of the mandible at an angle of about 45 degrees. Fractures through the coronoid process are quite rare and represent only 2% of all mandibular fractures. One reason for this is the good protection offered by the overlying zygomatic arch and the masseter muscle. Fractures of the coronoid process are caused either by direct trauma or by sudden contraction of the temporal muscle.

Usually fractures of the coronoid process heal uneventfully with no specific treatment. If other associated mandibular fractures occur, treatment should be in accordance with the proper management of the other fracture. In simple isolated fractures of the coronoid process, the normal occlusal relationship is generally undisturbed. Intermaxillary fixation may, however, be utilized to hasten healing and alleviate discomfort. This may be removed after 3 weeks.

Fractures of the Condylar Process of the Mandible (36%)

The condylar region is that portion of the mandible superior to, and separated from, the ramus by a line drawn posteroinferiorly from the inferior aspect of the mandibular notch and intersecting the posterior border of the ascending portion of the mandible at an angle of about 45 degrees. The condyle consists of a neck and an articular head.

Fractures in the condylar region are most often caused by indirect force, for the area is well protected by the zygomatic process and the muscles and ligaments associated with the temporomandibular joint. Force exerted in a posterior direction from sudden trauma upon the anterior mandible is transmitted along the mandibular arch to the temporomandibular joint. The weakest area is encountered at the neck of the condyle, which, consequently, is the most frequent region of the mandible to be fractured. Fractures in the condylar region represent 36% of mandibular fractures. These are generally referred to as intracapsular fractures if they involve the upper neck or head of the condyle and as subcondylar fractures if the fracture site is low on the neck of the condyle, near the junction of this region with the region of the ramus. In fractures of the condyle, the most likely displacement of the condylar fragment is in an anteromedial direction, following the pull exerted by the attached lateral pterygoid muscle. In *high fractures* (i.e., above the insertion of the lateral pterygoid), usually no displacement of the fracture fragment occurs.

Fractures in the condylar region should be suspected in patients with deviation of the mandible to one side (fractured side) when opening the mouth. This complication is caused by the loss of balanced protrusion by the lateral pterygoid muscles, the muscle on the fractured side being ineffective as a synergist with that on the unfractured side.

As a general rule, unilateral nondisplaced fractures of the condyle in adults with teeth require no specific therapy and can be managed with a soft diet and analgesics. If there is displacement, dislocation, or comminution of such a fracture, intermaxillary fixation will result in good occlusion and function. This is generally applied for 4 weeks except with bad dislocation or comminution, in which case earlier activity of the temporomandibular joint (after 2 or 3 weeks of immobilization) will do more to enhance molding of the fracture segment into a functional unit. Bilateral condylar fractures in adults with teeth should likewise be treated with intermaxillary fixation, even in nondisplaced cases.

Condylar fractures in children and in the edentulous mandible demand special consideration. In the pediatric age group, Leake, Doykos, Habal, and Murray have found increasing evidence that the best results can be obtained if no immobilization or surgical intervention is employed. In spite of severe dislocation, these condyles tend to remold and adjust until they function normally. Open or closed approaches to these fractures can only jeopardize the normal return of function that would otherwise result.

In the edentulous mandible, a unilateral fracture may be handled without immobilization, and satisfactory wearing of dentures may be expected once the pain and tenderness have resolved. In bilateral fractures, however, the mandible must be immobilized by intermaxillary fixation, using the patient's dentures to achieve a proper relationship between the alveolar processes. In these instances, extreme overriding of the fractures and a severe open bite deformity may serve as the only indication for open reduction of a condylar fracture in the acute phase. A good open reduction on one side often suffices.

Reduction of condylar fractures for the purpose of establishing intermaxillary fixation can often be achieved by first applying the arch bars and then placing the thumb upon the molar region of the fractured side(s) to exert downward pressure. At the same time, the surgeon places his fingers beneath the mentum to exert upward traction. By so doing, the open-bite deformity can often be corrected and the teeth then brought into good occlusion using intermaxillary fixation. If this reduction by manipulation is not possible, elastic traction can be applied to the arch bars, and the teeth will usually fall into good occlusion within a day or two.

Open Reduction of Condylar Fractures. Much controversy has revolved about the question of using an open approach to manage condylar fractures. The arguments against open reduction are strong. In the first place, it is generally known that satisfactory occlusion and good function usually result even in the face of malpositioned fragments or a pseudarthrosis. Next is the element of risk of damage to the facial nerve, the maxillary artery, and the remaining uninjured mandibular

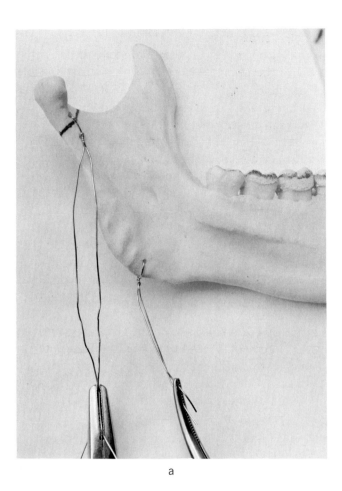 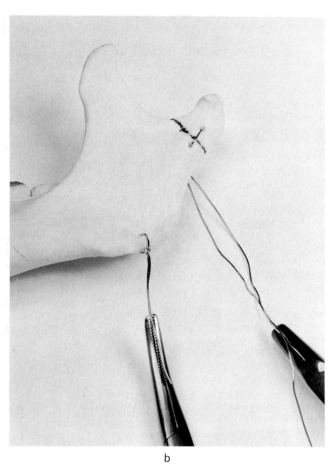

a   b

FIGURE 7.33. *Open reduction of condylar fracture.*

a. Technique from inner aspect of mandible. The open reduction and wiring of a fracture in the condylar region require two incisions for a direct approach to the fracture line—one in the region of the mandibular angle and a second in the preauricular region. For downward traction and reduction of the fracture, a drill hole is made through the region of the angle and a wire attached.

b. Lateral view. The wires are held away from the mandibular angle for purposes of demonstration. A subperiosteal plane is established along the inner aspect of the mandible. A drill hole is made on each side of this fracture. One end of a long piece of #25-gauge wire is placed through each drill hole and grasped from below with a hemostat. The wire is twisted from below and the ends cut. The wire through the drill hole in the angle of the mandible is removed prior to closure of the incision.

growth centers as a consequence of the operation. Finally is the extreme difficulty in obtaining adequate surgical exposure, a beneficial reduction, and satisfactory fixation of the fracture fragments without, at the same time, setting the stage for aseptic necrosis of the condylar head or temporomandibular joint ankylosis. It is not difficult to understand why an air of conservatism has prevailed in the management of these cases.

As mentioned previously, the only indication for open reduction of condylar fractures may be in the edentulous patient with bilateral subcondylar fractures and an open bite deformity. In these patients, a unilateral open reduction may suffice. Wiring of the reduced fragments is often unnecessary, and the trauma involved in trying to do so may be detrimental to the final result.

The auriculotemporal incision, for exposure of the temporomandibular joint, begins in the temporal hair, extending obliquely in a posteroinferior direction to the root of the helix. From this point, the second limb of the incision follows the preauricular skin crease to the inferior aspect of the tragus. The dissection is conducted along the anterior surface of the conchal cartilage to the fascia over the temporomandibular joint. The surgeon must be thoroughly familiar with the normal appearance, location, and course of the facial nerve in this region. The use of a nerve stimulator is recommended to help avoid facial nerve injury during the dissection. This incision and approach have been planned to avoid injury to the facial nerve, superficial temporal artery, and internal maxillary artery. The fascia over the temporomandibular joint is incised, the fracture site is identified, and the periosteum is elevated away from the line of fracture.

To aid in placing the mandible under downward traction, thereby opening the area of the temporomandibular joint, a second incision is made about 1 cm posterior and inferior to the mandibular angle. The angle is then exposed as described under the section on treatment of fractures in this region, and a #25-gauge stainless steel wire is placed through a drill hole in the angle (Fig. 7.33). The wire is left long and grasped with a needle holder so downward traction can be exerted as necessary. The fracture fragment is then located (usually lying anterior, inferior, and medial to the glenoid fossa) and is manipulated back into apposition with the fracture surface on the ramus. This procedure is accomplished against the pull of the lateral pterygoid upon this fragment. Once the mandible is reduced into this position of bony apposition, traction on the mandibular angle is released, intermaxillary fixation applied, and the soft tissues closed.

If reduction by the preceding method is so unstable that the fragment will not maintain osseous apposition, it is necessary to place an interosseous wire. A periosteal elevator is inserted to elevate the periosteum on the posteromedial aspect of the ramus of the mandible. The elevator is then held behind the fracture line to protect the soft tissues, and a drill hole is made through each fragment. A long piece of wire is placed through the drill holes and grasped by a hemostat, which has been inserted from below along the posteromedial aspect of the ramus of the mandible. The two ends of the wire are pulled through the incision at the angle of the mandible and twisted from this point. Wire cutters are inserted through this same route to cut the twisted ends of the wire. The soft tissues are then closed following application of the intermaxillary fixation.

Fractures of the Alveolar Region (3%)

Fractures of the alveolar process involve the teeth and the alveolar process immediately adjacent to them. These fractures may be an extension of fractures occurring in other regions or they may occur independently. In some cases a large segment of alveolar bone may be displaced by a direct blow.

Since soft tissue damage is usually associated with this type of fracture, the mucous membrane must be carefully reapproximated after the reduction has been accomplished. In alveolar fractures, immobilization may be accomplished by wiring the teeth of the fractured segment to adjacent teeth or by applying an arch bar. As a general rule, it is probably best to use arch bars and elastic traction to establish intermaxillary fixation and good dental occlusion.

External Skeletal Fixation

Although the vast majority of mandibular fractures can be adequately managed by the foregoing techniques of open or closed reduction and intermaxillary fixation, in some instances, satisfactory fixation is not so easily obtained. To handle these situations, the technique of external fixation has evolved.

Converse and Waknitz adapted the external skeletal pin fixation appliance of Roger Anderson to fractures of the mandibular angle. This appliance was then improved by Morris, with the introduction of a "biphasic" appliance utilizing Vitallium screws and quick-curing autopolymerizing acrylic as the connecting splint between the screws.

The indications for external skeletal fixation of mandibular fractures have been summarized by Converse in 1974. They include: (1) immobilization of edentulous fragments when other means are ineffective; (2) angle fractures when the body of the mandible immediately anterior to the fracture site is unsuitable for interosseous wiring; (3) comminuted mandibular fractures associated with maxillary fractures and loss of teeth, making dental appliances unsatisfactory; (4) immobilization of fragments during reconstructive bone grafting; (5) in rare cases when wiring of the jaws is medically contraindicated.

The technique of using the "biphasic" appliance was well described in the original article by Morris in 1949. It is broken down into two phases. The first entails dissection through small incisions down to the inferior mandibular margin, drilling of two holes into the mandible on each side of the fracture (5 mm above the margin), screwing in of the specialized Vitallium screws through both cortical plates, and, finally, manual reduction of the fracture and temporary fixation by means of special clamps and a connecting bar tightened to the screws. The second phase involves preparing the quick-curing acrylic, molding it to form a bar, placing it upon the Vitallium screws, securing it with lock nuts, allowing it to harden, and, finally, removing the temporary connecting bar and plates. The reader is referred to the original article by Morris in 1949 or the 1974 description by Converse for a more detailed account of the method.

Postoperative Management

Oral hygiene is essential when intraoral wires or appliances have been employed. The patient should keep his teeth and gums as clean as possible and free from foreign material. This prophylaxis can best be achieved with the aid of a Water Pik and warm saline solution. A small toothbrush may also be useful for removal of debris. Half strength hydrogen peroxide solution should be used frequently as a simple mouth rinse.

Antibiotics are usually administered, because most fractures of the mandible should be considered as open. They may be given orally in a liquid form or parenterally, and their use should be continued for at least 1 week.

Proper nutrition is essential. A high-protein diet with vitamin and mineral supplements is administered. With the advent of blenderized meals and commercially prepared liquid dietary supplements, this diet is not the problem it was in the past.

It is advisable to place the patient in a semi-sitting position and to apply cold compresses during the first day or two following either the injury or the surgery.

A careful follow-up of the patient is imperative, with examinations at approximately 1-week intervals, at which time the intermaxillary fixation apparatus is inspected. It may be necessary to tighten wires or to readjust their ends in order to protect the soft tissues. The rubber bands may become weakened or broken and should be replaced when necessary.

Approximately 4 weeks after the reduction, the elastic traction is removed from the arch bars and the stability of the mandible is tested. If the mandible feels stable, the patient is requested to bite down upon a throat stick placed between the occluding teeth on the side opposite the fracture. If this action elicits significant pain, the healing is incomplete and the elastics must be reapplied. If this test does not cause pain, the patient can go home with an appointment to return in a few days. At this time, if his teeth are still in good alignment, the arch bars are removed under local or general anesthesia. If it was necessary to replace the elastics because of instability or pain on biting, other attempts at removal are made at 2-week intervals until these signs of incomplete healing disappear. If a tooth has been involved in the fracture line, it is best to leave the intermaxillary fixation in place for 8 weeks.

REFERENCES

Adriani, J.: *Labat's Regional Anesthesia Techniques and Clinical Applications*, 3rd ed. Philadelphia, W. B. Saunders Co., 1967.

Aiello, L. M., and Myers, E. N.: Blowout Fracture of the Orbital Floor. Arch. Otolaryng. *82*:638–648, 1965.

Barclay, T. L.: Diplopia in Association with Fractures Involving the Zygomatic Bone. Brit. J. Plast. Surg. *11*:147, 1958.

Barclay, T. L.: Some Aspects of Treatment of Traumatic Diplopia, Brit. J. Plast. Surg. *16*:214, 1963.

Beyer, C. K., and Smith, B.: Naso-orbital Fractures: Their Complications and Treatment. In: P. Tessier et al. (Eds.): *Symposium on Plastic Surgery in the Orbital Region.* St. Louis, C. V. Mosby Co., 1976.

Brown, J. B., Fryer, M. P., and McDowell, F.: Internal Wire-pin Fixation for Fractures of Upper Jaw, Orbit, Zygoma and Severe Facial Crushes. Plast. Reconstr. Surg. *9*:276–283, 1952.

Codman, E. A.: Depressed Fracture of the Malar Bone: A Simple Method of Reduction. Boston Med. Surg. J. *162*:532, 1910.

Converse, J. M.: Orbital and Naso-orbital Fractures. In: P. Tessier et al. (Eds.): *Symposium on Plastic Surgery in the Orbital Region.* St. Louis, C. V. Mosby Co., 1976.

Converse, J. M., Cole, G., and Smith, B.: Late Treatment of Blowout Fracture of the Floor of the Orbit. A Case Report. Plast. Reconstr. Surg. *28*:183–191, 1961.

Converse, J. M., and Smith, B.: Enophthalmos and Diplopia in Fractures of the Orbital Floor. Brit. J. Plast. Surg. *9*:265–274, 1957.

Converse, J. M., and Smith, B.: Blowout Fracture of the Floor of the Orbit. Trans. Amer. Acad. Ophthal. Otolaryng. *64*:676–688, 1960.

Converse, J. M., and Smith, B.: Naso-orbital Fractures. Trans. Amer. Acad. Ophthal. Otolaryng. *67*:622–634, 1963.

Converse, J. M., and Smith, B.: Naso-orbital Fractures and Traumatic Deformities of the Medial Canthus. Plast. Reconstr. Surg. *38*:147–162, 1966.

Converse, J. M., Smith, B., Obear, M. F., and Wood-Smith, D.: Orbital Blowout Fractures: A Ten-Year Survey. Plast. Reconstr. Surg. *37*:20–36, 1967.

Converse, J. M., and Waknitz, F. W.: External Skeletal Fixation in Fractures of the Mandibular Angle. J. Bone Joint Surg. *24*:154, 1942.

Dickinson, J. T., Jaquiss, G. W., and Thompson, J. N.: Soft Tissue Trauma. Otol. Clin. N. Amer. *9*:331–360, 1976.

Dingman, R. O., and Natvig, P.: *Surgery of Facial Fractures.* Philadelphia. W. B. Saunders Co., 1964.

Edwards, W. C., and Riley, R. W.: Blowout Fracture of Medial Orbital Wall. Amer. J. Ophthal. *65*:248, 1968.

Fitz-Hugh, G. S., and Cole, J., Jr.: Some Observations in the Management of Recent Injuries to the Osseous Structures of the Midfacial Skeleton. Laryngoscope *72*:566–585, 1962.

Fomon, S.: *The Surgery of Injury and Plastic Repair.* Baltimore, The Williams & Wilkins Co., 1939.

Gill, J. A.: The Management of Latent Effects of Bony Orbital Injury. Virginia Med. Monthly *91*:232–239, 1964.

Gill, W. D.: Fractures About the Orbit. South. Med. J. *21*:527, 1928.

Gillies, H. D., Kilner, T. P., and Stone, D.: Fractures of the Malar-Zygomatic Compound, with a Description of New X-ray Position. Brit. J. Surg. *14*:651–656, 1927.

Goldthwaite, R. H.: Plastic Repair of Depressed Fracture of Lower Orbital Rim. J.A.M.A. *82*:628. 1924.

Harris, H. H.: Fixation of Fractures in the Middle Third of the Face, with Kirschner Wires. Laryngoscope *68*:95–108, 1958.

Hilger, J. A.: The Repair of Facial Fractures. Arch. Otolaryng. *72*:706–717, 1960.

Hollinshead, W. H.: *Anatomy for Surgeons,* Vol. 1. New York, Harper and Row, 1968.

Holmes, E. M.: Immediate Repair of Injuries of Face and Jaws. Laryngoscope *51*:1007–1015, 1961.

Huffman, W. C., and Lierle, D. M.: Zygomatic Fracture-Dislocations. Trans. Amer. Acad. Ophthal. Otolaryng. *56*:543–555, 1952.

Huffman, W. C., and Lierle, D. M.: The Treatment of Midfacial Fractures. Trans. Amer. Acad. Ophthal. Otolaryng. *62*:652–661, 1958.

Jones, D. E. P., and Evans, J. N. G.: "Blowout" Fractures of the Orbit: An Investigation Into Their Anatomical Basis. J. Laryng. Otol. *81*:1109–1120, 1967.

Jones, I. S.: Symposium: Midfacial Fractures. X-ray Findings. Trans. Amer. Acad. Ophthal. Otolaryng. *67*:635–642, 1963.

Jones, L. T.: New Concepts of Orbital Anatomy. In: P. Tessier et al. (Eds.): *Symposium on Plastic Surgery in the Orbital Region.* St. Louis, C. V. Mosby Co., 1976.

Kazanjian, V. H., and Converse, J. M.: *The Surgical Treatment of Facial Injuries,* 2nd ed. Baltimore, Williams & Wilkins Co., 1952.

Keen, W. W. (Ed.): *Surgery, Its Principles and Practice.* Philadelphia, W. B. Saunders Co., 1909.

Knight, J. S., and North, J. F.: The Classification of Malar Fractures: An Analysis of Displacement as a Guide to Treatment. Brit. J. Plast. Surg. *13*:325–339, 1961.

Lange, W. A.: Fractures of the Orbit. Their Anatomy, Diagnosis and Treatment. Plast. Reconstr. Surg. *35*:26, 1965.

Leake, D., Doykos, J., Habal, M. B., and Murray, J. E.: Long-term Follow-up of Fractures of the Mandibular Condyle in Children. Plast. Reconstr. Surg. *47*:127, 1971.

LeFort, R.: Étude Expérimentale sur les Fractures de la Machoire Supérieure. Rev. Chir. de Paris *23*:208–227, 360–379, 1901. (Trans. by P. Tessier) In Plast. Reconstr. Surg. *50*:497–506, 600–607, 1972.

Lewis, G. K.: Treatment of Old Depressed Fractures of the Zygoma. J. Oral Surg. *2*:101–104, 1953.

Lewis, G. K.: Middle Third Facial Fractures. Illinois Med. J. *30*:1–8, 1957.

Lothrop, H. A.: Fractures of the Superior Maxillary Bone, Caused by Direct Blows Over the Malar Bone. A Method for the Treatment of Such Fractures. Boston Med. Surg. J. *154*:8–11, 1906.

Manwaring, J. G. R.: Replacing Depressed Fractures of the Malar Bone. J.A.M.A. *60*:278–279, 1913.

Matas, R.: Fracture of the Zygomatic Arch. New Orleans Med. Surg. J. *49*:139, 1896.

McClurg, F. L., and Swanson, P. J.: An Orbital Roof Fracture Causing Diplopia. Arch. Otolaryng. *102*:497–498, 1976.

Millard, D. R., et al.: Immediate Reconstruction of the Resected Mandibular Arch. Soc. Head Neck Surg. *114*:605–613, 1967.

Morris, J. H.: Biphase Connector, External Skeletal Splint for Reduction and Fixation of Mandibular Fractures. Oral Surg. *2*:1382, 1949.

Patterson, R. F.: Treatment of Depressed Fractures of the Zygomatic (Malar) Bone and Zygomatic Arch. J. Bone Joint Surg. *17*:1069, 1935.

Petryshyn, W. A.: The Fractured Mandible. A Method of Treatment for the Otolaryngologist. Laryngoscope *70*:1060–1109, 1961.

Quickert, M. H., and Dryden, R. M.: Probes for Intubation in Lacrimal Drainage. Trans. Amer. Acad. Ophthal. Otolaryng. *74*:431–433, 1970.

Rowe, N. L. and Killey, H. C.: *Fractures of the Facial Skeleton,* 2nd ed. Baltimore, The Williams & Wilkins Co., 1968.

Shea, J. J.: The Management of Fractures Involving the Paranasal Sinuses. J.A.M.A. *96*:418, 1931.

Shumrick, D. A.: General Considerations in Cases of Maxillofacial Trauma. Otol. Clin. N. Amer. *2*:221–233, 1969.

Song, I. C., Bromberg, B. E., and Lane, F. L.: Anterior Fixation of Mandibular Fractures. Plast. Reconstr. Surg. *35*:317–321, 1965.

Tempest, M. N.: The Surgical Management of Displaced Fractures of the Malar Bone and Zygomatic Arch. A Review of 275 Consecutive Cases. Trans. Int. Soc. Plast. Surg., 2nd Congress. London, E & S Livingston, Ltd., 1959.

Tessier, P.: The Conjunctival Approach to the Orbital Floor and Maxilla in Congenital Malformations and Trauma. J. Maxillofacial Surg. *1*:3, 1973.

Weir, R. F.: On the Replacement of a Depressed Fracture of the Malar Bone. Medical Record *51*:335, 1897.

8

Surgery of the Nose

EPISTAXIS

Epistaxis is best classified according to its location: anterior, superior, or posterior (Fig. 8.1). *Anterior* bleeding occurs in Little's area on the anterior septum, from either a branch of the anterior ethmoid artery, septal branch of the superior labial artery, septal branch of the sphenopalatine artery, or the greater palatine artery. *Superior* bleeding occurs from either the anterior ethmoid artery, posterior ethmoid artery, or the superior nasal branch of the sphenopalatine artery. *Posterior* epistaxis results from rupture of the sphenopalatine artery or one of its branches.

Etiology

Trauma. Externally, any displacement of the cartilaginous or bony nasal framework may be compounded by a tear in the mucous membrane and result in epistaxis.

Internal trauma may result from sneezing, excessive nose-blowing, or nose-picking.

Infection. Acute inflammation of the nasal mucous membranes may lead to epistaxis. The superficial erosion and exposure of blood vessels, coupled with the irritation of nose-blowing, often results in nosebleed. This type of epistaxis is usually anterior and is easily controlled. Associated with chronic rhinitis, however, it can be most troublesome. It usually occurs in areas where there is crusting and ulceration of a mucous membrane, and often accompanies atrophic rhinitis or a septal perforation.

Pressure Changes. Epistaxis is not infrequently associated with the atmospheric pressure changes occurring during air or submarine travel and is more common in people living at higher altitudes than in those living in lower altitudes because of lower atmospheric pressure and lack of moisture.

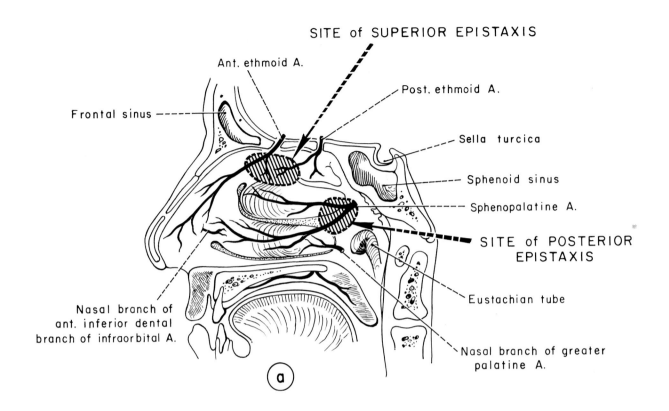

SITE of SUPERIOR EPISTAXIS

Ant. ethmoid A.

Post. ethmoid A.

Frontal sinus

Sella turcica

Sphenoid sinus

Sphenopalatine A.

SITE of POSTERIOR EPISTAXIS

Eustachian tube

Nasal branch of ant. inferior dental branch of infraorbital A.

Nasal branch of greater palatine A.

(a)

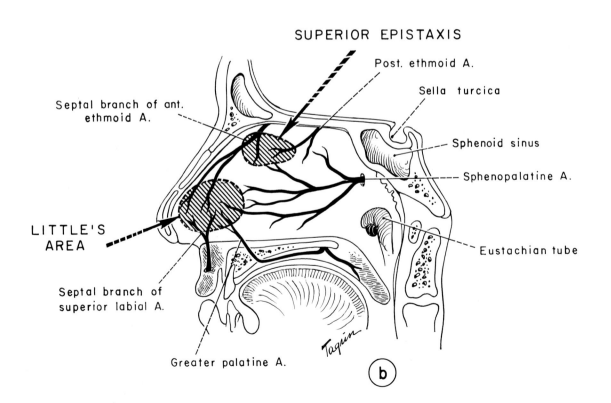

SUPERIOR EPISTAXIS

Post. ethmoid A.

Sella turcica

Septal branch of ant. ethmoid A.

Sphenoid sinus

Sphenopalatine A.

LITTLE'S AREA

Eustachian tube

Septal branch of superior labial A.

Greater palatine A.

(b)

Foreign Body. Epistaxis frequently is due to a foreign body in the nasal cavity. This is most common in children and mentally deranged patients. Nasal stuffiness or obstruction, accompanied by an odoriferous purulent discharge, is a manifestation of an intranasal foreign body.

Neoplasms. Benign lesions, such as angiofibroma, and malignant lesions are frequently complicated by epistaxis. The bleeding occurring with angiofibroma can be serious and difficult to manage. Each patient with epistaxis should be carefully examined to exclude the possibility of either benign or malignant neoplasm.

Familial Telangiectasia (Rendu-Osler-Weber Disease). The bleeding occurring with this disease usually begins during middle life. It can become so frequent and severe that it dominates the patient's life completely. The small cherry-red telangiectatic spots occur anywhere in mucous membrane or skin, but are most frequently found in the nasal cavity, mouth, pharynx, and skin of the face (see section on septal dermoplasty, p. 337).

Systemic Diseases. In most cases the exact cause of epistaxis is obscure. Epistaxis often occurs in patients with systemic diseases such as hypertension, arteriosclerosis, anemia, leukemia, deficiency states, hepatic cirrhosis, and chronic nephritis.

Vicarious Menstruation. Vicarious menstruation should be expected when epistaxis is experienced repeatedly during menstruation.

Coagulation Defects. The diagnosis of bleeding due to coagulation defects is made by means of tests such as blood counts, blood smears, determination of bleeding and clotting times, and platelet counts. Pseudohemophilia occurs more frequently in females than in males. In epistaxis due to this condition the only abnormality found is that of prolongation of the bleeding time.

FIGURE 8.1. *Anatomy of epistaxis.*

a. Lateral wall of the nasal cavity
From the internal carotid artery
    Anterior ethmoid artery from ophthalmic artery
    Posterior ethmoid artery from ophthalmic artery
From external carotid artery
    Sphenopalatine artery and its middle and inferior turbinate branches from the internal maxillary artery
    Nasal branch of the greater palatine artery from the internal maxillary artery
    Nasal branch of the anteroinferior dental branch of the infraorbital artery

b. Nasal septum
From the internal carotid artery via the ophthalmic artery
    Septal branch of the anterior ethmoid artery
    Posterior ethmoid artery
From the external carotid artery
    Sphenopalatine artery from the internal maxillary artery
    Greater palatine artery from the internal maxillary artery
    Septal branch of the superior labial artery from the facial artery

Anterior Epistaxis

It is fortunate that anterior bleeding is the most common type of epistaxis, for it is the easiest to control. Local measures to produce reflex vasoconstriction are helpful. These include placing an icebag on the back of the patient's neck, putting a wad of paper or cotton beneath his upper lip, and continuous irrigation of the nasal passage with ice water. Quite often anterior epistaxis will cease spontaneously if the patient remains calm and in a sitting position with his head slightly forward. He is instructed to breathe through his mouth and squeeze both nostrils shut. If these measures are not effective, a piece of moist cotton is placed in the anterior nasal cavity and compressed against the bleeding point by applying external pressure.

Cauterization. Cauterization may be necessary to control either a prolonged, solitary or repeated episode of anterior epistaxis.

Anesthesia is easily obtained by inserting 4% cocaine-impregnated cotton strips into the nasal cavity and waiting for 5 to 10 minutes. The vasoconstricting action of the cocaine slows down or controls the epistaxis which will facilitate the cauterization. Other topical anesthetic agents, such as 4% Xylocaine or 2% Pontocaine, with epinephrine solution added can be used as substitutes for the cocaine solution.

If it is impossible to control the bleeding by anterior packing, especially when dealing with an arteriosclerotic vessel, the area adjacent to the bleeding point should be injected with a local anesthetic agent, combined with epinephrine solution, prior to cauterization. Injection should be made with a #25 or #27 needle.

Chemical Cauterization. A silver nitrate stick is the most commonly used implement for chemical cauterization for epistaxis, but this provides superficial cauterization, which may not be efficient. A small chromic acid bead on the end of a wire produces excellent cauterization. A tiny cotton pledget dipped in 50% trichloroacetic acid solution is also very effective. The chromic acid bead is made by first heating a wire applicator so that it becomes cherry-red and then dipping it into chromic acid crystals. It is important that the chemical be placed only at the site of the bleeding; it should not be applied when the bleeding is profuse. The application of a dry cotton swab immediately after the cauterization prevents distribution of the chemical to adjacent areas of mucous membrane.

Electrocautery. Should chemical cauterization fail, the electrocautery may be utilized. Most types of instruments work well. The red hot tip cautery does not stick to the eschar produced as readily as do other types of electrocautery. Bleeding tends to occur as the eschar is pulled away by the cautery tip. Following cauterization, the patient is instructed to avoid straining, nose-blowing, and sneezing for a few days, and to insert a pea-sized piece of petroleum jelly on the septum, just behind the columella, each morning and evening for one week.

Packing. One-inch wide petrolatum-strip packing may be inserted into the anterior nasal cavity for treatment of troublesome anterior bleeding. In order to prevent its passing into the nasopharynx, it is important to secure the end of the packing in place externally with a piece of tape. The anterior packing should remain in place for from 1 to 3 days. Hemostatic agents, such as Gelfoam, oxidized cellulose, and topical thrombin, are of value when placed directly over the bleeding point. If the anterior packing is to remain in place for a number of days it is best to use antibiotic-impregnated iodoform gauze rather than petrolatum gauze, to help prevent secondary infection and odor.

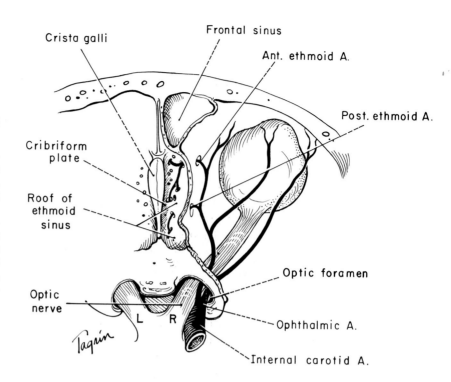

FIGURE 8.2a. *Relations of the ethmoid arteries from above.*

Note the internal carotid artery, ophthalmic artery, optic nerve, optic foramen, cribriform plate, crista galli, posterior ethmoid artery, anterior ethmoid artery, roof of the ethmoid sinuses.

The ethmoid arteries become extracranial as they enter the orbit by way of the optic foramen. They become intracranial again as they leave the ethmoid foramina and traverse above the bony roof of the ethmoid sinuses. The arteries become extracranial for the second time when they enter the nasal cavity.

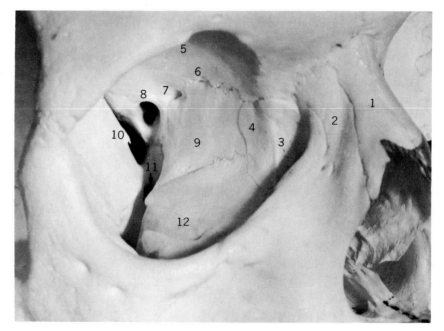

FIGURE 8.2b. *Relations of anterior and posterior ethmoid foramina in the medial wall of the orbit.*

1. Nasal bone
2. Ascending process of maxilla
3. Lacrimal fossa
4. Lacrimal bone
5. Orbital plate of frontal bone
6. Anterior ethmoid foramen
7. Posterior ethmoid foramen
8. Optic foramen
9. Lamina papyracea
10. Superior orbital fissure
11. Foramen rotundum (arrow)
12. Orbital plate of maxillary bone

Superior Epistaxis

Anterosuperior bleeding usually emanates from a medial or lateral branch of the anterior or posterior ethmoid artery (Figs. 8.1 and 8.2). Posterosuperior epistaxis is likely to come from a branch of the sphenopalatine artery. If the bleeding point can be seen it is cauterized after packing with a topical anesthetic agent and after a vasoconstrictor, as has been used for control of anterior bleeding. If the bleeding point cannot be located, then anterior packing must be utilized.

Anterior Packing. The patient is placed in a sitting position with his head tilted slightly backward and supported either by an assistant or a head rest. With a nasal speculum and bayonet forceps, iodoform gauze, which has been impregnated with antibiotic ointment, is carefully packed into both nasal cavities. The packing is begun posterosuperiorly and continued in a forward direction. The anterior ends of each strip of packing are tied together so that they will not be lost in the nasopharynx. The anatomy of the nose is such that this packing tends to become displaced inferiorly. Therefore, the inferior nasal cavity is packed with a finger-cot packing. If both nasal cavities are packed, a piece of rubber catheter is placed through the finger-cot packing, into the posterior nasal cavity, to prevent annoying interference with eustachian tube function during swallowing. This packing should remain in place for from 3 to 5 days.

Ligation of the Ethmoidal Arteries. Persistent superior bleeding is, on occasion, best treated by ligation of the anterior and posterior ethmoid arteries. These arteries are ligated just lateral to the point where they enter the medial wall of the orbit.

The anterior and posterior ethmoid foramina are situated in, or adjacent to, the frontoethmoidal suture line (between the orbital plate of the frontal bone and the lamina papyracea) (Fig. 8.2b). In some persons the foramina may be situated slightly above this suture line. According to Kirchner and associates the anterior ethmoid foramen is between 14 and 18 mm behind the maxillolacrimal suture line. The posterior ethmoid foramen is between 4 and 7 mm anterior to the optic foramen. The distance between the anterior and posterior ethmoid foramina averages 10 mm.

An external ethmoid incision is used for exposure (Fig. 8.3a). The lacrimal sac and orbital periosteum are retracted laterally as has been described for external ethmoidectomy (p. 52). The suture line between the orbital plate of the frontal bone and the lamina papyracea can easily be found. This is followed posteriorly until the anterior ethmoid artery is located. There are a number of ways to deal with the artery. A #3-0 silk suture can be looped around it with a hook-shaped needle carrier. A second method is that of cauterizing the artery just as it enters the anterior ethmoid foramen. This method is usually rapid and effective, except when the artery ruptures causing troublesome bleeding. A third method utilizes self-locking hemostatic clips (Figs. 8.3b and 8.10), which are applied after the artery is placed under tension by laterally retracting the orbital periosteum. The anterior ethmoid artery is divided so that the posterior ethmoid artery can also be identified and ligated. Closure and postoperative care are the same as described for external ethmoidectomy (p. 57).

Posterior Epistaxis

Posterior epistaxis can be severe, frightening, and difficult to control. It is the result of rupture of the sphenopalatine artery or one of its branches. Usually the patient gives a history of blood flowing profusely into the pharynx, as well as from the anterior nares. Much blood can be lost in a relatively short period of time. Often, much of this blood is swallowed, and the patient reports vomiting "coffee-ground" material.

Unless the patient shows signs of shock, he is placed in the sitting position. The nasal cavities are packed with cotton strips which are impregnated with 4% cocaine, or a topical anesthetic agent, plus epinephrine solution (1:1000). It is

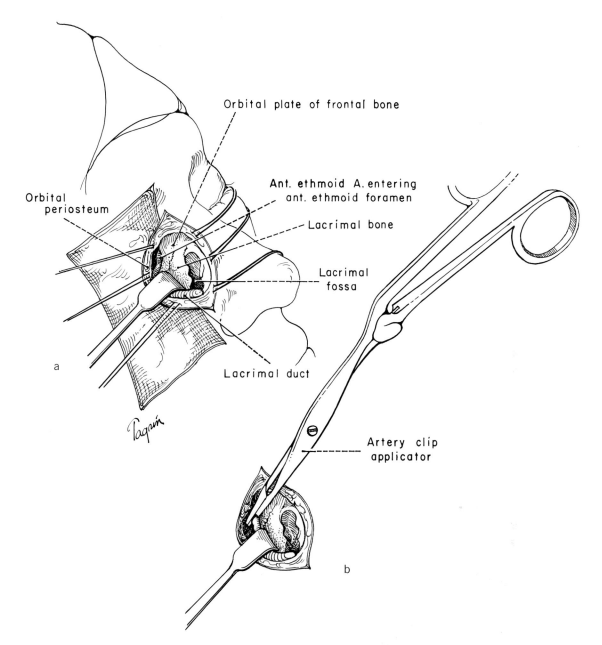

Orbital plate of frontal bone

Orbital periosteum

Ant. ethmoid A. entering
ant. ethmoid foramen

Lacrimal bone

Lacrimal fossa

a

Lacrimal duct

Artery clip
applicator

b

FIGURE 8.3

a. The anterior ethmoid incision exposes the lacrimal fossa, orbital plate of the frontal bone, lacrimal bone, and lamina papyracea.

Note the orbital plate of the frontal bone, orbital periosteum, anterior ethmoid artery entering the anterior ethmoid foramen, lacrimal bone, and lacrimal fossa.

b. The anterior ethmoid artery has been exposed and is being ligated with a hemostatic clip (Fig. 8.10).

important to place these strips behind both the middle and inferior turbinates. It may be necessary to fracture the middle or inferior turbinate medially in order to find the site of hemorrhage. If the bleeding site can be seen, it is worth the effort to attempt cauterization or to cover the area with a pledget of oxidized cellulose. The pledget can usually be wedged between the turbinate and the lateral nasal wall, in the inferior or middle meatus. If the bleeding cannot be controlled by such measures, then it is necessary to use anterior and posterior packing.

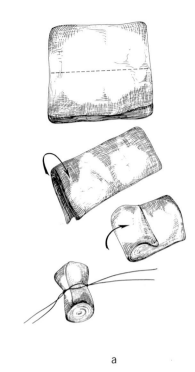

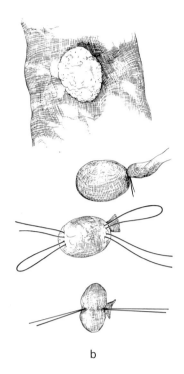

a

b

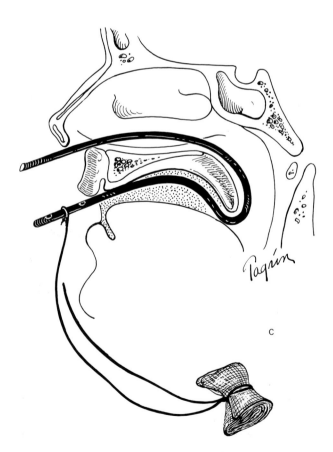

c

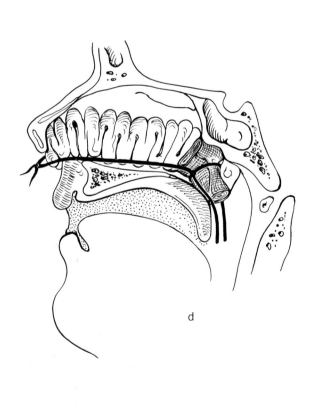

d

Anteroposterior Packing. The patient is sedated with either morphine or Demerol as soon as the decision to employ anteroposterior packing is made. Both the nasal cavity and soft palate are anesthetized topically with 2% Pontocaine or 4% cocaine solution. It is most important to tell the patient what is being done, for the experience of having postnasal packing inserted can be a frightening one. A soft rubber catheter is placed in the nasal cavity on the side of the epistaxis and advanced until it appears in the pharynx. The catheter is grasped with a bayonet forceps, or a Kelly clamp, and delivered through the mouth. One set of strings from the posterior pack is tied to the end of the catheter protruding from the mouth, as is shown in Figure 8.4a and b. The catheter is withdrawn from the nose, bringing the strings to the nasal orifice. The operator tenses these strings with one hand, while delivering the posterior pack into the nasopharynx with the index finger of the other hand, or with a Kelly clamp (Fig. 8.4c). An assistant can hold the strings protruding from the nasal orifice while the anterior packing is being inserted. This packing consists of one long strip of 1-inch antibiotic-impregnated iodoform gauze. One end is packed firmly against the anterior aspect of the posterior pack and then the entire nasal cavity is carefully filled with the gauze strip. The two strings protruding from the nostril are tied over a cotton dental roll or a rolled-up 2- x 2-inch gauze pad to pull the posterior pack forward and thereby exert anterior pressure against the intranasal packing. The strings protruding from the posterior aspect of the pack into the pharynx and out the mouth are cut flush with the uvula (Fig. 8.4d). It is not necessary to bring these out through the mouth and tape them to the cheek. If the uvula becomes excessively edematous, it should be incised.

A patient with an anteroposterior pack is kept in bed in a semi-sitting position for at least 24 hours. His feet, legs, and thighs are encased in elastic stockings. An ice collar is applied and ice packs are placed at the side of his nose. Tranquilizers and medication for relief of pain are given as needed. A soft diet is prescribed, and laxatives are administered to prevent constipation. As a general rule it is best to give antibiotics when anteroposterior packing is used in order to combat the inevitable sinusitis. Lost blood is replaced, as indicated, by transfusions. Daily hemoglobin and hematocrit determinations are essential. A general evaluation of the patient is conducted in order to detect any underlying cause of the epistaxis.

FIGURE 8.4. *Technique of posterior packing.*

a. A 4- x 4-inch gauze pad is impregnated with Aureomycin ointment, folded in half, and rolled up. Two lengths of heavy silk thread are tied around the center of this roll; the four ends of thread are not cut. The packing is put in place with two strands of thread protruding from the anterior nasal cavity and the other two either hanging into the pharynx or protruding from the mouth and taped to the cheek. The latter strands are for removal of the pack.

b. A more adequate posterior pack is made by opening a 4- x 4-inch gauze pad and folding it once. A ball of Aureomycin-impregnated iodoform gauze, 2 to 4 cm in diameter, depending on the size of the patient's pharynx, is placed upon the center of the gauze. The gauze is then folded around the packing and tied with heavy silk. With a large needle, heavy silk is threaded through the pack; the ends of the thread are left protruding from the pack as shown in the illustration. Because of its shape and smaller size, this pack is more effective and less uncomfortable than that described in "a." It also prevents or controls odor.

c. A soft rubber catheter has been inserted into the pharynx where it is grasped with a hemostat and pulled forward. Two ends of the silk thread are tied to the catheter. The catheter is pulled from the nose, and the thread grasped with one hand. The posterior pack is guided into the nasopharynx with the aid of a Kelly clamp or the opposite index finger.

d. The anterior nasal cavity is packed tightly with 1-inch Aureomycin-impregnated iodoform gauze. The two strings protruding from the nasal orifice are tied around a dental roll or a roll of gauze.

There are many disadvantages to anteroposterior packing. The patient is extremely uncomfortable, for mouth breathing results in a dry and sore throat. Deglutition is difficult. Complicating sinusitis often occurs. With the packing in place, blood may ascend by way of the nasolacrimal duct, and exit from the ocular punctum, or by way of the eustachian tube, causing hemotympanum and rupture of the tympanic membrane. Even after all this the bleeding may recur when the nasal packing is removed.

Transantral Ligation of the Internal Maxillary Artery. Posterior epistaxis from the sphenopalatine artery can be a serious medical problem, especially when bleeding persists during or following the removal of anterior and posterior nasal packing.

Ligation of the external carotid artery is not effective in many cases of posterior epistaxis. Ligation of the internal maxillary artery, on the other hand, has proven very effective for the control of sphenopalatine artery hemorrhage (Malcomson; Chandler and Serrins).

Anatomy of the Third Division of the Internal Maxillary Artery (Figs. 8.5, 8.6, and 8.7). The internal maxillary artery is the larger of the two terminal branches of the external carotid artery. It arises behind the neck of the mandible and is divided into three parts: the mandibular, pterygoid, and pterygopalatine (third division). The pterygopalatine division follows a tortuous course as it traverses the pterygomaxillary fossa where it gives off seven branches.

The description of the anatomy of the branches of the third division of the internal maxillary artery on page 332 is based on the microscopic dissection of a number of cadaver specimens.

FIGURE 8.5. *Contents of the pterygomaxillary fossa, after careful removal of adipose tissue.*

The entire posterior wall of the right maxillary sinus has been removed. A small portion of the internal pterygoid muscle can be seen. The unlabeled artery on the surface of this muscle is a branch of the second division of the internal maxillary artery, the buccal artery. Only a small portion of the infraorbital nerve can be seen. A view of the sphenopalatine ganglion and vidian canal is obstructed by the sphenopalatine artery. The greater palatine nerve can be seen as it descends to join the greater palatine artery.

1. Posterosuperior alveolar artery
2. Lesser palatine artery
3. Nasal accessory and superior pharyngeal arteries
4. Infraorbital artery
5. Foramen rotundum
6. Greater palatine artery
7. Sphenopalatine artery
8. Greater palatine nerve

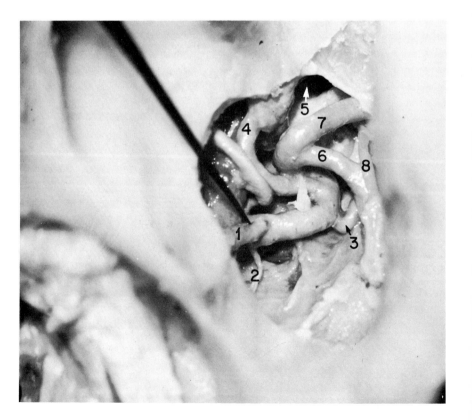

FIGURE 8.6

The infraorbital artery and nerve have been retracted laterally and the internal maxillary artery, antero-inferiorly, in order to expose the arteries to the foramen rotundum and the vidian canal. The foramen rotundum and a portion of the bony ridge between it and the vidian canal are seen. A better view of the infraorbital and greater palatine nerve has been obtained. The sphenopalatine artery obstructs the view of the underlying sphenopalatine ganglion and the vidian canal.

1. Posterosuperior alveolar artery
2. Lesser palatine artery
3. Nasal accessory and superior pharyngeal arteries
4. Infraorbital artery
5. Arteries to the foramen rotundum and vidian canal
6. Greater palatine artery
7. Sphenopalatine artery
8. Infraorbital nerve
9. Foramen rotundum
10. Greater palatine nerve

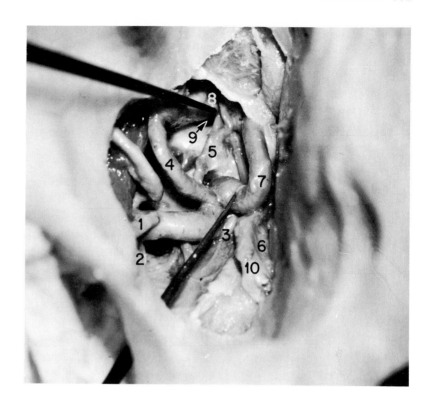

FIGURE 8.7

The greater palatine artery and nerve have been elevated superiorly and the internal maxillary artery retracted in a superior and lateral direction. Thus, the foramen rotundum, vidian canal, and bony ridge between these two are exposed. The rather indistinct sphenopalatine ganglion may be seen overlying most of the vidian canal and obstructing the view of the vidian nerve. The afferent connections between the sphenopalatine ganglion and the internal maxillary artery can be seen. The superior pharyngeal and accessory arteries have been reflected inferiorly.

1. Posterosuperior alveolar artery
2. Nasal accessory and superior pharyngeal arteries
3. Infraorbital artery
4. Arteries to foramen rotundum and vidian canal
5. Greater palatine artery
6. Sphenopalatine artery
7. Foramen rotundum
8. Greater palatine nerve
9. Afferent fibers
10. Sphenopalatine ganglion
11. Vidian canal
12. Bony crest between foramen rotundum and vidian canal

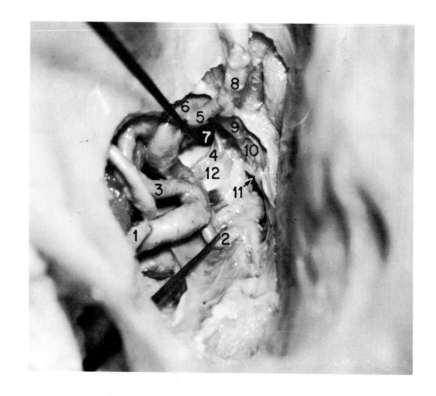

Posterosuperior Alveolar Artery. This vessel descends on the tuberosity of the maxilla and divides into numerous branches, some of which enter the alveolar canals to supply the molar and premolar teeth and the lining of the maxillary sinus, while others continue forward on the alveolar process to supply the gums. The posterosuperior alveolar artery may share a common trunk with the infraorbital artery.

Lesser Palatine Artery. In our cadaver dissections, the lesser palatine artery was found to originate from the superior aspect of the pterygomaxillary artery, directly medial to the origin of the posterior superior alveolar artery. It descends parallel to the greater palatine artery, supplying the posterior upper alveolus, gums, and hard and soft palate.

Nasal Accessory and Superior Pharyngeal Arteries. These arteries may have a common origin. The nasal accessory artery supplies the floor of the nose, inferior meatus, inferior turbinate, and lower middle meatus. The superior pharyngeal artery is distributed to the upper pharynx and the orifice of the eustachian tube.

Infraorbital Artery. The infraorbital artery passes anteriorly along the floor of the orbit, within the infraorbital canal, to emerge externally through the infraorbital foramen. It has numerous branches. Within the infraorbital canal, it supplies the inferior rectus and inferior oblique muscles, and the lacrimal sac. Anteriorly, its branches descend through the alveolar canals to supply the upper canine and incisor teeth and the mucous membrane of the maxillary sinus. Its terminal branches supply the tissues of the midface.

Arteries to the Foramen Rotundum and Pterygoid Canals. These arteries may arise separately or together in a common trunk. If they share a common trunk, they divide and pass into their respective foramina and are distributed to the enclosed nerves and connective tissues.

Greater Palatine Artery. The greater palatine artery descends through the pterygopalatine canal with the greater palatine branch of the sphenopalatine nerve, emerges from the greater palatine foramen, and extends forward on the medial aspect of the hard palate to the incisive canal. The terminal branch passes through this canal to anastomose with the branches of the sphenopalatine artery. Other branches are distributed to the gums, palatine glands, oral mucosa, soft palate, and palatine tonsils.

Sphenopalatine Artery. The sphenopalatine artery is the terminal branch of the internal maxillary artery. It passes through the sphenopalatine foramen into the nasal cavity behind the posterior tip of the middle turbinate. Here it gives off the posterior lateral nasal branches, which extend forward over the meatuses and turbinates to anastomose with branches from the ethmoid and palatine arteries and to assist in supplying the maxillary, ethmoid, and sphenoid sinuses. The terminal branches of the sphenopalatine artery cross the undersurface of the sphenoid and end on the nasal septum as the posterior septal arteries, which anastomose with the anterior and posterior ethmoids, and superior labial and greater palatine arteries, to supply the floor of the septum and the roof of the nose.

Surgical Technique of Transantral Ligation of the Internal Maxillary Artery. The operation may be performed with the patient under either general or local anesthesia. When local anesthesia is the choice, 2% Xylocaine with added epinephrine is injected into the gingivobuccal sulcus and around the infraorbital nerve.

A curved needle is inserted 2 cm into the greater palatine foramen, and 2 cc of the local anesthetic is slowly injected into the canal and pterygomaxillary fossa.

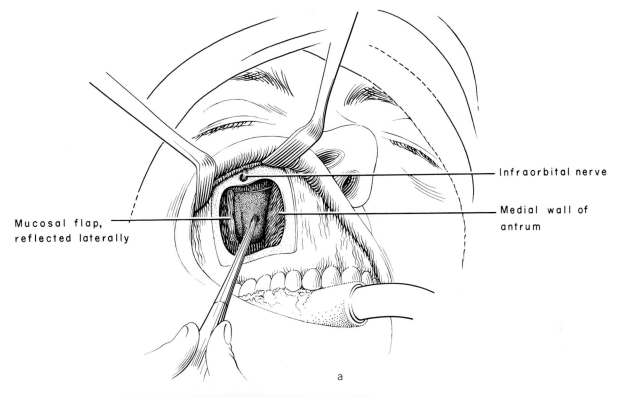

Infraorbital nerve

Medial wall of
antrum

Mucosal flap,
reflected laterally

a

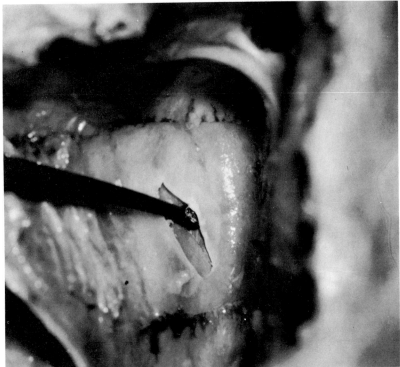

b

FIGURE 8.8   *Approach to the pterygomaxillary fossa.*

a. Most of the anterior wall of the right maxillary sinus has been removed with preservation of the infraorbital foramen and nerve. In this dissection the mucosal flap of the posterior wall is based and reflected laterally. A small opening is being made through the posterior wall of the maxillary sinus with care being taken to preserve the underlying periosteum.

b. An opening through the posterior wall of the maxillary sinus has been made with a sharp curette. This is enlarged sufficiently to admit a Hajek bone-cutting forceps. The entire posterior wall of the sinus is removed with the Hajek forceps, care being taken to preserve the underlying periosteum.

A Caldwell-Luc incision is used. The periosteum is elevated from the anterior wall of the antrum in the region of the canine fossa. The antrum is entered by using a curette, chisel, or rotating bur. As much of the anterior wall of the antrum is removed as is possible without damaging the infraorbital nerve (Fig. 8.5). This can be accomplished with Kerrison forceps, but is best done with a rotating bur.

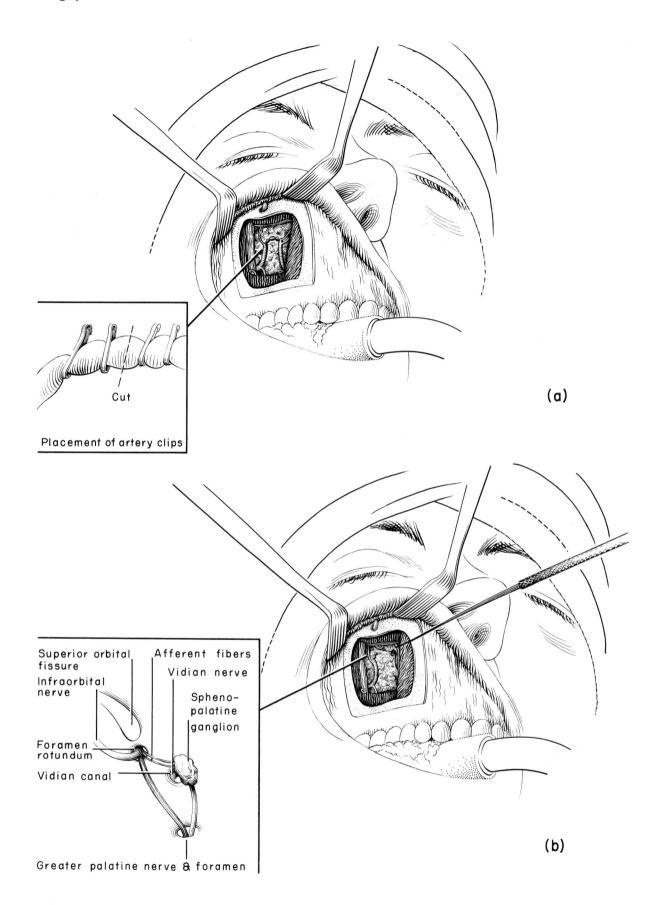

Cut

Placement of artery clips

(a)

Superior orbital fissure

Infraorbital nerve

Foramen rotundum

Vidian canal

Afferent fibers

Vidian nerve

Spheno-palatine ganglion

Greater palatine nerve & foramen

(b)

A cocaine pack is placed in the antrum for a few minutes to further anesthetize the antral mucosa and to decrease bleeding. A mucosal flap, based laterally or inferiorly, is elevated from the posterior wall of the antrum (Fig. 8.8a). A self-retaining retractor is applied.

The surgical microscope, with a 300-mm lens, should be used during the remaining dissection. The thin posterior wall is broken through with a curette or small chisel (Fig. 8.8b). The periosteum is carefully separated from the posterior sinus wall, which in turn is removed with Hajek bone-cutting forceps. It is important to extend this bony dissection as far medially as is possible, for the vidian canal is often found directly posterior to the medial wall of the antrum. There are a number of small blood vessels directly underneath the periosteum covering the pterygomaxillary fossa. The periosteum is best opened by using a spatula blade with electrocoagulation current to accomplish the cruciate incisions. The four flaps thus created are easily elevated, exposing the underlying adipose tissue.

Pulsations of the internal maxillary artery can often be seen, giving the surgeon some indication as to the location of this artery. Adipose tissue is carefully removed with dissectors, alligator and cup forceps, and suction tips, all especially designed for this purpose. As soon as the main artery is identified, it is elevated with an artery hook, so that its branches may be more readily dissected free.

The sphenopalatine artery is retracted anteriorly with an artery hook and doubly clipped as is shown in Figure 8.9a. I have found the various nonlocking hemostatic clips to be unsatisfactory, for they are gradually reopened by the strong pulsations of this artery. If possible, the infraorbital and greater palatine arteries should be identified so that the arterial occlusion can be accomplished medial to their origin.

It is not necessary to section the artery when using the self-locking clips. The sphenopalatine artery can be ligated with #3-0 silk suture material if the self-locking hemostatic clip and its applicators* are not available. The suture is passed beneath the artery with a ligature carrier, or small, curved or right-angle hemostat, and tied by hand or with the aid of a long, thin needle holder.

The posterior central mucosal flap is reflected over the pterygomaxillary fossa and covered with Gelfoam. Any intranasal packing is removed. Slight bleeding should not be of concern, for it will cease spontaneously. A nasoantral window is added for drainage only if bleeding has been a problem throughout the operation or if the patient has had intranasal packing in place for sufficient time for sinusitis to become a complication. If a nasoantral window is fashioned the antrum is packed with antibiotic-impregnated iodoform gauze, which is removed on the second or third postoperative day. The Caldwell-Luc incision is closed with loosely tied catgut sutures.

*The self-locking hemostatic clips (Fig. 8.10), with the dispenser and applicator, as well as the instruments used for pterygomaxillary surgery, may be purchased from Richards Manufacturing Company, 1450 Brooks Road, Memphis, Tennessee 38116.

FIGURE 8.9. *Section of internal maxillary artery.*

a. The internal maxillary artery is viewed by way of the right maxillary sinus. Four self-locking artery clips have been applied. The artery is sectioned with scissors.

b. Sectioned ends of the internal maxillary artery are reflected anteriorly and posteriorly giving a view of the foramen rotundum, bony ridge, vidian canal and sphenopalatine ganglion. A sketch showing the anatomic relationships appears in the lower left-hand corner.

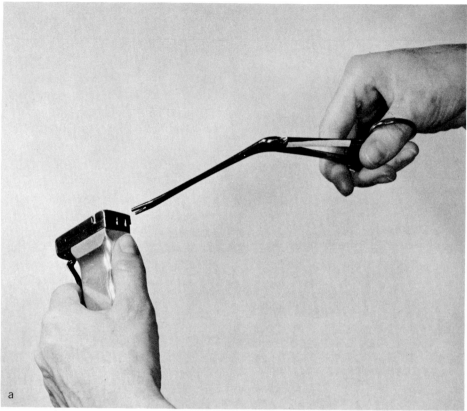

a

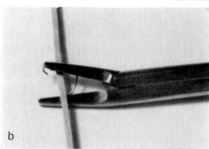

b

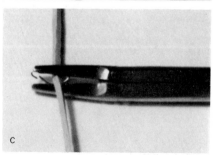

c

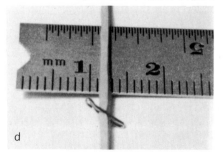

d

FIGURE 8.10.   *Artery clip dispenser and self-locking clip.*

a. The clip dispenser is used to insert the self-locking clip into the forceps. The two jaws of the clip applicator are inserted into their respective slots in the dispenser. The clip projects into the slots of the applicator as the trigger of the dispenser is compressed. The procedure should be carried out by the surgeon to prevent displacement of the clip from the applicator as might occur if the applicator were passed by a nurse or an assistant to the surgeon.

b. The upper loop is passed over and beyond the "artery."

c. As the forceps is compressed, the lower end of the clip bends so that it is extended into the upper loop.

d. As the clip is further compressed, it becomes locked and resembles a miniature safety-pin.

Postoperative Care. Postoperative care should include the administration of antibiotics, placing the patient in the semi-sitting position, and the application of an ice pack over the patient's face to prevent edema and ecchymosis. The ice pack should be applied as soon as the patient reaches the recovery room. It should remain in place for 24 hours.

Septal Dermoplasty for Hereditary Hemorrhagic Telangiectasia

In many cases the severe recurrent epistaxis associated with Rendu-Osler-Weber disease can be controlled by skin-grafting both sides of the anterior nasal septum (Figs. 8.11–8.15) as outlined by Saunders. The epistaxis associated with this systemic disease can be a most severe problem. In some cases, daily hemorrhages dominate the patient's entire existence. Gastrointestinal bleeding and hemorrhage from the lips, tongue, and gums also occur.

The telangiectatic lesions may be found on any epithelial surface. They are bright red, usually about a millimeter or two in diameter, slightly raised, and blanch with pressure. Microscopically the vessels in the telangiectatic lesions are superficial, thin-walled, and void of muscular or elastic tissue. Thus bleeding with minimal trauma occurs with a lack of spontaneous cessation of hemorrhage.

Septal Dermoplasty Technique. Approximately 30 cc of 1% Xylocaine solution are required to anesthetize the donor site on the thigh for a split-thickness skin graft. The upper lip, columella, nasal septum, and nasofacial sulcus are also anesthetized with 1% Xylocaine solution (Fig. 8.11b).

A split-thickness skin graft, approximately 2.5 by 4 inches in size and 0.016 to 0.020 inch in thickness, is sufficient to cover both sides of the anterior nasal septum and the floor and tip of the inferior turbinate. The skin-graft donor site is covered with petrolatum gauze, or Telfa or Owen's silk, and then with an overlying pressure dressing.

A nasofacial incision (Fig. 8.12a) is made to acquire better exposure of the anterior nasal cavity. This incision should extend slightly into the floor of the nose. One suture through the ala, weighted with a heavy hemostat, serves for retraction (Fig. 8.12b).

A vertical postcolumellar incision is made anterior to the mucocutaneous junction. This incision is made along the full vertical dimension of the anterior nasal septum, but not through the mucoperichondrium. The mucous membrane is resected, preserving the perichondrium, with a knife, scissors, and sharp curettes (Fig. 8.13a). It is essential that all mucous membrane be removed so that mucus-secreting epithelium will not be present under the skin graft. Bleeding is controlled with cautery and topical epinephrine solution.

The skin graft is halved, one half to be used for the anterior third of the nasal septum, the other for the anterior portion of the lateral wall and inferior turbinate. The skin graft is secured in place (Fig. 8.13b) anteriorly with #4-0 chromic catgut sutures and then pushed posteriorly so that it covers all areas which have been denuded of mucous membrane (Fig. 8.14a). The graft may be tacked in place with a few additional sutures if necessary. If indicated, the operation is repeated on the contralateral side. The nasal cavity is loosely packed with antibiotic-impregnated iodoform gauze. The nasolabial incision is approximated subcutaneously with #4-0 chromic catgut and the skin is closed with #5-0 dermal suture material (Fig. 8.14b).

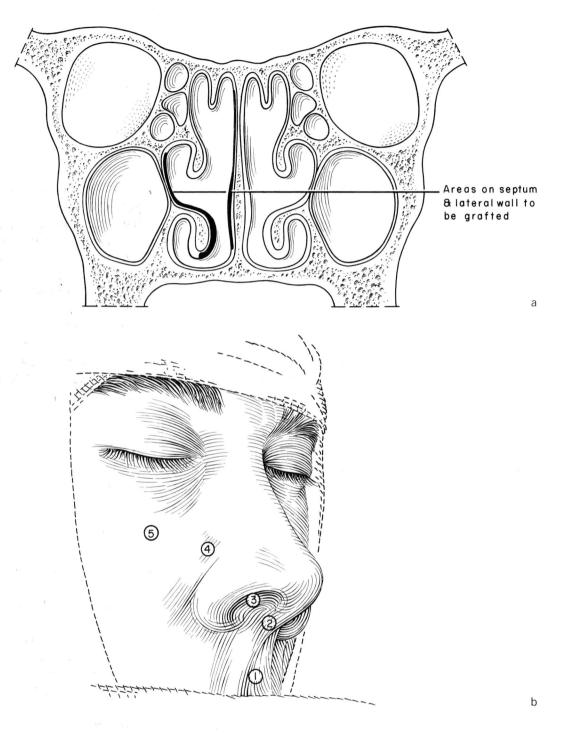

Areas on septum
& lateral wall to
be grafted

a

b

FIGURE 8.11.   *Septal dermoplasty.*

a. A coronal section through the nasal cavities showing the usual areas to be grafted. The graft may be extended around the lateral aspect of the inferior turbinate and include the inferior meatus as well as the floor of the nose.

b. The sites for injecting local anesthetic solution: (1) upper lip; (2) columella; (3) nasal septum; (4) nasofacial sulcus; (5) infraorbital nerve. The nasal cavity is packed with 4% cocaine-impregnated cotton pledgets.

The skin graft donor site is injected with local anesthetic solution.

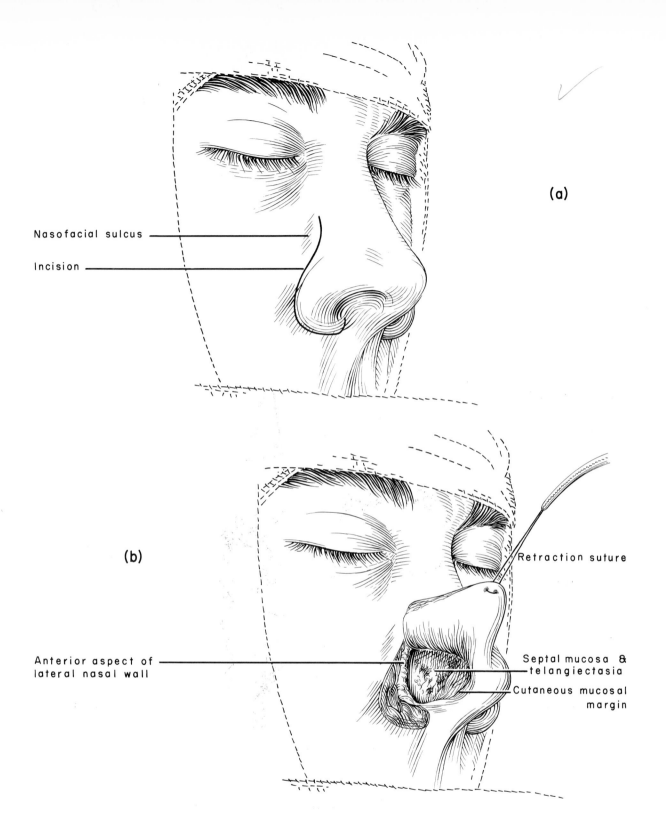

Nasofacial sulcus

Incision

(a)

(b)

Retraction suture

Anterior aspect of
lateral nasal wall

Septal mucosa &
telangiectasia

Cutaneous mucosal
margin

FIGURE 8.12. *Septal dermoplasty (continued).*

    a. The incision is extended through the nasal mucosa to the level of the bony piriform aperture. The incision begins superiorly halfway between the nasofacial crease and the nasal dorsum. It is continued directly inferior to the alar sulcus and around to the nasal orifice inferiorly.

    b. The incision is extended through the nasal mucosa to the level of the bony piriform aperture. One or two sutures are placed to retract the ala superiorly and to the opposite side. Telangiectatic spots can be seen on the septum.

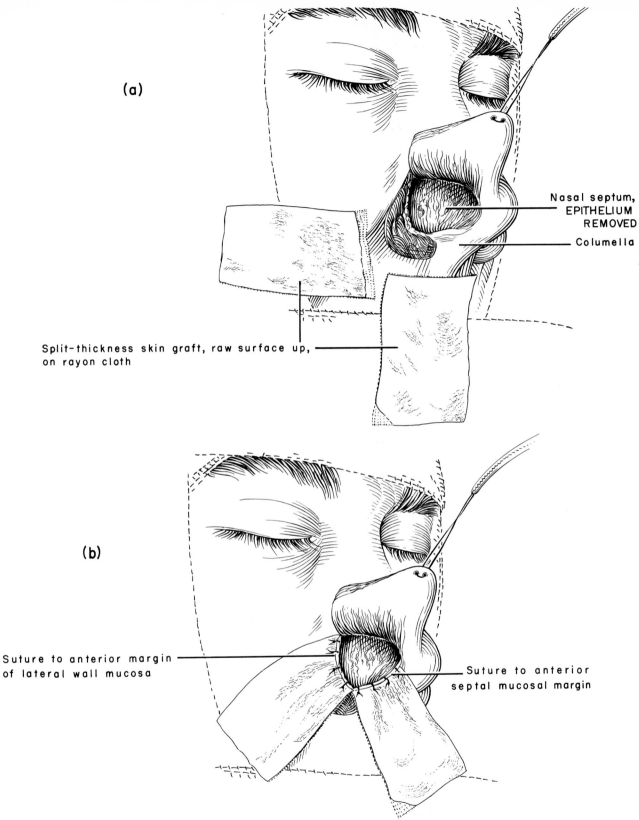

(a)

Nasal septum, EPITHELIUM REMOVED

Columella

Split-thickness skin graft, raw surface up, on rayon cloth

(b)

Suture to anterior margin of lateral wall mucosa

Suture to anterior septal mucosal margin

FIGURE 8.13. *Septal dermoplasty (continued).*

a. The mucous membrane is dissected from the anterior septum and the lateral wall, including that on the medial aspect of the inferior turbinate. The perichondrium is to remain undisturbed as much as is possible. A split-thickness skin graft is placed on rayon cloth with the raw surface facing free.

b. One edge of each skin graft is sutured to the anterior margin of the mucous membrane of the septum and lateral wall. The grafts are to be reflected into the nasal cavity and packed in place.

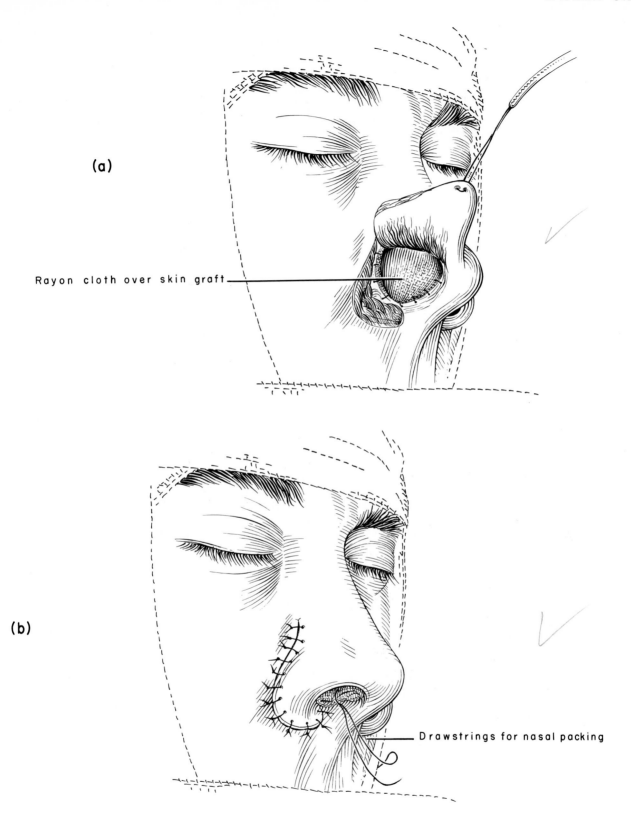

(a)

Rayon cloth over skin graft

(b)

Drawstrings for nasal packing

FIGURE 8.14. *Septal dermoplasty (continued).*

a. After the skin grafts have been reflected into the nasal cavity the rayon cloth can be seen covering the grafts.

b. The subcutaneous layer is sutured with #4-0 catgut and the skin incision with #5-0 or #6-0 suture material. The nasal cavity is loosely packed with antibiotic-impregnated iodoform gauze.

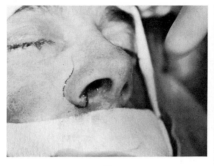

a

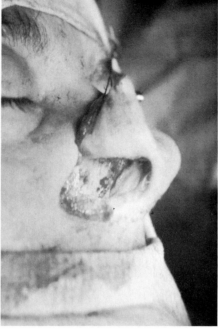

b

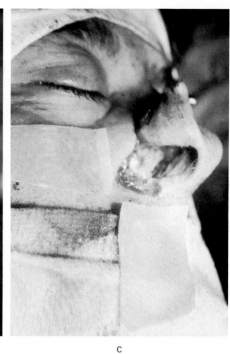

c

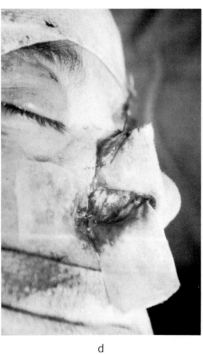

d

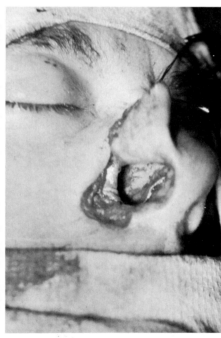

e

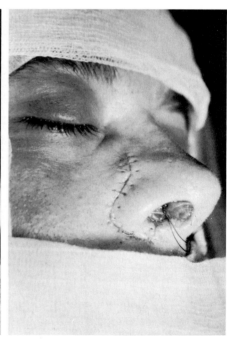

f

FIGURE 8.15. *Septal dermoplasty.*

a. Incision for exposure of anterior nasal cavity and septal dermoplasty.

b. The ala has been retracted superiorly and to the opposite side. The mucous membrane has been dissected from the septum and lateral nasal wall.

c. Split-thickness skin grafts on rayon cloth are in readiness to be sutured anteriorly.

d. The skin grafts have been sutured to the anterior margin of the mucous membrane of the septum and lateral wall.

e. The skin grafts have been reflected into the nasal cavities.

f. The nasal cavity has been packed loosely with antibiotic-impregnated iodoform gauze and the incision closed in layers.

The intranasal packing remains in place for 4 or 5 days. The nasolabial skin sutures are removed after one week. The patient is instructed to apply petrolatum or mineral oil to each side of the nose several times a day. The nasal cavity should be examined once a week, at which time crusts and excessive skin graft are removed. Instructions for long-term nasal care are necessary, for some degree of crusting will persist. This can be controlled with saline irrigations and the application of petrolatum.

NASOSEPTAL PERFORATION

The symptoms associated with nasoseptal perforation can be distressing. The crusting and epistaxis accompanying a large perforation are usually controlled by topical agents which effect lubrication. On the other hand, the noisy respiration (whistle) produced by the small anterior perforation is quite annoying for the patient and for those who surround him. It is usually this symptom which prompts the patient to seek aid.

The causes of septal perforations have been thoroughly reviewed by Seeley. The structural abnormality consists of a bilateral mucosal dehiscence coupled with the absence of septal cartilage, and, at times, bone. Most commonly the limits (margins) of the perforation are covered with mucous membrane which has extended over the exposed cartilage. Chemical agents, such as those used with cauterization of blood vessels in the treatment of epistaxis, are probably the most common cause of perforations. Metabolic disorders, particularly diabetes mellitus, are predisposing factors to septal perforations because of impaired vasculature and greater susceptibility to infection. Infection, either directly by necrosis of tissue or indirectly following incision and drainage of a septal abscess, can result in a septal perforation. Trauma to the septum—accidental, iatrogenic (nose-picking), or surgical—occasionally results in a septal perforation. Congenital perforations, although rare, have been reported.

Ballenger has stated that large nasoseptal perforations are not amenable to surgery. Small defects, usually 1.5 cm in diameter or less and located anteriorly in the septum, are the most common and happily the easiest to repair. As would be expected, there have been many techniques introduced for the repair of these perforations. Most methods utilize unilateral or bilateral sliding flaps of septal mucous membrane.

After the inner rim of mucous membrane has been removed, simple primary closure of septal perforation with through-and-through sutures usually results in failure (Fig. 8.16).

Hazeltine's method, as described by the Ballengers, represents the principle of sliding mucosal flaps (Fig. 8.17). With small perforations, the advantage of this procedure is that both sides are covered; thus the chances for a permanent closure are greatly enhanced. A unilateral septal flap, described by Berson, has been noted to have a rather high incidence of failure.

Autogenous septal cartilage grafts have been used to lend support to the septal flaps. Central necrosis and curling of the graft is described by Goldman, and by Huffman and Lierle. These authors noted that cartilagenous grafts, inserted during submucous resection of the nasal septum, underwent resorption as a late complication. Missal reported a rejection of five out of seven Ivalon septal implants. He speculated that the rejection was secondary to specific hyperimmunity of nasal

FIGURE 8.16

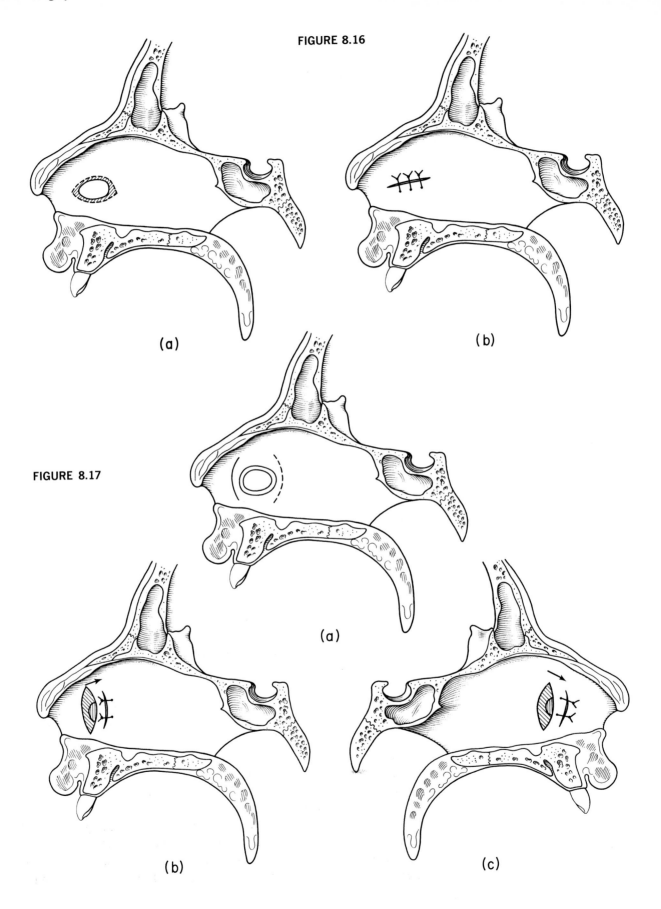

(a)

(b)

FIGURE 8.17

(a)

(b)

(c)

tissue to foreign substances. Behrman reported three cases of fascia lata grafts in which the fascia lata was sandwiched between septal mucosal flaps. In two of the three patients, infection occurred, but healing eventually took place in all three.

An entirely different approach to repair of the septal perforation is Seiffert's method as described by Aubry. The septum is tented toward the largest middle turbinate until direct approximation occurs. Both the inner rim of the perforation and the adjacent area of middle turbinate must be denuded of epithelium. The nasal septum is held against the middle turbinate with a tamponade in the opposite nasal cavity until union has been made between the septum and middle turbinate. The union is then divided by resecting a portion of the middle turbinate (Fig. 8.18). It would seem that this method of repair is rather uncomfortable for the patient, as well as quite difficult for the surgeon.

Ismail, in 1964, presented 13 cases of septal perforation repair made by utilizing a free full-thickness graft from the middle turbinate. The procedure is described as being technically easy, and the results are creditable.

Meyer has presented the possibility of the use of an acrylic or nylon obturator in the treatment for septal perforation. No report of the results was published. It might be speculated that long-term usage of an obturator could lead to such complications as secondary infection and epistaxis.

An inferiorly based flap fashioned from the anterior lateral nasal mucous membrane was advocated by McGivern. The mucous membrane flap is reflected medially and inferiorly so that its lateral, or raw, surface can be sutured to the nasal septum surrounding the perforation (Fig. 8.19). The flap must traverse the nasal cavity and be subsequently divided after the perforation has been closed. It would seem that such a pedicled flap would be difficult to create and maintain.

Goldstein (Ballenger, 1947) presented a technique using a pedicled flap of the septal mucous membrane directly behind the perforation (Fig. 8.20). This flap is based just posterior to the perforation. It is rotated through the perforation and inserted between the septal cartilage and the mucous membrane on the opposite side of the septum. In preparation for the mucosal flap, the mucous membrane is removed from the inner margin of the perforation, and the septal mucous membrane is separated from the cartilage surrounding the perforation on the opposite side of the septum.

FIGURE 8.16. *Simple primary closure of nasoseptal perforation.*

   a. The perforation is prepared by removing the mucous membrane on its inner margin.
   b. The perforation is closed with transfixion sutures.

FIGURE 8.17. *Hazeltine's method of closure of nasoseptal perforation.*

   a. A slightly curved, vertical incision is made anterior to the perforation on one side and posterior to the perforation on the opposite side. The mucous membrane is removed from the inner margin of the perforation.
   b. The mucous membrane on the side with the anterior vertical incision is reflected posteriorly as this side of the perforation is closed.
   c. The mucous membrane on the opposite side migrates anteriorly, and thus the suture lines are not on opposing sides of the nasal septum.

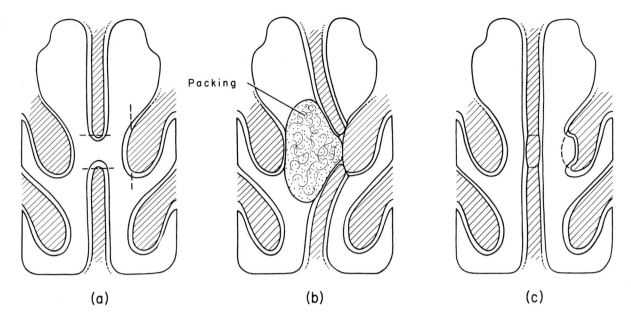

FIGURE 8.18. *Seiffert's method of closure of nasoseptal perforation.*

a. A coronal section showing the septal perforation and the turbinates.

b. The mucous membrane has been removed from the inner rim of the perforation and the opposing portion of the middle turbinate. The septum is packed and placed against the middle turbinate.

c. When healing has taken place (approximately 2 weeks) a portion of the middle turbinate is removed and the septum replaced to the midline.

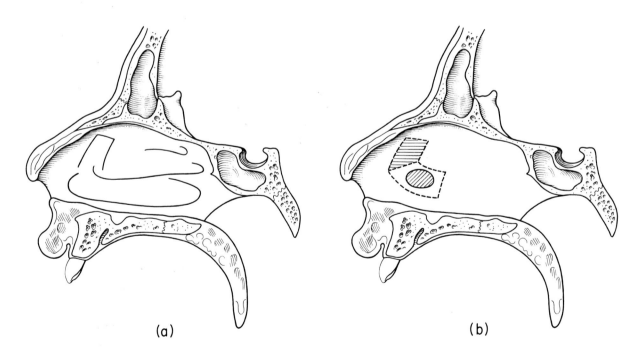

FIGURE 8.19. *McGivern's method of closure of nasoseptal perforation.*

a. An inferiorly based flap of anterosuperior lateral wall nasal mucous membrane is elevated.

b. The flap is reflected medially and inferiorly so that its raw surface can be sutured to the area surrounding the perforation. It is necessary to remove mucous membrane surrounding the perforation on this site to receive the pedicle flap. The flap is separated at a later date when all healing has taken place (approximately two to three weeks).

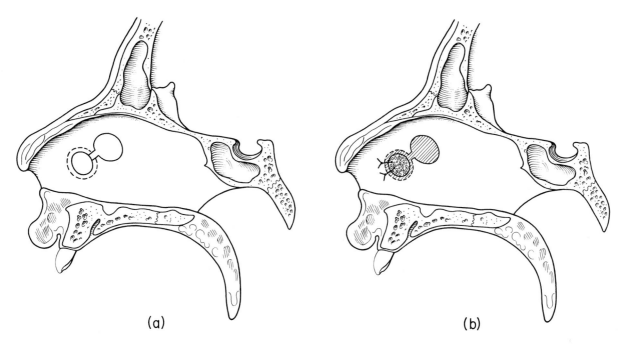

FIGURE 8.20. *Goldstein's method of closure of nasoseptal perforation.*

    a. An anteriorly based flap of nasal mucous membrane is elevated anteriorly and reflected through the perforation. A circumferential incision is made around the perforation on the opposite side of the septum. The mucous membrane and the inner margin of the perforation are also removed.

    b. The flap is held in place with one or two transfixion sutures.

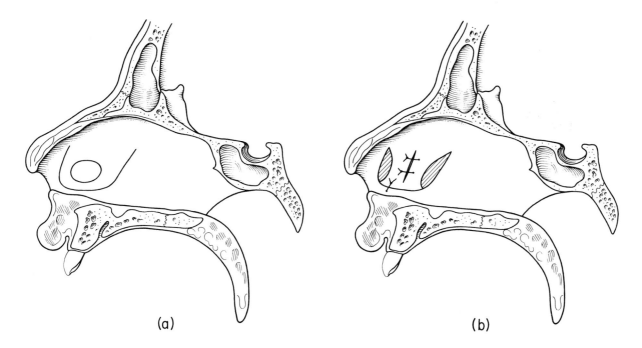

FIGURE 8.21. *Seeley and Climo's method of closure of nasoseptal perforation.*

    a. A superiorly based flap is elevated on one side of the septum after routine rhinoplasty incisions have been made in an attempt to eliminate all tension on the suture line.

    b. The perforation is then closed, creating a denuded area anterior and posterior to the flap.

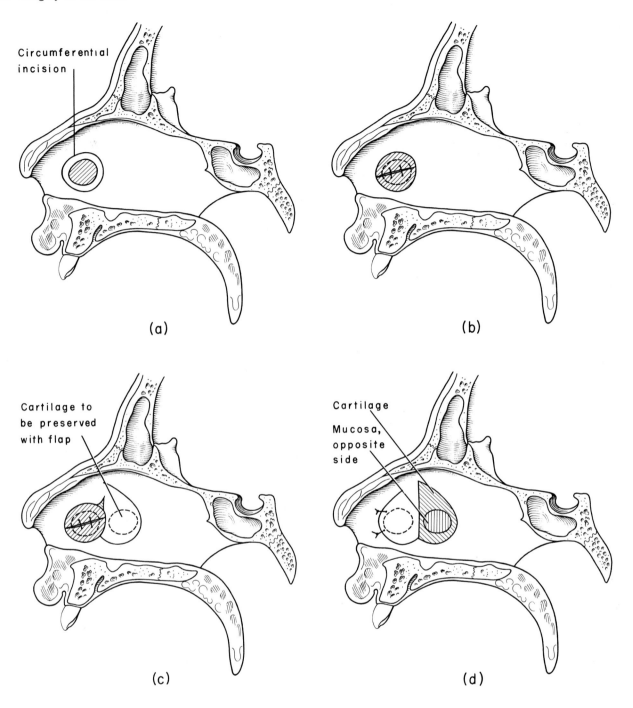

FIGURE 8.22. *Method of closure of nasoseptal perforation preferred by author.*

a. A circumferential incision is made around the perforation approximately 3 mm from its edge. The mucous membrane is elevated toward the perforation and also from the inner rim of the perforation.

b. Usually enough mucous membrane is acquired so that the perforation can be closed from the opposite side with two #4-0 chromic catgut sutures.

c. A superiorly based pedicle flap is fashioned posterior to the perforation. As the flap is elevated, cartilage remains attached to the lower half of the pedicle flap. The upper half of the flap is elevated in the plane between the cartilage and the mucoperichondrium. The cartilage is fashioned so that it is exactly the size of the perforation.

d. The flap is advanced forward and held in place with one or two #3-0 chromic catgut transfixion sutures.

Seeley and Climo have presented a more extensive and involved approach to the problem. Both authors advocate the standard rhinoplasty incision because of the greater visibility it permits at the time of operation and because of the more extensive mucosa available for approximation. The posterosuperiorly based flap (Fig. 8.21) enjoys an excellent blood supply.

Another method of closure found to be most useful is that which employs a superiorly based pedicle flap on the nasal septum, to which is attached a piece of septal cartilage the size of the perforation (Fig. 8.22). This procedure is in concert with the thoughts of Huffman and Lierle that, "if the cartilage could be left attached to at least one side of the septal membrane as part of a compound flap," there is a higher incidence of success. The repair can be accomplished from either side of the nasal septum. A circumferential incision is made approximately 3 to 4 mm around the edge of the perforation (Fig. 8.22a). The mucous membrane is carefully raised toward the perforation and elevated away from its inner margin. This maneuver affords enough epithelium so that it may be approximated with #4-0 chromic catgut on a very small, cutting, curved needle, thus closing the perforation on the contralateral side of the septum (Fig. 8.22b).

A superiorly based mucoperichondrial flap, which is large enough to cover the perforation and the surrounding defect, is fashioned (Fig. 8.22c). The inferior half of this pedicle flap is made through the cartilage, whereas the upper half is elevated in a place between the perichondrium and the cartilage. The cartilage attached to the lower half of the pedicle flap is then trimmed so that it is just the size of the septal perforation. The flap is swung anteriorly into the defect and sutured in place with #3-0 chromic catgut sutures (Fig. 8.22d). Keogh has described a similar procedure with apparently good results. He has chosen to cover the exposed cartilage of the pedicle flap with a free skin graft, rather than invert the nasal mucosa through the perforation.

Rubber finger-cot packs covered with Aureomycin ointment are inserted into both nasal cavities. These should remain in place for at least 2 days. The patient should be instructed to avoid blowing or picking his nose during the early postoperative period. Thus far, results from this method have been quite encouraging.

ABSCESS OF THE NASAL SEPTUM

Abscess of the nasal septum most commonly follows hematoma secondary to trauma or an operation upon the septum. It can also occur secondary to intranasal or sinus infection. It occasionally follows a furuncle of the upper lip or nose. Its most common site is the anterior cartilaginous area.

Signs and Symptoms

An abscess of the nasal septum usually develops over a period of several days. The patient complains of chills, fever, pain, and increasing unilateral or bilateral nasal obstruction. There may or may not be erythema and swelling of the external nose. On examination, either one or both sides of the nasal septum are seen to be swollen and red. There may be a loss of cartilaginous septum when the purulent discharge accumulates between the mucoperichondrium and cartilage and remains there for some time (Fig. 8.23a). Thus, early, adequate drainage is of great importance.

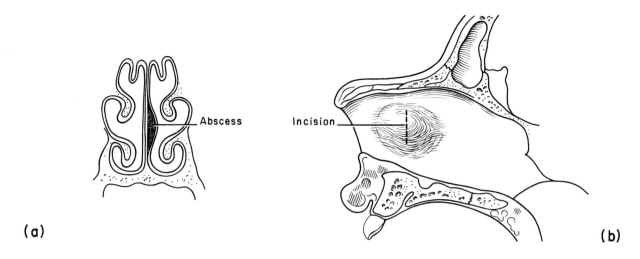

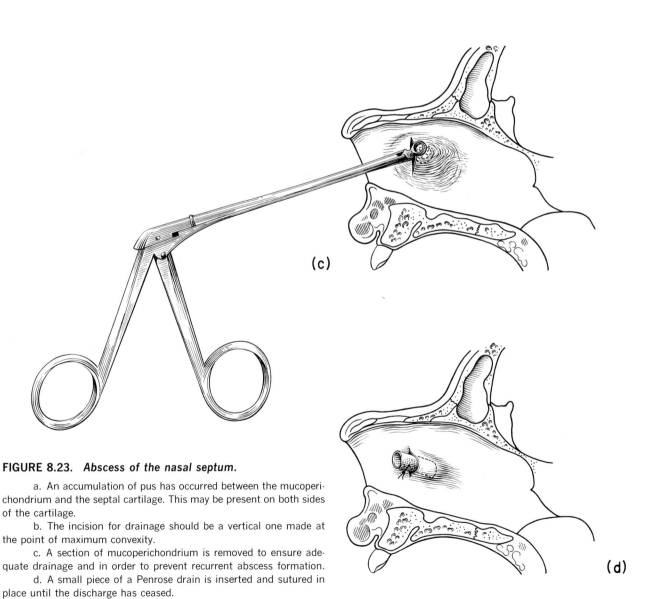

FIGURE 8.23.   *Abscess of the nasal septum.*

a. An accumulation of pus has occurred between the mucoperichondrium and the septal cartilage. This may be present on both sides of the cartilage.

b. The incision for drainage should be a vertical one made at the point of maximum convexity.

c. A section of mucoperichondrium is removed to ensure adequate drainage and in order to prevent recurrent abscess formation.

d. A small piece of a Penrose drain is inserted and sutured in place until the discharge has ceased.

Diagnosis

Usually the diagnosis of abscess of the nasal septum is obvious when there is a history of trauma, surgical procedure, or intranasal infection. There is unilateral or bilateral nasal obstruction due to swelling of the medial wall of the nasal cavity. The fluctuation may be palpated with a cotton applicator. On occasion the development of a septal abscess may be insidious and difficult to diagnose. In such an instance, aspiration of the area with a #20-gauge hypodermic needle will be required to determine its presence. A topical anesthetic should be applied prior to the aspiration.

Treatment

Adequate drainage and antibiotic therapy constitute the treatment of choice. Cocaine solution (4%) is applied to the nasal cavity, first by spray, and then by packing with cotton strips. With a #11 or #15 surgical blade, a vertical incision is made in the area of maximum convexity (Fig. 8.23b). Pus is removed by aspiration and sent to the bacteriology laboratory for culture and sensitivity tests. A section of mucoperichondrium is removed with a ring punch to ensure adequate drainage (Fig. 8.23c). A small section of Penrose drain is then secured in place with catgut suture (Fig. 8.23d). When the swelling is bilateral, incision and drainage are carried out on both sides of the septum. These incisions should not be apposing so as to avoid a complicating septal perforation. The drain or drains remain in place until discharge has subsided (2 to 3 days). Specific antibiotic therapy is continued for at least 10 days to prevent recurrence of the abscess and loss of cartilage.

NASAL POLYPECTOMY

Nasal polyps develop from a prolapse of overloaded edematous respiratory epithelium. The stimulus for this reaction is an irritant, which may be an allergen— bacterial or chemical. Polyps develop in areas in which tissue constructions are delicate, such as in the middle meatus and sinuses. The common sites of origin are the crest of the uncinate process, the sinus ostia, the anterior surface of the ethmoid bulla, and the mucous membrane of the sinuses, especially of the ethmoid and maxillary sinuses.

Signs and Symptoms

Nasal polyps almost invariably occur bilaterally and are quite often associated with chronic allergic or bacterial sinusitis. The symptom which brings the patient to his doctor is a gradually increasing nasal stuffiness which can terminate in complete nasal obstruction. Some patients tolerate the nasal obstruction and do not seek medical attention until they have widening of the external nose or until the polyps protrude from the nostrils. Other symptoms are those of chronic, allergic, or bacterial sinusitis.

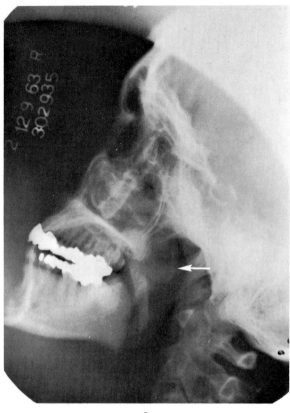

a

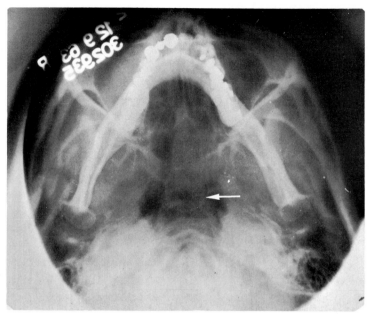

b

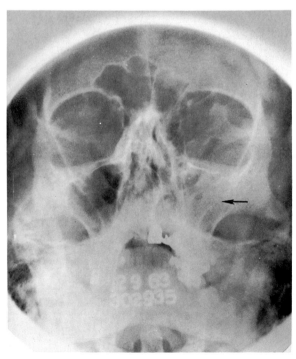

c

FIGURE 8.24. *Choanal polyp.*

a. The most obvious abnormality shown in this x ray is the large choanal polyp (arrow). Also of note is the decalcification and loss of cell partitions in the ethmoid region.

b. A base-of-skull view, showing the outline of the choanal polyp in the left nasal cavity and nasopharynx.

c. This x ray of the same patient demonstrates some increased density in the ethmoid regions. Both nasal cavities are partially obstructed by polyps. Thickened membrane can be seen in the right maxillary sinus. The left antrum is dense, indicating the site of origin of the left choanal polyp. In this situation, a Caldwell-Luc operation is performed to ensure against the possible recurrence of the lesion.

Diagnosis

Nasal polyps are smooth, glistening, grapelike masses, yellowish or pink in color. They are rarely found in one nasal cavity only. The patient has a history of gradually increasing nasal stuffiness. As a rule, the symptoms are not seasonal and the patient has signs and symptoms of chronic sinus disease. Sinus x rays (Fig. 8.24) will show that the nasal cavities are partially or completely occluded. The ethmoid cell partitions are washed out, and there is usually increased density in the ethmoid labyrinth. The maxillary sinuses may show evidence of either thickened membrane or polyps. A choanal polyp may be present.

Surgical Technique of Polypectomy

The removal of nasal polyps as an office procedure is an art. An improperly conducted polypectomy is a most unpleasant experience, both for the patient and for the surgeon. If the patient seems apprehensive, slight sedation or a tranquilizer, given one half hour before the procedure, is quite helpful.

For anesthesia, the nasal cavities are packed with cotton strips impregnated with 4% cocaine solution or 2% Pontocaine solution, with added epinephrine. The packing is removed after 10 minutes. Fresh cotton strips, impregnated with the anesthetic agent, are inserted at least one additional time, until adequate anesthesia is obtained. The areas usually missed during a first attempt are in the superior and posterior nasal cavity and middle meatus.

A nasal snare with a loop, 1 inch in diameter, is used. It is adjusted to a size that can be inserted into the nasal cavity without producing pain. The operator grasps the shaft of the snare in its midsection as one would grasp a pencil. He inserts the loop in a vertical plane and then rotates it to the horizontal plane below the level of the polyps. He then slowly manipulates it over the polyps in an upward and lateral direction, toward the middle meatus, which is the usual site of polyp origin. He grasps the handle to close the wire loop while steadying the snare at its center with his free hand. The polyps are removed with forceps or metal suction tips.

This procedure is repeated until all polyps have been removed. If bleeding becomes troublesome at any time the nasal cavity is packed with cotton strips impregnated with epinephrine solution, and the operator proceeds to remove the polyps in the opposite nasal cavity. Smaller polyps are removed with Brownie, Takahashi, or ring forceps. It is best not to use traction on polyps having their origin in the superior meatus, for these may extend to the olfactory slit. Trauma in this region can produce a defect in the cribriform plate resulting in cerebrospinal fluid leakage and its complications.

All tissue, regardless of the number or size of the polyps, or of the number of past polypectomies, should be sent to the pathology laboratory for sectioning and diagnosis. Many malignant tumors are masked by overlying nasal polyps.

Those patients who have had repeated polypectomies and in whom x rays show evidence of either chronic polypoid ethmoiditis or maxillary sinusitis, or both, should be admitted to the hospital for both polypectomy and the appropriate sinus operation, i.e., intranasal ethmoidectomy or the Caldwell-Luc operation. These procedures are quite gratifying, for a significant percentage of the patients will either not have recurrence of the polyposis or will have a remission of several years' duration.

Choanal Polyp

The choanal polyp is a separate clinical entity. This polyp is most often unilateral and can attain enormous size. The symptom which troubles the patient is nasal obstruction. The obstruction is at first unilateral, and then, as the choanal polyp increases in size, it obstructs the entire nasopharynx. On occasion a choanal polyp may appear below the level of the uvula.

The patient should be admitted to the hospital for removal of the choanal polyp and a Caldwell-Luc operation. Simply removing the polyp is unwise, for unless the condition responsible for its origin, chronic maxillary sinusitis, is treated, a recurrence is probable.

To remove the choanal polyp, a piece of #5 snare wire, about 1 foot in length, is doubled upon itself to form a loop which is inserted into the nasopharynx by way of the nasal cavity. The ends of this snare wire are held with the surgeon's left hand. The surgeon's right hand is inserted into the nasopharynx by way of the patient's mouth. The tip of the surgeon's finger palpates the end of the wire loop and maneuvers it up over the dome of the choanal polyp. Traction is then applied with the surgeon's left hand, and the wire loop is pulled forward in contact with the stalk of the choanal polyp in the middle meatus as it exits from the ostium of the maxillary sinus. The ends of the wire are then inserted into, and attached to, the snare apparatus. The stalk of the choanal polyp is sectioned, and the polyp is removed from the nasopharynx by way of the mouth.

A Caldwell-Luc operation (see p. 211) is then performed, removing all polyps and diseased membrane.

Postoperative Care

Hemorrhage rarely occurs following a polypectomy. If it does it should be handled as any other epistaxis. It is best to tell the patient that in all probability the polyps will return and that it is impossible to predict when. If purulent secretion is noted at the time of polypectomy, this should be cultured and the appropriate antibiotics administered. Sinus x rays are indicated at this time. Many surgeons elect to institute short-term steroid therapy (10 days) following polypectomy in an attempt to reverse the process completely or to prolong the remission.

INTRANASAL TUMORS

Tumors of the nasal cavity vary from small, benign lesions to massive, destructive, and invasive malignant tumors. Benign lesions tend to be smooth, firm, localized, and covered with mucous membrane. Malignant lesions are usually friable, granular, infiltrating, and susceptible to bleeding.

Signs and Symptoms

The signs and symptoms of intranasal tumors are as follows:
1. Nasal stuffiness or obstruction, usually unilateral
2. Nasal discharge, either mucoid or purulent
3. Bleeding, scanty or profuse, usually unilateral

4. External deformity (an expanding lesion may displace the nasal bones laterally and cause widening of the nose; masses may appear externally after eroding through bone, especially in the region of the inner canthus; destruction of bone can cause depression deformities)

5. Polypoid change, which may be associated with other tumors, benign or malignant, and may mask the underlying pathologic condition in spite of repeated polypectomies and histologic examinations (thus, when suspicious of a tumor, a thorough examination [x ray, etc.] is most important as well as admission to the hospital, where more adequate biopsies may be obtained with the patient under general anesthesia if necessary; any complication, such as hemorrhage, can be best managed at the hospital)

6. Pain (this may be severe when the tumor is accompanied by cellulitis or osteomyelitis)

7. Tearing (caused by invasion of the lacrimal sac, lacrimal duct, or obstruction of the nasolacrimal duct orifice by a lesion in the inferior meatus)

8. Such symptoms as pain in the teeth, exophthalmos, diplopia, paresthesia, or anesthesia of the cheek, which may indicate extension of disease to the sinuses or orbit

Diagnosis

Diagnosis is established by means of anterior and posterior rhinoscopy, x-ray study (planograms), or biopsy.

Classification

Lesions found in the nasal cavities may be classified as follows:

	Benign Lesions	Malignant Lesions
ECTODERMAL		
	Glioma	Olfactory esthesio-
	Encephalocele	neuroblastoma
	Neurofibroma	Malignant schwannoma
	Meningocele	
EPITHELIAL		
	Dermoid cyst	Squamous cell carcinoma
	Sebaceous cyst	Basal cell carcinoma
	Epidermoid cyst	Transitional cell carcinoma
	Papilloma	Adenocarcinoma
	Inverted papilloma	Malignant melanoma
MESODERMAL		
	Hemangioma	Ameloblastoma
	Lipoma	Fibrosarcoma
	Mixed tumors	Chondrosarcoma
	Chondroma	Osteogenic sarcoma
	Fibroma	Plasmacytoma
	Osteoma	Lymphoblastoma
	Angiofibroma	
	Ossifying fibroma	

Certain of the benign lesions are classified as clinically malignant, either because of their location or their rapidly progressive growth and tendency to recur after removal. The inverted papilloma, mixed tumor, and chondroma are classified as such and should be treated as malignant tumors.

Principles of Treatment

Chondroma, Chondrosarcoma, Malignant Mixed Tumor, and Inverted Papilloma. The recurrent chondroma, chondrosarcoma, and malignant mixed tumor should be treated by wide resection, for they are multiple, sessile, friable, and very susceptible to bleeding. Inverted papillomas which recur rapidly, show signs of early malignant change, or demonstrate extensive recurrence or invasion should be treated by resection followed by a full course of postoperative radiation therapy. Repeated biopsies are often misleading, for the malignant portion of the lesion may be deep. The malignant inverted papilloma (papillary squamous carcinoma) tends to metastasize to the lungs and submaxillary lymph nodes.

Ossifying Fibroma. Ossifying fibroma is considered to be a localized manifestation of fibrous dysplasia. It may appear first as an intranasal tumor and is frequently noted in childhood. It usually involves the anterior ethmoid bone, sphenoid bone, nasal bone, orbit, and base of the skull. Surgical treatment is usually unsatisfactory, incomplete, and complicated by hemorrhage.

It is now well known that the less spectacular form of fibrous dysplasia (i.e., that of a solitary monostotic lesion) is not associated with any known physiologic changes and is by far the more common than the polyostotic form, the ratio being about 40:1. The monostotic form is considered by some to be an entirely different entity from the polyostotic form with non-bony manifestations.

The clinical characteristics of ossifying fibroma may be described briefly as follows:

1. The lesion has a definite female preponderance (3:1).
2. The bone lesions usually have their inception in childhood, although they may not become clinically evident until later. Occasionally, however, the onset may not be until later in life.
3. The facial bones, femur, tibia, and ribs are the bones most commonly involved.
4. The tumor usually is a slow-growing asymptomatic tumor which ceases to grow, or very markedly slows in growth rate, after adolescence.
5. There are no diagnostic laboratory findings, although, in patients with an actively growing lesion, there is an elevation of serum alkaline phosphatase (apparently derived from the abnormal elevation of this substance in the connective tissue cells of the tumor).
6. The roentgenographic picture is one of replacement of bone tissue outward, from within, toward the cortex, producing the typical "ground-glass" appearance. In the facial bones particularly, the lesions are generally sclerotic and, therefore, radiopaque.
7. The lesions, if multiple, are usually unilateral.

The prognosis is excellent. Complete removal is desirable and offers the best chance for permanent cure. Recurrence is usually the price of incomplete removal. There are, however, reports of patients who had incomplete excision without subsequent recurrence during a number of years of follow-up study. If the tumor is not symptomatic in an adult and does not appear to be growing, no therapy may be necessary. It would seem that, as with most benign tumors, individual consideration should be given to each patient in regard to the growth rate of the tumor, location of the lesion, extent of the surgical defect which would be produced by excision, and the age of the patient, since, as stated previously, growth rate generally slows or ceases with increasing age. The physician should be alert for signs of malignant change such as pain or sudden acceleration of growth.

The fact that malignant degeneration of fibrous dysplasia does occur is still not universally accepted. To date there have been 29 cases of malignant degeneration of fibrous dysplasia involving the nose reported. These cases all appear to be well substantiated, and several are histologically confirmed.

There is no appreciable difference in the incidence of degeneration between the monostotic and polyostotic lesions when one considers the number of lesions in the individual with the polyostotic form.

The influence of prior radiation is not clear, but radiation therapy does appear to have a predisposing propensity to malignant degeneration, as 12 of the 29 patients had received radiation therapy on an average of about 14 years prior to the onset of signs of malignant change. Conversely, it can be stated that radiation therapy is not necessarily a prerequisite for malignant degeneration, as 16 of the 29 patients had none at all. Certainly, radiation therapy should be avoided if practically possible, as it is not only implicated in the malignant degeneration of fibrous dysplasia, but is also believed to be the most significant factor in the production of bone sarcoma. Many patients with fibrous dysplasia have received radiation therapy without having malignant degeneration; therefore it is most important that consideration be given to each patient individually and all factors evaluated carefully.

Any lesion of fibrous dysplasia which suddenly exhibits an accelerated growth rate or causes severe pain must be suspected of having undergone malignant degeneration. Once the diagnosis is established, the treatment is the same as that for any bone sarcoma. Complete surgical excision of the lesion with a wide margin of uninvolved bone and soft tissue is the treatment of choice. There is a great tendency for local implantation and recurrence. Regional node dissection is not routinely advocated, as metastasis is usually by the hematogenous route. The most frequent site of metastasis is the lung. The prognosis of osteogenic sarcoma is actually not as bad as is generally believed, and occasionally patients with solitary pulmonary metastasis, in whom the entire metastatic lesion has been removed by lobectomy or pneumectomy, have experienced 5-year survivals. Radiation therapy is also frequently beneficial. It should be emphasized that osteogenic sarcoma is not a hopeless condition and that surprisingly good cure rates have been reported.

Treatment of Intranasal Tumors

Very small lesions of the anterior nasal septum or nasal vestibule, whether malignant or benign, can be resected with adequate surgical margins by way of the nostril. Electrosurgical excision is certainly of great value when removing these small lesions. For malignant lesions involving the septal mucosa, the resection should include the mucoperichondrium and cartilage. All other lesions should be approached by using the lateral rhinotomy incision.

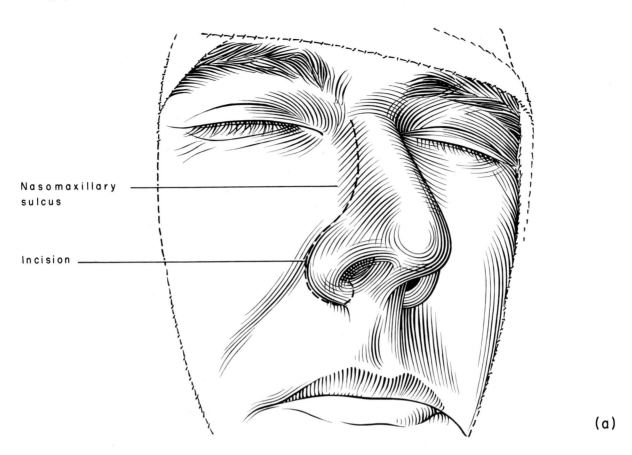

Nasomaxillary sulcus

Incision

(a)

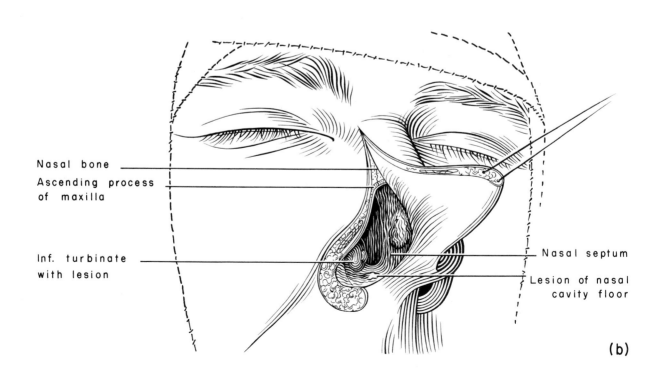

Nasal bone

Ascending process of maxilla

Inf. turbinate with lesion

Nasal septum

Lesion of nasal cavity floor

(b)

Technique of Lateral Rhinotomy. The entire face is prepared for the operation and draped. The eyelids are closed through the tarsal plates with #5-0 or #6-0 suture material.

The patient is placed in the supine position with his head and face parallel to the floor and supported by a rubber doughnut pillow. His head is placed above the level of his chest to reduce venous pressure.

A local anesthetic agent, with epinephrine added, is infiltrated into the line of incision.

The skin incision (Fig. 8.25a) begins, as does the external ethmoid incision, half way between the inner canthus and the nasal dorsum. A #15 blade is used for making this incision. The skin is carefully incised to the subcutaneous layers and blood vessels. The angular artery and vein are identified, clamped, and ligated. If they are inadvertently incised, bleeding can be quite troublesome. Smaller vessels can be cauterized. The incision extends down along the side of the nose rather than in the nasomaxillary skin crease until it reaches the superior aspect of the alar crease (Fig. 8.25a). It is then continued in the alar crease to the nostril.

The alar incision is extended through all layers and into the nasal cavity. This is continued until the maxilla (pyriform crest) is reached. A traction suture of #00 chromic catgut, weighted with a heavy hemostat (Fig. 8.25b), is placed subcutaneously to provide better exposure. If the tumor is fairly anterior on the nasal septum or in the nasal cavity, additional exposure may not be necessary.

The periosteum is elevated from the nasal bone and ascending process of the maxilla with a broad square-ended periosteal elevator. Sufficient nasal bone and ascending process of the maxilla are removed for proper visualization of the nasal cavity (Fig. 8.26). This exposure usually is sufficient for resection of a fairly anteriorly placed lesion or is at least adequate for evaluation and plan of attack.

Malignant lesions of the *nasal septum* should be handled by septectomy with as large a margin as is possible. Skimpy surgical margins or attempts to preserve the opposite mucoperichondrium or periosteum only invite recurrent disease which may be impossible to cure.

Lesions of the floor of the nasal cavity are, in essence, lesions of the palate. Malignant lesions in this area require wide excision. X rays may demonstrate evidence of bone destruction. If the malignant lesion has not invaded the bone of the hard palate, the lesion and the underlying hard palate are resected with an adequate margin (Figs. 8.27b and 8.28). The mucosal incision can be made with the electrosurgical knife and the bone removed with the tangential Stryker saw, preserving the underlying mucosa and thus preventing a palatal defect.

FIGURE 8.25. *Lateral rhinotomy.*

a. The lateral rhinotomy incision begins just above the level of the inner canthus, half way between the latter and the nasal dorsum. For best cosmesis it is continued anterior to the nasomaxillary sulcus (otherwise the scar is likely to be depressed). It then follows the alar sulcus to the nasal vestibule as shown. Rather than make the incision directly from skin to bone, a better technique is to take each layer in an orderly fashion, identifying and ligating vessels as they are encountered.

b. The alar incision is carried through all layers including the nasal mucosa until the bony edge of the maxillary process is encountered. At this time, a traction suture is placed subcutaneously in the lateral alar region and weighted by a heavy hemostat.

This exposes the nasal vestibule and the anterior nasal cavity. Lesions of the anterior septum, floor of the nasal cavity, and inferior turbinate can be seen. The periosteum over the nasal bone and ascending process of the maxilla is elevated so that bone and underlying nasal mucosa can be removed for additional exposure.

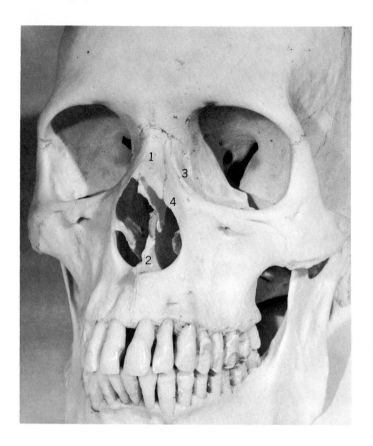

FIGURE 8.26. *Lateral rhinotomy.*

a. The bones involved with the lateral rhinotomy exposure of the nasal cavity include the nasal bone, ascending process of the maxilla, and, on occasion, the lacrimal bone.

1. Nasal bone
2. Nasal septum
3. Lacrimal fossa
4. Ascending process of maxilla

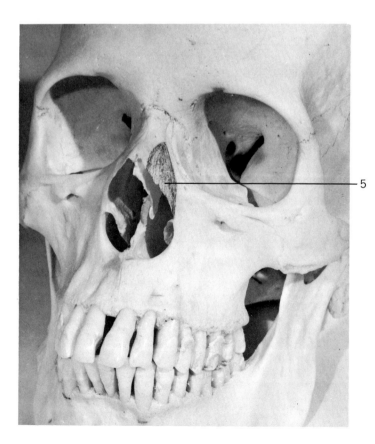

b. The amount of ascending process of maxilla and nasal bone to be removed for adequate exposure of the nasal cavity is indicated (5). If additional exposure is required the bony dissection may be extended to include a portion of the lacrimal bone. Kerrison and "duck-bill" forceps are used for bone removal.

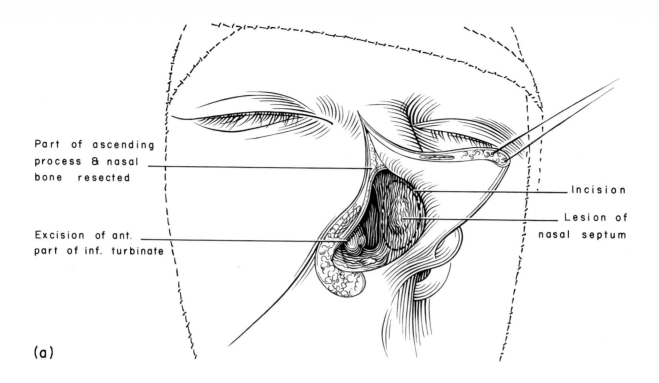

Part of ascending
process & nasal
bone resected

Excision of ant.
part of inf. turbinate

Incision

Lesion of
nasal septum

(a)

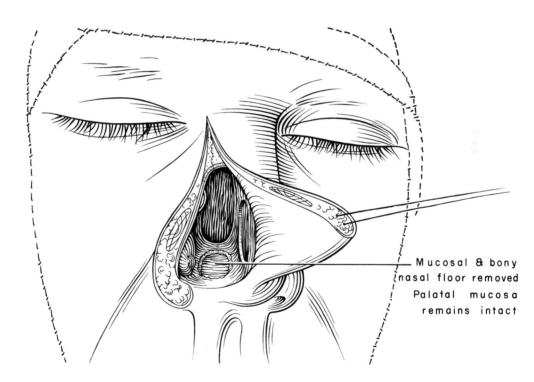

Mucosal & bony
nasal floor removed
Palatal mucosa
remains intact

(b)

FIGURE 8.27. *Lateral rhinotomy.*

a. A portion of the ascending process of the maxilla and nasal bone has been removed. A lesion of the nasal septum and floor of the nose is illustrated to show the exposure acquired by this approach. Even benign lesions should be removed with a good margin of normal mucous membrane.

The underlying bone or cartilage is removed with malignant lesions. The opposite muco-perichondrium or periosteum remains intact. It is not necessary to cover the defect on the septum by grafting.

b. An anterior view of the lateral rhinotomy exposure. A lesion of the floor with the surrounding mucosa and bony floor has been removed. The palatal mucosa is left intact when there is no involvement of the bone. A combined transpalatal approach is best for lesions of the posterior half of the nasal cavity.

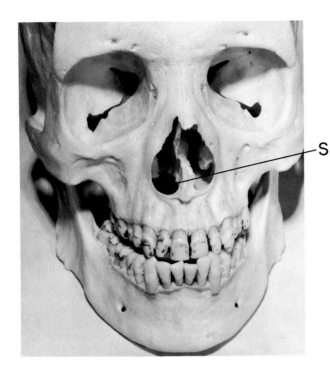

FIGURE 8.28. *Lateral rhinotomy.*

a. Photograph of a skull showing the amount of nasal cavity floor (hard palate) which can be practically removed by way of the lateral rhinotomy exposure. S indicates the surgical defect in the floor of the right nasal cavity.

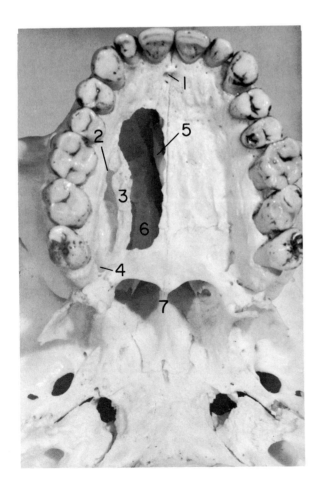

b. A view of this defect from below. The bony palate can be removed piecemeal with Kerrison forceps, or in one piece, using the Stryker saw. The anterior and posterior palatine foramina should be avoided.

1. Anterior palatine foramen
2. Lateral margin of excision
3. Undersurface of inferior turbinate
4. Greater palatine foramen
5. Nasal septum
6. Undersurface of middle turbinate
7. Posterior aspect of nasal septum dividing the choanae

If the malignant lesion has invaded bone, then all layers of the nasal floor are removed (Fig. 8.28), leaving a palatal defect. The defect is blocked temporarily with gauze or cotton packing. After healing is complete, a dental prosthesis can be made.

Often it is difficult to block out a specimen from above. In these cases the procedure is combined with a palatal approach (Fig. 8.29). A flap is elevated and reflected laterally and the bony hard palate removed (Fig. 8.30a). The antero-posterior incision is made to the contralateral side of the midline so that there will be bone under the suture line (Fig. 8.30b).

There are a number of operations for *lesions of the lateral wall,* depending upon their origin (Figs. 8.31 and 8.32). As a rule the operation involves either removing the upper half (middle turbinate), lower half (inferior turbinate), or both.

With lower half lesions, the periosteum is elevated laterally, exposing the anterior wall of the antrum. The incision in the anterior wall of the antrum is made with a tangential Stryker saw (Figs. 8.32 and 8.33). The incisions above and below the inferior turbinate are made with either heavy turbinate scissors or with a chisel. The specimen is transected posteriorly, with either a snare (preferably one that is insulated so that cautery can be used) or right-angle scissors.

The technique for resecting the upper half or entire lateral nasal wall is very similar, except that superiorly the lacrimal fossa and lamina papyracea must be exposed. The ethmoid bone is transected superiorly, just below the plane of the anterior and posterior ethmoid arteries. For malignant lesions—or potentially malignant lesions—the operation should also include a complete ethmoidectomy.

Benign and small malignant lesions of the *superior nasal cavity* can be resected with a good margin by using the lateral rhinotomy incision (Figs. 8.32 and 8.33). It is quite often necessary to reflect the nasal bone of the involved side to the opposite side, or it may be necessary to remove this bone with the specimen. A cerebrospinal fluid leak may occur. This can be repaired with either a septal mucosal flap (see p. 205) or a skin graft.

Lesions which invade the *cribriform area or roof of the ethmoid sinus* present a serious problem. Most often they are recurrent lesions (cylindroma). The best chance for cure is by means of a combined intracranial-intranasal procedure. The floor of the anterior cranial fossa is exposed by way of the frontal flap. A block including the cribriform plate and roof of the ethmoid sinus (crista galli and roof of orbit, if necessary) is outlined from above. A similar block is outlined from below by way of a lateral rhinotomy which may be extended as shown in Figures 8.35 and 8.36. The two approaches are connected and the specimen removed. The defect is repaired from above with fascia lata. A split-thickness skin graft is used intranasally. A mucosal flap from the septum cannot be used, for at least the upper portion of the septum is removed with the specimen. To accomplish a complete rhinotomy the skin incision is extended superiorly across the nasal dorsum (Fig. 8.35). Inferiorly, the incision does not extend into the ipsilateral nasal cavity but just below it—across the base of the columella and into the opposite nasal cavity. Lateral osteotomies are made on each side with a chisel (Fig. 8.36a). These are connected superiorly at the nasofrontal suture line. The nasal septum is divided with straight scissors in the same plane as the osteotomy incisions, and the nose is reflected to one side (Fig. 8.35b). In addition to the superior nasal cavity, the frontal, maxillary, and ethmoid sinuses are easily accessible by this approach. When closing the wound, the nasal septum should be carefully reapproximated. The skin incision is closed with #4-0 chromic silk suture and #5-0 or #6-0 dermal suture.

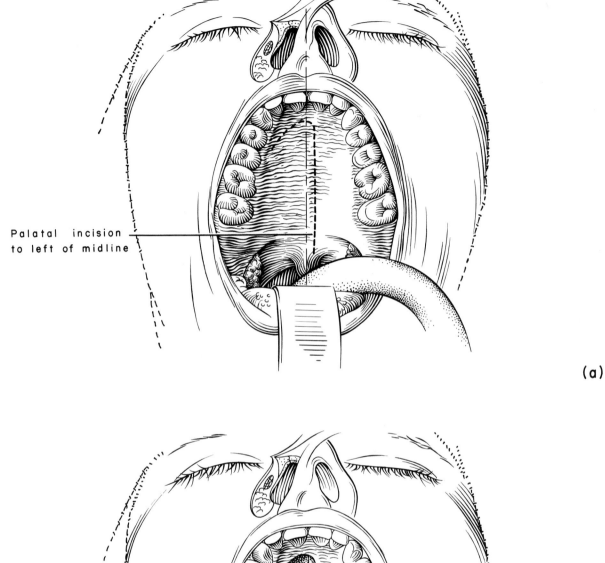

Palatal incision
to left of midline

(a)

Hard palate

Soft palate

(b)

FIGURE 8.29. *Lateral rhinotomy.*

a. Quite often a combined approach—lateral rhinotomy and intraoral—is necessary to remove a lesion of the floor of the nasal cavity. The anteroposterior incision of the mucous membrane and periosteum is made to the left of the midline so that there will be bone underlying the suture line. The incision is directed laterally, immediately posterior to the anterior palatal foramen.

b. A flap consisting of mucosa and periosteum is elevated, exposing the bony hard palate. Traction sutures either weighted by heavy hemostats or tied around the teeth are used for retraction. The mucoperiosteum is easily reflected from the hard palate with flat square-ended periosteal elevators. Elevation of the flap over the soft palate requires a sharp dissection immediately superficial to the muscle layer.

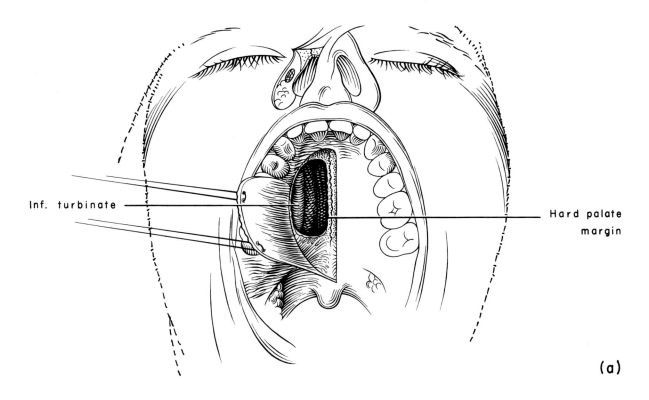

Inf. turbinate

Hard palate margin

(a)

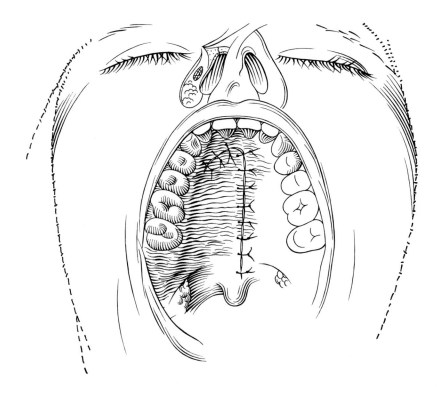

(b)

FIGURE 8.30. *Lateral rhinotomy.*

a. The hard palate has been removed along with the lesion and surrounding nasal mucosa. The nasal mucosal incision is best made from above, with an electrosurgical knife, to ensure an adequate surgical margin. The inferior turbinate is visible.

b. The repaired palatal incision with a one-layer closure. Carefully applied sutures (of #00 chromic catgut) with three knots will guard against development of an oronasal fistula.

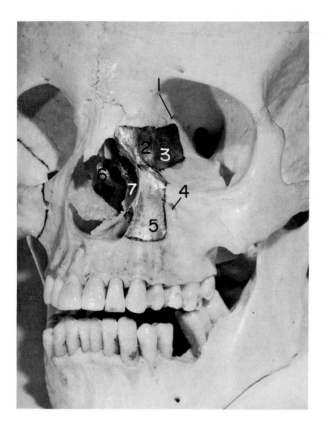

FIGURE 8.31. *Lateral rhinotomy.*

a. The skull is rotated slightly to the right to show the structures to be removed in the upper half and lower half resection of the lateral nasal wall. The upper resection includes a portion of the nasal bone and ascending process of maxilla, the lacrimal bone, and entire ethmoid labyrinth, including the middle turbinate. The lower resection includes a portion of the anterior wall of the antrum (medial to the infraorbital nerve), and the entire inferior turbinate.

1. Anterior ethmoid foramen
2. Lacrimal fossa
3. Lamina papyracea
4. Infraorbital foramen
5. Anterior wall of antrum
6. Right middle turbinate
7. Nasal septum

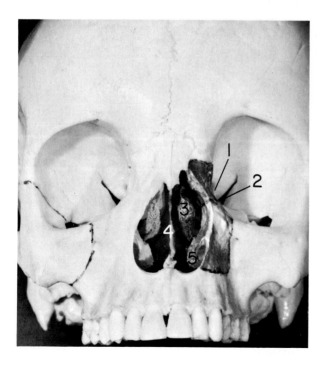

b. A front view of the skull demonstrating the upper and lower half resections of the lateral nasal wall. The middle turbinate and outline of the ethmoid sinus can be seen superiorly on the left. The inferior turbinate, lateral nasal wall, and the amount of anterior wall of the antrum to be resected medial to the infraorbital foramen are indicated below.

1. Optic foramen
2. Superior orbital fissure
3. Middle turbinate
4. Nasal septum
5. Inferior turbinate

FIGURE 8.32. *Lateral rhinotomy.*

a. A medial view of the lateral nasal wall showing the upper and lower resections. The middle turbinate and its upper extension (i.e., medial wall of the ethmoid labyrinth) are included in the upper half resection of the lateral nasal wall. The inferior turbinate and medial wall of the maxillary sinus are included in the lower half resection of the lateral nasal wall.

1. Cribriform plate
2. Roof of ethmoid
3. Probe in left frontal sinus
4. Probe in left nasolacrimal duct
5. Left middle turbinate
6. Probe in left sphenoid ostium
7. Probe from left frontal sinus
8. Inferior turbinate

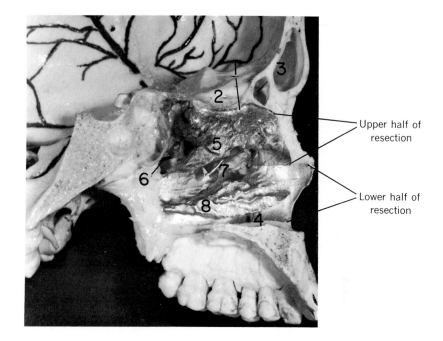

b. An upper resection of the lateral nasal wall is seen on the left side of this skull. The roof of the ethmoid, attachment of the upper extension of the middle turbinate, and a small portion of the anterior wall of the sphenoid sinus can be seen. Note the close relationship of the posterior ethmoid cell and the optic foramen. A lower half resection has been done on the right side and is viewed from the left. This transects the nasolacrimal duct. Note the amount of anterior maxillary sinus wall which has been resected.

1. Sphenoid ostium
2. Perpendicular plate of ethmoid
3. Right antrum
4. Vomer bone
5. Roof of ethmoid
6. Optic foramen
7. Superior orbital fissure

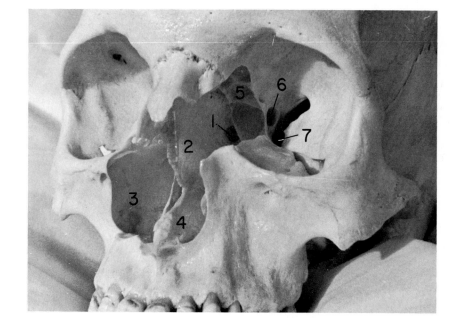

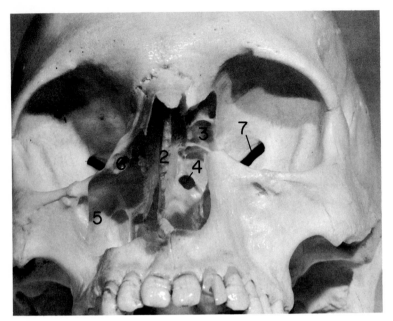

FIGURE 8.33. *Lateral rhinotomy.*

a. The skull is rotated slightly to the right showing the end result of an upper half resection of the lateral nasal wall. The remaining portions of the nasal bone and ascending process, the anterior and posterior ethmoid foramina, optic foramen, roof of ethmoid sinuses, and anterior wall of the sphenoid, outline this resection. Note the size of the bony sphenoid sinus ostium.

It may be necessary to transect the lacrimal duct. If so, the medial wall of the lacrimal sac is removed to ensure proper drainage.

1. Cribriform plate
2. Nasal septum
3. Roof of ethmoid
4. Sphenoid ostium
5. Right maxillary sinus
6. Transected nasolacrimal duct
7. Superior orbital fissure

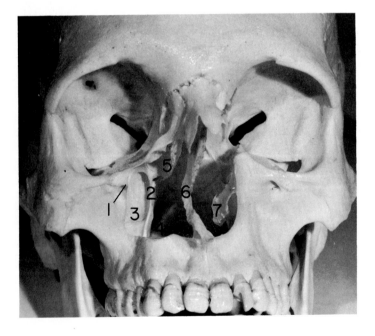

b. The skull is rotated slightly to the left showing the end result of a lower half resection of the lateral nasal wall on the right side. The infraorbital nerve must be identified and carefully retracted before the anterior wall of the antrum is removed. The entire inferior turbinate and anterior wall of the antrum to the level of a vertical line through the infraorbital foramen have been resected. A view of this resection from the left side can be seen in Figure 8.32b. It is necessary to transect the nasolacrimal duct with this resection. This should be cut atraumatically with a sharp blade to prevent stenosis.

1. Infraorbital foramen
2. Posterior aspect of lateral nasal wall
3. Maxillary sinus
4. Floor of nasal cavity
5. Middle turbinate
6. Nasal septum
7. Inferior turbinate

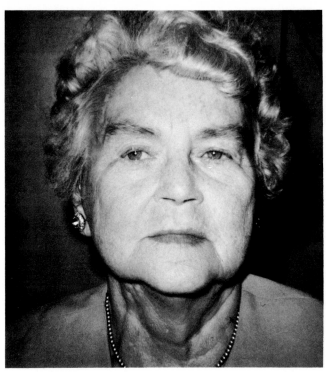
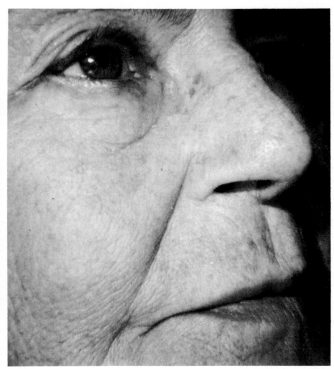

a   b

FIGURE 8.34. *Lateral rhinotomy.*

Mrs. E. G., a 58-year-old widow, was referred because of uncontrollable bleeding following an attempt to remove a tumor of the medial wall of the right antrum. No tissue was taken for biopsy during this procedure. The presenting symptom had been mild swelling of the right cheek of 3 months' duration. There had been no history of nasal obstruction, epistaxis, or pain. X rays of the sinuses showed destruction of the medial aspect of the floor of the orbit and of the lateral nasal wall.

A lateral rhinotomy was performed in which the anterior wall of the antrum and orbital floor medial to the infraorbital foramen, the entire lateral nasal wall, and the ethmoid sinuses were removed. The histologic diagnosis of removed tissue was "metastatic renal-cell carcinoma" (hypernephroma). An intravenous pyelogram revealed a large mass in the left kidney which was removed by nephrectomy. Postoperative radiation therapy was administered to the right maxilla. The patient is alive and well 4½ years after surgery.

a and b. The patient is shown 3½ years after lateral rhinotomy. There is no external deformity—even following extensive bone removal. The lateral rhinotomy scar is barely visible. The photographs emphasize the importance of a properly placed incision.

Intranasal portions of encephalocele which do not atrophy after intracranial section of the stalk are best approached by this exposure.

When the diagnosis of glioma is established by intranasal biopsy, a bifrontal craniotomy is performed prior to resection of the intranasal tumor. If intracranial connections are found, they are removed along with the nasal mass by the lateral rhinotomy exposure. If no connections are found, the lateral rhinotomy is performed at a later date.

For large malignant lesions which may be radiosensitive there is some value in combined preoperative x-ray therapy. If adequate surgical margins are not obtained, a full course of postoperative radiation therapy is indicated.

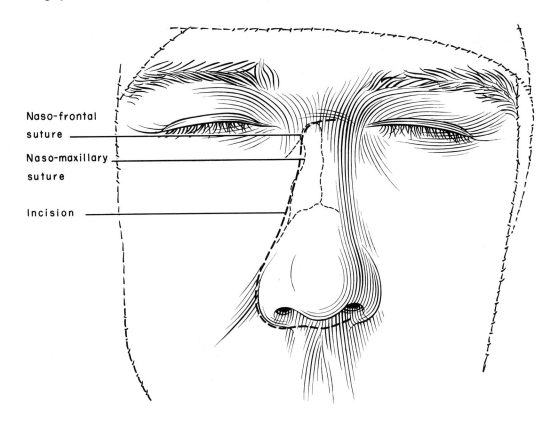

Naso-frontal suture

Naso-maxillary suture

Incision

(a)

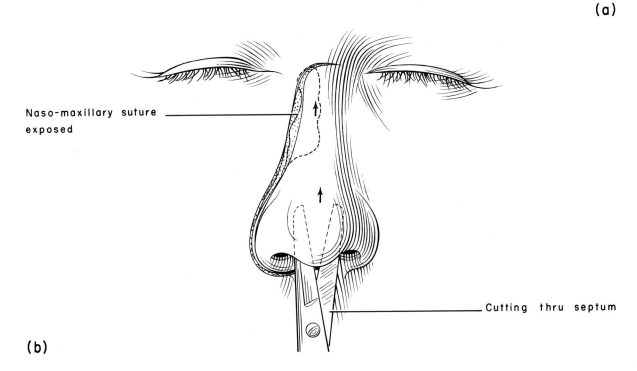

Naso-maxillary suture exposed

Cutting thru septum

(b)

FIGURE 8.35. *Complete rhinotomy.*

a. Incision for complete rhinotomy. The lateral rhinotomy incision (Fig. 8.25) is extended across the root of the nose and across the base of the columella to the opposite nostril.

b. One blade of a scissors is placed in each nostril to divide the nasal septum. The tips of the scissors are placed as superiorly and anteriorly as is possible. The nose can then be swung to the opposite side exposing both nasal cavities.

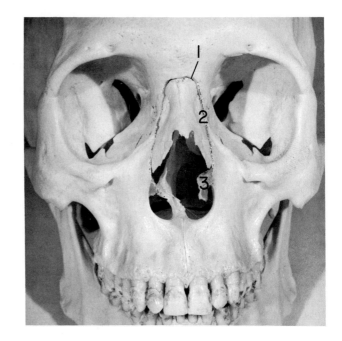

FIGURE 8.36. *Complete rhinotomy.*

a. A lateral osteotomy is performed on each side with a chisel. A bone incision is then made superiorly in the nasofrontal suture line, with a chisel or, preferably, a tangential Stryker saw, connecting the two osteotomy openings.

1. Nasofrontal suture
2. Bone incision
3. Inferior turbinate

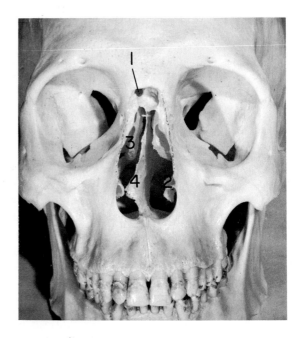

b. The exposure obtained by a complete rhinotomy. The dissection can be extended into all sinuses from this approach. The bony flap, consisting of nasal bones and ascending processes, has been removed to show the interior of both nasal cavities.

1. Right nasofrontal orifice
2. Inferior turbinate
3. Middle turbinate
4. Nasal septum deviated to right

RHINOPHYMA

A rhinophyma is a slowly growing tumor usually involving the lower half of the nose. It may, however, involve the entire nose and part of the cheeks. Cases have also been reported in which the ear and chin are affected. The lesion is said to be an advanced stage of acne rosacea (Anderson and Dykes).

Basically the process is an inflammatory one with an associated hypertrophy of the subcutaneous and sebaceous tissues. The sebaceous glands become markedly enlarged and the dilated ducts are filled with sebum and keratotic debris. Masses of hypertrophic skin having large pores develop. Sebum accumulates between the masses of tissue. Superficial vessels invade the surface of the rhinophyma, giving it the reddish color.

The main complaint of a patient with a rhinophyma is the unsightliness of the nose. On occasion the growth may become large enough to obstruct the nostrils. A foul odor is usually present when the growth is large and ovulated. Occasionally, the rhinophyma becomes large enough to interfere with vision (Fig. 8.37).

Rhinophyma is usually thought to be associated with alcoholism. Actually, there is no basis for this belief, since there is no consistent relationship. Other factors such as rich diet, gastrointestinal disorders, exposure to sunlight, and vitamin deficiency have also been indicated as etiologic possibilities without any real basis.

Treatment

If acne rosacea is the precursor of rhinophyma, possibly intensive care by the dermatologist would prevent its development. Once the rhinophyma has developed, surgical treatment is the only effective therapy. There are two basic methods of surgery. One consists in excision of the rhinophyma within the sebaceous gland layer so as to leave remnants of glandular epithelium which will undergo metaplasia to form the skin covering of the nose.

This procedure may be conducted with either local or general anesthesia and entails sculpturing, by means of a straight razor, #10 surgical blade, a small electric dermatome, or, as I prefer, an electric knife. Bleeding can be quite profuse and is controlled by electrocoagulating the larger vessels and packing the surface of the nose with epinephrine solution-impregnated gauze sponges. The incision around the rhinophyma should be beveled in order to eliminate the sharp demarcation between the surrounding skin and the limit of the rhinophyma. Blood loss during the procedure usually does not exceed 500 cc.

The area is dressed with petrolatum gauze or Aureomycin-impregnated conforming gauze covered by a bulky dry dressing if postoperative bleeding occurs. If not, no dressing is applied and the nose is swabbed with Betadine solution three times a day. The dressing should be changed at the end of 5 or 6 days. Re-epithelialization is usually complete by the end of 8 weeks (Fig. 8.37a), and the cosmetic result, although not perfect, is satisfactory to most patients. Figures 8.37a–f and 8.38a–k show the details of the healing process following excision with an electrical knife and also the 5-year result.

The second method of surgical treatment for rhinophyma is total excision in the areolar layer between the disease and the supporting structures of the nose. Some form of skin grafting is, of course, necessary. Split-thickness grafts obtained

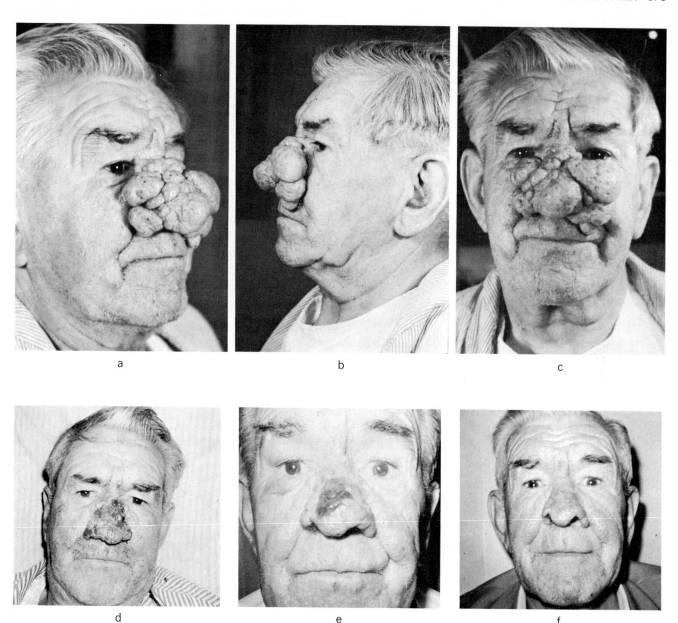

FIGURE 8.37. *Rhinophyma.*

a, b and c. Oblique, lateral, and front face views of a patient with a huge rhinophyma. The appearance of the lesion did not particularly bother this patient. He sought medical aid only after the lesion became large enough to interfere with his reading.

d. Appearance of the patient 1 week after operation.

e. Appearance of the patient 4 weeks after operation.

f. Appearance of the patient 2 months after operation.

from the lateral neck are said to be superior to those taken from the thigh (Anderson and Dykes). Excellent results have been reported by Macomber and by Smith through the use of full-thickness skin grafts obtained from the supraclavicular region. Matching skin grafts are taken from both supraclavicular areas for each half of the nose. The skin grafts must be very carefully sutured in place and covered by a dressing similar to the one just described. Healing is usually complete at the end of 1 week.

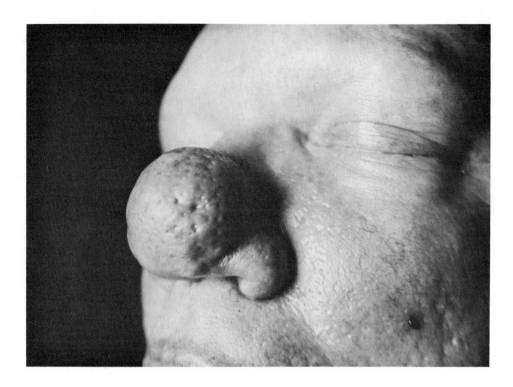

FIGURE 8.38.

 a. This rhinophyma developed over a period of 4 years in a 53-year-old patient with no history of alcohol consumption and total alopecia of sudden onset 10 years previously.

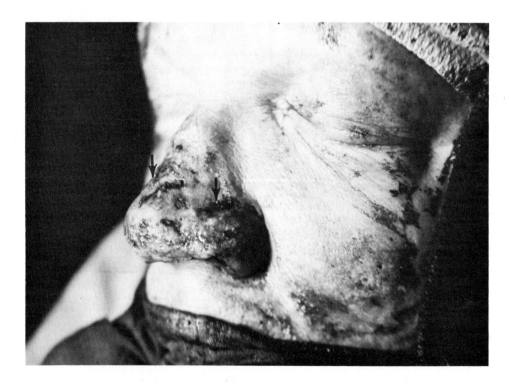

 b. The rhinophyma was resected using an electric knife. At the end of this sculpturing procedure, it is important to emphasize the supratip dip and the alar creases (arrows).

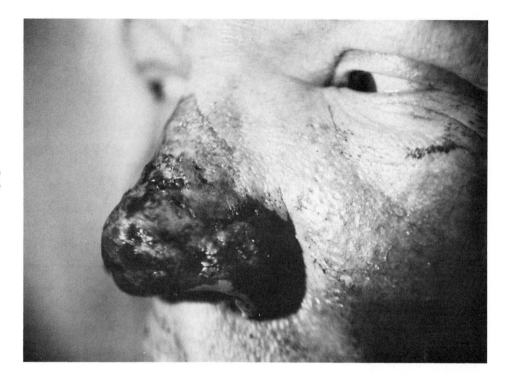

c. Four days postoperative there is moderate edema and some oozing but as yet no crusting.

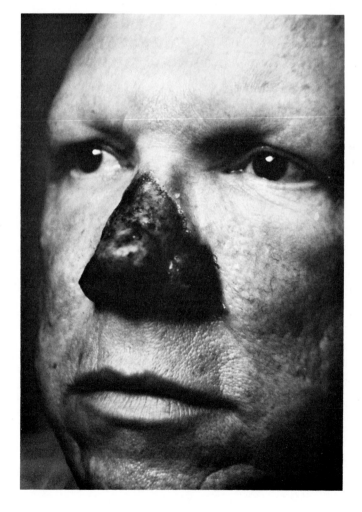

d. At the end of 2 weeks there is almost complete crusting. Postoperative treatment consisted only of three t.i.d. applications of Betadine.

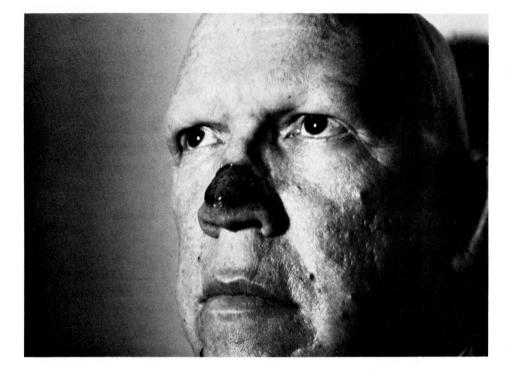

FIGURE 8.38. Continued

e. In 1 month the periphery of the dissection has begun to epithelialize.

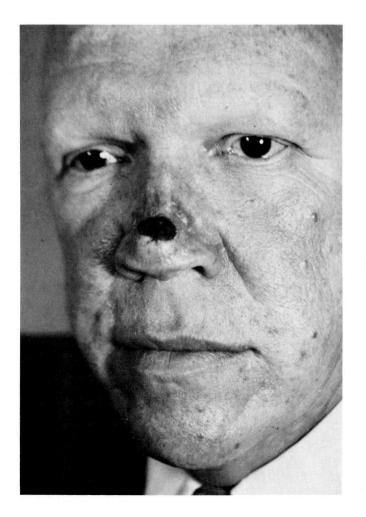

f. At the end of 6 weeks the area of crust has been reduced to the supratip region.

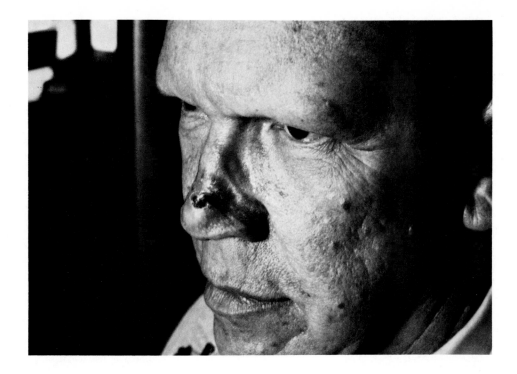

g. After 8 weeks the almost complete epithelialization has occurred.

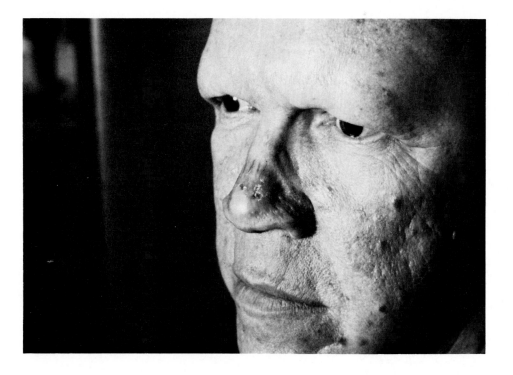

h. Ten weeks after surgery the process of healing is about complete.

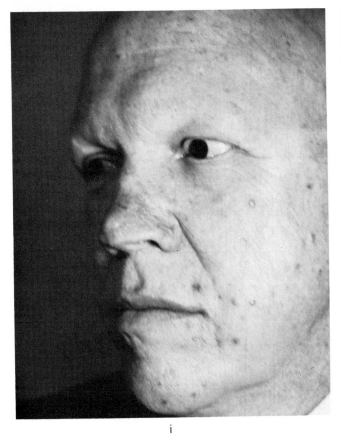

i

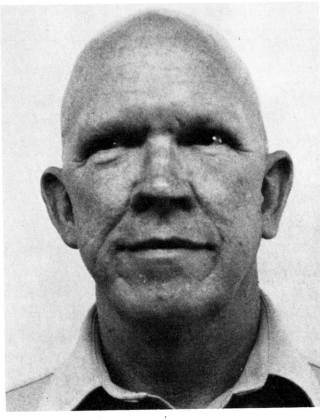

j

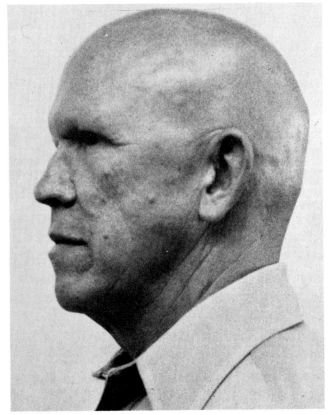

k

FIGURE 8.38. Continued

    i. The appearance of the nose 6 months following resection of the rhinophyma.

    j and k. The appearance of the patient's nose 5 years following the surgical procedure. There has been no recurrence of his rhinophyma.

ATROPHIC RHINITIS (OZENA)

Atrophic rhinitis is a chronic, inflammatory disease involving the nasal mucous membrane with atrophy and fibrosis of all layers. The epithelium undergoes metaplasia to the squamous type. The cilia are destroyed, and there is a decrease or complete absence of glandular structures. The vascular supply to the mucous membrane undergoes obliterative endarteritis. The condition is referred to as "ozena" when an odor is present.

The etiologic basis of this condition has not been established. Although bacteria are usually found associated with the disease, infection is not accepted as the primary cause. Endocrine and metabolic factors have been labeled as possible causes. Cultures usually show mixed infection. Klebsiella ozaenae, Perez bacillus, Proteus vulgaris, and coliform-group bacilli are the organisms responsible for the odor associated with this condition.

Signs and Symptoms

The signs and symptoms of atrophic rhinitis are:
1. Crusting
2. Foul odor
3. Complaint of nasal stuffiness, especially when crusting is extensive
4. Wide nasal passages
5. Bleeding mucous membrane
6. Atrophy of mucous membrane
7. Thick, greenish, purulent discharge
8. Extension of the disease to the nasopharynx, pharynx, and larynx

Medical Treatment

The nasal discharge is cultured, and specific antibiotic therapy instituted locally and systemically. The nasal cavities are irrigated with warm normal saline solution or Alkalol at least twice daily. The irrigation container is placed well above the patient's head. The nozzle is inserted into one nasal cavity. The patient is then asked to lean forward over a washbasin, breathing quietly through his mouth. The irrigating solution will enter by one nostril and leave by way of the other. Frequent visits to the rhinologist, at least during the early phase of treatment, may be necessary for removal of crusts. Such medication as vitamin A, given in high doses; nicotinic acid tablets, 50 mg three times a day; and syrup of hydriodic acid, 1 teaspoonful in half a glass of water three times a day, are well worth a trial. A lubricating nasal spray or one containing iodine can be used after irrigations.

Surgical Management

Surgical treatment is designed to narrow the abnormally patent nasal passages. Basically, there are two techniques for implantation of substances such as bone chips from the iliac crest, deproteinated bovine chips, dolomite, and silicone. These are: implantation through a sublabial incision and implantation by way of an incision into the nasal vestibule. There have also been reports of beneficial effects following the submucosal injection of silicone or Teflon paste.

The sublabial incision is made just anterior to the canine fossa in the gingivo-buccal sulcus. A small amount of pyriform crest is removed for better access to the periosteum of the lateral wall and to reduce the incidence of mucosal tearing when the implant is inserted. The periosteum is elevated lateral to the inferior turbinate as far superiorly as is possible. The pocket between the periosteum and bone is then packed with the chosen implant. It is most important that there be no communication between the nasal cavity and the implant, for if a communication exists, infection and extrusion of the implant are inevitable. The sublabial incision is closed tightly without drainage. No intranasal packing is required.

Postoperatively, there will be complete nasal obstruction on the side operated upon for approximately one week, after which the swelling will gradually subside.

Implants inserted by way of incisions into the nasal vestibule can be positioned subperiosteally in the lateral wall, in the floor of the nose, or in the nasal septum. The sharp anterior margin of the pyriform crest is the guide to the periosteum of the lateral wall. Because of the pathogens that are present in the nasal cavity in association with atrophic rhinitis, infection is slightly more prone to follow implants positioned through this route than those inserted through a sublabial incision.

RECONSTRUCTIVE NASAL SURGERY

For centuries man has been quite conscious of the size, shape, and color of the structure projecting anteriorly from his face. His, and the attention of his fellows, is immediately focused on the slightest defect of his nose.

Nasal defects are caused by trauma, infection, or operation for tumor removal. Surgical repair of these defects dates back many centuries and probably represents man's first attempt at reconstructive surgery. Surgeons have not only utilized the surrounding tissues for repair of nasal defects, but have also employed

FIGURE 8.39. *Repair of lower lateral nasal defect.*

a. An incision, in the shape of an inverted V, approximately 0.5 cm above the small notchlike defect is shown.

b. The surrounding area, including the ala, is extensively undermined so that the inferior margin of the incision can be retracted downward with a skin hook.

c. The resulting surgical defect is repaired in a linear vertical suture line.

d. This type of defect can also be repaired by a V-Y advancement technique. The inverted V incision is made as is shown, again undermining the surrounding area, including that of the alar margin.

e. The notchlike defect is erased as the defect is repaired, creating a 'Y' suture.

f. Incision 'a' is made in the nasolabial sulcus. The flap is elevated in the subcutaneous plane and the area posterior to the defect is undermined. The flap is then rotated anteriorly, so that point 'b,' after being tailored to conform with the deformity, is sutured to point 'b'.'

g. The flap has been sutured in place. The skin of 'c' is sutured to the mucous membrane margin 'c'.' A better cosmetic result and alar contour can be accomplished by rolling the skin margin 'a' laterally, to form the inferior margin of the ala.

h. A full-thickness postauricular skin graft is obtained, fashioned, and sutured in place, so that it covers the external nasal defect.

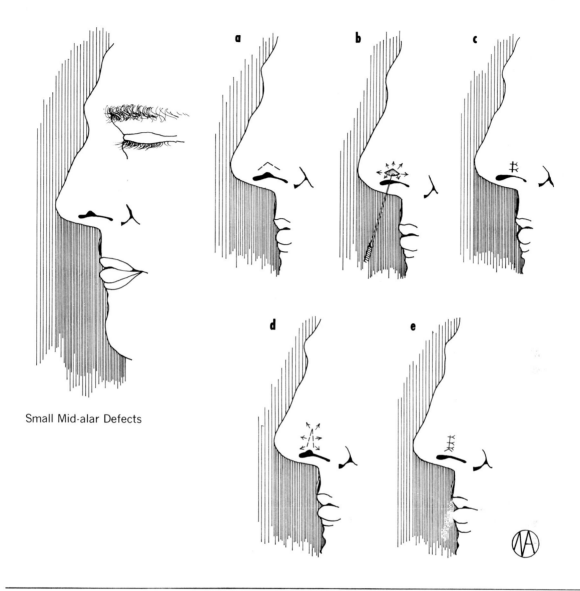

Small Mid-alar Defects

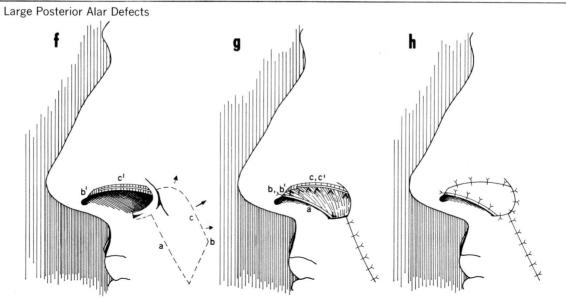

Large Posterior Alar Defects

remote, pedicled and free autografts. In the following paragraphs are presented descriptions of those procedures best suited for repair of defects in the various anatomic sites on the nose, and, finally, the technique for total nasal reconstruction.

Repair of Lower Lateral Nasal Defects

On occasion, a small notchlike defect in the central lower lateral region of the nose can be repaired by means of a simple advancement procedure (Fig. 8.39a–e).

A large, posterior, lower lateral alar defect can be repaired by using a superiorly based pedicle flap which is based posteriorly and inferiorly to the nose (Fig. 8.39f, g, and h). A modification of this technique is that of obtaining a composite graft from the conchal region consisting of the conchal cartilage and the overlying postauricular skin. During a first-stage procedure, the conchal cartilage and skin are buried beneath the end of the flap shown in Figure 8.39f. The cartilaginous part of the composite graft faces the subcutaneous layer. After a few weeks the flap is elevated, tailored, and sutured to the alar defect. In so doing, the postauricular skin forms the external layer of the repair.

A defect of the lower lateral nose may be repaired by creating a defect above the deformity, which, in turn, is repaired by using a composite graft (Fig. 8.40a, b, and c).

A notchlike defect in the anterior aspect of the lower lateral nose can be repaired by rotating an inferiorly based flap in a postero-inferior direction (Fig. 8.40d, e, and f).

Deformities of the lower lateral nose can also be repaired with composite auricular grafts (Fig. 8.41). The graft is measured to be slightly larger than the nasal defect. The postauricular side of the composite graft is used for the external nasal surface. The skin-to-mucosa membrane layer is completed before the external dermal sutures are applied.

An anterior, lower lateral, nasal alar defect is repaired by means of a two-stage procedure, using a posteriorly based full-thickness nasal pedicle flap as shown in Figure 8.42a–e.

A defect in the lower lateral nose above the alar region can be repaired by using an inferiorly based pedicle flap (Fig. 8.42f and g). A superiorly based nasofrontal pedicled flap can also be used to repair this defect.

A malignant infiltrative lesion in the region of the ala and lower lateral nasal wall should be widely resected as shown in Figure 8.43a. This resection includes all layers of the lateral nasal wall. Repair is made with a long nasolabial flap. The tip of this flap is folded in to repair the defect in the nasal lining. The cosmetic result following this repair is quite good (Fig. 8.43f, g, and h). A cartilage graft may be used to support the lateral alar rim.

Repair of Nasal Tip Defects

There are a number of techniques for repair of a defect of the nasal tip. A free full-thickness postauricular skin graft is probably the most popular. For this type of repair a pattern is made from the defect so that the full-thickness graft will fit exactly into place. The graft is sutured with one layer of fine dermal suture material

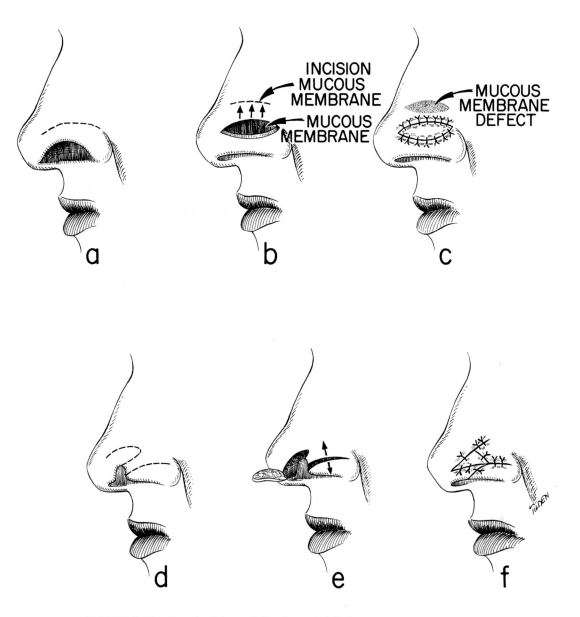

FIGURE 8.40. *Repair of lower lateral nasal defect.*

a. An incision is made as shown. This must be slightly curved in the shape of an inverted U. The incision is carefully carried through the subcutaneous layer to the level of the intranasal mucous membrane.

b. A plane is established just external to the mucous membrane. Undermining is carried out in all directions, especially superiorly, to form an ellipse. The elliptic defect develops as the lateral alar margin is depressed. It is usually necessary to incise the mucous membranes intranasally as is shown, to lower the lateral alar margin, and also to make certain that the mucous membrane is present in the floor of the defect.

c. A postauricular full-thickness graft is fashioned so that it accurately fills in the defect. Intranasal packing is inserted, and an external pressure dressing is applied.

d. The incisions to construct the flap are shown as is the incision superior to the remaining portion of the ala, which is to receive the triangular-shaped flap.

e. The anterior flap has been elevated in a plane, just above the nasal mucous membrane. Undermining is carried out on the same plane, above and below the horizontal incision, as is indicated by arrows.

f. The anterior flap is rotated in a postero-inferior direction and sutured in place. If the defect is small, it may be possible to close it without grafting. Usually, however, to avoid elevation of the alar margin, it is necessary to utilize a composite postauricular graft. Again, the nasal cavity is carefully packed, and a dry dressing is applied externally.

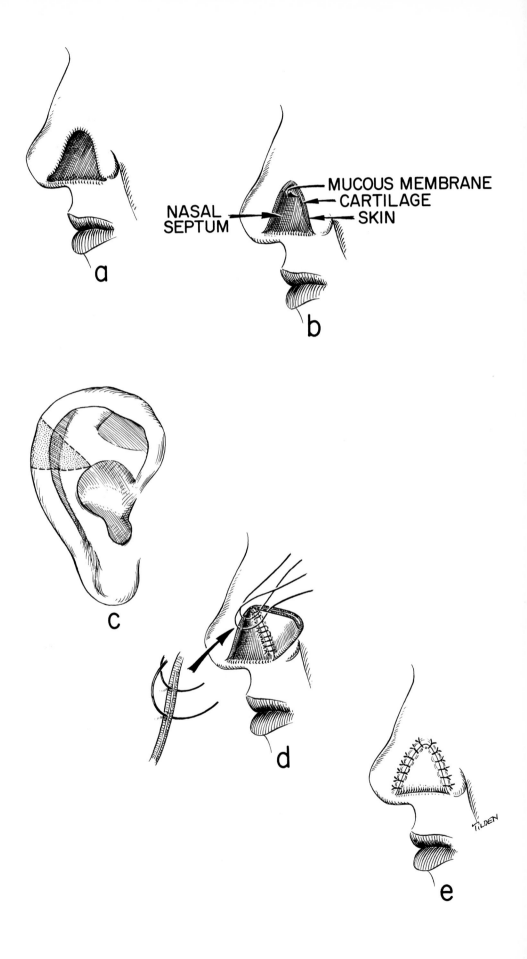

MUCOUS MEMBRANE
CARTILAGE
SKIN
NASAL
SEPTUM

a

b

c

d

e

FIGURE 8.41. *Repair of lower lateral nasal defect.*

a. A defect in the lower lateral alar region.

b. The skin on the inner margin of the defect, as well as all scar tissue, is resected. It is most important to remove this scar tissue in order to obtain an adequate blood supply for the composite graft.

c. The posterior margin of the auricle, just inferior to the beginning of the triangular fossa, is usually the best site from which to obtain the full-thickness graft. If the graft is not too large, the auricular defect may be repaired in a straight line. For repair of larger and irregular defects, refer to otoplasty, pages 524–528.

d. The skin is sutured to the intranasal mucous membrane with #4-0 chromic catgut. It is important to make certain that the skin is in contact with the mucous membrane in all areas.

e. The composite graft is sutured in place. A very fine polyethylene or silk suture material is used for external closure. The nasal cavity is packed lightly, but usually no external dressing is necessary.

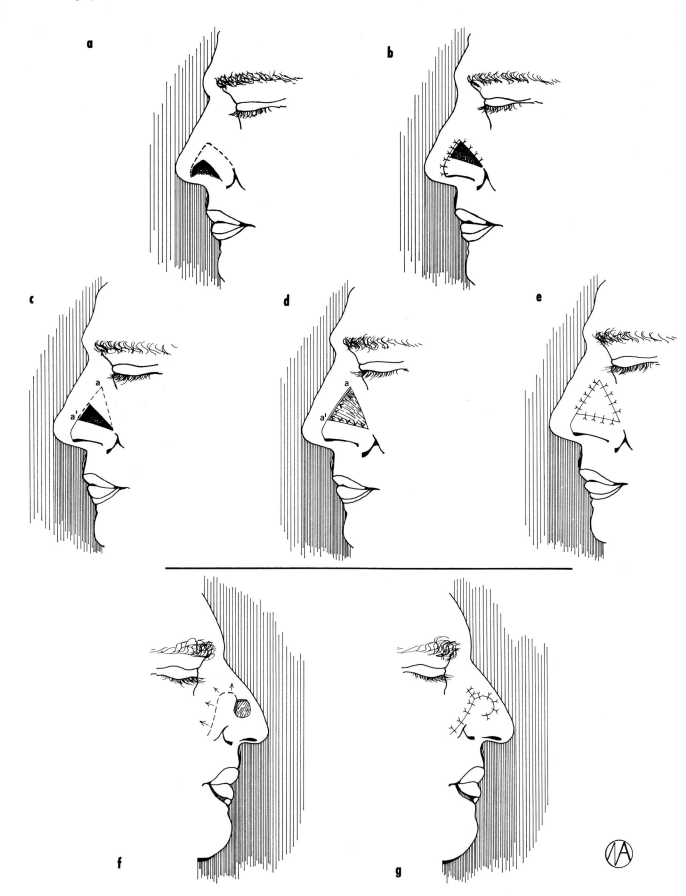

and covered with a pressure dressing. The postauricular full-thickness graft technique (Fig. 8.44a and b) is by far the simplest one, but on occasion the color and texture match is not good.

A second method for repair of the nasal tip involves the use of bilateral nasolabial skin flaps (Fig. 8.43), which are sutured together in the midline. This technique is most satisfactory if the nasal tip defect is large and not suitable for a postauricular composite graft or a rotational flap as described below. The cosmetic result and color match with bilateral nasolabial flaps are excellent.

In a third technique for repair of defects of the nasal tip, a local advancement flap is employed. This procedure (Fig. 8.44c, d, and e) is somewhat more difficult than that utilizing the postauricular full-thickness graft, but the color match and texture are considerably better.

Repair of Lateral Nasal Defects

Large lateral nasal defects are repaired by using superiorly or inferiorly based nasofacial skin flaps. As a rule, the superiorly based flap (Fig. 8.45a and b) gives the best cosmetic result.

Smaller lateral nasal defects can be repaired with either the advancement technique (Fig. 8.45c and d) or with a postauricular composite graft (Fig. 8.41).

Repair of Nasal Root Defects

Operations for repair of defects in the root of the nose are numerous. A technique which gives an excellent cosmetic result, unless the patient has scanty eyebrows, is outlined in Figure 8.46a, b, and c. A small inferiorly based glabellar flap is useful for lateral defects of the nasal root (Fig. 8.46d, e, and f).

FIGURE 8.42. *Repair of lower lateral nasal defect.*

a. An anterior, lower lateral, nasal alar defect can be repaired by a two-stage procedure, in which a posteriorly based full-thickness nasal pedicle flap obtained from the lateral nasal wall superior to the defect is used.

b. The pedicle flap is sutured in place anteriorly. The superior and anterior margins of the through-and-through defect into the nasal cavity are carefully repaired.

c. A triangular incision is made above the through-and-through defect as is shown, as the first step of the second stage.

d. The skin flap thus formed is reflected inferiorly and sutured to the intranasal mucous membrane anteriorly and inferiorly. In so doing, point 'a' is sutured to point 'a'.'

e. A full-thickness postauricular skin graft is used to repair the superficial defect.

f. An alternate method of repair for the second stage. The pedicled flap is elevated and reflected antero-inferiorly. The skin superior and posterior to the defect is undermined.

g. The inferiorly based pedicle flap has been rotated to cover the defect, and the donor area is eliminated by primary repair.

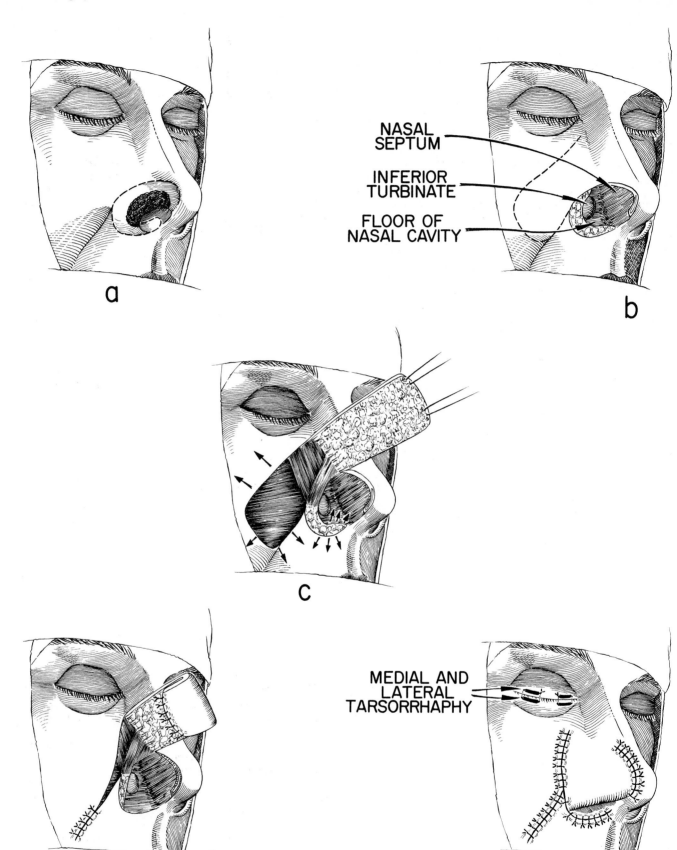

a

NASAL
SEPTUM

INFERIOR
TURBINATE

FLOOR OF
NASAL CAVITY

b

c

d

MEDIAL AND
LATERAL
TARSORRHAPHY

e

TILDEN

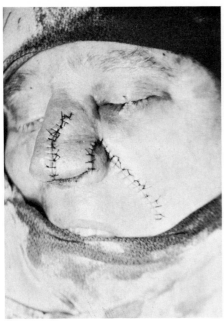
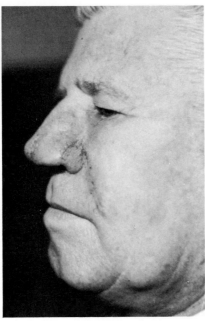
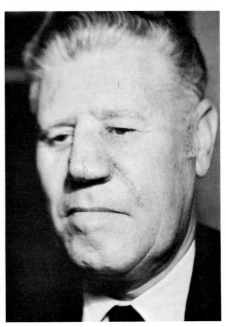

f   g   h

FIGURE 8.43. *Repair of lower lateral nasal defects.*

    a. The resected area includes a portion of the inferior nasal vestibule and anterior aspect of the floor of the nasal cavity. Bleeding should be controlled by either electrocoagulation or catgut suture.

    b. A superiorly based nasofacial flap is quite suitable for repairing this defect, which is too large to nourish a composite graft from the auricle. The length of the flap is determined by measuring the external defect and adding the required length for the intranasal lining. This flap should, of course, not be longer than twice the width of its base. Following resection of the lower lateral nasal wall, the nasal septum, anterior tip of the inferior turbinate, and floor of the nasal cavity can be seen.

    c. The flap is elevated in a plane which includes the fascia covering the muscles of facial expression. The skin is elevated superiorly, laterally, and inferiorly so that the defect lateral to the nose can be closed. Subcutaneous #3-0 or #4-0 chromic catgut and dermal #5-0 polyethylene or #6-0 silk suture material are used for this repair. In order to close the defect in the floor of the nasal orifice, the mucous membrane posterior to the defect and the skin inferior to the defect are undermined sufficiently so that there is very little tension in the suture line. This defect is closed with a single layer of dermal sutures.

    d. A goodly portion of the defect lateral to the nose has been closed. This causes some elevation of the upper lip and tends to pull the lower lid downward. If it is apparent that an ectropion will result, then it is best to perform a medial lateral tarsorrhaphy, leaving the sutures in place until the tissues have relaxed. The defect in the floor of the nasal vestibule has been repaired. The tip of the nasofacial flap is reflected onto itself after the length necessary to cover the lower lateral nasal defect has been measured carefully. Chromic catgut suture material (#4-0) is used.

    e. The flap has been sutured in place with a single layer of dermal suture material. The extra width of the superior portion of the flap causes an outward bulge or convexity which roughly approaches a normal contour. The nasal cavity is loosely packed anteriorly with petrolatum-impregnated iodoform gauze. A dry, external pressure dressing is applied to the right eye, right face, and lateral surface of the nose. This remains in place for 48 hours. The intranasal packing can be removed after 3 or 4 days. If the cosmetic result and contour of the repair are not satisfactory, a cartilage graft can be inserted in the alar region at a later date.

    f. Postoperative result. A tarsorrhaphy was not necessary.

    g and h. Result, 8 days after surgery.

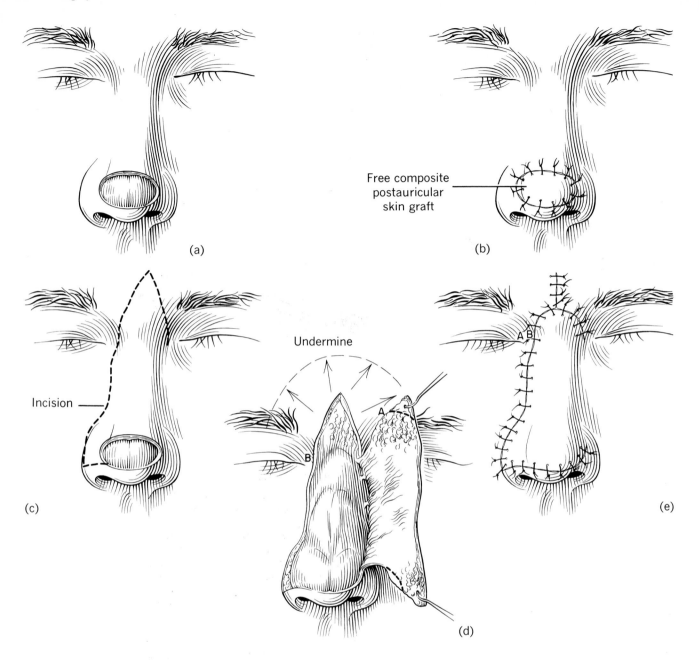

FIGURE 8.44. *Repair of nasal tip defect.*

a. A moderate-sized defect of the nasal tip is shown. This defect extends to or through the lower lateral cartilages. An exact pattern of the defect is made and placed in the postauricular region from which a full-thickness skin graft, slightly larger than the pattern, is obtained.

b. The postauricular full-thickness graft is carefully placed in the defect and sutured with one layer of fine dermal suture material. A pressure dressing is applied over the graft and left in place for 48 hours.

c. The incisions for construction of a flap consisting of skin and subcutaneous layers, overlying the nasal dorsum and root, are shown.

d. The flap is carefully elevated over the perichondrium of the upper lateral cartilages and over the fascia overlying the frontalis muscles superiorly. A rather extensive undermining is required superiorly in all directions. As the flap is advanced inferiorly, tip A is rounded and sutured to point B just above the level of the inner canthus. Superiorly, the defect is closed in a vertical suture line.

e. The repair and advancement are continued from above, downward. A small "dog ear" may occur at the base of the flap as a result of this inferior rotation. If this has not disappeared after a few months, it can be excised. A pressure dressing is applied over the entire nose and forehead and left in place for at least 24 hours. The cosmetic result following this procedure is surprisingly good.

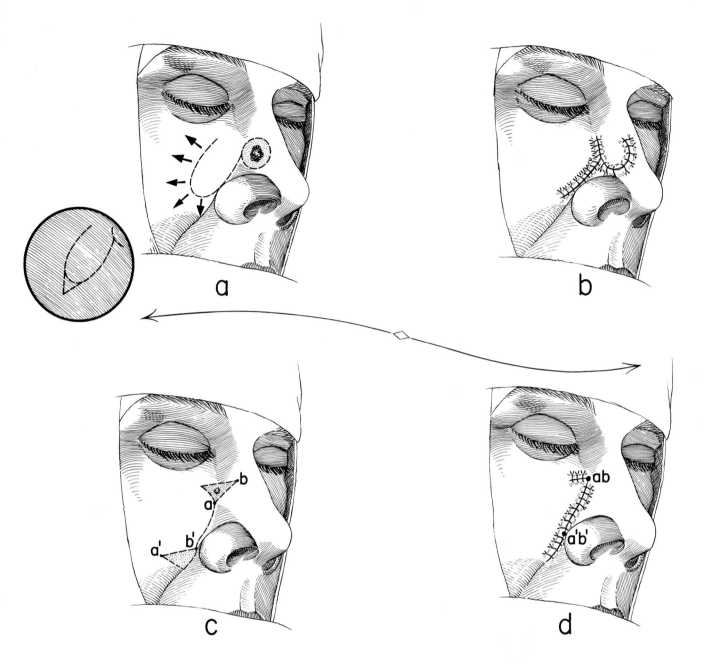

FIGURE 8.45. *Repair of lateral nasal defects.*

a. Defects on the side of the nose can be repaired with a superiorly based cheek flap as outlined. The flap is based near the lateral aspect of the nose. The medial incision for the flap is in the nasofacial crease, and the tip of the flap is pointed to facilitate closure. A triangular segment of skin is removed from the tip so that it can conform with the lateral nasal defect. Laterally, rather extensive undermining is necessary.

b. The flap is advanced and sutured into place. The defect is closed so that the resultant scar will simulate the nasofacial sulcus. Since tension is not particularly in an inferior direction, a medial and lateral tarsorrhaphy is usually not necessary.

c. A smaller defect on the side of the nose can be repaired by means of an advancement technique. This operation is especially feasible if the defect can be converted to a triangular shape. An incision is made from the inferior angle of the defect to the nasolabial sulcus. A triangular piece of skin approximately the size of the defect is removed just lateral to the alar sulcus. Segment a′–b′ should be the same length as segment a–b.

d. After the skin has been undermined rather widely over the cheek, creating a flap which can be advanced superiorly, point a′ is sutured to point b′, and point a is sutured to point b.

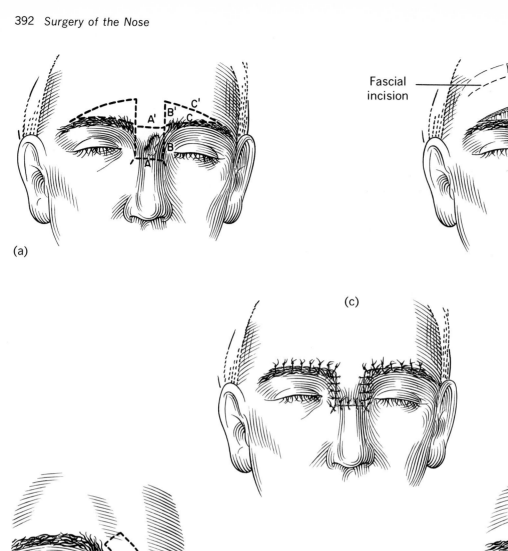

(a)

(b)

Fascial incision

Undermine

(c)

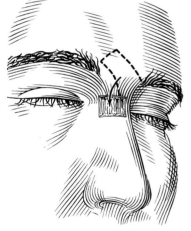

(d)

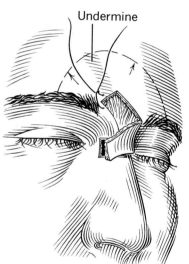

Undermine

(e)

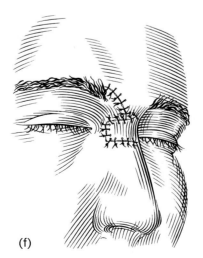

(f)

Subtotal Nasal Reconstruction

Subtotal nasal reconstruction is necessary for repair of defects following resection of a large lesion of the nose. These defects are not difficult to repair, even when most of the nasal dorsum has been removed, provided sufficient bony and cartilaginous support remains.

It is usually not necessary to cover the defect with split-thickness skin graft following resection of a large lesion of the nasal dorsum, nor is this required for observation for recurrent tumor, provided careful frozen sections are made of the skin margins at the time of resection. Secondary repair after skin grafting is technically more difficult, and the cosmetic result is not very satisfactory. Large defects of the nasal dorsum which do not involve the cartilage and bone can be repaired by using the Indian type of pedicled forehead skin flap (Fig. 8.49) or the island forehead flap (Figs. 8.47 and 8.48). An alternate method for repair of a large defect of the nasal dorsum is by means of bilateral nasofacial flaps (Figs. 8.43, 8.45, and 8.51).

A thorough knowledge of the blood supply to the bases of the various pedicled skin flaps used to accomplish subtotal and total nasal reconstruction is essential (Fig. 8.47a).

FIGURE 8.46. *Repair of nasal root defect.*

a. The incisions for the repair of the defect remaining after resection of a lesion at the root of the nose are indicated. The measurements of the flap to be reflected from the forehead to the root of the nose are made according to the width and height of the defect (a and b). Incision c is made in the upper margin of the eyebrow. This is a most important incision, for if the scar is even 1 mm above the eyebrow, it can become an unsightly one. The incision c' approaches incision c and abuts at a very sharp angle laterally.

b. The triangular piece of skin (b', c, and c') is removed, exposing the fascia over the frontalis muscle in this area. The skin is undermined superiorly in a plane over the frontalis muscle so that the flap a', b' can be pulled into the defect a, b without too much tension. If the defect at the root of the nose is large, and the skin of the forehead is taut, it may be necessary to elevate the superior flap in a plane between the frontalis muscle and the periosteum of the frontal bone. In such cases it is usually also necessary to make a horizontal incision through the fascia underlying the frontalis muscle as is indicated.

c. The flap and defects above the eyebrows are sutured subcutaneously with multiple, carefully placed, #4-0 chromic catgut. The skin is then repaired with #5-0 polyethylene or #6-0 silk suture material.

d. A small defect in the side of the root of the nose can be repaired by using a pedicled flap in the glabella region. The flap, based on one frontal artery, is oblique, as shown.

e. The flap has been elevated and transposed to cover the defect. Rather extensive undermining is necessary to close the defect in the glabella region.

f. The defect in the glabella region is repaired by subcutaneous suturing with #00 catgut and approximating the skin edges with fine dermal suture material. This flap is rotated less than 90 degrees and has an excellent blood supply.

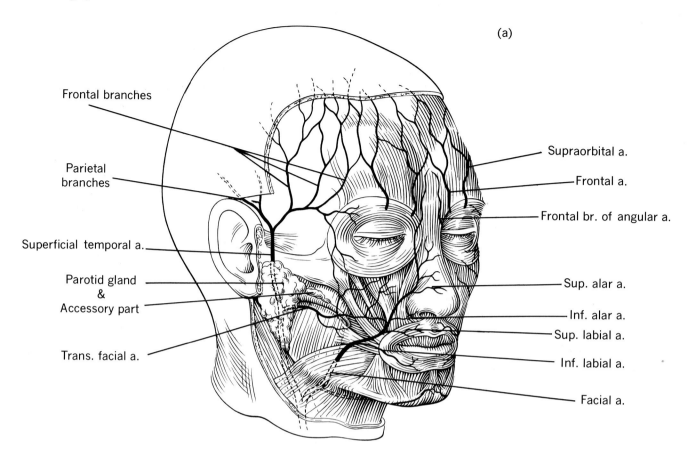

(a)

Frontal branches

Parietal branches

Superficial temporal a.

Parotid gland & Accessory part

Trans. facial a.

Supraorbital a.

Frontal a.

Frontal br. of angular a.

Sup. alar a.

Inf. alar a.

Sup. labial a.

Inf. labial a.

Facial a.

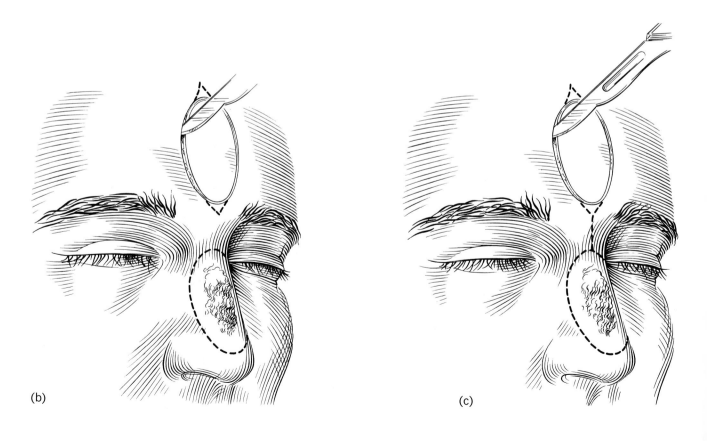

(b)

(c)

FIGURE 8.47. *Subtotal nasal reconstruction.*

a. Blood supply to the face. Forehead flaps used for reconstructive surgery are based on the frontal branches of the superficial temporal artery, the supraorbital artery, frontal artery, or frontal branch of the angular artery. The large forehead flap used for total nasal reconstruction is based on all of these arteries.

The Island Forehead Flap

b. After the lesion and its margins are resected, a pattern of paper or cloth is carefully made of the defect. This pattern is transferred to the median forehead. Following the outline of the pattern an incision is carried through skin and subcutaneous layers to the fascia over the frontalis muscle. It is then carried through the frontalis muscle laterally and superiorly, but *not* inferiorly, exposing the periosteum over the frontal bone. A wedge of skin and subcutaneous tissue are resected superiorly and inferiorly in order to facilitate the vertical midline closure of the defect.

c. An incision connecting the inferior aspect of the forehead defect and the upper margin of the nasal defect facilitates exposure and dissection of the subcutaneous vascular pedicle. It also aids the rotation of the island flap, as it is reflected inferiorly to cover the nasal defect.

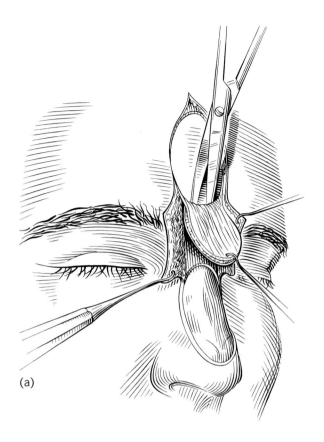

(a)

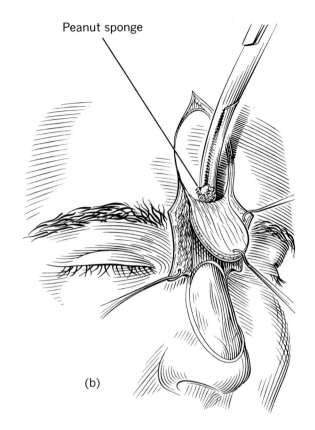

Peanut sponge

(b)

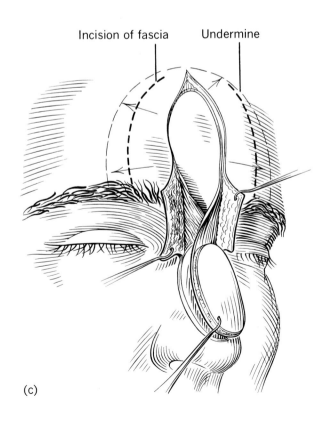

Incision of fascia   Undermine

(c)

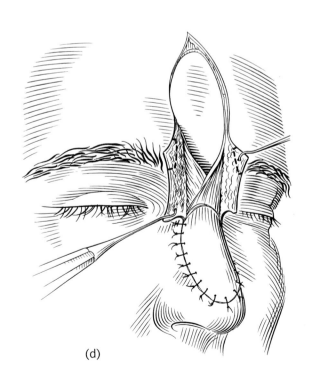

(d)

FIGURE 8.48. *Subtotal nasal reconstruction.*

The Island Forehead Flap (continued)

a. The flaps have been elevated in a subcutaneous plane between the nasal and forehead defects. The subcutaneous vascular pedicle is dissected posteriorly between the frontalis muscle and the frontal periosteum, in the region of the glabella.

b. Using a "peanut" sponge the posterior aspect of the vascular pedicle is dissected further without jeopardizing the blood supply of the island flap.

c. The island flap is rotated 180 degrees into position to cover the nasal defect. By exposing the area between the nasal and forehead defects, rather than tunneling, the vascular pedicle can be more neatly arranged to prevent kinking and interruption of the blood supply. The carefully repaired vertical defect that results is a small price to pay for prevention of such sequelae. Rather extensive undermining is necessary over the periosteum of the frontal bone in order to close the forehead defect. Vertical incisions through the fascia underlying the frontalis muscle on each side of the defect may be necessary in order to effect a primary closure.

d. The island flap has been sutured into place. The forehead defect is then repaired, and the incision between the two defects sutured. A dressing applied with moderate pressure over the dorsum of the nose and forehead, which necessitates having both eyes covered, is left in place for 24 hours.

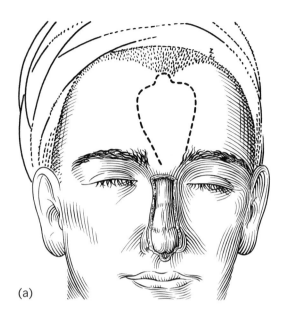

(a)

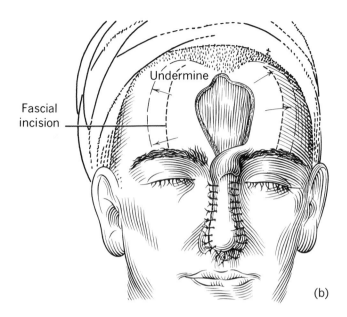

Undermine

Fascial
incision

(b)

(c)

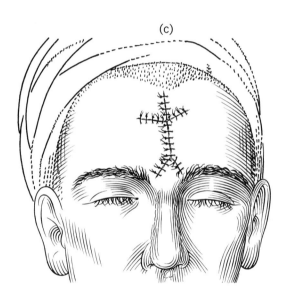

(d)

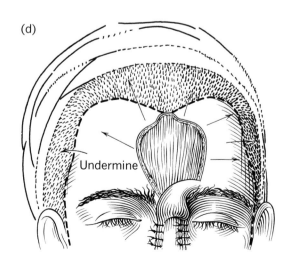

Undermine

(e)

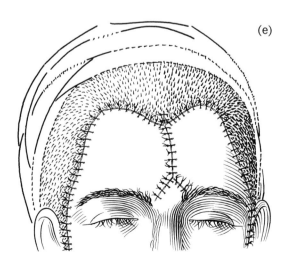

FIGURE 8.49. *Subtotal nasal reconstruction.*

a. Most of the epithelial covering of the nose has been lost, including that of the columella. The cartilaginous and bony areas of the nasal pyramid remain intact. The midline Indian forehead flap, as popularized by Dr. V. Kazanjian, probably provides the most practical method for repairing this defect. This flap is based on the medial and lateral frontal arteries.

b. The forehead flap is rotated 180 degrees forward and sutured to the nasal defect. If the columella is absent a superiorly based pedicled skin flap is elevated from the midline of the upper lip and sutured to the inner posterior surface of the distal end of the forehead flap. A mucous membrane flap from the midline of the inner aspect of the upper lip may also be used for this purpose. This is also based superiorly and brought out through the buttonhole incision in the base of the columella.

c. If the forehead donor site is 2 cm or less in width, it may be closed by extensive undermining over the periosteum. Vertical incisions as indicated through the fascia underlying the frontalis muscle are usually necessary to accomplish this closure. The portion of the defect used for construction of the columella is closed in a vertical suture line. The defects representing the portion of the forehead flap used for the nasal alar region are closed with an oblique suture line. The remainder of the defect is closed in the vertical midline, with heavy subcutaneous sutures as well as dermal sutures.

d. If the defect is wider than 2 cm, it is necessary to use a large rotational scalping flap on each side of the forehead. The flaps are rotated medially and sutured in the midline. The coronal incisions are made along the hairline to the level of the external auditory canals. Care should be taken to preserve the frontal branches of the superficial temporal arteries.

e. The final repair following advancement of bilateral scalping flaps, which are based on the frontal branches of the superficial temporal artery, is shown. If the entire nose is devoid of epithelium, then the midline flap is not practical, and the scalping flap, as shown in Figure 8.53, must be used.

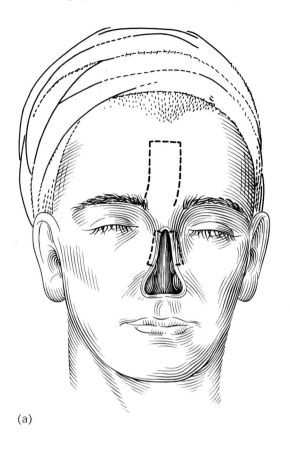

(a)

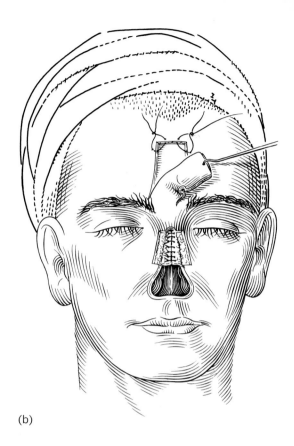

(b)

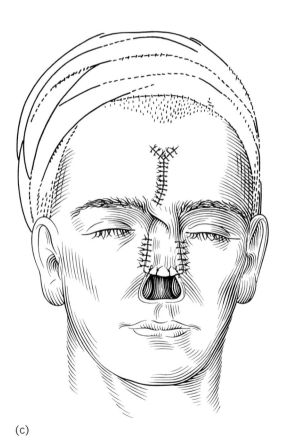

(c)

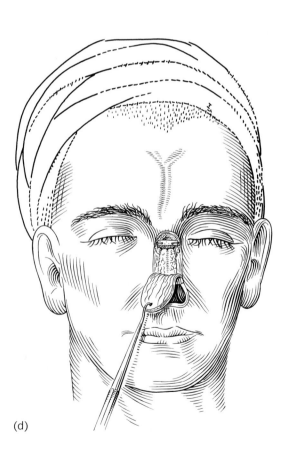

(d)

Total Nasal Reconstruction

Total reconstruction of the nose is a complicated and technically difficult undertaking as is manifested by the numerous techniques presented in the literature. When planning this multi-procedure reconstruction the surgeon must outline a schedule for the following:

1. Lining of the nasal cavity
2. Bony support of the nasal pyramid
3. Outline of forehead flap for covering of nose
4. Reconstruction of the columella and alae
5. Repair of the forehead
6. Touch-up procedures to accentuate alae, narrow the bridge, and thin the columella

Lining. The lining for a total nasal reconstruction can be obtained from remaining mucous membrane on the lateral nasal walls, forehead flaps, or paranasal pedicled skin flaps. These various flaps have a high percentage of take, for the blood supply to these areas is more than adequate with the numerous branches of the facial, sphenopalatine, and anterior ethmoid arteries.

A medial forehead flap can be used for the lining of the nasal cavity (Fig. 8.50). This will not interfere with the forehead flap to be used for the covering of the reconstructed nose. The fulcrum for the bony cantilever support can be wired in place when the median forehead is detached.

When using a combination of local and nasolabial flaps (Fig. 8.51) to construct the lining of the nasal cavity, it is possible to apply the bony support and nasal covering at the same operation.

Bony Support. The technique of constructing a cantilever shaft of rib bone, as reported by Millard, is the best means of providing support for a total nasal reconstruction because of the simplicity of the technique itself and the resulting strength and stability. The beam of rib bone extends from the glabella to the nasal tip and is supported by a fulcrum between the two maxillary bones to finally resemble the gnomon of a sundial (Fig. 8.52).

FIGURE 8.50. *Total nasal reconstruction—lining for nasal cavities.*

a. Flaps consisting of skin and mucous membrane are constructed on each side of the upper nasal cavity. These are turned in from each side and sutured in the midline.

b and c. A small "Indian" midline forehead flap, based on a frontal artery, is reflected inferiorly to cover the flaps shown in a.

d. After approximately 6 weeks, the midline flap is divided at its base and dissected from the underlying lining of the upper nasal cavity. A piece of rib bone is bridged between the two maxillary bones. This bone, which is to function as a fulcrum for the bony cantilever support of the reconstructed nose, is mortised and wired to the maxillary bones. The flap is sutured back into place to cover this bony fulcrum. The final stage of the nasal reconstruction is performed at a later date. The flap is again reflected inferiorly to form the lining of the anterior aspect of the lower nasal cavity during the operation for construction of the bony support of the nose and rotation of the forehead flap for the nasal covering.

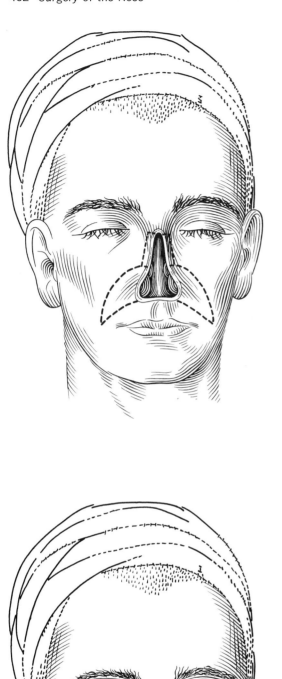

(a)

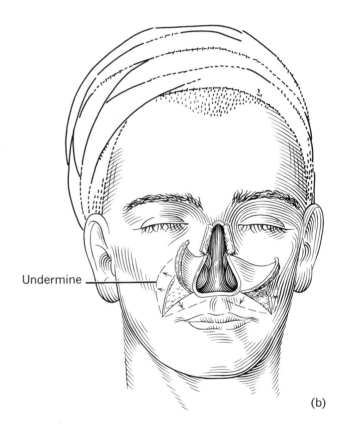

Undermine

(b)

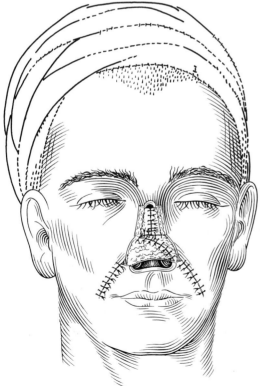

(c)

The fulcrum to support this beam is made by mortising and wiring a piece of rib bone to the maxillary bones on each side of the nasal defect. Wire holes are then drilled through the fulcrum and the maxillary bones. After the wires on each side are twisted, one end is left long so that it can be used to attach the cantilever to the fulcrum (Fig. 8.52a).

The cantilever shaft is also constructed of rib bone. It is rounded on one end and notched at the other (Fig. 8.52b). Prior to its application the soft tissue is elevated in the superior aspect of the nasal defect, exposing the nasal process of the frontal bone. The frontal bone is notched inferiorly to receive the notched end of the cantilever strut. After the cantilever strut has been mortised in place, it is wired to the fulcrum as shown in Figure 8.52c and d.

Covering. A scalping forehead flap provides the best covering for a total nasal reconstruction. This flap is based on the frontal artery and the frontal branches of the superficial temporal artery. Some surgeons prefer to delay this flap for at least 2 weeks.

As a first stage, in addition to delaying the forehead flap, the portion of the flap which is to form the alae and the columella may be raised and lined with split-thickness skin graft (Fig. 8.53a).

The forehead flap is elevated in a plane above the periosteum of the frontal bone. It is folded on its pedicle, rotated into position, and sutured into place.

In some cases, the recipient area for the tip of the columellar portion of the forehead flap may have an inadequate blood supply. Tubing this portion of the forehead flap adds to its viability, but, on the other hand, can cause sufficient thickening of the columella so as to interfere with the airways. There are two methods which will both increase the blood supply of this columellar portion of the forehead flap and line its posterior surface. The first is that of forming a superiorly based skin flap from the upper lip. This flap is elevated subcutaneously in the midline as is shown in Figure 8.53b. An alternate method is that of lining the inner aspect of the columella with a superiorly based mucous membrane flap from the midline of the inner aspect of the upper lip. This flap is reflected superiorly through a buttonhole incision in the region of the columellar base (Fig. 8.53c).

FIGURE 8.51. *Total nasal reconstruction—lining for nasal cavities.*

a. The superior nasal cavity is lined by constructing a flap of skin and mucous membrane on each side of the nose. As small an amount of skin as possible is used in this flap, in order that the lateral defect in this area will be as little as possible. Triangular-shaped nasolabial flaps are constructed on each side in the nasolabial sulcus.

b. Both the superior and nasolabial flaps are elevated in the subcutaneous plane. The skin lateral to the nasolabial defect is undermined sufficiently to provide for a linear closure.

c. The superior flaps have been sutured to each other in the midline. Nasolabial folds are advanced superiorly and medially and sutured to each other and to the superior flaps. The nasolabial defect is sutured in a straight line. The scar will simulate a nasolabial sulcus.

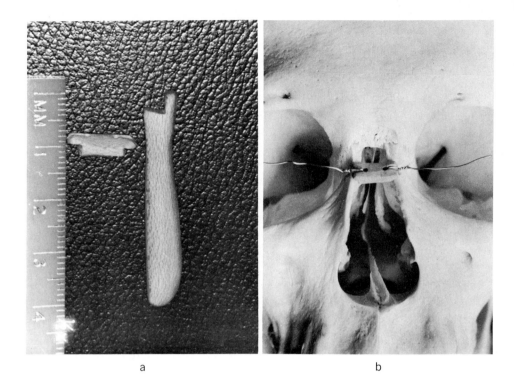

a   b

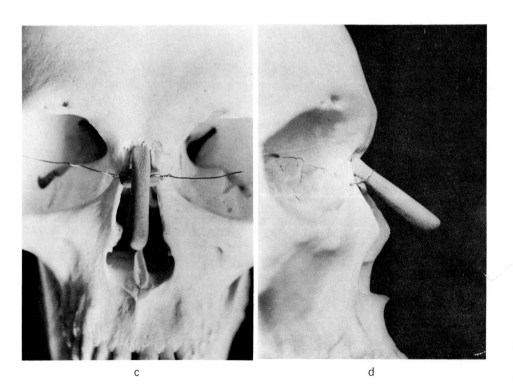

c   d

FIGURE 8.52. *Total reconstruction of the nose—bony support.*

a. On the left is a small piece of rib bone, notched at both ends. Two holes are drilled in this bone to make a fulcrum which bridges across the upper aspect of the nasal defect between the two maxillary bones. On the right is a cantilever strut which is notched at one end and rounded at the other. The notch fits posterior to the nasal process of the frontal bone.

b. The fulcrum is bridged between the two maxillary bones, and then mortised and wired in place. One end of each of the two wires is left long. These ends will be used to secure the cantilever strut to the fulcrum.

c. The cantilever strut has been mortised to the nasal process of the frontal bone and wired to the fulcrum. The mortising of the fulcrum to the maxillary bone and of the cantilever strut to the nasal process of the frontal bone adds great strength and stability to this bony support.

d. A lateral view of the cantilever strut and the fulcrum. An additional wire can be placed around the fulcrum and cantilever strut if necessary.

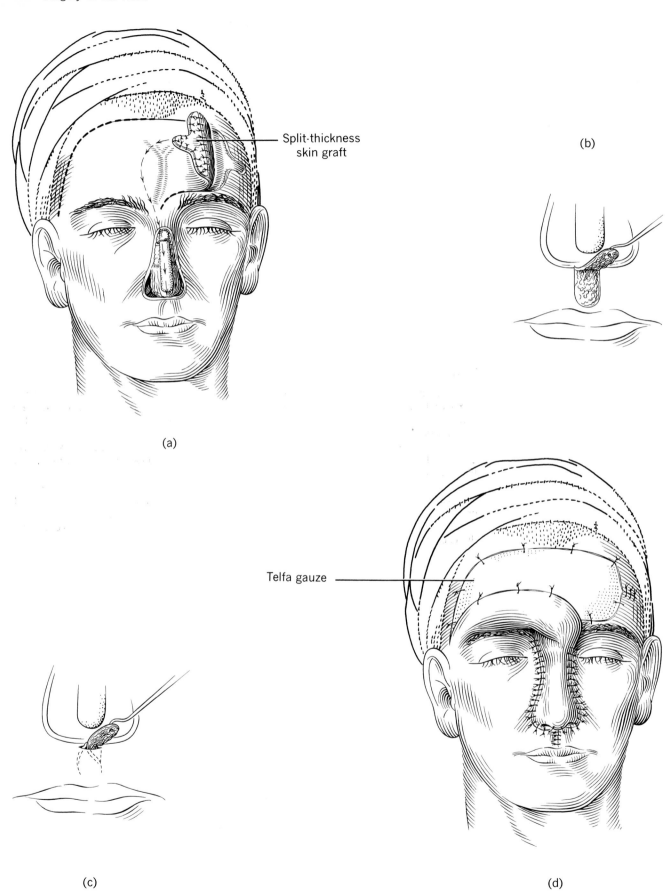

Split-thickness skin graft

(b)

(a)

Telfa gauze

(c)

(d)

FIGURE 8.53. *Total reconstruction of the nose—covering.*

a. A scalping forehead flap is used for covering in a total reconstruction. The entire forehead is utilized. The flap is based on the frontal artery and the frontal branches of the superficial temporal artery on one side. If the flap is to be delayed, the areas to form the alae and columella are lined with split-thickness skin graft. Elevation of the flap is accomplished in a plane above the periosteum of the frontal bone.

b. The posterior surface of the columellar portion of the forehead flap can be lined by using a superiorly based pedicled skin flap from the midline of the upper lip.

c. An alternate method for lining the posterior surface of the columella is that of fashioning a superiorly based mucous membrane flap from the inner aspect of the upper lip. This flap is advanced through a buttonhole incision in the region of the columellar base.

d. The forehead flap is folded on its pedicle, rotated to form the nasal covering, and sutured in place. The forehead defect is carefully dressed and the dressing kept in place for from 3 to 5 weeks, until the forehead flap is divided at the root of the nose. That portion of forehead which remains unsurfaced is covered with a split-thickness skin graft.

The periosteum of the frontal bone which is uncovered remains exposed and is covered with ointment-impregnated gauze or Telfa gauze. The portion of the defect supplying the columella for the reconstruction is closed in a horizontal, linear suture line (Fig. 8.53d). An external dressing of moderate pressure is applied both to the forehead and to the reconstructed nose.

The forehead flap is divided in the region of the root of the nose after 3 to 5 weeks and is reflected to its anatomic position on the forehead. That portion of the forehead remaining uncovered can be covered with a split-thickness skin graft or with scalp flaps rotated into this area.

Touch-up procedures may be added at a later date to narrow the nose and to form a lateral alar crease. The nose can be narrowed by incisions in the nasofacial creases. A Z-plasty can be used to form nasoalar creases in this area.

REFERENCES

Alexander, F. W.: Malignant Melanoma of the Nasal Septum. Laryngoscope *64*:123–129 (Feb.) 1954.

Anderson, R., and Dykes, E. R.: Surgical Treatment of Rhinophyma. Plast. Reconstr. Surg. *30*:397–402 (Oct.) 1962.

Aubry, G. J.: La Chirurgie Correctrice des Perforations de la Cloison. Ann. Otolaryng. (Paris) *75*:5–15, 1958.

Ballenger, J. J.: *Diseases of the Nose, Throat and Ear*, 11th ed. Philadelphia. Lea & Febiger, 1969, pp. 71–73.

Behrman, W.: Perforatio Septi Nasi—Free Transplantations. Acta Otolaryng. *39*:78, 1946.

Bernstein, J. M., Montgomery, W. W., and Balogh, K., Jr.: Metastatic Tumors to the Maxilla, Nose and Paranasal Sinuses. Laryngoscope *76*:621–650 (April) 1966.

Berson, M. T.: *Atlas of Plastic Surgery*. New York, Grune & Stratton, 1948, pp. 144–145.

Birrell, J. F.: *The Ear, Nose and Throat Diseases of Children*. Philadelphia, F. A. Davis Co., 1960, p. 113.

Blumenfeld, R., and Skolnik, E. M.: Intranasal Encephaloceles. Arch. Otolaryng. *82*:527–531 (Nov.) 1965.

Bordley, J. E., and Cherry, J.: The use of the rhinotomy operation in nasal surgery. Case Reports. Laryngoscope *70*:258–270 (March) 1960.

Chandler, J. R., and Serrins, A. J.: Transantral Ligation of the Internal Maxillary Artery for Epistaxis. Laryngoscope *75*:1151–1159 (July) 1965.

Climo, S.: The Surgical Closure of a Large Anterior Perforation of the Nasal Septum. Plast. & Reconstr. Surg. *17*:410–414, 1956.

Conley, J. J.: Malignant Schwannoma of Tip of Nose. Arch. Otolaryng. *62*:638–640 (Dec.) 1955.

Crone, R. P.: Malignant Amelanotic Melanomas of the Nasal Septum and Maxillary Sinus. Laryngoscope *76*:1826–1833 (Nov.) 1966.

Deutsch, H. J.: Carcinoma of the Nasal Septum. Report of a Case and Review of the Literature. Ann. Otol. *75*:1049–1057 (Dec.) 1966.

Fitz-Hugh, G. S., Allen, M. S., Jr., Rucker, T. N., and Sprinkle, P. M.: Olfactory Neuroblastoma. Arch. Otolaryng. *81*:161–168 (Feb.) 1965.

Frazell, E. L.: The Surgical Treatment of Cancer of the Paranasal Sinuses. Laryngoscope *65*:557–567, 1955.

Frazell, E. L., and Lewis, J. S.: Cancer of the Nasal Cavity and Accessory Sinuses. Report of the Management of 416 Patients. Cancer *16*:1293–1301 (Oct.) 1963.

Goldman, I. B.: Problems Relating to Nasal Implants and Grafts. Eye, Ear, Nose, Throat Monthly *35*:798, 1956.

Huffman, W. C., and Lierle, D. M.: Progress in Septal Surgery. Plast. Reconstr. Surg. *20*:185–198, 1957.

Hutter, R. V. P., Lewis, J. S., Foote, F. W., Jr., and Tollefsen, H. R.: Esthesioneuroblastoma. Amer. J. Surg. *106*:748 (Nov.) 1963.

Ismail, H. K.: Closure of Septal Perforations. A New Technique. J. Laryngol. *78*:620–623, 1964.

Jackson, C., and Jackson, C. L.: Diseases of the Nose, Throat and Ear, 2nd ed. Philadelphia, W. B. Saunders Co., 1959, p. 42.

Keogh, C. A.: Affections of the Nasal Septum. *In:* W. G. Scott-Brown, J. Ballantyne, and J. Groves (Eds.): *Diseases of the Ear, Nose and Throat* Vol. 1, 2nd ed. London, Butterworths, 1965, Chapter 7, p. 155.

Kirchner, J. A., Yanagisawa, E., and Crelin, F. S., Jr.: Surgical Anatomy of the Ethmoidal Arteries. A Laboratory Study of 150 Orbits. Arch. Otolaryng. 74:382–386 (Oct.) 1961.

Larchenko, R. M.: Abscesses of the Nasal Septum in Children. Vestn. Otorinolaring. 23:45 (Mar.–Apr.) 1961.

Lederer, R. L., Snitman, M. F., Skolnik, E. E., and Soboroff, B. J.: Tumors of the Nasal Cavity. Laryngoscope 67:592–604 (June) 1957.

Letterman, G., and Schurter, M.: Split Thickness Skin Graft in the Management of Hereditary Hemorrhagic Telangiectasia Involving the Nasal Mucosa. Plast. Reconstr. Surg. 34:126–135 (Aug.) 1964.

Lewis, J. S., Hutter, R. V. P., Tollefsen, H. R., and Foote, F. W., Jr.: Nasal Tumors of Olfactory Origin. Arch. Otolaryng. 81:169–173 (Feb.) 1965.

Mabery, T. E., Devine, K. D., and Harrison, E. G.: The Problem of Malignant Transformation in a Nasal Papilloma. Arch. Otolaryng. 82:296–300 (Sept.) 1965.

Macomber, D. W.: Surgical Cure of Acne Rosacea and Rhinophyma. Rocky Mountain Med. J. 43:466, 1946.

Malcomson, K. G.: The Surgical Management of Massive Epistaxis. J. Laryng. 77:299–314, 1963.

Matton, G., Pickrell, K., Huger, W., and Pound, E.: The Surgical Treatment of Rhinophyma. An Analysis of 57 Cases. Plast. Reconstr. Surg. 30:403–414 (Oct.) 1962.

McGivern, C. S.: A Simple Method for Closing Septal Perforations. Med. Rec. 151:267, 1940.

Meyer, R.: Neuerungen in der Nasenplastik. Prac. Otorhinolaryngol. 13:373–376, 1951.

Millard, D. R.: Total Reconstructive Rhinoplasty and a Missing Link. Plast. Reconstr. Surg. 37:167–183 (March) 1966.

Missal, S. C.: Ivalon as a Nasal Septal Implant. Laryngoscope 69:268–283, 1959.

Pratt, L. W.: Midline Cysts of the Nasal Dorsum: Embryologic Origin and Treatment. Laryngoscope 75:968–980 (June) 1965.

Rogers, K. A., and Walker, E. A., Jr.: Primary Epidermoid Carcinoma of the Nasal Septum. J. Okla. Med. Assoc. (Oct.) 1963, p. 458.

Saunders, W. H.: Septal Dermoplasty for Control of Nosebleeds Caused by Hereditary Hemorrhagic Telangiectasia or Septal Perforations. Trans. Amer. Acad. Ophthal. Otolaryng. 64:500–506 (July–Aug.) 1960.

Schall, L. A.: Cancer of the Nose and Nasal Sinuses. Laryngoscope 53:3 (April) 1943.

Schall, L. A.: Malignant Tumors of the Nose and Nasal Accessory Sinuses. J.A.M.A. 137:1273 (Aug. 7) 1948.

Seeley, R. C.: Repair of the Septal Perforation, a Rhinologic Problem. A Rhinoplastic Approach (Author's Technique). Laryngoscope 59:130–146, 1949.

Smith, A. E.: Correction of Advanced Rhinophyma by Means of Plastic Reconstructive Surgery. Amer. J. Surg. 96:792, 1958.

Soboroff, B. J., and Lederer, F. L.: Chondrosarcoma of the Nasal Cavity. Ann. Otol. 64:718 (Sept.) 1955.

Van Alyea, O. E.: Nasal Polyps and Sinusitis. Ann. Otol. 75:881–887 (Sept.) 1966.

Walker, E. A., and Resler, D. R.: Nasal Glioma. Laryngoscope 73:93–107 (Jan.) 1963.

Wallenborn, W. M., and Fitz-Hugh, G. S.: Abscess of the Posterior Nasal Septum. Arch. Otolaryng. 77:3–5 (Jan.) 1963.

9

Rhinoplasty

By Edgar Holmes

SURGICAL ANATOMY

The surgeon's familiarity with the structure of the nose invites smooth, easy operating. The lack of it invites anxiety, awkwardness, poor results, and complications.

Over the nasal bones and lateral cartilages the skin is thin and fairly freely movable. The skin is much thicker, contains more glands, and is firmly adherent over the alar cartilages. The blood supply is mainly in the soft tissues. The dissection should lie in planes of cleavage whereby vessels are avoided and bleeding is minimized. The bony nose consists of paired nasal bones which are thin in their lower half to two thirds, and solid in their upper third (Fig. 9.1c, d, and e). These bones rest upon the frontal spine (nasal process) of the frontal bone and are held, as if in a vise, between the two frontal (ascending) processes of the superior maxilla. The frontal (ascending) process of the maxilla forms the lateral aspect and lower two thirds of the nose. The maxilla also forms the floor of the anterior nasal cavities (Fig. 9.1f and g).

Description of the Cartilages

The cartilages of the nose are basically five. They form the support of the flexible portion of the nose. The septum lies in the midline, and firmly attached to it are the two lateral cartilages which in some persons are apparently fused (Fig. 9.2a and d). Below these cartilages, and resting upon them, are the lateral wings of the paired alar cartilages. When feeling one's nose, it is easily noticeable that the mid-portion can be moved freely from side to side, but can be depressed only slightly. The tip, which is formed by the alar cartilages, can be moved quite freely upward, downward, and in and out. It also will be noted that the lateral

411

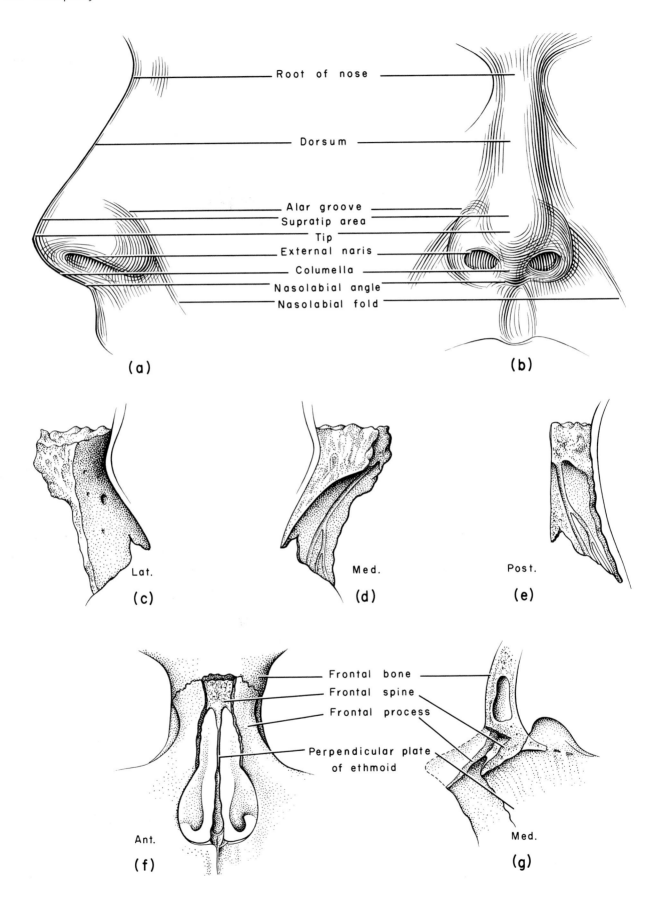

Root of nose

Dorsum

Alar groove
Supratip area
Tip
External naris
Columella
Nasolabial angle
Nasolabial fold

(a)   (b)

Lat.   Med.   Post.

(c)   (d)   (e)

Frontal bone
Frontal spine
Frontal process

Perpendicular plate
of ethmoid

Ant.   Med.

(f)   (g)

cartilages go beneath the nasal bones and are quite firmly attached to them for a varying distance of from 2 mm to 1 cm (Fig. 9.2a, b, c, and e). This relationship is extremely important if there is a fracture of the septum which deviates the cartilaginous portion of the nose to one side. When this occurs, the lateral cartilages, after having been torn loose from the nasal bone at the time of injury, will heal in this new angulated position. One may straighten the septum to create a nose which is aligned in the midline, but it will migrate back again unless the lateral cartilages are freed from the undersurface of the nasal bones, permitting them to re-align also. The septal cartilage extends up beneath the nasal bones, at least as far as the lateral cartilages, where it joins the perpendicular plate of the ethmoid, and here it thickens (Fig. 9.4c). Just beneath the dorsum the nasal septum becomes thicker and tends to bifurcate, or flare to its edge, where it comes in contact with the lateral cartilages (Fig. 9.2d). The septal cartilage and the lateral cartilages do not fuse in this area, although they appear to do so. A section through this area will show that the perichondrium is continuous around the septum and around each lateral cartilage. The edges of the cartilages are bound together with dense connective tissue.

The paired alar cartilages are the supporting skeleton of the nasal tip. Each cartilage has a lateral and a medial crus, or what is really an irregularly shaped U. The medial crura come together in the midline, and their lower portions flare slightly into each nostril (Fig. 9.3a and b). The lateral crura are bulbous, sometimes irregular at the tip, with a tendency to flare and flatten out laterally. The skin of the undersurface of the lateral cartilage is quite readily separated from it, but at the medial crus, the skin is adherent and difficult to separate. The alar cartilages move freely over the lateral and septal cartilages.

There are muscles attached to the lateral and alar cartilages which control the size of the vestibular opening. On close observation it will be noted that the nose is quite animated (Fig. 9.3c). Stand before a mirror and make facial expressions of surprise, disgust, and move the lips from side to side and appreciate the extent of this mobility. Next grasp the tip of the nose and observe that it is freely movable and not attached to the septum or lateral cartilages. When the planes of cleavage are not adhered to by the surgeon, and the muscles are cut through or torn, the nose will become quite motionless and appear lifeless.

FIGURE 9.1. *Surgical anatomy of the nose.*

a and b. The anatomic parts and terms used in the text.

c, d and e. Drawings of the disarticulated right nasal bone. Note that the upper third of the nasal bone is thick and solid. The lower two thirds are thinner and concave on the undersurface. The groove on the undersurface in d and e is for the anterior ethmoidal nerve and its corresponding arteries.

f and g. The nasal bones have been disarticulated to illustrate the bed in which they rest. The frontal spine is a shelf which prevents inward displacement in the region of the root of the nose. If a fracture associated with inward displacement should occur, the perpendicular plate of the ethmoid would be involved, and one must assume that the cribriform plate of the ethmoid is fractured unless otherwise proven.

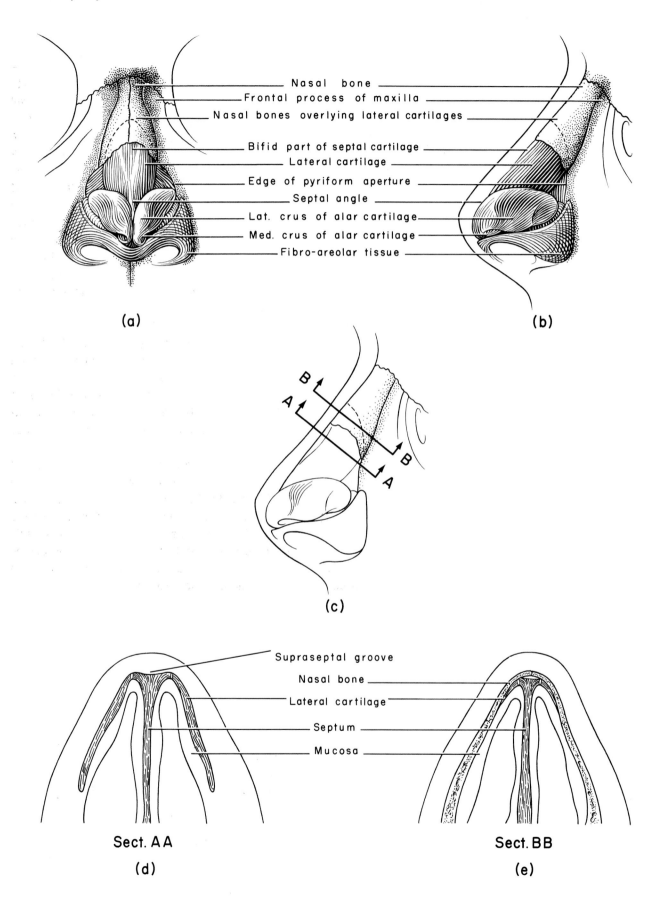

Nasal bone

Frontal process of maxilla

Nasal bones overlying lateral cartilages

Bifid part of septal cartilage

Lateral cartilage

Edge of pyriform aperture

Septal angle

Lat. crus of alar cartilage

Med. crus of alar cartilage

Fibro-areolar tissue

(a)

(b)

(c)

Supraseptal groove

Nasal bone

Lateral cartilage

Septum

Mucosa

Sect. AA

(d)

Sect. BB

(e)

FIGURE 9.2.   *Surgical anatomy of the nose—the cartilages.*

a and b. Note that, in addition to the customary anatomic findings, the lateral cartilages extend beneath, and are attached to, the under-surface of the nasal bones. The dotted line beneath the nasal bone illustrates the extent to which this sometimes occurs.

c, d and e. In section AA, it will be noted that the septum comes to the surface, flares out, and grossly appears to be continuous with the lateral cartilages. On microscopic examination, however, these cartilages are found to be fused with connective tissue at the apex of the nose. Section BB illustrates the relationship of the lateral cartilages to the under-surface of the nasal bone. This emphasizes the point that if these cartilages have been torn loose, and have healed in a distorted position, they must be separated from the nasal bone before they can be re-aligned.

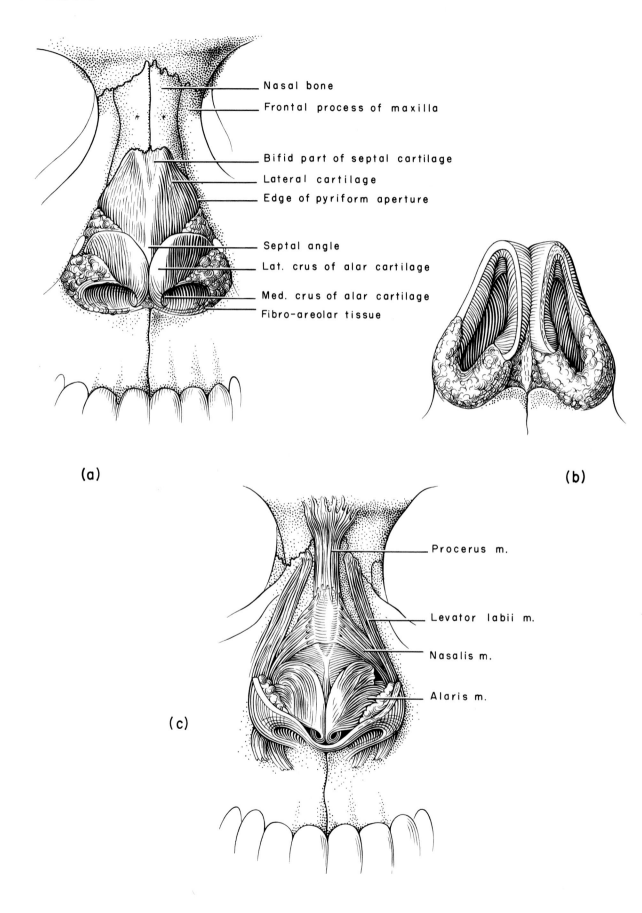

Nasal bone

Frontal process of maxilla

Bifid part of septal cartilage

Lateral cartilage

Edge of pyriform aperture

Septal angle

Lat. crus of alar cartilage

Med. crus of alar cartilage

Fibro-areolar tissue

(a)

(b)

(c)

Procerus m.

Levator labii m.

Nasalis m.

Alaris m.

FIGURE 9.3. *Surgical anatomy of the nose—the cartilages.*

a. Note that the upper one third to one half of the nose is solid due to the nasal bones. The lower half to two thirds is mobile. The alar cartilages are freely movable over the lateral cartilages and septum and actually rest on top of the lateral cartilages.

b. The alar cartilages are supported partially by the septum and also by fibro-areolar tissue which permits motion in all directions.

c. Nasal motion is accomplished through these muscles, which can lift the alae as well as flare them. The muscles of the cheek (not shown) can move the tip of the nose from side to side.

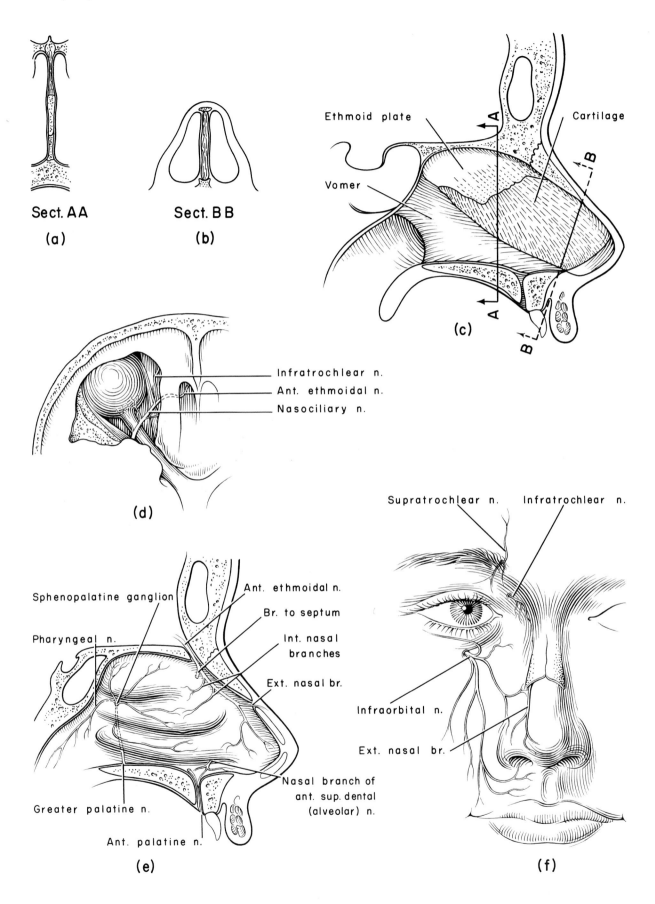

Sect. AA

(a)

Sect. BB

(b)

Ethmoid plate

Cartilage

Vomer

A

B

A

B

(c)

Infratrochlear n.
Ant. ethmoidal n.
Nasociliary n.

(d)

Sphenopalatine ganglion

Pharyngeal n.

Greater palatine n.

Ant. palatine n.

Ant. ethmoidal n.
Br. to septum
Int. nasal branches
Ext. nasal br.
Nasal branch of ant. sup. dental (alveolar) n.

(e)

Supratrochlear n.   Infratrochlear n.

Infraorbital n.

Ext. nasal br.

(f)

The Septum

The septum is extremely important in rhinoplasty, particularly when it is post-traumatically bent and causes an external deformity, and obstructs the nasal airways as well. The quadrilateral cartilage of the septum forms a part of the nasal dorsum. If the septum is broken and thus depressed or deviated, the cartilaginous dorsum will become depressed or angulated. This cartilage is held firmly between the nasal bones and the groove in the premaxillary spine and vomer and also in its articulation with the perpendicular plate of the ethmoid bone (Fig. 9.4a, b, and c). A blow to the tip of the nose which bends it sharply to one side will create a common deformity by fracturing the cartilage between the two fixed points, the tip of the nose and the premaxillary spine (Fig. 9.4c, line BB). If the blow is on the dorsum of the cartilaginous tip, the cartilage may disarticulate from the vomer groove and in so doing will depress the dorsum. This is observed following trauma with or without nasal bone fractures (Fig. 9.14.c). If observed soon after injury, the cartilage should always be replaced and immobilized in position until healing occurs. This replacement of a broken and displaced septum will also maintain the support of the nasal bones once they have been reduced. However, this is sometimes extremely difficult to do, because of the marked lacerations, multiple fractures, and swelling of the soft tissues resulting from the trauma.

ANESTHESIA

The external nose is supplied by branches of the infraorbital nerve, the nasociliary nerve, and a nasal branch of the superior alveolar nerve (Fig. 9.4d, e, and f). The lining of the nasal cavities is supplied by the anterior ethmoid nerve, the nasal branch of the superior dental nerve, and branches from the spheno-palatine ganglion, which also supply the septum and the lateral wall of the nose.

Local anesthesia is preferable in most cases not only for plastic operations upon the nose, but also for most intranasal procedures. Combined with correct preoperative medication, local anesthesia permits the surgeon to operate in a

FIGURE 9.4. *Surgical anatomy of the nose—the septum and nerves.*

a, b and c. Section AA shows solid bone on the top and bottom of the septum. In between the upper third is the thin perpendicular plate of the ethmoid. This broadens out at the junction with the quadrilateral cartilage to form the tubercle; frequently the latter is quite broad. The bottom third is the vomer, which is firm bone. Where the quadrilateral cartilage rests in the vomer groove, the perichondrium completely surrounds the cartilage and at the same time is firmly adherent to the periosteum. (See Fig. 9.13 [a], Sect. BB.)

d. The origin of the nasociliary nerve with its branches, the infratrochlear nerve, and the anterior ethmoidal nerves.

e. Nerves that supply the interior of the nose.

f. The area supplied by the infraorbital nerve.

comparatively dry field on an unapprehensive patient. The inside of the nose should first be shrunk and superficially anesthetized with the combination of a vasoconstrictor and a topical anesthetic. A good combination is 2 cc of 1:1000 epinephrine solution in 100 cc of 2% Pontocaine or 4% topical Xylocaine, which may be made up as a stock solution. The nose is sprayed with this solution before the patient is brought to the operating room. Once the patient is "prepped" and draped, the inside of the nose is ready to receive cotton moistened with the anesthetic. Cocaine (4%) is also very satisfactory, because it is a vasoconstrictor as well as an anesthetic. When a barbiturate is used for premedication there is practically no risk of a cocaine reaction. The topical anesthetic is placed in the region of the anterior ethmoidal nerve and the sphenopalatine ganglion either by a cotton-tipped applicator or by strips of cotton about 2 inches long, $\frac{1}{2}$ inch wide, and $\frac{1}{8}$ inch thick.

The external nose may be anesthetized either by a block or an infiltration anesthetic. The combination of the two is most satisfactory. Here, again, the choice of anesthetic may be left to the operator. Either procaine or Xylocaine with epinephrine 1:50,000 to 1:100,000 works well. The epinephrine, by its vasoconstricting action, holds the anesthetic in location and controls capillary bleeding.

There are several methods of injecting. The one I find most satisfactory is as follows: A 24-gauge needle, $1\frac{1}{2}$ inches long, attached to a 5-cc Luer Lok syringe is used. Choosing an injection site on the dorsum of the nose, about the level of the inner canthus, infiltration is carried out slowly, so as not to cause ballooning of the tissues, down to, and including, the infraorbital nerve, first on one side, and then on the other. By fanning the direction of the needle (Fig. 9.5a), the region of the glabella and the entire dorsum of the nose may be infiltrated. The upper lip and buttresses may be blocked by injecting into the infraorbital foramen. This may readily be performed by directing the needle through the skin adjacent to the ala of the nose, but $\frac{1}{4}$ inch from it and then up to $\frac{1}{4}$ inch below the infraorbital rim. A finger placed on the infraorbital rim is of assistance in locating the foramen. For the entire external nose, 4 to 5 cc is adequate. The next site of injection is at the base of the left ala, if the operator is right-handed. The injection is carried beneath the columella to the opposite side. Pulling the needle back, it may be directed into the base of the columella, and, by tipping the nose to one side, the needle may be directed up, in front of the septum. This will usually give complete anesthesia of the outside of the nose although additional injection into the vestibule is occasionally advisable to control bleeding. The dorsum of the nose may now be skeletonized completely in preparation for removal of the hump. Before doing this, I inject both sides of the septum beneath the dorsum and laterally on the undersurface of each nasal bone. If a submucous resection of the septum is necessary, topical anesthesia is combined with infiltration anesthesia, primarily for hemostasis.

With careful injection technique, tachycardia, palpitations, anxiety, or nervousness rarely follows, particularly when adequate preoperative sedation has been given. Of course, it is impossible to have a set anesthesia schedule, because no two people respond identically to medication. A routine preoperative medication may be employed, but, when the patient is in the operating room, supplementary anesthesia may also be prescribed at the surgeon's discretion. For basic anesthesia, 100 mg of Nembutal are given by mouth 2 hours before the operation. One hour preoperatively, another 100 mg of Nembutal, plus 50 or 75 mg of Demerol, and 0.4 mg of scopolamine are administered intramuscularly. This may be varied to suit the individual patient and is not prescribed as the only or ultimate preoperation medication.

RHINOPLASTY TECHNIQUE

Exposure of the Nasal Skeleton

The basic incision for exposure of the nasal skeleton, called the intercartilaginous incision, is made between the alar and lateral cartilages. This incision exposes the outer surface of the lateral cartilage where a dissection plane is encountered (Fig. 9.5b and c). Utilizing traction of the ala, the soft tissues are dissected away from the lateral cartilage with either a double-edged Joseph knife or a very flat, nearly pointed scissors. This may be done under direct vision, and getting out of the plane of dissection into the overlying muscles will be avoided. The dissection is carried up to the lower border of the nasal bones and to the edge of the frontal process of the maxilla, but not up over the bone. With a sharp blade, an incision is made through the periosteum over the nasal bones as near their lower border as practical. This bony edge is usually serrated, and it is necessary to make the incision 2 or 3 mm above the margin. This can be done under direct vision, but it is easier to do by touch (Fig. 9.5e). The blade is inserted on top of the nasal bones, brought down on its edge, and then raised and brought up to the point of incision. Starting laterally, near the frontal process, and using only the tip of the blade, the periosteum is incised up to the midline. A thin and narrow periosteal elevator may be inserted beneath the periosteum at the lower end of the incision and carried up to the root of the nasal bones. The entire elevator can then be brought broadside to the dorsal midline (Fig. 9.5f). It is quite difficult to separate the median raphe from the dorsum. A pair of scissors may be used to effect the separation, cutting close to the bone and cartilage (Fig. 9.5g).

The transfixion incision is next made with either a curved button knife or a #15 Bard-Parker knife blade. Holding the nasal tip up with a double-hooked instrument and pulling the columella away from the septum, the knife is pushed through the soft tissue just in front of the septal cartilage. The incision is carried down in front of the cartilaginous septum to the premaxillary spine (Fig. 9.6a and b). If it is desirable to extend this further, the columella is retracted and the muscles dissected away from the maxilla either with a periosteal elevator, knife, or scissors. The transfixion incision is next extended upward to communicate with the previously made intercartilaginous incisions.

The nasal framework is now exposed. Strands of tissue attaching the skin to the framework should be cut.

Removal of Nasal Hump

There are several ways of removing a nasal hump, which consists of both bone and cartilage. The three main methods employ (1) the nasal hump rongeur, (2) the osteotome, (3) the nasal saw.

Rongeur Technique. The sharpness of the surgeon's instruments for this procedure is very important. A nasal hump rongeur, as purchased, is rarely sharp enough and must be re-sharpened. If the hump is small, the instrument may be placed at the level that one wishes to remove the hump, and one closure of the instrument will cut the cartilage and bone straight through without much more having to be done. If the hump is large and particularly broad, it is necessary to uncap it by merely removing its top. This exposes each nasal bone and the septum as separate entities. Next the lateral cartilages are separated from the septum by using scissors and making certain that the cut is made adjacent to

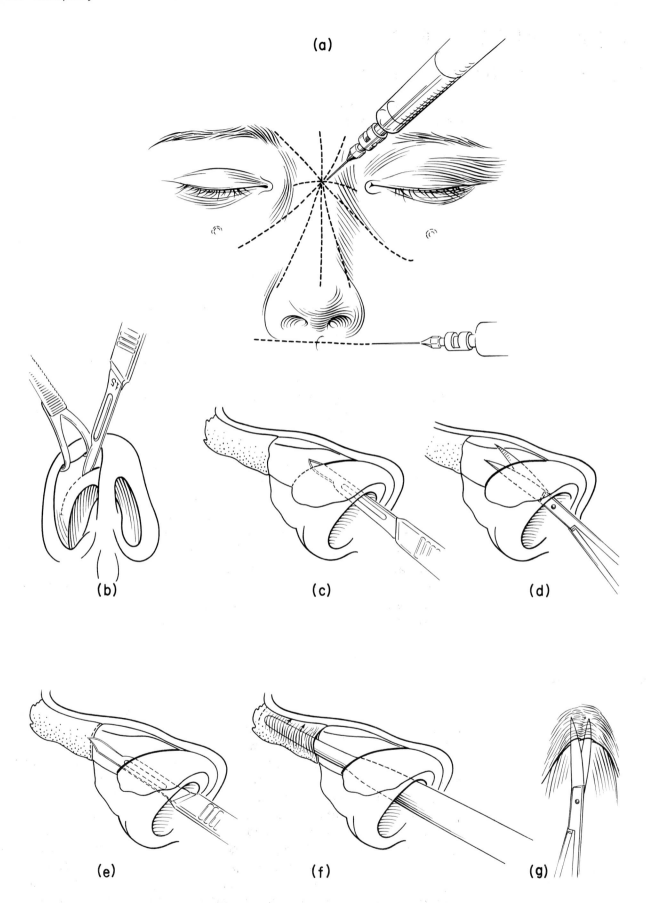

(a)

(b)

(c)

(d)

(e)

(f)

(g)

the septum (Fig. 9.7a). Under direct vision, each side of the nasal dorsum is removed down to the desired level. This is followed by trimming the septum (Fig. 9.7b). In this way, fracture of the nasal bone in an undesirable place is avoided; such a fracture may occur if removal of a large hump is attempted with only one cut of the rongeur. With the rongeur the surgeon is able to cut not only the cartilage, but also the membrane. It is easier to cut the membrane and cartilage in this manner than with a knife or scissors. Once the nasal dorsum is lowered to the desired level, it may be necessary to lower the bone near the glabella, where it is solid, by using a rasp or osteotome (Fig. 9.7c and d). Care must be taken that the plane of the rasp is parallel to the desired dorsal profile. The level to which the dorsum is lowered may be predetermined by a set of ideal aesthetic angles, but in reality it is up to the surgeon's aesthetic judgment to decide when enough has been done. It is always advisable to remove too little at first, because more can always be removed if this seems necessary. The reverse is not true, and the insertion of cartilage to restore the dorsum to the desired level is never as satisfactory as lowering the dorsum in an exact manner.

The rongeur method of removal of the nasal hump, as well as the two methods described below, requires practice before perfection is attained. The rongeur technique is my preference.

Osteotome Technique. The osteotome must be broad enough to include the entire width of the hump to be removed and sharp enough to cut through the cartilage without buckling or deforming it. The instrument must be knife-sharp prior to each use. Once the cartilaginous portion has been cut through, the osteotome, propelled with a mallet, is carried through the nasal bone (Fig. 9.7f). If the bone is hard and brittle, as is frequently found in older patients, an osteotome cut may result in a fracture ahead of the instrument and not in a desired location. For this reason I do not use this method even though it is easy and fast in most cases.

Removal of Hump with Bone Saw. In this method first one side of the bony hump is cut through with a bone saw and then the other. The remaining cartilage is cut with a knife (Fig. 9.7e).

FIGURE 9.5. *Local anesthetization and exposure of nasal skeleton.*

a. Infiltration of local anesthetic. To avoid distortion of soft tissue, a minimum of solution is used to infiltrate the entire area of the nose. The infraorbital nerves may be blocked as they exit from their foramina.

b. This is known as the intercartilaginous incision. It is made between the lateral and alar cartilages.

c. The blade is inserted at the septum and is carried laterally to the lower border of the lateral cartilage.

d. Through this incision, and adjacent to the perichondrium of the lateral cartilages, the soft tissue, including the perichondrium, may be elevated to the nasal bones.

e. The blade is placed through the undermined area up to the nasal bones, where an incision is made through the periosteum along the line indicated.

f. The periosteum is elevated from the upper and lateral surface of the nasal bones, but the surgeon may find that he cannot separate the median attachment to the nasal bones because of the firm, fibrous union found here.

g. This fibrous attachment may be cut with curved scissors.

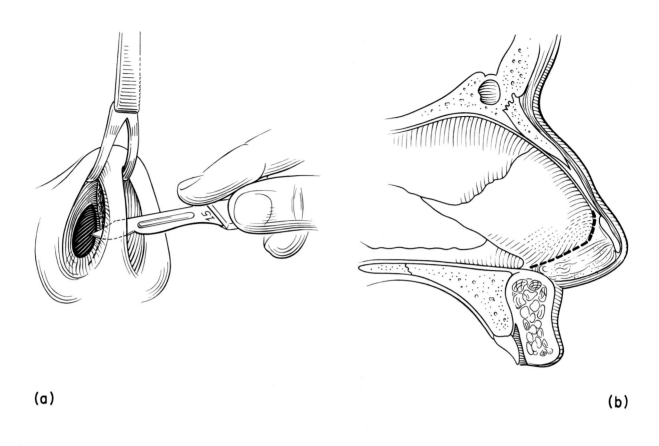

(a)

(b)

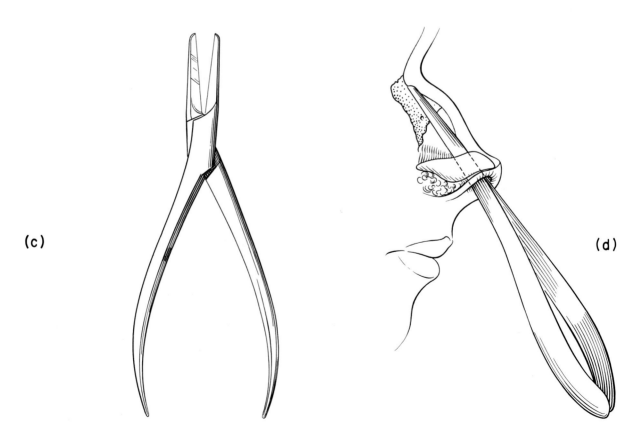

(c)

(d)

FIGURE 9.6. *Transfixion incision; nasal hump rongeur.*

a and b. To make a transfixion incision, the tip of the nose is lifted up and forward with some form of a double-pronged, blunt-tipped retractor. With the knife-blade at right angles to the surface of the septum, the columella is cut free in a plane just anterior to the septal cartilage and behind the medial crura of the ala. The incision is carried down as far as necessary, which is usually to the premaxillary spine (dotted line in b).

c and d. The Kazanjian-Holmes rongeur designed to remove the nasal hump. This rongeur should be sharp enough to cut membrane as well as bone. The cutting blades are flush with the undersurface of the instrument and this surface is placed on a level with the area to be cut. The tip of the instrument must never be placed below the contour of the profile. If this is done the instrument will dig into the bone and create an unwanted fracture.

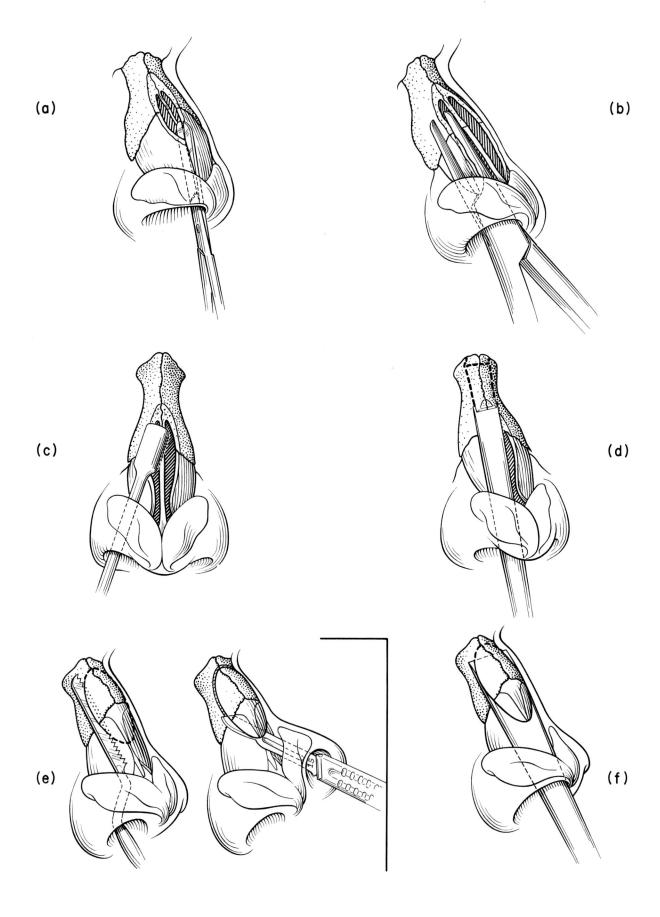

(a)

(b)

(c)

(d)

(e)

(f)

FIGURE 9.7. *Removal of nasal hump.*

a. Once the hump is removed, the distal portion of the lateral cartilages, still adherent to the septum, may be cut adjacent and parallel to the septum with scissors.

b. The septum, each lateral cartilage, and the nasal bones may now be seen and lowered or smoothed with the rongeur.

c. The solid portion of the nasal bones and the remaining surface of the bone may be smoothed and lowered by using a rasp.

d. If the amount of bone to be removed is extensive, a chisel may be employed.

e. The dorsal hump is removed with a nasal saw and a knife. The nasal saw is first used from one side and then from the other, cutting through the bone. If the cartilage is not cut with the saw, a knife is used.

f. The hump is removed with a very sharp osteotome.

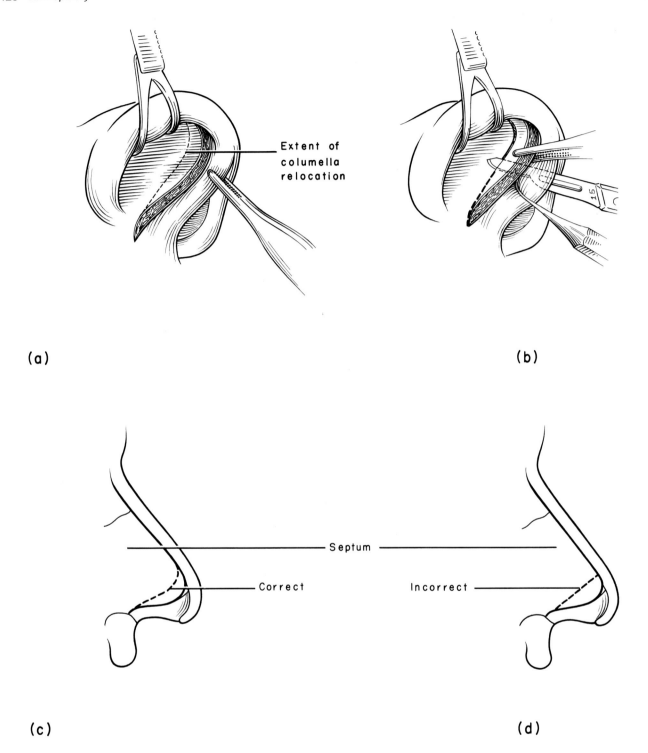

(a)

(b)

(c)

(d)

FIGURE 9.8. *Shortening length of nose.*

a. To determine the extent of excision of the lower border of the septum, the columella is grasped gently with forceps and pushed inward so that it overrides the septum.

b. When the desired contour of the nose is obtained, the location of the columella on the septum is noticed. This marks the line of the cut to be made.

c. The incision should be perpendicular to the flat surface of the septum and conform to the contour of the inferior border of the septum.

d. The incision should not be in a straight line as is shown here.

Shortening Length of Nose

As soon as the hump has been removed it is always advisable to feel the dorsum, as well as to evaluate it visually. Sometimes an irregularity that is not visible can be felt, because the soft tissues and skin, a little swollen at the time of the operation, may obscure any irregularity.

It is now usually necessary to shorten the length of the nose so that the nasolabial angle and tip are in a satisfactory relationship. When the hump is lowered, it automatically makes the nasal tip too pointed in the profile view, and the nasolabial angle is prone to be too acute. The amount to be removed may be determined by grasping the columella with forceps, pushing the tip up into its proper position, and ascertaining how far the columella overlaps the septum (Fig. 9.8a). It is at this level that the septum must be excised. This may readily be done by grasping the septum and cutting through the cartilage and its overlying membrane on each side. A scalpel is more satisfactory than scissors for this procedure (Fig. 9.8b). It is important to round the septal tip prior to trimming the lower border (Fig. 9.8c and d). If this is not done, a sharp point sticking up between the alar cartilages may be the result. This excision should leave the lower border curved as it was prior to removal.

Mobilizing the Lateral Walls of the Nose

With the hump removed and the septum shortened, the profile of the nose is now final. However, the front view may present a very flat, broad nose, because the nasal bones and septum are separated. To create a narrow, more normal-looking dorsum, it is necessary to mobilize the bony lateral walls of the nose so that they may be hinged or replaced until the dorsal portions are in contact with the septum. There are three separate procedures which must be employed to accomplish this: (1) a lateral osteotomy, (2) removal of bone at the solid angle, and (3) a superior osteotomy connecting the lateral osteotomy and the bone excision at the solid angle.

Lateral Osteotomy. The lateral osteotomy should be performed through the ascending or frontal process of the maxilla, laterally so that the nasal contour will have the desired proportions. If the base of the nasal pyramid is narrow, the lateral walls may be hinged along the osteotomy to permit the nasal bones to come in contact with the septum, and a pleasing contour will result. If the base is broad, it may be necessary to slide the freed ascending process and attached nasal bones medially, creating a step at the osteotomy. This will create the desired nasal contour and the bony irregularity will not be apparent, as it will be covered with soft tissue in the concave area. The step will be obvious by palpation only. The osteotomy may be done either with nasal saws or with a thin, narrow osteotome, either plain or with a blunt guiding tip. I use a saw, except when reducing an old fracture, because, if the bone is brittle, it may fracture in a line that will not be desirable. With an old fracture the surgeon may feel his way and cut through the old fracture line. In the majority of nasal fractures healing takes place more by fibrosis than by callus formation.

To perform the osteotomy, an incision is made through the nasal vestibule, just anterior to the attachment of the inferior turbinate and directly over the sharp edge of the piriform aperture of the bone (Fig. 9.9a and b) which may be first palpated with the handle end of the knife. With the cutting blade facing superiorly, a stab wound is made to the edge of the bone. The tip of the blade is carried

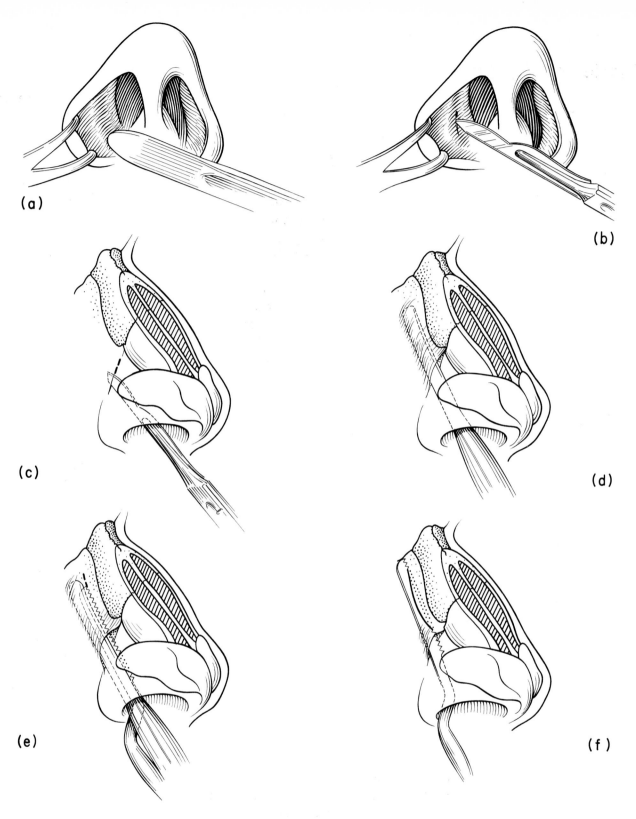

FIGURE 9.9. *Lateral osteotomy.*

    a. A knife handle is used for palpation to locate the bony margin of the piriform aperture.
    b. An incision is made to the bone.
    c. The incision is carried through the periosteum on the lateral surface of the bone.
    d. A periosteal elevator is inserted up to the level of the inner canthus.
    e. An elevator is employed as a retractor to permit insertion of a saw.
    f. The saw is in the correct position for cutting through the ascending process of the maxilla.

laterally and on the external surface of the bone a millimeter or two, where an incision is made through the periosteum just long enough to introduce the periosteal elevator which is to be employed (Fig. 9.9c). As the blade is withdrawn, a cut is made equal to the periosteal cut through the tissues and the skin of the vestibules. A flat and narrow periosteal elevator is next inserted through this incision beneath the periosteum, and directed up along the bone to the level of the inner canthus (Fig. 9.9d). This brings the elevator just medial to the attachment of the medial canthal ligament. The elevator may be used as a retractor to permit the tip of the saw to be introduced into the tunnel thus constructed (Fig. 9.9e). As the saw is introduced, with its flat surface on the bony surface, the elevator is removed. The saw is pushed up to the extent of the tunnel and rotated into a cutting position. It is important that the plane of the cut be exact, not only in its relationship to the dorsum, but also in its relationship to the surface which is to be cut (Fig. 9.9f).

With the saw in position, the bone incision is usually made at a right angle to the surface of the ascending process. Controlled short strokes will result in rapid engagement of the saw in the bone. The engagement is readily determined by pressing on the skin over the saw blade and releasing the saw handle. If the saw is engaged it will retain its position when its handle is flicked; if not engaged, flicking of the handle will cause the saw to fall loose. There is usually a convex bulge in this area of bone, therefore the saw may cut through in the middle before doing so at the lower end. Attention should be paid to the upper end where the bone is thick; the saw may not penetrate through this area as rapidly as the rest of the bone. As the bone incision nears completion, the saw is removed. If any "saw dust" remains, it should be removed by cannula suction through the subperiosteal incision.

Removal of a Wedge of Solid Bone between the Septum and Nasal Bones. In order to narrow the nose as high as desired and rule out the possibility of a bulge between the narrowed dorsum and the glabella, it is necessary to remove a wedge of bone from the solid upper third of the nasal bones (Fig. 9.10a–e). The removal of this wedge of bone will prevent the lateral upper surface of the bone from protruding laterally when the vault is narrowed. This piece of bone, when removed, can no longer act as a fulcrum, thus permitting the entire lateral wall to be hinged in its uppermost part.

I use a pointed cutting rongeur to remove the wedge of bone. The male blade is inserted beneath the nasal bones, the female blade rests on the surface and extends as high as one wishes to narrow the nose. The bone is then removed with one closure of the instrument (Fig. 9.10a and b). If this instrument is not available, the same result may be obtained with a flat osteotome at least one third of an inch wide. A cut is made parallel to the outer surface of the nasal bone up to the midline along the dorsum (Fig. 9.10c). A second cut is made parallel and adjacent to the septum, up to the first cut (Fig. 9.10d). The bone thus freed may be removed with a straight mosquito hemostat (Fig. 9.10e).

Osteotomy Connecting the Two Cuts. The apexes of the two cuts just described are now connected by employing a narrow osteotome, which is introduced through the skin just lateral to the midline. The skin incision is made with the osteotome (Fig. 9.10f). By using the corner of the osteotome, and pointing the instrument diagonally toward the nasal tip, the bone may be scored down through to the cut made previously in the ascending process (Fig. 9.10f). The bone may now be hinged into position with the fear of an undesirable fracture eliminated.

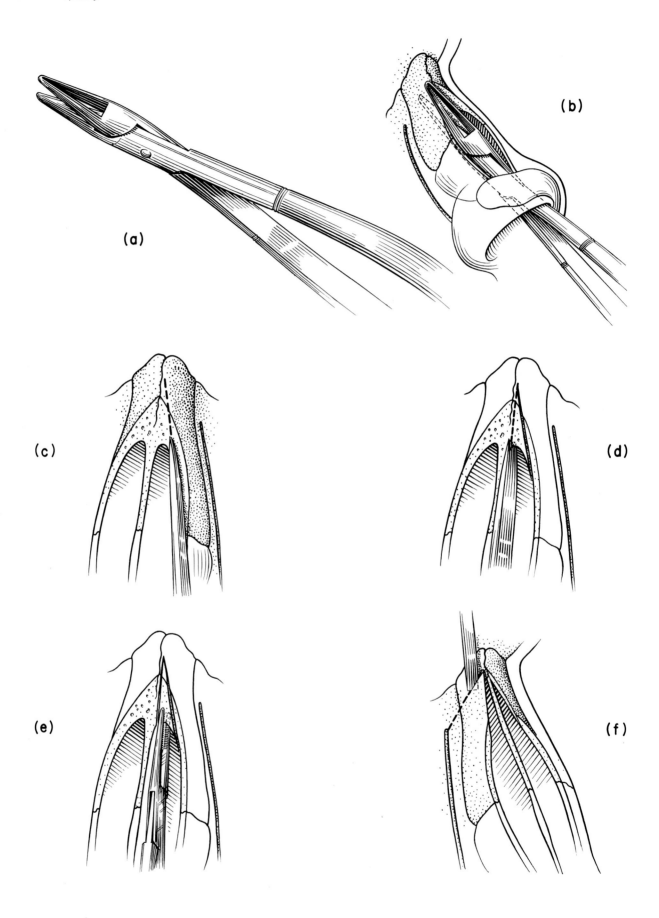

(a)

(b)

(c)

(d)

(e)

(f)

FIGURE 9.10.   *Removal of bone at solid angle.*

a. A through-and-through cutting rongeur employed to remove the wedge of bone shown in e.

b. The male blade is inserted beneath the nasal bone, parallel and adjacent to the septum. The female blade is placed on top, and, with a firm, slow, steady closure, the desired wedge of bone may be removed.

c and d. If an osteotome is used, it should be thin and about a third of an inch wide. The first bone incision is parallel to the outer surface of the nasal bone, and the cut is carried up to the midline. The blade is then withdrawn and placed parallel to, and flat with, the septum. This cut is extended to meet the superior end of the first.

e. The wedge of bone is now free, and may be removed with a pointed hemostat.

f. The lateral wall remains attached by a portion of the nasal bone and ascending process. This must be scored with a chisel, not more than 3 mm wide.

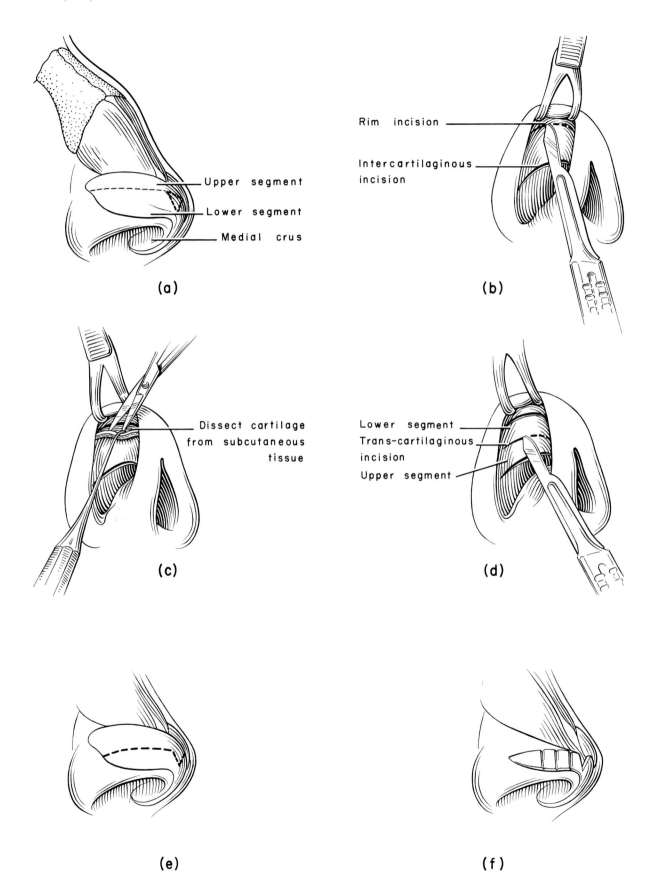

(a)

Upper segment
Lower segment
Medial crus

(b)

Rim incision
Intercartilaginous incision

(c)

Dissect cartilage from subcutaneous tissue

(d)

Lower segment
Trans-cartilaginous incision
Upper segment

(e)

(f)

Some surgeons fracture the bone and ascending process laterally before bringing it into the midline. Others attempt to fracture it indirectly, hoping that the fracture line will be to their liking. This is never a safe method because the fracture line may result in undesirable irregularity.

Surgery of the Tip of the Nose

It is rare when a plastic alteration of the nasal tip is not necessary with a plastic procedure on the dorsum. Once the dorsum is altered and the nose narrowed, the shape of the tip, which depends on the contour of the lateral wings of the alar cartilages, will invariably be too broad and rounded. There are many procedures for altering the shape of the tip, but they all have in common the fact that there are certain areas where cartilage must be removed and other areas where the spring of the cartilage must be broken to permit adequate and permanent re-shaping. The basic surgical procedure to alter the shape of the tip was described by Joseph, and most other methods involve variations of his technique.

The lateral wing of the alar cartilage may be divided into an upper third and lower two thirds. This division varies, depending on the size of the tip and the amount of alteration to be made (Fig. 9.11a). When the upper segment is removed, the tip rests closer to the lateral cartilages, and, in some cases, this is all that needs to be done. In most patients, however, it is necessary to remove a wedge from the apex, permitting the ala to hinge near its free border and allowing the lateral crura to come nearer the midline. To expose the alar tip an incision is made along the free margin of the alar cartilage. Small round-tipped scissors are introduced, separating the overlying soft tissues from the perichondrium of the cartilage (Fig. 9.11b and c). After complete exposure of the lateral wing, a transcartilaginous incision is made to separate the upper from the lower segments (Fig. 9.11d). The vestibular skin is then separated from the undersurface of the upper segment, thus freeing it and permitting its resection and removal.

I have found that the same end result may be obtained by making only one vestibular incision. In order to employ this technique, it is essential to determine how much of the alar cartilage should be removed to correct the tip deformity before any incision is made. Once this is accurately estimated, a primary incision is started at the apex of the triangular piece of cartilage to be removed. This

FIGURE 9.11. *Surgery of tip of nose.*

a. The upper and lower segments are those portions of the lateral crus of the alar cartilage. The transverse dotted line represents the incision through the cartilage frequently made for exposure of the dorsum. The dark triangular dotted area represents a segment removed to permit narrowing of the bulbous tip.

b. The intercartilaginous incision is made between the alar cartilage and the lateral cartilages. The rim incision is made on the anterior margin of the alar cartilage.

c. By pulling down on the alar cartilage with blunt-tipped scissors, the alar cartilage may be freed from the upper surface.

d. The trans-cartilaginous incision is made at the level predetermined, depending on the amount of lateral wing of alar cartilage to be removed.

e. The dotted line represents the incision that the author prefers to make to expose the dorsum when a bulbous ala is to be corrected. Through this incision, not only may the hump be removed, but the excess cartilage may also be excised, and only one incision, instead of three, is made in the vestibule.

f. When the tip is to be narrowed further, the remaining cartilage is everted adjacent to the overlying skin, and two or three cuts are made as shown.

incision is made through the vestibular skin and cartilage and angulated laterally at the dividing line between the upper and lower segments which have been described (Fig. 9.11e). Coming back to the apex, the incision is carried diagonally toward the midline and up to the upper and medial border of the alar cartilage at the midline. Through this incision and by scissors dissection, the upper segment of the lateral wing is separated from the overlying skin. When its upper border is reached, the lower border of the lateral cartilage is encountered. Adhering to the lateral cartilage, the dorsum is exposed as previously described in a routine rhinoplasty. Once the dorsum is exposed, the transfixion incision is completed, and the hump operation and shortening of the septum are carried out.

At this point, to complete the tip operation, the vestibular skin is separated from the upper lateral segment and the segment is removed. If there is still too much convexity to the tip, or not enough of a wedge has been removed, further alar cartilage may be excised until the desired contour is obtained. This excision may be made by everting the lower segment to view where it may be readily trimmed with scissors.

If the lateral arm of the ala creates too much of a bulge the cartilage may be separated from the overlying skin, everted, and two or three cuts made perpendicular to the vestibular margin, breaking the spring and permitting the convexity to become a concavity if need be (Fig. 9.11f). This results in only one incision in the vestibule instead of two or three so that, in closing the wound and splinting the nose, there is only one incision to be closed with interrupted sutures. If all the vestibular skin is retained and the incisions are sutured, webs or an atresia of the nares will not result.

I usually employ two or three interrupted through-and-through sutures to secure the columella to the septum. Plain gut sutures (#3-0 threaded through a small straight cutting or non-cutting needle) are satisfactory. While pushing the needle through the septum or columella the surgeon must not grasp the tissues with forceps, as this causes unnecessary trauma. The needle is positioned on one side; partially opened forceps are placed on the other side, thus creating a firm surface, immobilizing the tissues, and permitting the needle to go through. To close the vestibular incisions, #5-0 plain gut, with a small swedged curved cutting needle, is used.

Splinting the Nose

Splinting is employed basically to avoid subcutaneous accumulation of blood and tissue fluid. It will also prevent accidental displacement of the movable parts of the nose when the patient is asleep. Pressure is not necessary, but diffuse splinting over the entire operative field does reduce postoperative swelling and provides protection.

If a submucous resection of the nasal septum has been performed, surgical gloved fingers or large finger cots, with tips removed, are ideal for packing. A catheter is put through the cot, so that when inserted into the nose the patient has an airway, and the marked discomfort created by swallowing with the nose tightly closed is avoided. By using a Killian speculum, the rubber finger cot may be gently filled with strips of gauze. The finger cot packing may extend back to, but not into, the choanae.

The outside of the nose is taped with ½-inch adhesive tape. The strip is started just beneath the tip to hold the columella up and the alar cartilages together (Fig. 9.12h). Two or three pieces of tape are placed over the bridge of the nose, but need not extend onto the cheeks. This adhesive splinting is extremely important and must be performed with extreme care as it molds the tip. Wrinkling of the skin must be avoided. Petrolatum gauze is placed over the taped nose and forehead, wherever the dental composition mold is expected to come into contact with the skin. This will protect the skin from the heat of the melted composition and facilitate easy removal. A soft metal form (White's dental form) is cut to act as a carrier for the composition. There are other materials which may be used for splinting, but dental composition seems to be the one most universally employed because of its ease in acquisition and use. It melts in hot water and solidifies at around body temperature. After melting the composition in hot water, it may be molded and applied over the metal form. When moderately cooled, it still may be molded and shaped over the nose with the metal facing externally. It is then chilled with ice water. The splint is held in place with adhesive strips which go completely around the head. The strips should adhere to the forehead and cheeks, but the portion that is to be placed over hair must be backed with adhesive tape so that it will not adhere to the hair (Fig. 9.12i).

The nasal packing may be removed the day following the operation. The external splint may be removed 1 or 2 days postoperatively, depending upon the amount of postoperative reaction, but the adhesive splinting should be allowed to remain for 3 or 4 days.

It is very difficult to overcome the tendency of round and bulbous tips to remain round because of the pad of subcutaneous fat beneath the skin. This pad may be excised using a plane of cleavage adjacent to the under-surface of the skin, instead of adjacent to the cartilage. An overly rounded tip may also result if the mucous membrane of the septum and lateral cartilages were not cut flush when the dorsum was lowered.

Correction of the Wide Base and Long Ala

When the main rhinoplastic procedure is completed, the nostrils may be found to have too broad a base. The operator must decide how much tissue should be removed to accomplish the desired adjustment of the alae. The amount of narrowing or shortening necessary may be estimated or it may be measured with calipers. If only slight narrowing is required, a wedge resection of skin from the floor of the vestibule may suffice (Fig. 9.12a). Should more extensive alteration be required, the ala is cut free from the lip and a wedge removed, along with some of the alar buttress (Fig. 9.12b and c). The incision is closed with buried sutures of #5-0 plain catgut and #5-0 or #6-0 silk or nylon dermal sutures.

A prominent columella is the result of too much septal cartilage and premaxillary spine. Once the nose as a whole has been corrected, this prominence may be removed by excising the free border of the septum and the premaxillary spine.

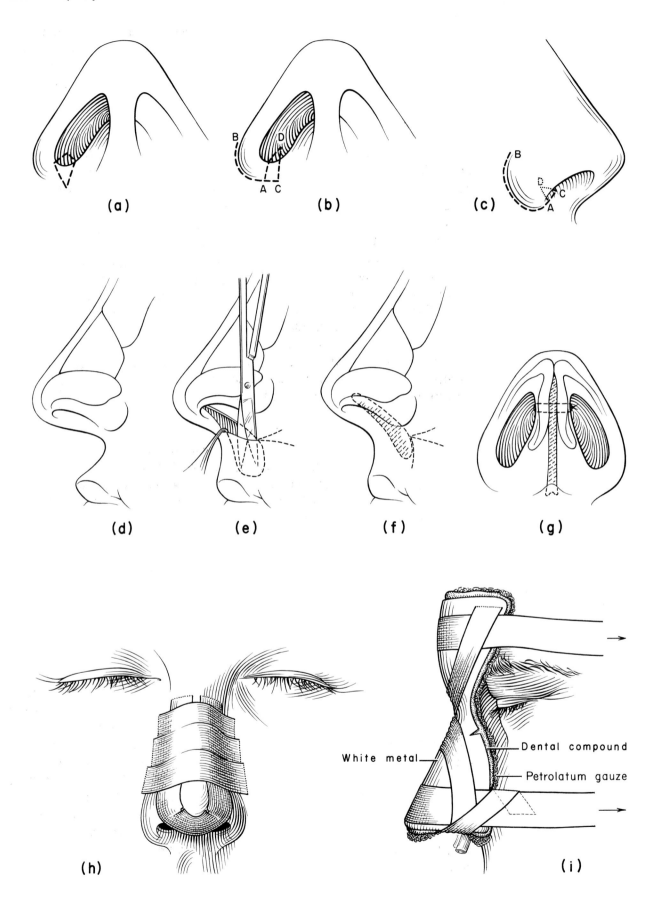

(a)

(b)

(c)

(d)

(e)

(f)

(g)

(h)

White metal

Dental compound

Petrolatum gauze

(i)

FIGURE 9.12. *Correction of wide base and long ala and splinting of nose.*

a. To narrow a broad base, a section of the ala and floor of the nose is removed without creating a secondary deformity.

b and c. If there is a very broad, flaring nostril, much more must be excised and the entire alar buttress freed and rotated into position.

d. An acute angulation of the columellar-lip angle, due to retraction of the base of the columella secondary to lost cartilage.

e. A pocket is constructed in front of the remaining cartilage and in front of the premaxillary spine.

f. The cartilage graft is sutured in front of the maxillary spine.

g. A piece of septal cartilage, if available, is shaped and sutured between the medial crus of the alar cartilage.

h. If septal surgery has been performed, finger cots or fingers of a glove, with catheters inserted through them, are filled loosely with gauze before introduction into the nostril. The outside is then carefully splinted with adhesive tape. This is extremely important in shaping the tip. Wrinkling of the skin should be avoided.

i. Petrolatum gauze is shaped and placed over the nose and the forehead. Dental compound is next molded on top of this. Adhesive strips are placed over the forehead and around the occiput or neck. The adhesive areas which would come in contact with the hair are covered with gauze or adhesive strips.

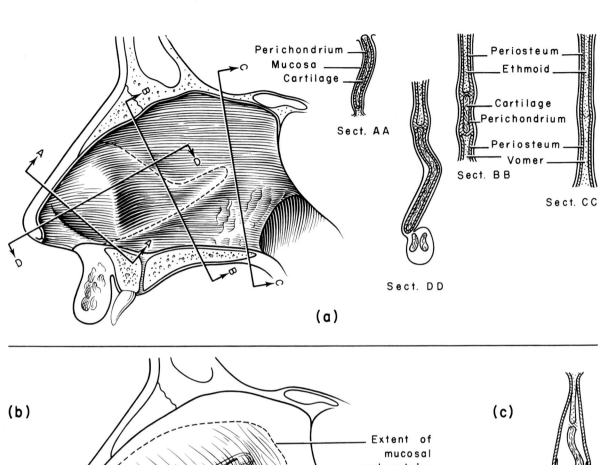

Perichondrium
Mucosa
Cartilage

Sect. AA

Periosteum
Ethmoid

Cartilage
Perichondrium

Periosteum
Vomer

Sect. BB

Sect. CC

Sect. DD

(a)

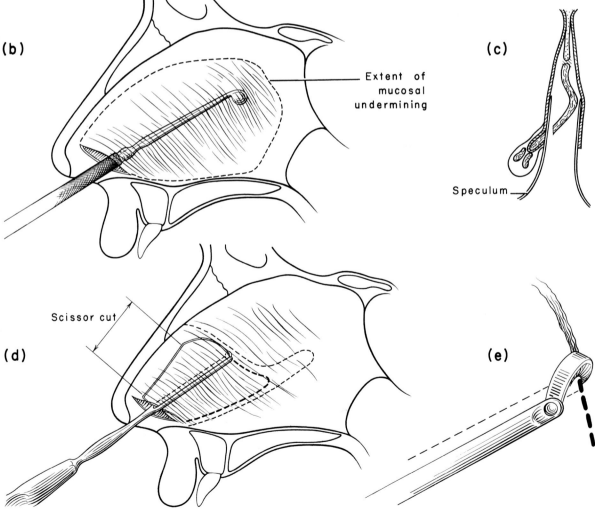

(b)

Extent of mucosal undermining

(c)

Speculum

Scissor cut

(d)

(e)

SUBMUCOUS RESECTION OF THE SEPTUM

Etiology of Septal Deviations

The nose has two fixed points, the tip of the nasal bones and the tip of the premaxillary spine (Fig. 9.4c). The quadrilateral cartilage of the septum is in contact with these two points and fixed from them inward. The part anterior to line BB, in Figure 9.4c, represents the portion outside of the skull. When the tip of the nose is hit violently, it will invariably deflect to one side or the other and, in most cases, the cartilage has sufficient spring and will not break. If it should break, it does so along a line corresponding to BB. This is one of the most common nasal deflections. It is usually associated with a deviation of the entire nasal dorsum below the tip of the nasal bone.

If the blow is from above, so that the distance between the cartilaginous dorsum and the vomer ridge is decreased, the cartilage has a tendency to become dislocated from the vomer groove and displaced to one side or the other. This may or may not involve a fracture of the cartilage. Whether it does or not, the cartilaginous dorsum is depressed because of lack of support. If the patient is seen immediately after the injury, it is possible to lift the cartilaginous septum into position, where it may be splinted until it heals. This same principle holds true with a fracture of the nasal bones along with a fracture of the septum. With a very comminuted fracture, the components will invariably be found broken, twisted, or duplicated, as well as displaced from the vomer groove. If careful attention is paid to the reduction of the septum and its immobilization, the nasal bones will maintain their reduced position without complicated splinting.

FIGURE 9.13. *Submucous resection of nasal septum.*

a. Sections through septum to demonstrate planes of separation during a submucous resection. In section AA, one will note that the cartilage is completely surrounded by perichondrium.

In section DD the periosteum over the perpendicular plate of the ethmoid tends to fuse with the perichondrium of the cartilage, so that separation is easily accomplished in this area. In section BB, where the cartilage rests into the groove of the vomer the perichondrium completely surrounds the cartilage and the periosteum goes around and over the vomer. This creates a barrier so that it is difficult to separate the mucous membrane from the cartilage extending over the vomer ridge to the vomer.

In section CC the periosteum is continuous over the perpendicular plate of the ethmoid and the vomer, making separation very easy.

b. With a Pierce elevator or similar instrument, separation is extended from an anterior direction moving posteriorly to beneath the dorsum, over the perpendicular plate and the vomer, and then forward.

c. This is a view looking down onto a cross section similar to that shown in DD (in a). It shows the incision through the membrane on the patient's left continued at a diagonal cut through the cartilage, and separation of the membrane on both sides of the deviation.

d. Control of the initial cut through the cartilage beneath the nasal dorsum is facilitated by using scissors as indicated and then employing a Ballenger swivel knife to complete the excision of cartilage to be removed.

e. A magnified drawing of the swivel knife in use.

A blow to the nasal tip may dislocate the quadrilateral cartilage from the vomer ridge and fracture it from the tip of the nasal bones perpendicular to the dorsum (Fig. 9.14c). Line AA (in Figure 9.14c) represents the perpendicular section which is shown to the right. In this view, it will be observed that the dorsum would be depressed the distance between the vomer groove and the lower margin of the displaced cartilage. Between the cartilage and the membrane is a pad of fibrous tissue which in some cases will be as thick as 3 to 4 mm (Fig. 9.14d and e, Black Section, AA).

Surgical Technique

Incision. In operating on most deviated septums, I find an incision on the convex side at the mucocutaneous junction, or just behind it, to be the most convenient approach (Fig. 9.13b). If the deviated septum is associated with a nasal deformity which will require a rhinoplasty as well, the septum is approached through the transfixion incision.

In making the incision in the membrane, care should be taken to cut to, but not through, the cartilage. The perichondrium is dissected from the cartilage with a semi-sharp flat elevator. In this step, care should be exercised to ensure that the elevator is under the perichondrium as it is easy to start the separation between the mucous membrane and perichondrium. Such a separation soon becomes difficult and results in bleeding, tearing of membrane, and frustration. Once the plane of separation is obtained, a blunt instrument should be used. A Pierce elevator is an excellent one as it is well shaped, light, and the operator may readily feel what the instrument is doing. The elevation is usually easily accomplished in a non-fractured septum except along the vomer ridge (see Fig. 9.13a). In cross section BB (of Figure 9.13a) the perichondrium is continuous around the bottom of the cartilage in the vomer groove and in this area the periosteum lines the bony grooves so that there is no plane of separation along this line. In the area of the tubercle, however, the perichondrium and periosteum seem to blend into one another. This, plus the fact that the membrane is thicker in this area than in others, makes elevation easy. Continuing the elevation back over the perpendicular plate of the ethmoid bone the operator can readily progress down over the vomer. By using the Pierce elevator as shown in Figure 9.13b, elevation along the vomer ridge can usually be accomplished without tearing the membrane.

In noses having old fractures with a marked ridge plus scarring and thinning of the membrane, this separation may be impossible without tearing. If tearing does occur, the operator should not be concerned as long as the membrane on the other side is left intact.

An incision is next carried through the cartilage parallel to the first membrane incision with the blade held at an angle of about 40 degrees to the surface of the cartilage. Care must be taken to avoid cutting through the membrane on the concave side, as to do so invites a postoperative perforation. A semi-sharp instrument which will cut cartilage without cutting bone is useful. With this type of incision it is usually easy to separate the membrane on the concave side without tearing it.

It is essential to leave the membrane in contact with one side of the cartilage which is to be left in place. This maintains nutrition to the cartilage and holds the cartilage in position when it is cut to correct a bend or angulation. The membrane should be left attached to the concave side. With all the deflected and obstructive cartilage and bone exposed these tissues may then be removed. It is not necessary to remove all of the vomer bone if it is not causing obstruction. In my experience, in the majority of the cases justifying a submucous resection of the septum a complete removal of the component parts is required before adequate alignment can be made.

While the obstructing cartilage and bone are being removed, care must be taken to leave an adequate amount of cartilage to create a supporting strut between the premaxillary spine and tip of the nasal bones. This strut will continue beneath the dorsum to the perpendicular plate of the ethmoid bone so that the dorsum will not become depressed by the natural contraction in the area of the removed cartilage and bone. Usually 4 to 5 mm of cartilage are adequate, although more may be left if there is no obstruction. If the surgeon is not careful, he is apt to separate the quadrilateral cartilage from the perpendicular plate of the ethmoid at the tubercle (just beneath the nasal bones), thereby causing a depression of the cartilaginous dorsum. If depression occurs, it is quite difficult to hold the dorsum in its proper position until healing takes place. The easiest way to support the dorsum is to employ a stainless steel wire threaded to a straight cutting needle. The wire is inserted from the outside through the thin lateral cartilages and through the septal cartilage, that is held up in position, and out through the other side. The ends of the wire are then cut, leaving sufficient length so that they will not be lost in the tissues. When there is adequate healing the wires may be removed. This requires 4 or 5 days.

To avoid these pitfalls, a straight scissors is the safest instrument to use in making the first cut under direct vision, keeping the plane of the cut parallel to the plane of the nasal dorsum (Fig. 9.13d). The Ballenger swivel knife is next used to follow this first cut. With a firm, controlled, inward-downward pressure, the cut is extended to the perpendicular plate of the ethmoid bone and then downward to the vomer bone. When the vomer bone is encountered a straight pull downward and forward completes the cut. The freed piece of cartilage may then be grasped with a forceps and removed. If the external deformities are extreme and there is loss of dorsal support, the cartilage may be saved for future grafting.

To avoid dislocating the supporting cartilage from the perpendicular plate of the ethmoid bone, it is always advisable to use a through-and-through cutting forceps such as Jensen's (Fig. 9.14a and b). Once the obstructing cartilage and bone have been removed back to the thin portion of the perpendicular plate, a grasping rocking instrument may be used. Such an instrument must be employed where the bone is too thick to permit the use of the cutting forceps.

Some operators prefer using an osteotome to separate the deviated vomer ridge from the palate, but I have found that more bleeding tends to follow this procedure than when cutting forceps are employed, particularly if the anterior palatine artery is cut across. When the bone is broken and the artery is torn, bleeding is less.

If the anterior and dorsal cartilaginous septum (Fig. 9.14d) that is left as support to the dorsum and nasal tip is angulated and creates obstruction or an external deviation, it must be mobilized and placed into proper alignment. First the pad of fibrous tissue which fills in the vomer groove must be cut out (Fig. 9.14c, [Section AA] and e). The membrane is cut away from this tissue with a knife under direct vision. The pad is then easily separated from the cartilage and removed. This will allow 3 to 4 mm more room on the preoperative concave side

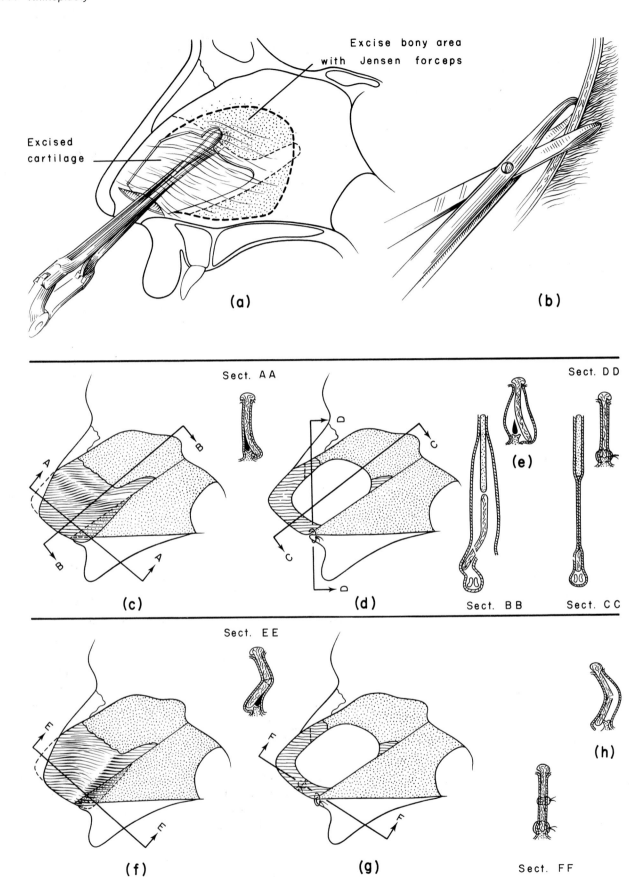

Excise bony area with Jensen forceps

Excised cartilage

(a)

(b)

Sect. AA

(c)

Sect. DD

(d)

(e)

Sect. BB

Sect. CC

Sect. EE

(f)

(g)

(h)

Sect. FF

and eliminate the possibility of obstruction when the cartilage is repositioned in the midline. Sometimes the displaced cartilage can be freed from the vomer groove by blunt dissection. If this is impossible, a sharp dissection is the best alternative.

Once the dislocated cartilage is completely freed and a new bed on which it may be placed is prepared, it is elevated and sutured in place with a mattress suture that goes through the entire septum and back beneath the premaxillary spine (Fig. 9.14d and DD).

Before sewing the cartilage in place, it is necessary to break up any angulation beneath the tip of the nasal bones. This may readily be done by making a cut through the cartilage beneath the tip of the nasal bones where the membrane is still in contact with one side of this cartilage. Care must be taken not to cut the membrane as it will act as a splint to hold the mobilized distal cartilage in place. The cut through the cartilage should be perpendicular to its surface and yet form a 45-degree angle to the dorsum. This permits the cartilage to hinge at the tip of the nasal bones. The shelving projection which is left supports the distal cartilage and prevents it from slipping into the nose, which would result in a depression of the dorsum below the nasal bones (Fig. 9.14d, dotted line). Figures 9.14f and g represent an angulation of the cartilage in a plane parallel to the vomer ridge. Here, again, the same principles are employed in correcting the deviated and displaced cartilage. The obstructed, deviated cartilage and bone are removed. The cartilage which must be saved is straightened by removing a trough of cartilage parallel to the bend on its convex side, so that when straightened, there will be a square butt without further tendency to angulate (Fig. 9.14f [Section EE] and h). The membrane is not disturbed on the concave side of the remaining cartilage. The cartilage is freed and replaced, the angulation is corrected at the tip of the nasal bones, and the remaining mobilized cartilage is sutured in place (Fig. 9.14g and FF).

FIGURE 9.14. *Submucous resection of nasal septum.*

a. Through-and-through cutting forceps should be used to cut through the upper shaded area to avoid fracture of the perpendicular plate and separation of the cartilage from the bone.

b. Jensen cutting forceps in use.

c. A fracture of the septal cartilage from the tip of the nasal bones down to the vomer. This results in dislocation and depression of the anterior part of the quadrilateral cartilage downward from the vomer groove shown in section AA. BB represents the horizontal section after the membranes have been elevated at operation.

d and e. In d are demonstrated the amount of obstructing cartilage removed and replacement of the remaining cartilage. The dotted line beneath the tip of the nasal bone indicates the direction and area of a cut made through the cartilage to permit the tip to be brought to the midline and elevated into position. Note the suture holding the displaced anterior cartilaginous strut to the premaxilla, shown also in sections DD and AA and in e. The solid black area represents a pad of fibrous tissue and e shows the flaps elevated from the pad, ready to be removed. Section CC shows the replaced anterior strut and the flaps in apposition.

f. A fracture secondary to a blow to the cartilaginous dorsum with a fracture parallel to the dorsum and a secondary displacement of the cartilage from the vomer ridge into the nasal vestibules.

Section EE shows this angulation and displacement. The dotted line at the angulation of the fracture represents cartilage which is to be removed and also the pad of fibrous tissue.

g. The finished realignment.

h. Pad of fibrous tissue and the wedged-out cartilage removed, ready for replacement.

Section FF shows replacement and through-and-through suturing.

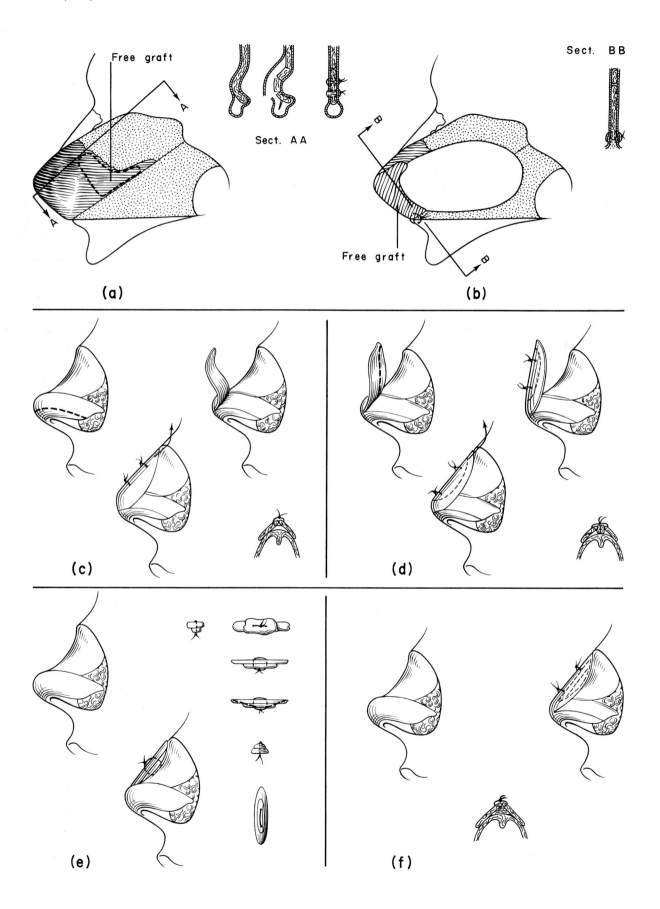

Free graft

Sect. AA

Sect. BB

Free graft

(a)

(b)

(c)

(d)

(e)

(f)

So far, cartilage which has been primarily angulated or displaced has been considered. Not infrequently, cartilage which is markedly curved, not only in one plane but in two planes, is encountered, so that it is difficult to free and realign the strip which is normally saved for support in the midplane (Fig. 9.15a). If an attempt is made to realign the cartilage in situ this is done as diagrammed in AA (Fig. 9.15a). When cartilage is found behind the deviation, which is fairly flat, most of the septum can be removed, including that which should be saved for support. The flatter cartilage is then shaped, reinserted, and sutured to support the dorsum and the columella (Fig. 9.15b). This should be done as a last resort, for a free graft will occasionally be absorbed even though it consists of autogenous septal cartilage. In certain cases, it is possible to utilize some of the vomer or even the perpendicular plate of the ethmoid for support. However, bony implants are rigid and very easily fractured.

CORRECTION OF DEPRESSION OF NASAL DORSUM

Depression of the nasal dorsum is frequently encountered when there has been an injury to the nasal septum, either traumatic, infectious, or postoperative. When there is septal destruction due to infection and loss of support because of the removal of too much cartilage, the surgeon's only alternative is to add something to the existing dorsum to create the desired contour. I have always found it expedient to use living autogenous material when available. Discussion of the use of inert implants may be found in the literature.

The depression of the cartilaginous dorsum is due to loss of septal support secondary to destruction of the cartilage itself. Careful analysis of the anatomy will frequently indicate that if the depression of the dorsum and the tip of the nose are brought into alignment with existing nasal bones, the resulting profile is the one to be obtained. Not infrequently, it will be observed that individual alar cartilages are more developed than desirable and there is slight flaring or bulbousness of the tip. This makes an ideal situation because adequate cartilage is present to form a restoration.

FIGURE 9.15. *Submucous resection; alar swing.*

a and b. A severely angulated septum is illustrated in a. The middle view in section AA shows a method of correcting this curved trough and anterior supporting cartilage with a replacement of the free border of cartilage in the columella. If it is physically impossible to realign the cartilage and a flat piece of cartilage can be obtained to use as a free graft (as in a), all the cartilage can be removed and employed as a free graft as shown in b and section BB.

c. Alar swing. The heavy dotted line represents the vestibular incision through the vestibular skin and alar cartilage. After exposing the dorsal surface of the alar cartilage, lateral cartilages, and nasal bones, the upper three fourths of the lateral alar cartilage is freed from the underlying skin. Both alar cartilages are then swung into the middle and sutured as illustrated. A stay suture (indicated by the arrow) may be placed through the alar cartilages and brought up through the skin near the glabella to hold the pedicled grafts in the midline.

d. If more bulk is needed, the same procedure is performed, but, in addition, each alar cartilage is scored on its top surface, as indicated by the heavy dotted lines. The cartilages are then folded along this line before being brought to the middle and sutured together.

e. When the tip is in position and there is a depression of the cartilaginous dorsum, septal cartilage may be obtained and the pieces sutured together and sculptured to fit the defect.

f. The combination of alar swing and cartilage graft beneath it.

Alar Swing

The incision employed to expose the cartilage of the dorsum is made from the tip of the vestibular apex parallel to and about 2 to 3 mm from the anterior border of the alar cartilage all the way to its lateral portion. This incision extends through the cartilage. At the apex the incision is carried backward, so that the medial crus is not involved, to the anterior border of the septum where a transfixion incision is made (Fig. 9.15c). The outer or top surface of the alar cartilage is then freed subperichondrally by blunt dissection. The separation is continued adjacent to the lateral cartilage to the nasal bone as for exposure for a rhinoplasty. The nasal bones are then exposed subperiosteally, if there is work to be done on them, although in this case it is usually not necessary. The skin must be separated over the nasal bones to the glabella.

With fine, blunt-edged scissors the alar cartilage is now separated from the vestibular skin, but it is left attached to the vestibular skin at the apex. This attachment maintains a fixed relationship in this area plus a small viable attachment (See Fig. 9.15c, upper right drawing.) With the tip and the columella freed, the alar cartilages which have also been freed may be brought out through one nostril. Their upper edges are sewed together with interrupted sutures. A #5-0 plain catgut eye suture on a small curved needle is quite satisfactory for this purpose.

To be certain that the cartilages remain in the proper position during splinting, a suture of nylon, threaded to a straight needle, is placed through the lateral-most portions of the alae. This suture will take the uppermost position when the alae are placed over the dorsum adjacent to the nasal bone. The suture material may then be brought beneath the skin and to the surface while the skin is elevated with a rhinoplastic skin retractor. After one end of the suture material is brought through the skin, the needle is rethreaded on the other end and brought through the skin; a snap is clamped onto the suture material to provide traction. This traction stitch is indicated by the arrow in Figure 9.15c.

Once brought into position, the tip is elevated, the dorsum shortened, and the bulging portion of the ala alleviated. The transfixion incision is then closed with interrupted sutures as are the vestibular incisions. Intravestibular packing for closure of vestibular incisions cannot be relied upon because improper healing will result in web formations.

When the depression is too great to be filled by a single layer of alar cartilage, the alar cartilage may be folded upon itself to create more bulk (Fig. 9.15d). To execute this procedure the alar cartilages are freed, delivered through the vestibule, and placed upon the skin of the nasal tip. The dorsal surface of the ala is then cut through to a very thin layer of perichondrium which is almost always present. This permits the cartilage to be folded along the cut line. The cut and folded surfaces of each ala are then sutured together and held in position as already described. The cross section of an end view in Figure 9.15d illustrates the relative position and added bulk of the cartilage used.

If septal cartilage is present, and the depression is the result of buckling of the septum, a submucous resection may be performed and large sections of the cartilage obtained, cut, sutured together, and sculptured to fill the defect (Fig. 9.15e).

In certain cases I have found it expedient to employ a combination of these last two methods, using the alar swing and septal cartilage to provide the support. This is shown in Figure 9.15f.

Grafting Techniques

It is sometimes impossible to obtain sufficient local cartilage in a nose which has lost both its cartilaginous and bony support and in which a saddle-back deformity is present. In such an instance, in order to provide support, transplant material must be obtained from a source that will offer an adequate supply. Many materials have been employed to supplement an inadequate supply of bone and cartilage in the restoration of a nasal framework; a word is in order concerning these substances. The materials fall into two main groups, organic and inorganic. Gold, silver, tantalum, Vitallium, and the plastics are several of the inorganic, while ivory, cartilage, bone, fibrin, and fascia are the organic materials used. With most of these materials the chance of a foreign-body reaction is very high. In recent years, the use of tantalum (Fox), a completely inert basic metal, and the alloys (Pressman), Vitallium and stainless steel, have been introduced. These substances, when employed in their solid form and buried beneath the skin, may be well tolerated. They can be anchored to the tissues when multiple perforations exist permitting fibrous tissue to grow through. Or, these materials can be screwed into place if in contact with bone. In a dorsal implant in the nose, there is a constant, light pressure of the metal beneath the skin. This creates a very slow avascularization and pressure necrosis, necessitating the removal of the material. My first successful attempt at implanting tantalum occurred when the implant was inserted so that the alar cartilages were between it and the skin directly over it, so there was a wide distribution of pressure. Tantalum wool and other metals are mentioned only to be condemned, for, in my experience, they are poor materials for reconstruction of the dorsum of the nose.

Ivory, the product of living tissue, has been used as an implant for many years (Salinger). I have seen a patient in whom it had been retained for 25 years, until a slight blow to the tip of the nose caused a foreign-body reaction requiring its removal. Today, however, ivory is rarely employed as a rhinoplastic implant. Several plastic substances (such as the acrylic resins [Rapin], polyethylene [Heanley], Teflon, and the silicones) were found experimentally to be well tolerated by body tissues. If improperly shaped or inserted they will initiate a foreign-body reaction, and removal will be necessary.

Polyethylene sponge (Johnson and Grindlay), and silicone rubber are similar to cartilage in that they are flexible and can be readily tooled at the operating table with a sharp knife. The fact that they will not curl or change shape makes them more ideal than cartilage as inserts. There have been few reported failures, and these materials appear to be fairly good substitutes for autogenous cartilage and bone.

Let us consider some of the organic materials which may be used for nasal implants. Autogenous cartilage (Peer), transplanted into a vascular field, will usually be incorporated as living cartilage. If, on the other hand, this same cartilage should be buried in a scarred or avascularized area, it may atrophy as it is infiltrated and replaced by fibroblasts which, in turn, may greatly diminish in size so that for practical purposes the mass may disappear completely. It is my experience that this is more prone to happen in the young child than in the adult.

Large blocks of rib cartilage, which can provide all the cartilage needed for nasal operations, have the great disadvantage of curling soon after being cut. This problem is not only annoying to the surgeon, but disastrous to his reconstructive work. Septal and auricular cartilage very rarely curls. Three or more pieces may

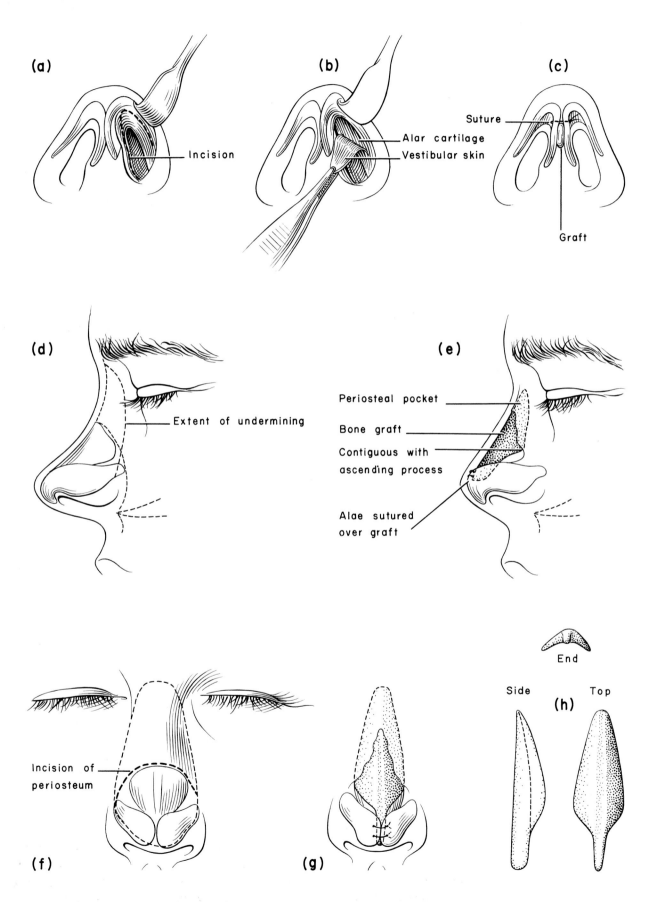

(a) Incision

(b) Alar cartilage
     Vestibular skin

(c) Suture
     Graft

(d) Extent of undermining

(e) Periosteal pocket
     Bone graft
     Contiguous with
     ascending process
     Alae sutured
     over graft

(f) Incision of
     periosteum

(g)

(h) End
     Side   Top

be sutured together to create sufficient bulk, and then shaped. This gives the surgeon an ideal material for the replacement of the lost dorsal support.

Attempts have been made to obtain ideal materials which could be had in large amounts and banked. Homologous (Spangler) and bovine (Cottle, Quilty, and Buckingham) cartilage come under this group of substitutes. Many of these implants are replaced by fibrous tissue invasion; so many, in fact, that I discarded bank cartilage several years ago.

Many implants of heterogenous cartilage are apparently well tolerated up to one year postoperatively, but long-term results have been discouraging because these grafts disappear.

It is recognized that autogenous bone, buried in contact with bone and surrounded by good blood supply, will become incorporated as living bone (Cannon and Murray; Cottle et al.). Obtaining this result is not quite as simple as it sounds. The grafted bone first dies; osteoclasts invade its structure and destroy its framework. At the same time, osteoblasts start laying down new bone, so that by the time the process of destruction is completed the entire bone has been replaced by a living structure firmly adherent to the recipient bone by a callus. Homologous bone, which is dead when buried in the host, goes through the same process of absorption and regeneration. The grafted bone merely acts as a framework through which the new bone is laid down. Bone, therefore, is an ideal medium for repairing large defects of the nasal skeleton and may be obtained from several sources.

Some operators prefer the tibia, which is accessible and already has a surface which needs little changing to form a desirable implant. Occasionally, removal of bone for a graft weakens the tibia, so that precaution must be taken against fracture. The rib and scapula have also been employed, but the source which is considered best by most surgeons is the crest of the ilium. Here large quantities of cortical and medullary bone may be obtained without affecting function, and the resulting scar may be covered by clothing.

What type of bone graft, cortical or medullary, is best for nasal implants has long been a matter of general discussion. It is conceded today that myelogenous

FIGURE 9.16. *Bone graft to dorsum.*

a. The incision through the skin extends only to a point near the anterior border of the alar cartilage. At the apex it goes back to the posterior border of the medial crus of the alar cartilage, then through and through for the transfixion incision.

b. The vestibular skin is freed from the undersurface of the alar cartilage. From there, dissection continues over the lateral cartilage as in rhinoplasty.

c. The medial crura are sutured over the tip of the bone graft.

d. The extent of the exposure of the nasal bones and ascending process.

e. A bone graft is in position beneath the periosteum and in contact with the ascending process and nasal bones.

f. The extent of the incision through the periosteum to permit adequate elevation over the nasal bones.

g. Looking down on the nose, with the graft in position, the alar cartilages are seen sutured over bone (see also c and e).

h. Three views of the graft illustrating the contouring required.

bone may be received and integrated quicker than cortical, but cortical bone will make a better shaped graft which will be maintained. Whether or not a strut is employed to maintain an elevation of the tip of the nose, roentgenography has shown that the bone assumes a new architectural structure. One may see a cortex which corresponds to the contour of the nose and will withstand the stresses which are placed on it. The opponents of the use of autogenous bone as a nasal implant maintain that plastics or bank cartilage or bone do just as well and that they avert the need for another operation. These claims are partially just; yet, when a solid graft is indicated, autogenous bone gives the best results. The additional operative procedure which the opponents dislike is really minor, as it takes little time to expose the ilium and obtain the graft. While an assistant is closing the wound, the surgeon may be sculpturing the insert; thus, little added time is needed.

In summary, what the surgeon should strive for is an implant which is completely tolerated by its recipient host. Autogenous bone fulfills this end better than any other material and is preferred as an implant when a large skeletal defect of the nose is to be corrected.

There are several incisions through which the dorsum of the nose may be approached to prepare it for the reception of a graft. An incision through the skin of the nasal tip or the columella creates a direct view of the dorsum, yet it may be difficult to obtain an opening of sufficient size to permit the passage of a large graft. In addition to this, this incision leaves a visible scar. In order to overcome these objections, I have found the following approach to be satisfactory.

An anterior incision is made through the vestibular skin parallel to, and $\frac{1}{8}$ inch from, the margin of the lateral wing of the alar cartilages. When the medial crura are reached, the incision is directed back to their posterior border and carried through and through as a transfixion incision (Fig. 9.16a). The vestibular skin is dissected free from the lateral crura of the alar cartilage up to the lateral cartilages, which are then exposed up to the nasal bones (Fig. 9.16b). An incision is made parallel to the piriform aperture and through the periosteum, which is elevated from the nasal bones up to the glabella (Fig. 9.16d and f). Usually the median raphe must be cut to permit elevation of the periosteum in the midline, but it is always possible to create a pocket to receive the upper end of the graft in the region of the glabella (Fig. 9.16e and g). The nasal periosteum is elevated laterally down over the ascending processes, to permit the skin to form a normal-appearing lateral side for the nose. The medial crura of the alar cartilages are freed from one another by blunt dissection. This step is important, for the medial crura are sutured over the graft at its tip and are to be dealt with later (Fig. 9.16e and g). If the columella is to be brought forward, the dissection of the medial crura of the alar cartilages is continued down through the soft tissues to the region of the premaxillary spine. A graft may be placed in this pocket. It may also be advisable to make a pocket in the free border of the septum. The nose is now ready for the reception of the graft.

The crest of the ilium is exposed. With a thin, broad osteotome, the cortex is sculptured in situ to form the exact contour desired for the dorsal support. It is very easy to tool the bone while it is in this position as it is completely immobile. Once the dorsum and the bone which will correspond to the lateral sides of the nose and the lost ascending processes are sculptured, the graft is removed as a block, with a good margin of bone in all directions. If there is a possibility that bone will be needed to fill out the columella, it may be taken at this time. Bleeding is controlled and the wound closed.

Once removed from the ilium, the bone is sculptured so that the finished product will completely fill the defect into which it is to be inserted. Sculpturing is performed with rongeurs, rasps, and high-speed burs. If any groove or space is left between the graft and ascending processes, an external depression in that area will result when the skin is pulled in as healing progresses. If the operator is unable to tool the graft exactly to size, bone chips or cancellous bone can be used to fill in these small areas. Best results are obtained when the graft fills the entire defect (Fig. 9.16e, g and h). The solid upper half of the graft is carved so that it will rest securely upon the nasal bones. Care is taken so that its upper end will insert into the pocket at the glabella. This should hold it firmly in contact with the bone. The lateral wings will then rest either upon the nasal bones or the ascending processes and, in turn, by cantilever action, will support the tip. This procedure eliminates the use of a columellar strut. The graft is tapered gradually from its contact with the lower border of the nasal bones until it comes to the region of the alar cartilages. Here it is thinned from the lateral aspect and permitted to come between the medial crura, which are sutured on top of it for support (Fig. 9.16e and g). This elevates the tip above the graft, giving the profile a more normal appearance.

The original incisions are closed, and the nose is packed intranasally. A routine type of external pressure bandage is applied. This autogenous bone graft has the advantage of being in contact with a large surface of living bone. It is immobile, takes well, becomes an integral part of the nasal framework, and supports the tip of the nose in a normal anatomic relationship without resorting to a strut of bone between the anterior premaxillary spine and the undersurface of the tip of the graft. If the columella needs to be more prominent, a piece of bone may be inserted for this purpose, but not to act as a support for the tip.

REFERENCES

Cannon, B., and Murray, J. D.: Plastic Surgery: Tissue and Organ Homotransplantation. New Eng. J. Med. 255:900–904 (Nov.) 1965.

Cottle, M. H., Loring, R. M., Cohen, H., and Kirschman, R.: Cancellous Bone Grafts in Nasal Repair. Ann. Otol. 58:135–146 (March) 1949.

Cottle, H., Quilty, J., and Buckingham, A.: Nasal Implants in Children and in Adults; with Preliminary Note on the Use of Ox Cartilage. Ann Otol., 62:169–175 (March) 1953.

Fox, L.: Tantalum in Rhinoplastic Surgery. Ann Otol., 58:40–54 (March) 1949.

Heanley, C. L.: Restoration of Nasal Contour, with a Note on Use of Polythene Block. J. Laryng. 68:112–113 (Feb.) 1954.

Johnson, H. A., and Grindlay, J. H.: Experimental Alteration of Nasal Contour by the Use of Polyvinyl Sponge. Plast. Reconstr. Surg. 14:293–297 (Oct.) 1954.

Joseph, J.: Nasenplastik und soustige Gesichtplastik. Leipzig, Kabitzsch, 1931, pp. 498–842.

Peer, L. A.: Fate of Autogenous Septal Cartilage after Transplantation in Human Tissues. Arch. Otolaryng. 34:696–709 (Oct.) 1941.

Pressman, J. J.: Nasal Implants. Laryngoscope 62:6:582–600 (Aug.) 1952.

Rapin, M.: Eight Years Experiment with Synthetic Acrylic Resins in Rhinoplastic Practice. Arch. Otol. 11:425–427, 1949.

Salinger, S.: Ivory Implants: Survival after Twenty-Three Years. Arch. Otolaryng. 63:419–420 (April) 1956.

Sheehan, J., and Swanker, A.: Gelatinized Bone for Repair of Skeletal Losses. Brit. J. Plast. Surg. 2:268–273 (Jan.) 1950.

Spangler, S.: A New Treatment for Pitted Scars. Arch. Derm. 76:708–711 (Dec.) 1957.

Vidaurre, S.: Saddle Noses; Their Treatment with the Semilunar Cartilage of the Knee Joint. Plast. Reconstr. Surg. 10:35–38 (July) 1952.

10

Surgery of the Nasopharynx

TUMORS OF THE NASOPHARYNX

Benign Tumors

In the nasopharynx benign tumors are less common than malignant growths. They include: (1) pseudotumors (choanal polyp [Fig. 1.17]), (2) cystic tumors (Thornwaldt's cyst, Rathke's pouch, mucous cyst [Fig. 1.17]), (3) solid tumors (juvenile angiofibroma, benign mixed tumor, fibroma, chondroma, ossifying fibroma, sarcoid neurofibroma, xanthoma, glioma, teratoma).

Signs and Symptoms. The signs and symptoms of benign tumors of the nasopharynx include nasal obstruction, epistaxis, anterior and posterior nasal discharge, voice change, otalgia, and hearing loss.

Treatment of Benign Tumors of the Nasopharynx. The choanal polyp is resected with a snare inserted by the nasal route. Following this a Caldwell-Luc operation is performed to ensure against recurrence. The technique for the Caldwell-Luc procedure is described on page 211.

Cystic tumors of the nasopharynx, such as Thornwaldt's cyst, Rathke's pouch, and a mucous cyst, are left undisturbed unless they present symptoms. The outstanding symptoms indicating surgery are: repeated infections, interference with the nasopharyngeal airway, and discharge. Therapy consists of marsupialization or removal of the anterior wall of the cyst. This is accomplished with an adenotome.

Solid tumors of the nasopharynx are resected by the transpalatal route unless they are completely asymptomatic and are not increasing in size. Those benign tumors which have a tendency to undergo malignant change should be resected, even when attended with no symptoms.

NASOPHARYNGEAL ANGIOFIBROMA

The juvenile nasopharyngeal angiofibroma, by far the most common benign tumor of the nasopharynx, warrants special emphasis. It almost invariably occurs in adolescent males. It is highly vascular, not encapsulated, and locally invasive. It is said to undergo spontaneous regression when the patient is between the ages of 20 and 25 years. The lesion has its origins from the posterosuperior nasopharyngeal vault. There are many theories as to its pathogenesis. The most logical is its derivation from embryologic cartilage between the basiocciput and the body of the sphenoid. The fact that there is ossification between the sphenoid and occiput at about 25 years of age somewhat substantiates this theory.

The histopathologic appearance of the juvenile angiofibroma varies considerably. The tumor may be smooth or lobular; in consistency it varies from firm to hard; it is usually reddish in color, with occasional areas of ulceration and exudation. Microscopically it is seen to have a fibrous capsule, and its vascular network varies in number, size, shape, and distribution of the vessels. The vessel walls consist of a simple endothelial lining and closely resemble those of the cavernous hemangioma or erectile tissue. The variation in the number of vessels is apparent during surgical resection, epistaxis and hemorrhage being severe in some patients and minor in others. The stroma of the tumor is made up of fibrous tissue consisting of fine and coarse collagenous fibrils.

The signs and symptoms of the juvenile angiofibroma are nasal obstruction; recurrent epistaxis (often alarming); progressive deformity of the palate, face, and pharynx; otalgia and hearing loss; rhinolalia; and anosmia.

Treatment of Juvenile Nasopharyngeal Angiofibroma. There are numerous treatments for juvenile angiofibroma of the nasopharynx.

Chemical Therapy. Superficial chemical cauterization with such agents as phenol, trichloroacetic acid, and chromic acid has been used for many decades. The use of sclerosing agents such as sodium morrhuate has been reported as being successful in reducing the size of these tumors. The injection sites, however, tend to slough; this ultimately increases the bleeding surface of the tumor.

Radiation Therapy. External radiation is reported to decrease the amount of angiomatous tissue. Doses up to 2500r have been employed. Maximum radiation should not be used because of its probable effect upon facial growth.

Radium Therapy. Reports of excellent resolution of the angiofibroma through radium therapy have appeared in the literature. Radon seeds of 1.5 mμ are placed in the tumor, approximately 1 cm apart. With the use of radon seeds there is very little chance for interference with the facial growth centers.

Thermal Therapy. Diathermocoagulation of the juvenile angiofibroma has been popular but currently has fallen into disuse, except for electrocoagulation of the site of origin following resection. The feasibility of cryosurgery for resection of the juvenile angiofibroma is still doubtful. The freezing of a small or recurrent angiofibroma and allowing the tumor to remain in place and slough off may prove to be effective.

Hormone Therapy. Hormone therapy for juvenile angiofibroma has been in use for many years. For the most part the response is not marked and not lasting. Long-term hormone therapy in patients of this age group is decidedly detrimental. Preoperative use of stilbestrol is of great value, however, for the prevention of hemorrhage during surgery.

Surgical Treatment. Surgical removal of angiofibromas is still the treatment of choice. A careful hematologic work-up is indicated, for many of these patients are anemic. Whole blood or packed red blood cells are administered several days before the operation. The hematocrit value should be as near normal as is possible at the time of the operation. The patient's blood is typed and cross-matched for six units of whole blood, and the laboratory should be alerted that additional blood may be necessary.

Hormone therapy, consisting of 2.5 mg of stilbestrol given three times a day for 2 weeks prior to the operation will reduce the amount of hemorrhage during the surgical procedure. Breast tenderness and nipple enlargement will be noted after approximately 10 days of this therapy. These should be of little concern, for both disappear during the immediate postoperative period after the administration of stilbestrol has been discontinued.

Carotid arteriography contributes considerably to the diagnosis and surgical management. The carotid arteriogram is taken in the usual fashion. If the tumor extends beyond the midline, bilateral carotid arteriography is of value. The subtraction technique is helpful in outlining the vessels since these tumors are fairly well surrounded by bone. The vascular nature of the nasopharyngeal tumor is typical and fairly well establishes the diagnosis. The arteriograph will also outline the extent and size of the tumor, the origin of its major arterial supply, and the site of its vascular pedicle.

Hypothermia or hypotensive techniques during the operation are of questionable value and add to the risk. Preoperative Gelfoam embolization of the tumor vessels has markedly reduced the blood loss during surgery. Surgery is performed 2 to 3 days following embolization rather than the following day so that any complications following embolization can be evaluated.

Numerous techniques for surgical resection of angiofibroma of the nasopharynx have been reported in the literature. Those which seem most practical are the transpalatal (see p. 460) and the transantral procedures (p. 232). The transpalatal approach allows for better control of hemorrhage than does the transantral approach and provides direct access to the site of origin. The transantral approach, following resection of the posterior and bony medial walls of the maxillary sinus, gives an excellent view of the posterior nasal cavity, upper nasopharynx, and pterygomaxillary space. A combination of both the transpalatal and transantral approaches is used for those tumors which extend into both the nasal cavity and the pterygomaxillary fossa.

Malignant Tumors

Malignant tumors of the nasopharynx are relatively rare (0.05% of all malignant tumors). They are more common in men than in women (3 to 1). Their incidence is increased in populations which are predominantly oriental (0.3 to 0.5% of all malignant lesions).

A histopathologic classification of malignant tumors of the nasopharynx is somewhat confusing because of the variance in nomenclature. One is as follows:

1. Transitional cell carcinoma
2. Squamous cell carcinoma
3. Undifferentiated carcinoma
4. Lymphoepithelioma
5. Lymphosarcoma
6. Reticulum cell sarcoma
7. Angiofibrosarcoma
8. Chemodectoma

Transitional cell carcinoma is the most common. Most of the others rarely occur in the nasopharynx.

Signs and Symptoms. The signs and symptoms of carcinoma of the naso-pharynx are divided into four main groups: (1) nasopharyngeal, (2) otologic, (3) ophthalmoneurologic, and (4) cervical metastatic.

The nasopharyngeal symptoms include obstruction of one or both sides of the nose, a change in speech due to hyponasality, anterior and posterior nasal discharge, and bleeding.

The otologic manifestations are due to obstruction of the eustachian tube. A conductive hearing loss is not an uncommon sign of carcinoma of the naso-pharynx. This may be associated with either serous or purulent otitis media.

The ophthalmoneurologic signs are due to the extension of the tumor from the nasopharynx into the surrounding spaces. Nearly all the cranial nerves are vulnerable when the tumor extends. The sixth cranial nerve is the one most commonly involved; diplopia due to paralysis of the lateral rectus muscle results. The third, fourth, and fifth cranial nerves are next in order for implication.

The most common site of metastatic extension of a nasopharyngeal malig-nant lesion is the neck and usually cervical metastasis provides the initial sign of the disease. The lymphatic drainage from the nasopharynx is by the way of the retropharyngeal glands to the upper deep cervical lymph nodes. Tumor of the cervical glands is most commonly palpated between the mastoid process and the angle of the mandible.

The signs and symptoms of malignant disease of the nasopharynx in order of their frequency are:

1. Enlarged cervical lymph nodes
2. Blockage of the ear(s)
3. Bloody nasal discharge
4. Nasal obstruction
5. Change in speech
6. Diplopia

Diagnosis. The diagnosis is made by careful history-taking, physical exami-nation, x-ray study of the nasopharynx, and exploration and biopsy. If there is clinical and radiographic evidence of carcinoma of the nasopharynx, one biopsy study showing no abnormality will not be conclusive evidence that a malignant lesion is not present. The tumor can occur submucosally and thus biopsy speci-mens must be obtained from a deep-down area in order to obtain a positive diagnosis.

Treatment. External radiation is the primary therapy for malignant tumors of the nasopharynx. Surgical treatment is rarely indicated except for a low-grade, encapsulated malignant growth such as a malignant mixed tumor or a cylin-droma. Complete extirpation of a malignant lesion of the nasopharynx is usually impossible. The midline transpalatal route is preferred if surgery is indicated (Fig. 10.2). When the disease is limited to the nasopharynx, a 5-year survival rate of more than 50% can be expected. This drops to approximately 10% if there is extension of disease beyond the confines of the nasopharynx. A second course of radiation therapy is indicated for recurrent tumor at the primary site in the nasopharynx. This is administered by either external radiation or radium in a nasopharyngeal mold. It is of interest that the longer the time elapse between the initial radiation therapy and the recurrence, the better the prognosis after the second course of therapy.

RESECTION OF TUMORS OF THE NASOPHARYNX

The incisions for the transpalatal approach for nasopharyngeal tumors are identical to those for the repair of choanal atresia (see Figs. 10.1–10.4). After the horizontal incision has been made through the nasopharyngeal mucous membrane at the junction of the hard and soft palate the nasopharynx can be inspected. Usually at least the posterior aspect of the lesion can be seen. As much of the bony hard palate at the site of the lesion is removed as is necessary for proper exposure of the tumor. Unless the tumor is large and extends anteriorly into the nasal cavity and laterally into the pterygomaxillary fossa, it can be readily resected at its site of origin. This area is tightly packed for a few minutes. Following removal of this packing, the bleeding can be gradually controlled by electrocoagulation. The insulated suction tip is valuable in accomplishing this coagulation. It is best to insert a posterior and anterior pack consisting of iodoform gauze impregnated with Aureomycin ointment. Even though the bleeding appears to be controlled at the termination of the procedure, this packing should remain in place for at least 3 days.

If the tumor is a large angiofibroma extending anteriorly into the nasal cavity and laterally into the pterygomaxillary fossa, none of the lesion is resected after the transpalatal exposure of its nasopharyngeal portion until a Caldwell-Luc procedure has been executed to expose the portion of the tumor that extends into the pterygomaxillary fossa and nasal cavity. Having acquired a good view of the entire lesion from two angles by the transantral and transpalatal approaches, the tumor can be readily resected, and the site of origin quickly packed, thus markedly reducing the amount of hemorrhage. The site of origin is treated as has been described. If necessary, the pterygomaxillary fossa and maxillary sinus can be packed in addition to the anterior and posterior nasal packing.

CHOANAL ATRESIA

Choanal atresia may be membranous or bony, unilateral or bilateral. Approximately 90% are of the bony type (Flake).

Unilateral choanal atresia often eludes diagnosis because of the absence of subjective symptoms in the neonatal period. In fact, it may be overlooked until adulthood when the patient complains of an inability to breathe through one side of his nose and of a thick, unilateral nasal discharge. The discharge may be purulent if the sinuses are chronically infected.

Complete bilateral atresia of the choanae presents as a neonatal emergency. If the infant having bilateral choanal atresia begins life crying, he is able to breathe through his mouth and thus asphyxiation is prevented. As soon as he stops crying and closes his mouth his airway is obstructed and he then becomes cyanotic. If the correct diagnosis is not made immediately and an oral airway is not inserted, the condition can be fatal. Choanal atresia probably accounts for a number of neonatal asphyxiations of undetermined cause. Thus, it is most important that the obstetrician and pediatrician be well aware of this deformity. If the infant survives the neonatal period with the aid of an oral airway, gastric feeding tube, McGovern nipple, or, possibly, a tracheotomy, he will have the classic signs and symptoms of bilateral choanal atresia. These are: (1) constant mouth-breathing, (2) bilateral, thick nasal discharge, (3) absence of taste and smell, (4) undernourishment, and (5) defective speech. In addition there are secondary complications such as chronic sinusitis and conductive hearing loss.

Examinations for the diagnosis of unilateral or bilateral choanal atresia include (1) attempt at passing a rubber catheter or probe through the patient's nose, (2) mirror examination of the nasopharynx, (3) digital examination of the nasopharynx, and (4) x-ray examination including a lateral and base view of the nasopharynx after installation of radiopaque material into the nasal cavity with the patient in the supine position.

Surgical Treatment of Unilateral Choanal Atresia

The surgical repair of unilateral choanal atresia is usually made when the patient is an adult. The simplest method consists in removal of the posterior portion of the nasal septum. This is accomplished by making a vertical incision in the mucous membrane of the septum, on the side of the atresia, approximately 1.5 cm anterior to the site of the atresia. The incision is best made with a right-angle knife. It is continued through the perpendicular plate of the ethmoid bone and the mucous membrane on the opposite side of the nasal septum. With ring punch forceps, the nasal septum posterior to the incision is totally removed. Following this a horizontal incision is made through the mucous membrane on the superior and inferior aspect of the atresia; the mucous membrane is then elevated and based laterally. The bony choanal atresia, with the mucous membrane on its posterior surface, is resected with Kerrison forceps. The laterally based mucous membrane flap is then reflected posteriorly and packed in place with one large finger-cot. The packing is left in place for 2 or 3 days. This intranasal procedure usually enjoys a high incidence of success, and therefore a transpalatal approach for repair of unilateral choanal atresia is rarely necessary.

Surgical Treatment of Bilateral Choanal Atresia

Some surgeons prefer to treat bilateral membranous choanal atresia by simply breaking through the obstructing membrane with an instrument such as a long, curved hemostat and inserting rubber or plastic tubing into the nasopharynx. The tubes are anchored anteriorly, just behind the columella, with a suture. Of course, this procedure is impossible for correction of a bony atresia.

Transpalatal Approach to the Nasopharynx. The transpalatal approach is the preferred method for repairing either a membranous or a bony bilateral choanal atresia, since it provides a direct route, thus permitting an exacting reconstruction. It also is used for the removal of nasopharyngeal tumors such as juvenile angiofibrous and mixed tumors.

There are a number of palatal incisions for this approach to the nasopharynx (Fig. 10.1). The midline incision (Fig. 10.2a) is the simplest, and if properly executed, is rarely complicated. The anterior palatal flap approach is also widely used.

For repair of bilateral choanal atresia the operation may be performed in the immediate neonatal period, as soon as the infant is able to withstand general

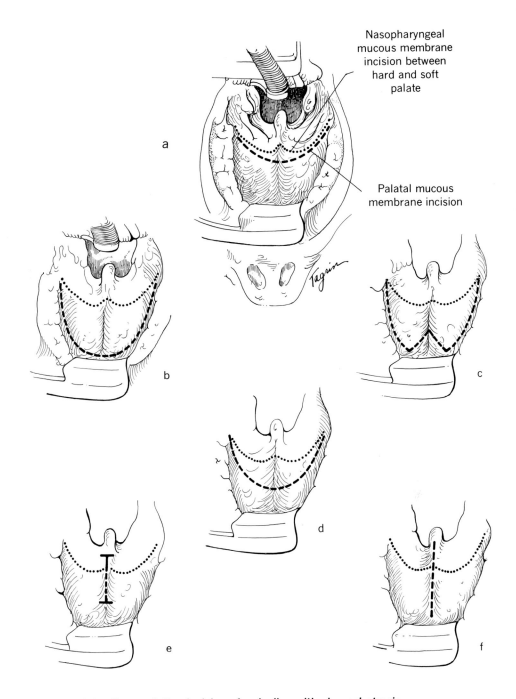

Nasopharyngeal
mucous membrane
incision between
hard and soft
palate

Palatal mucous
membrane incision

FIGURE 10.1. *Transpalatine incisions for dealing with choanal atresia.*

    a. Precechtel incision
    b. Owens incision
    c. Steinzeug incision
    d. Ruddy incision
    e. Schweckendiek-Neto "I" incision
    f. Midline incision

———— Broken lines indicate palatal mucous membrane incision.
• • • • Dotted lines indicate incisions of the nasopharyngeal mucous membrane between the hard
    and soft palate.

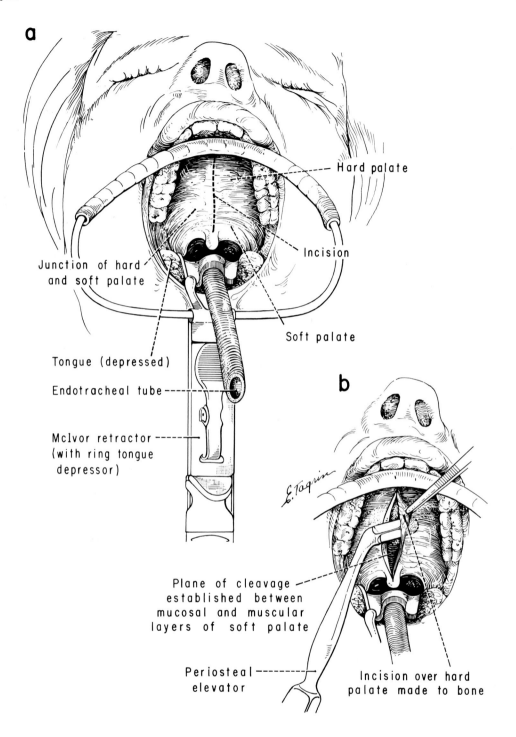

FIGURE 10.2. *Repair of choanal atresia.*

a. Exposure of the hard and soft palate is obtained with a McIvor retractor. The midline incision over the hard palate is made to the bone, but the incision in the soft palate is made only to the muscular layer.

b. A flap is made on each side by elevating the periosteum over the hard palate and by establishing a plane of cleavage between the mucosal and muscular layers of the soft palate.

anesthesia. McGovern states that the use of his specially designed nipple permits delay of the operation for one year when the operative field is doubled in size as compared with that at birth. A tracheotomy is not necessary when the McGovern procedure is employed.

Technique of Operation. The patient is placed in the supine position with the head extended. The surgeon sits at the head of the operating table working with the palate "in his lap." Exposure is acquired with a McIvor, Brown-Davis, or Digman self-retaining retractor.

Infiltration of a local anesthetic with added epinephrine along the line of incision may be used for hemostatic purposes and to supplement the general anesthesia. The incision is made in the midline along the entire length of the hard and soft palate, to the base of the uvula (Fig. 10.2a). The incision over the hard palate is made down to the bone, whereas the incision in the soft palate is made only to the muscular layer. The mucosa and periosteum over the hard palate are readily elevated with right and left palatal dissectors (Fig. 10.2b). A plane of cleavage is established between the mucosal and muscular layers of the soft palate as shown in Figures 10.2b and 10.3a.

The mucosal flaps (Fig. 10.3a) are reflected laterally by using #00 chromic catgut sutures for retraction. These sutures are either anchored around a molar tooth or weighed with heavy hemostats. The dissection proceeds with care in the region of the greater palatine foramina. It is most important that the blood supply not be disturbed after the flaps have been reflected laterally. A horizontal incision is made at the junction of the hard and soft palates (Fig. 10.3a). The soft palate retracts slightly in a posterior direction, exposing the nasopharynx and the choanal atresia (Fig. 10.3b). The posterior aspect of the hard palate extends in a postero-superior direction forming the choanal atresia. If the atresia is not bony, the reflected tissue will, of course, be mucous membrane. The dashed lines (Fig. 10.3c) represent the area of bone to be removed. The area of bony atresia is removed with a mallet and chisel, Kerrison and Citelli forceps (Fig. 10.3d). When this has been accomplished, the posterior aspect of the nasal septum can be seen along with the membranous atresia. Figure 10.4a shows the incisions for relief of the obstruction and the formation of the mucous membrane flaps.

The mucosal flaps are elevated (Fig. 10.4b) and tubing is inserted into the nasopharynx from the anterior nares. This tubing should be of a soft material such as Portex, polyvinylacetate, or silicone.

At this point (Fig. 10.4c) the operation has been completed with the exception of closure of the initial incision. A tube has been inserted through each choana and the mucosal flaps are placed on the inferior surfaces of the tubes.

The midline palatal incision (Fig. 10.4d) is closed with #3-0 chromic catgut, and the tubes are anchored in place by a postcolumellar suture of #4-0 silk or polyethylene.

Postoperative Care. No intranasal care is required other than keeping the tubes patent. This can be done with a flexible cotton-tipped applicator saturated with hydrogen peroxide solution. Oral hygiene is important during the first post-operative week to prevent contamination of the palatal incision. After a few days, the tubes are well tolerated. They should remain in place for approximately 4 weeks following the operation. If the operation has been performed after infancy, there may be some disturbance of speech and reflux of liquids into the nasal cavities for a short period following removal of the tubes. The parents can be reassured that this phenomenon is transient.

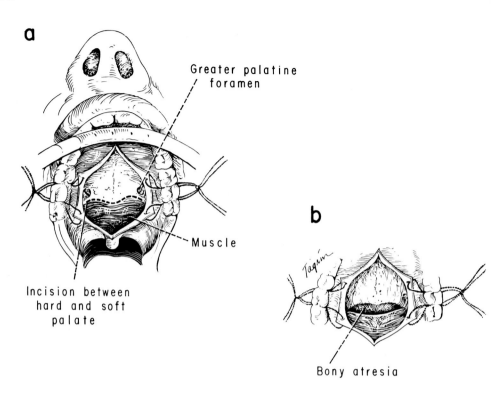

a

Greater palatine
foramen

Muscle

Incision between
hard and soft
palate

b

Tagim

Bony atresia

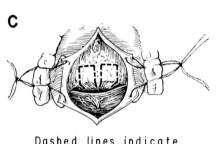

c

Dashed lines indicate
areas of bone to
be removed

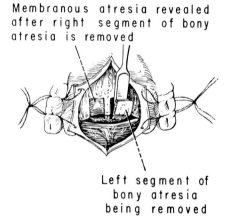

d

Membranous atresia revealed
after right segment of bony
atresia is removed

Left segment of
bony atresia
being removed

FIGURE 10.3.   *Repair of choanal atresia (continued).*

a. The mucosal flaps have been elevated laterally, sutures being used for retraction. The dashed line indicates the incision between the hard and soft palate.

b. The soft palate retracts posteriorly exposing the choanal atresia and nasopharynx.

c. The bony atresia is removed by use of chisels and various bone-cutting forceps. This should be accomplished with care in order to avoid injury to the underlying mucoperiosteum.

d. The bony atresia has been removed on the right side and is being elevated on the left.

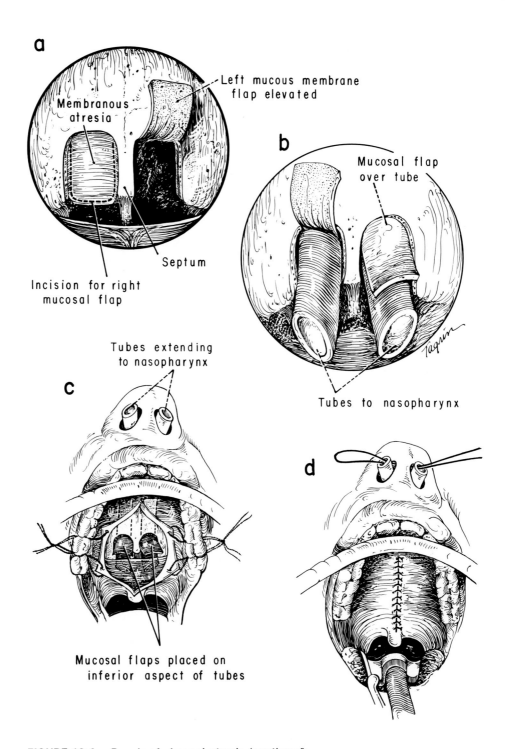

Left mucous membrane
flap elevated

Membranous
atresia

Septum

Incision for right
mucosal flap

Mucosal flap
over tube

Tubes to nasopharynx

Tubes extending
to nasopharynx

Mucosal flaps placed on
inferior aspect of tubes

FIGURE 10.4. *Repair of choanal atresia (continued).*

a. The technique for obtaining a mucoperiosteal flap from the membranous atresia is illustrated.

b. The mucosal flaps have been elevated and tubes inserted into the nasopharynx by way of each nostril.

c. The mucosal flaps are placed on the inferior aspect of each tube before the palatal flaps are replaced and sutured. The purpose of the mucosal flaps is to assist in the prevention of subsequent stenosis.

d. The operation has been completed. One suture through the nasal septum behind the columella prevents displacement of the tubes.

VELOPHARYNGEAL INSUFFICIENCY

Velopharyngeal incompetence renders a person incapable of speaking without a noticeable nasality. The emission of excessive air by way of the nasal cavity during speech results in a disturbance in quality and articulatory accuracy of the voice. Velopharyngeal closure is necessary to prevent regurgitation of liquids from the oropharynx into the nasopharynx during deglutition.

Closure of the oropharynx and the nasopharynx is accomplished by a rather complex coordinated contraction of both the palatal and pharyngeal muscles. The elevator palatine muscle contracts to pull the soft palate upward and backward. The superior constrictor muscle contracts to narrow the pharynx. The posterior wall of the pharynx is also displaced anteriorly during this contraction, especially in the region of Passavant's ridge.

Etiology. The most common causes for velopharyngeal insufficiency are listed below:

1. Cleft palate
2. Paralysis of the palate
3. Congenital shortening of the palate or excessive depth of the pharyngeal vault due to basilar skull deformities
4. Injudicious removal of adenoid tissue in children with unrecognized submucous cleft palate
5. Defects in the soft palate resulting from injury or from surgical procedures, as well as scarring of the soft palate

It is gratifying that the improved techniques for repair of cleft palate have reduced the incidence of velopharyngeal insufficiency. Hypernasality, however, persists in nearly 40% of patients who have undergone cleft palate repair.

Diagnosis. A thorough ear, nose, and throat examination and an audiometric evaluation are, of course, essential. The patient is also tested for level of speech maturity. His speech is recorded on tape and evaluated as to articulation and nasality. The degree of velopharyngeal insufficiency is also measured by comparing air pressures obtained when the nasal cavity is open with those obtained when the nares are closed.

Lateral and basal x rays of the pharynx and nasopharynx are secured both while the patient is at rest and while he is speaking. Before these x rays are taken, 1 cc of barium suspension is instilled into each nasal cavity. The vocalization of the letters U and S is shown in Figure 10.5. If the apparatus for determining pressure readings is not available, a simple comparison can be made by having the patient blow an easily inflatable balloon with and without the nares occluded. Cinefluorographic study of velopharyngeal function during speech, blowing against pressure with and without the nares occluded, and swallowing are sometimes necessary for an accurate evaluation of the velopharyngeal incompetency. The incompetency during swallowing can be most accurately evaluated by making the contrast study with the patient in the supine position.

Treatment. *Speech Therapy.* Speech therapy is the treatment of choice if the velopharyngeal incompetence is minimal. Surgery may not be necessary.

Dental Prosthesis. A dental prosthesis in the form of an obdurator or an elevator is effective in some adult patients with velopharyngeal insufficiency.

Injections. Injections of the posterior pharyngeal wall are often adequate for restoration of normal speech when there is a minimal velopharyngeal insufficiency (Fig. 10.6).

FIGURE 10.5. *Velopharyngeal insufficiency. (From Bernstein, L.: Treatment of Velopharyngeal Incompetence. Arch. Otolaryng. 85:69–70 (Jan.) 1967.)*

a. Lateral radiogram of normal person at rest (left) and vocalizing the letter S (right).

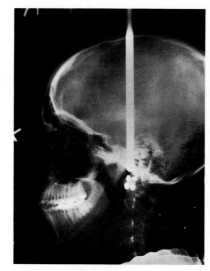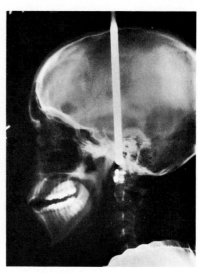

b. Lateral radiograms of patient with velopharyngeal incompetence secondary to cleft palate repair, (left) vocalizing the letter "u," (right) "s." Note marked pad formation on posterior pharyngeal wall.

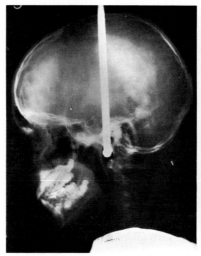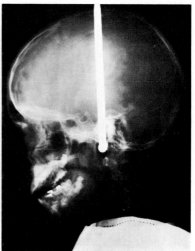

c. Lateral radiograms of patient with congenital short palate, (left) vocalizing "u," and (right) "s."

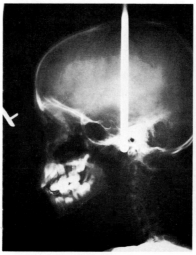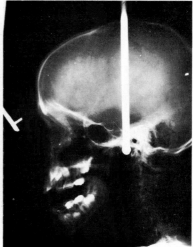

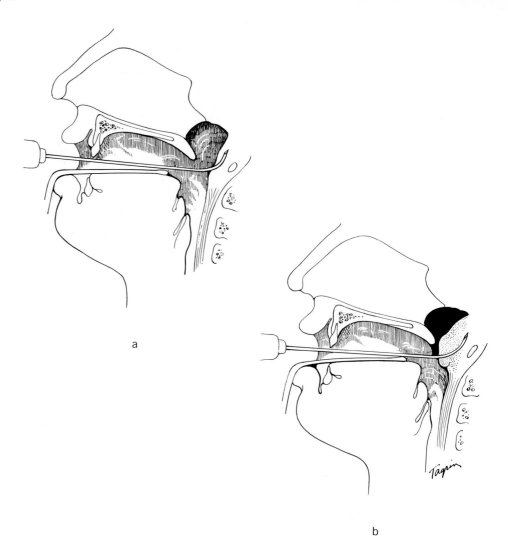

a

b

FIGURE 10.6.   *Injection of spaceoccupying substance into posterior epipharyngeal wall.*

a. Diagrammatic representation of a sagittal section of a human head with a short palate, showing Teflon being injected into the posterior pharyngeal wall. The hump created by the Teflon enables the short palate to touch the posterior pharyngeal wall, closing the velopharyngeal space.
b. The palate after injection.

Liquid Silastic can be injected into the posterior pharyngeal wall. According to Blocksma's experience in a series of cases, its use appears quite promising. The liquid Silastic (4 to 8 cc) is injected after either a local or general anesthetic has been administered. Immediately prior to its injection, three drops of stennous octoate catalyst are added to 10 cc of the fluid Silastic. The material is agitated briefly and rapidly poured into a 10-cc Luer lock syringe to which is attached a #15-gauge needle with a curved end. It is injected beneath the mucosa of the posterior pharyngeal wall, just above the protuberance of the atlas (Fig. 10.6a and b). The material vulcanizes in 10 minutes into an inert rubbery mass. To prevent it from migrating caudally as it vulcanizes, a tongue depressor is pressed into the posterior pharyngeal wall, just below the site of injection.

Teflon paste (Ethicon PTFE paste) has also been used for augmentation of the posterior pharyngeal wall. The paste is placed in a 10-cc Luer lock syringe, to which is attached an #18-gauge needle with a curved end. The needle is inserted just above the prominence caused by the tubercle of the atlas, and the paste is injected until an adequate prominence can be seen. The material is placed in the submucosal layer. Caudal spread can be prevented by applying pressure, with a tongue depressor, just below the site of injection. The amount of Teflon paste necessary to effect an adequate closure is usually 5 to 15 cc. In some cases, additional amounts can be injected at a later date. The velopharyngeal space can be closed further by injecting 1 or 2 cc of Teflon paste into each side of the posterior margins of the palate. Smith and McCabe report 60% success when treating velopharyngeal incompetency by injecting Teflon into the posterior nasopharyngeal wall.

Implants. In the treatment of velopharyngeal insufficiency, implants of cartilage, adipose tissue, and fascia into the posterior pharyngeal wall were for a time reported to be quite promising. However, the long-range results are unpredictable because of varying degrees of resorption. The use of solid implants of silicone rubber has been pretty much abandoned because of migration or extrusion of the implant. Possibly a soft, solid implant will be developed that will neither extrude through the mucous membrane nor migrate from its site of implantation.

Lengthening of the Soft Palate (Palatal Pushback). The soft palate can be lengthened by making a simple U-shaped mucosal incision (Fig. 10.7a, b and c) or executing a V-Y Wardill pushback over the hard palate (Fig. 10.7d and e). A mucoperiosteal flap is elevated and displaced posteriorly after the nasal mucosa at the junction of the hard and soft palates has been incised.

Posterior Pharyngeal Mucosal Flap. The pharyngeal flap procedure is indicated for those patients with moderate to severe velopharyngeal insufficiency for whom procedures designed for augmentation of the posterior pharyngeal wall are not suited. This group especially includes those with a congenitally short soft palate or paralysis of the soft palate, as well as those having various defects of the soft palate.

The posterior pharyngeal mucosal flap operation should not be performed on children under 7 years of age because of the frequency with which tracheotomy is required for these patients. The optimal age for patients undergoing this procedure is between 7 and 9 years.

The operation is performed with the patient under general endotracheal anesthesia and in the Rose position. The palate and pharynx are exposed with the aid of a Brown-Davis mouth gag as for a tonsillectomy. A soft palate retractor or traction sutures applied to the soft palate are used to expose the posterior epipharyngeal wall (Fig. 10.8a). Submucosal infiltration of a local anesthetic agent, with epinephrine added, supplements the general anesthesia, reduces the amount of bleeding during the procedure, and facilitates the dissection in a plane between the constrictor muscle and the prevertebral fascia. A vertical incision is made on

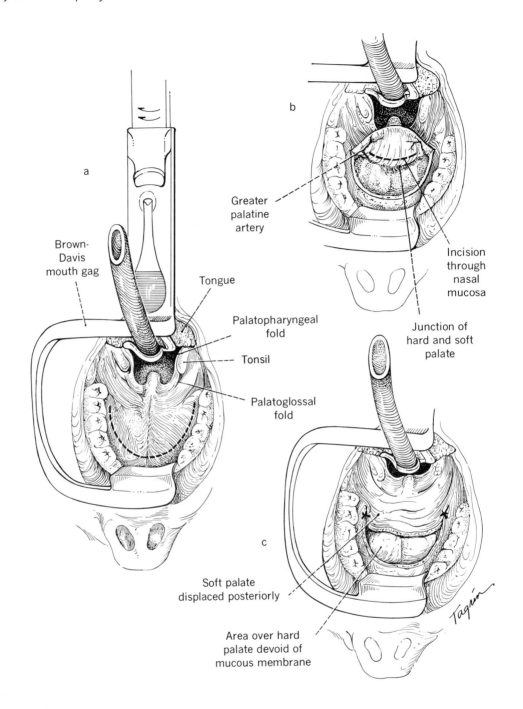

a

Brown-
Davis
mouth gag

Tongue

Palatopharyngeal
fold

Tonsil

Palatoglossal
fold

b

Greater
palatine
artery

Incision
through
nasal
mucosa

Junction of
hard and soft
palate

c

Soft palate
displaced posteriorly

Area over hard
palate devoid of
mucous membrane

FIGURE 10.7.   *Lengthening of the soft palate.*

a. Exposure for the operation is obtained by using a Brown-Davis mouth gag with a Ring attachment so that the endotracheal tube will not be in the way during the operation. The patient is placed in the Rose position. A U-shaped incision is employed, as is shown. This should avoid both the greater palatine foramina and the incisive foramen anteriorly. The mucoperiosteum over the hard palate is elevated with right and left palatal elevators until the pos-

terior margin of the hard palate can be palpated. The incision is extended on each side to include the lateral soft palate posterior to the greater palatine foramen.

b. The mucoperichondrium has been elevated to the level of the junction of the hard and soft palates. The greater palatine arteries are identified and preserved. An incision is made through the membrane of the mucosa on the nasal side of the palate at the junction of the hard and soft palates.

The hamulus is dissected free on each side. A small segment of bone is removed in the posterior medial aspect of the greater palatine foramen so that the artery may be displaced posteriorly along with the palate.

c. The soft palate has been displaced posteriorly leaving, anteriorly, an area over the hard palate devoid of mucous membrane. This area will fill in rapidly during the immediate postoperative period.

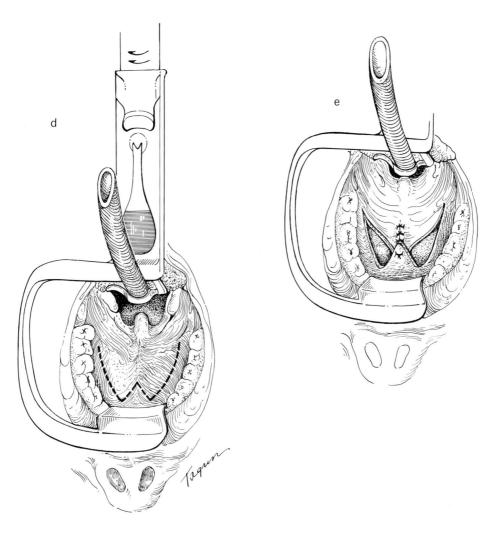

FIGURE 10.7 (Continued).

d. The modified V-Y push-back technique is preferred by some surgeons because the anterior palatine foramen is more easily avoided by this method and the resulting mucous membrane defect over the hard palate is less than that following the procedure described in a–c. The incision is made as is shown, and the palate is elevated, avoiding injury to the greater palatine arteries.

e. The palatal push-back has been accomplished. The anterior "V" defect in the soft palate flap is sutured with #3-0 chromic catgut. The anterior aspect of the palatal flap is then sutured to the tip of the "V" defect anteriorly.

each side of the posterior pharyngeal wall. This should include most of the width of the wall (Fig. 10.8b). Dissection is carried through the mucosa, pharyngeal fascia, and constrictor muscle. The prevertebral fascia is identified, and a plane of cleavage is established with either curved or right-angled scissors. It is most important to acquire a flap of adequate length. The inferior horizontal incision connecting the two vertical incisions is thus made just at the level of the superior aspect of the epiglottis (Fig. 10.8c). The flap retracts superiorly as this dissection is completed. A moist gauze pack is placed against the posterior pharyngeal wall and also in the nasopharynx to control bleeding, while the soft palate is prepared to receive the inferior margin of the pedicled flap (Fig. 10.8d).

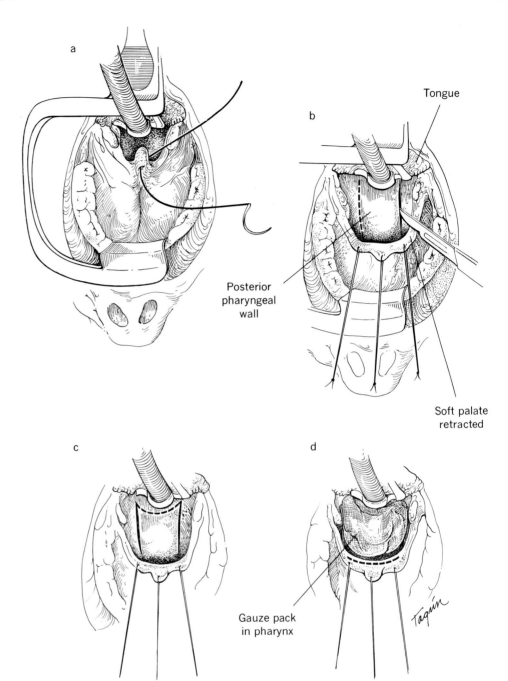

FIGURE 10.8.   *Superiorly based posterior pharyngeal flap.*

a. The exposure of the palate and posterior pharynx is accomplished with a Brown-Davis mouth gag with a Ring attachment so that the endotracheal tube will not be in the way during the operation. The soft palate is retracted forward by using traction sutures.

b. The soft palate is retracted, exposing the epipharynx. A vertical incision has been completed on one side and a second is being made on the opposite side. The width of this flap should be nearly the same as that of the entire posterior pharyngeal wall.

c. A horizontal incision is made inferiorly, connecting the two vertical incisions at the level of the superior margin of the epiglottis. As this incision is completed the posterior pharyngeal flap retracts superiorly.

d. The nasopharynx and posterior pharyngeal wall have been packed to control bleeding. A horizontal incision is made on the posterior surface of the soft palate between the bases of the palatal pharyngeal folds.

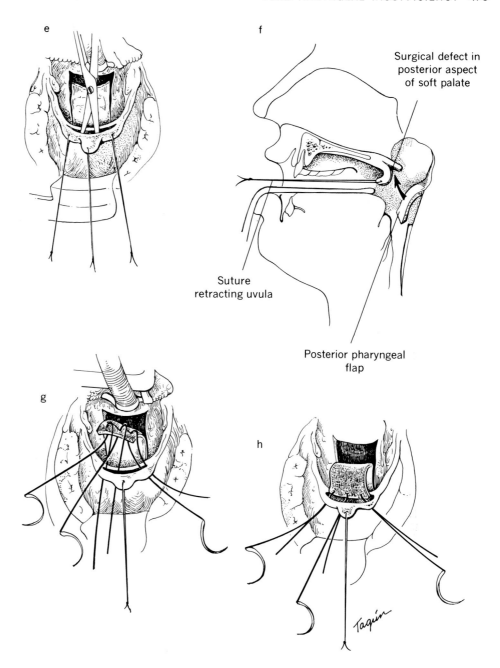

FIGURE 10.8 (Continued).

     e and f. Either right-angle or curved scissors are used to create a bed in the posterior aspect of the soft palate, which is to receive the inferior end of the posterior pharyngeal flap.

     g. Three sutures are placed through the end of the posterior pharyngeal flap. These sutures are then carried through the mucous membrane on the oral surface of the soft palate by way of the bed in the posterior or nasal surface of the soft palate.

     h. The sutures are placed into the defect and out the oral surface of the soft palate. The other ends of these sutures are placed at a distance of a few millimeters.

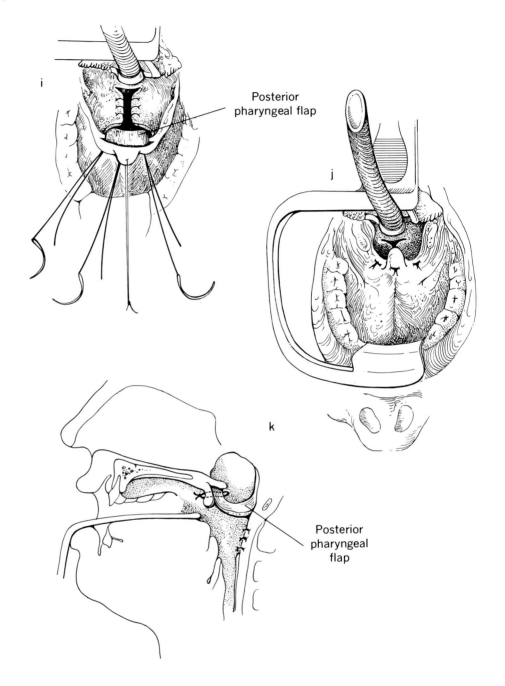

Posterior
pharyngeal flap

Posterior
pharyngeal
flap

FIGURE 10.8 (Continued).

i. The lateral edges of the pharyngeal defect are partially approximated to the underlying fascia. The end of the posterior pharyngeal flap has been drawn into the surgical defect in the posterior aspect of the soft palate.

j. The sutures are loosely tied so as to prevent their cutting through the mucous membrane as edema develops during the postoperative period.

k. A midsagittal view of the completed operation. The undersurface of the posterior pharyngeal flap will be covered by mucous membrane migrating from both an anterior and a posterior direction.

The uvula is grasped with atraumatic forceps, or secured with three traction sutures of #2-0 chromic catgut, and retracted anteriorly. This exposes the immediate posterior aspect of the soft palate and the palatal pharyngeal fold. A horizontal incision is made on the posterior aspect of the soft palate between bases of the palatal pharyngeal folds (Fig. 10.8d). The soft palate is then split horizontally, creating a bed for the inferior aspect of the posterior pharyngeal flap (Fig. 10.8e,f). Three sutures of #2-0 chromic catgut are placed at the end of the pharyngeal flap (Fig. 10.8g). All three are passed through the bed created in the soft palate before they are tied (Fig. 10.8h). The end of the pharyngeal flap is then drawn onto the bed by pulling on the sutures (Fig. 10.8i). The knots are tied loosely so that they will not cut through mucous membrane when postoperative edema occurs (Fig. 10.8j).

The superiorly based posterior pharyngeal flap is far superior to the inferiorly based flap, for dissection is simpler. It is much more suitable for patients in whom the distance between the palate and the posterior pharyngeal wall is great, and in whom the flap can be sutured without tension and the posterior pharyngeal defect can be at least partially closed.

The lateral edges of the posterior pharyngeal defect are undermined, and the defect is at least partially closed by suturing the lateral margins to underlying fascia (Fig. 10.8i). By this technique not only is the postoperative discomfort reduced, but also the superior pharynx is narrowed, thus assisting with the velopharyngeal closure.

Complications of this operation are infrequent. Postoperative bleeding may occur. This can be avoided by careful dissection and either ligating or cauterizing bleeding vessels. If persistent bleeding does occur, it may be necessary to perform a tracheotomy and insert a pharyngeal pack. On occasion, the flap may become detached from the palate. This usually occurs within one week after the operation, and it is, of course, essential that it be re-attached to the soft palate. If nasal respiration is inadequate following this procedure, revision of the lateral gutters must be undertaken at a later date. A late complication of this operation is shrinkage of the pharyngeal flap due to scar-tissue contraction, resulting in an insufficient velopharyngeal closure. This can often be remedied by tissue augmentation such as with the injection of Teflon paste.

Combined Procedures. A combination of the palatal pushback and the posterior pharyngeal flap is necessary for the treatment of moderate to severe velopharyngeal insufficiency. Either a U-shaped or V-Y pushback procedure is accomplished as has been described. The result is a mucosal defect on the nasopharyngeal surface of the palate (Fig. 10.9a). The posterior pharyngeal flap is elevated and sutured to this defect (Fig. 10.11b and c).

Repair of Palatal Defects. Defects of the soft palate are a cause of velopharyngeal incompetency. They may be congenital or the result of neoplasm, surgical procedure, or trauma.

The technique for repair of a unilateral defect through the hard palate is shown in a and b of Figure 10.10; c and d of this figure show the technique for repair of a central defect through the hard or soft palate.

Repair for a defect involving nearly one half of the soft palate is shown in Figure 10.11.

The procedure for repair of the postero-central defect of the soft palate with the uvula absent is demonstrated in Figure 10.12.

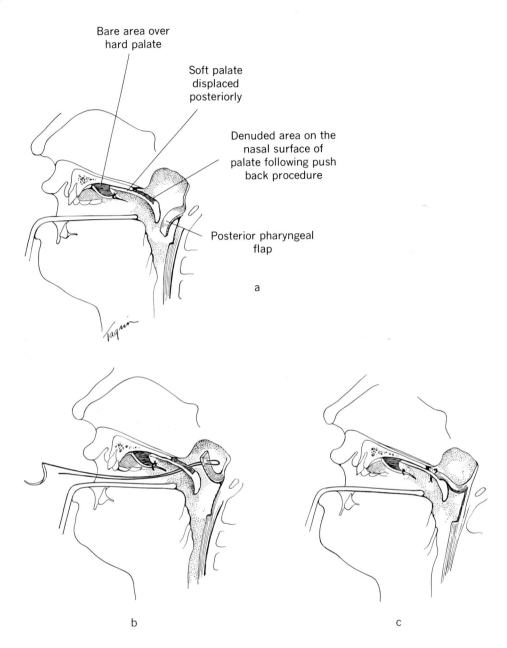

Bare area over
hard palate

Soft palate
displaced
posteriorly

Denuded area on the
nasal surface of
palate following push
back procedure

Posterior pharyngeal
flap

a

b

c

FIGURE 10.9.   *Combined push-back and pharyngeal flap.*

     a. A U-shaped palatal incision is used to construct a palatal flap for a push-back procedure (see Fig. 10.7b). A V-Y push-back procedure may also be used (see Fig. 10.7d). The mucoperiosteum is elevated over the hard palate with the right and left palatal elevators. The greater palatine artery is preserved on each side and the posterior margin of the hard palate is dissected free. An incision is made through the mucous membrane on the nasal side of the palate at the junction of the hard and soft palates.

     b. The palatal dissection has been completed. The superiorly based posterior pharyngeal flap has been elevated and sutures of #2-0 chromic catgut have been placed through its inferior end. Each end of these sutures is placed through the mucoperichondrium on the oral surface of the palate.

     c. The sutures through the inferior end of the posterior pharyngeal flap and oral surface of the palatal mucoperiosteum are tied loosely. One suture is placed on each side to secure the flap in place. The end of the pharyngeal flap is in contact with the denuded area on the nasal surface of the palate as a result of the palatal push-back procedure.

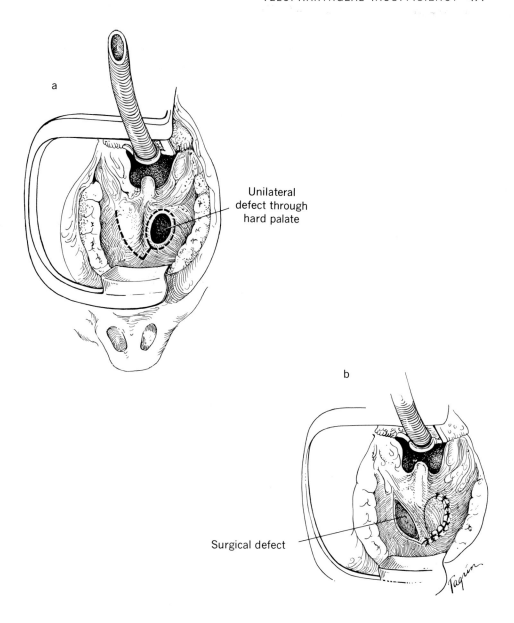

FIGURE 10.10. *Repair of defects of the palate.*

a. A unilateral defect through the hard palate is repaired by first making a circumferential incision through the mucous membrane around the defect. The inside margins of mucous membrane are carefully reflected in the direction of the nasal cavity.

b. The outline of the mucous membrane incision for construction of a flap to cover the unilateral defect is illustrated. The mucous membrane flap is reflected to the right, covering the palatal defect. It is sutured in place with #3-0 chromic catgut. There remains a mucosal defect on the left side over the hard palate which needs no covering for it rapidly becomes covered by mucous membrane.

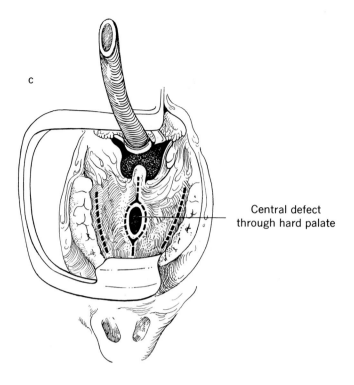

Central defect
through hard palate

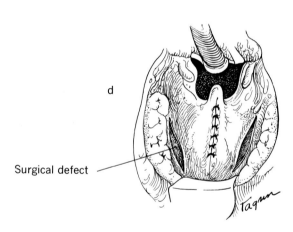

Surgical defect

FIGURE 10.10 (Continued).

c. The incisions for repair of a central defect through the hard or soft palate are shown. A circumferential incision is made around the defect as shown in a. The incisions are extended anteriorly and posteriorly so that the defect may be closed in a straight line. An anteroposterior incision is made just medial to the alveolar ridge on each side. Care must be taken not to injure the greater palatine arteries. The mucous membrane between the lateral incision and the medial incisions must be extensively elevated so that the resulting bipedicled flaps may be advanced medially without lateral tension.

d. The completed repair is shown. A defect over the hard palate laterally on each side results as the midline defect is closed. A strong suture, such as #2-0 chromic catgut, is preferred for this repair. The incidence of breakdown and recurrent perforation is negligible, if the bipedicled flaps have been sufficiently undermined so that there is no lateral tension, because the blood supply to these flaps is excellent.

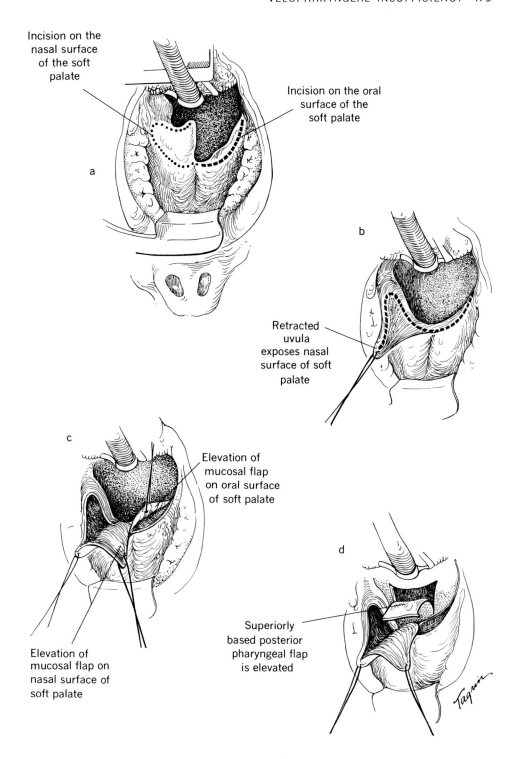

Incision on the nasal surface of the soft palate

Incision on the oral surface of the soft palate

a

b

Retracted uvula exposes nasal surface of soft palate

c

Elevation of mucosal flap on oral surface of soft palate

Elevation of mucosal flap on nasal surface of soft palate

d

Superiorly based posterior pharyngeal flap is elevated

FIGURE 10.11. *Repair of defects of soft palate.*

a. Nearly one half of the soft palate is missing. The heavy interrupted line indicates the incision on the oral surface of the soft palate. The dotted lines indicate the incisions on the soft palate's nasal surface.

b. The uvula is retracted anteriorly to expose the nasopharyngeal side of the left soft palate. This facilitates the elevation of the mucosal flap.

c. The mucosal flaps have been elevated on each side.

d. A superiorly based posterior pharyngeal flap is elevated. This is to serve as a mucosal lining for the posterior soft palate and to assist in reducing the nasopharyngeal insufficiency.

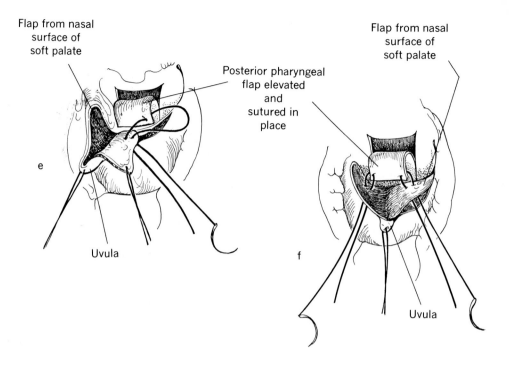

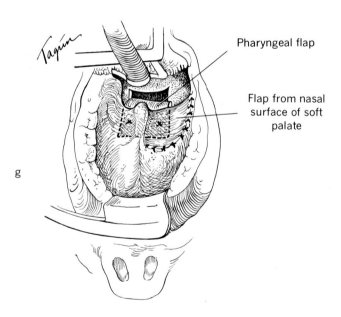

FIGURE 10.11 (Continued).

   e. The right side of the posterior pharyngeal flap is sutured to the posterior aspect of the flap of the left soft palate. This results in a double layer closure of the right palatal defect.

   f. The left side of the posterior pharyngeal flap is sutured to the posterior surface of the left soft palate.

   g. The sutures attaching the posterior pharyngeal flap to the posterior surface of the soft palate are tied on the oral side of the soft palate. The soft palate flap is sutured in place to the marginal defect on the right side.

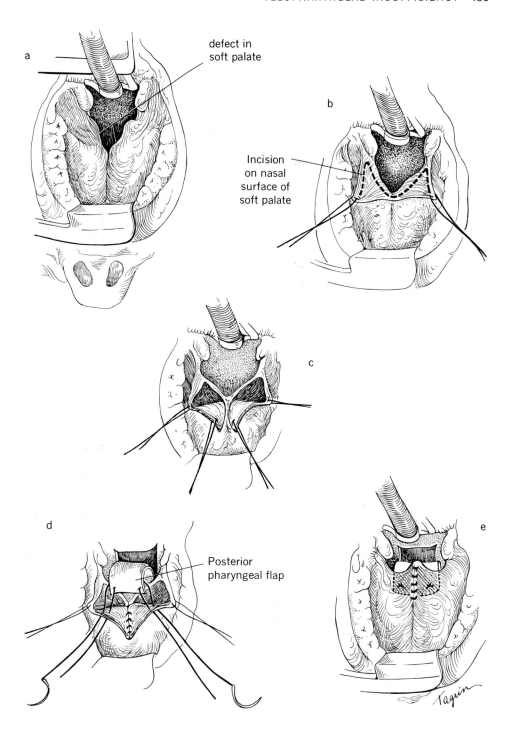

FIGURE 10.12. *Repair of defects of soft palate.*

a. A postero-central defect is present in the soft palate. The uvula is absent.

b. Both sides of the soft palate are retracted anterolaterly with a traction suture so that the incision can be made on the nasal surface.

c. Anteriorly based mucosal flaps are elevated on each side from the posterior surface of the soft palate.

d. The paired flaps from the posterior surface of the soft palate are sutured together in the midline. A superiorly based posterior pharyngeal flap is elevated. This is sutured to the normal surface of the soft palate as is shown.

e. The posterior pharyngeal flap serves to cover and support the nasal surface of the soft palate. The completed operation is shown.

STENOSIS OF THE NASOPHARYNX

The most common cause of nasopharyngeal stenosis is the ingestion of caustic material. Other possible causes are trauma, severe infection, and sequelae of surgical procedures. The stenosis, which involves adherence of the soft palate to the epipharyngeal wall, may be partial or complete. The patient complains of hyponasality. There may be a conductive hearing loss due to interference with eustachian tube function. Simple excision of the adhesions or the use of electrocautery is usually ineffective. Skin grafting and the use of stents often result in gradually recurring stenosis.

Technique of Repair. The operation for repair of stenosis between the oropharynx and nasopharynx is performed with the patient in the Rose position. Exposure is obtained with a Brown-Davis mouth gag with a Ring attachment for an endotracheal tube. The procedure is then carried out as described in the legend of Figure 10.13.

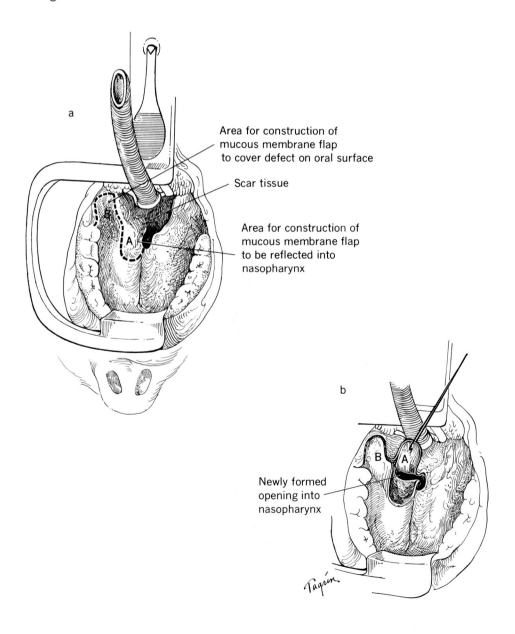

a

Area for construction of
mucous membrane flap
to cover defect on oral surface

Scar tissue

Area for construction of
mucous membrane flap
to be reflected into
nasopharynx

b

Newly formed
opening into
nasopharynx

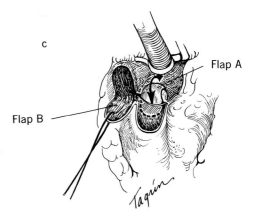

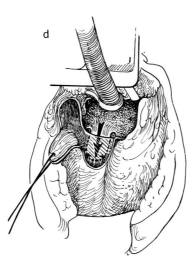

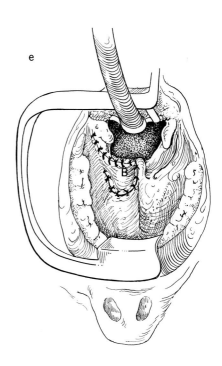

FIGURE 10.13.   *Stenosis of the nasopharynx.*

a. A mucosal incision is made on the oral surface of the soft palate to fashion a mucous membrane flap which is to be reflected into the nasopharynx to cover the denuded posterior epipharyngeal wall. The incision for the construction of a buccal mucosal flap (B) which is to cover the defect on the oral surface of the soft palate is outlined.

b. The mucous membrane flap (A) has been elevated from the oral surface of the soft palate and reflected inferiorly. This leaves a denuded area on the oral surface of the soft palate.

c. The newly formed opening into the nasopharynx is now apparent. The mucosal flap (A) has been reflected into the nasopharynx to cover the denuded area on the posterior epipharyngeal wall. This flap is sutured in place with #4-0 chromic catgut as the margin of the soft palate is reflected anteriorly. The mucous membrane flap (B) has been elevated from the inside of the cheek in preparation for its rotation to cover the denuded oral surface of the soft palate.

d. The buccal mucosal flap (B) has been further dissected and the palatal flap (A) sutured in place.

e. The buccal mucous membrane flap has been rotated into place and sutured with #3-0 or #4-0 chromic catgut. The defect inside of the cheek is closed by first undermining the surrounding buccal mucosa and closing it in a straight line.

ADENOIDECTOMY AND TONSILLECTOMY

The decision to perform a tonsillectomy and/or adenoidectomy can be quite perplexing. With local and general nasal decongestants, biochemotherapy, and minor procedures such as myringotomy for serous otitis media, the surgeon can procrastinate and play for time. Each case must be individualized, reviewing a carefully taken history and the physical findings. At times it is difficult to overrule the persistence of the parent or referring physician who insists that the tonsils and adenoids be removed.

The following are a few positive indications which can be used as ground rules.

Indications and Contraindications for Adenoidectomy

1. Large adenoids obstructing the eustachian tubes and causing repeated or persistent ear disease and hearing loss.
2. Sufficient obstruction from the adenoids to cause chronic sinus infection.
3. Obstruction of the nasopharynx associated with chronic mouth-breathing and "adenoidal" abnormal facial appearance.
4. A short palate or submucous cleft of the palate are most often contraindications for an adenoidectomy.

Indications for Tonsillectomy

1. Repeated episodes of acute tonsillitis
2. Peritonsillar abscess and a history of past tonsillitis
3. Unusual tonsil hypertrophy that interferes with swallowing and respiration. The tonsils at times can become so large that they meet in the midline.
4. Should the tonsils be removed when there is only indication for an adenoidectomy? As a rule the answer is no, for only a small percentage of these patients will require a subsequent tonsillectomy. The postoperative course following an adenoidectomy is quite benign as compared to that following a tonsillectomy.
5. Tumor of tonsil.

Technique of Surgery

The adenoidectomy and tonsillectomy are best performed with the patient in a supine position with his head extended (Rose position) (Fig. 10.14a). The surgeon can sit comfortably at the head of the table during the operation. Excellent exposure of the pharynx can be acquired by use of a Brown-Davis mouth gag which has a Ring attachment for the endotracheal tube. The McIvor mouth gag is used with the Ring attachment if the incisor teeth are either very loose or absent. An endotracheal tube is used to give the anesthesiologist better control of the airway and to facilitate the administration of the anesthetic. With an endotracheal tube in place, there is very little chance for aspiration of blood or other substances.

If both adenoidectomy and tonsillectomy are to be performed, the adenoidectomy is carried out before the tonsillectomy because bleeding from the site

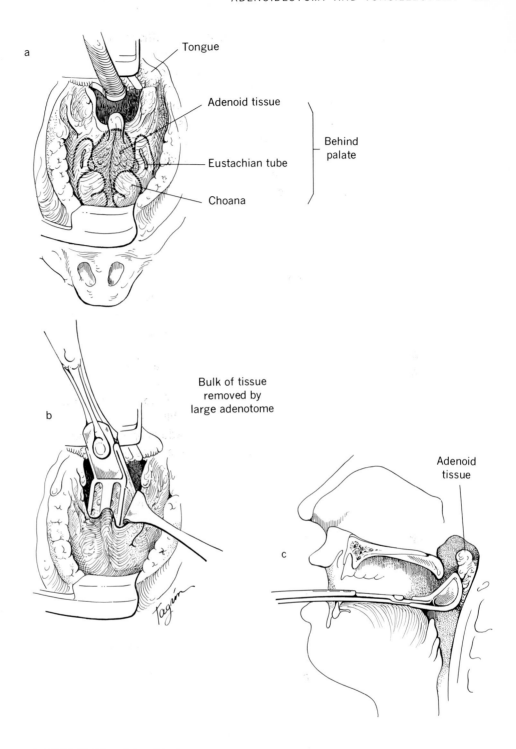

FIGURE 10.14.   *Adenoidectomy.*

a. A view of the pharynx obtained by placing the patient in the Rose position (hyperextension) and after inserting a Brown-Davis mouth gag with a Ring modification for placement of the endotracheal tube. The relative positions of the adenoid tissue, eustachian tubes, and choanae are illustrated.

b. The adenotome is inserted into the nasopharynx with the blade in the closed position. It may be necessary to retract the soft palate anteriorly while inserting the adenotome.

c. A side view of the nasopharynx with the large adenotome in place. The adenotome is positioned, over the adenoid, the blade is opened, slight posterior pressure is exerted, and the blade is closed. If too great a posterior pressure is exerted or if the head is hyperextended, there is a chance that the underlying fascia will be injured.

of the adenoids is more difficult to control than that from the tonsil area. Keeping a nasopharyngeal pack in place until the completion of the tonsillectomy is usually all that is necessary to control bleeding from this location. The nasopharynx is exposed with a soft palate retractor in order to determine the amount of adenoid tissue present. The instruments used to remove adenoid tissue include various-sized adenotomes, Ring punches of varied shape, and adenoid curettes.

Adenoidectomy. If the patient's head is in hyperextension, it is slightly flexed so that the bodies of the cervical vertebrae and prevertebral fasciae will not be too convex. An adenotome, with a width slightly less than the distance between the eustachian tube orifices, is inserted, pressed slightly in a posterior direction, and closed to remove the main mass of adenoid tissue (Fig. 10.14b and c). Before closing the blade of the adenotome, the position of the uvula must be determined so that it will not be resected. Even though the absence of a uvula usually causes no dysfunction, it can cause considerable apprehension to both the parents and the patient.

The soft palate is again retracted and the nasopharynx suctioned with a Yankauer suction tip. If any of the main mass of the adenoid in the lower nasopharynx is still present, it is removed by a second application of the large adenotome. The surgeon's index finger is inserted into the vault of the nasopharynx, palpating first one choana, the posterior margin of the nasal septum, and then the opposite choana. Quite often a mass of adenoid tissue will be palpated just below the choana (Fig. 10.15a). A smaller adenotome with closed blade is inserted with the index finger still in place. The adenotome is guided by this finger to the mass of tissue, the blade is opened, slight posterior pressure is exerted, and the blade is closed. Multiple bites with the adenotome may be necessary to remove the mass.

With the patient's head in hyperextension, the soft palate is again retracted in order to obtain a view of the torus tubarius and eustachian tube orifices. Lymphoid tissue in these areas is removed with Ring punches having both rounded and flat ends (Fig. 10.15b).

When the operator is satisfied that all adenoid tissue has been removed, the nasopharynx is packed with two or more dental rolls previously moistened with saline solution to which has been attached black silk suture material. The black silk suture is essential, for it is very easy to inadvertently leave a packing in the nasopharynx.

The nasopharyngeal packing remains in place until the completion of the tonsillectomy. As soon as the tonsillectomy is completed and the tonsillar fossae are packed with dental rolls, the nasopharyngeal packing is removed, and the nasopharynx inspected with the soft palate retracted. If bleeding is absent, the nasopharynx is left undisturbed. A bleeding vessel high in the nasopharynx can be detected by flexing the patient's head so that the nasopharynx is no longer dependent. The site of the bleeding will become obvious as blood trickles down the posterior pharyngeal wall. Bleeding points in the nasopharynx can be cauterized with a silver nitrate stick or electrocoagulated with an insulated suction tip. The exposure for this cautery is acquired by either retracting the soft palate or inserting a Yankauer nasopharyngoscope.

If there is any question that there may be bleeding from the nasopharynx in the immediate postoperative period, a nasal-oral string is inserted in case a nasopharyngeal pack is needed. To accomplish this a catheter is inserted into the pharynx by way of the nasal cavity. The tip of the catheter is grasped as it

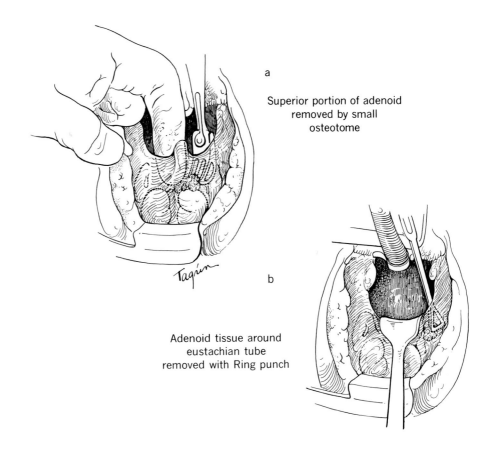

a

Superior portion of adenoid
removed by small
osteotome

b

Adenoid tissue around
eustachian tube
removed with Ring punch

FIGURE 10.15. *Adenoidectomy.*

a. The technique for removing adenoid tissue from the posterosuperior aspect of the naso-pharynx. The tissue is palpated with the surgeon's index finger. The smaller adenotome is inserted and guided into position over the adenoid tissue with this finger. The finger is removed, and the blade of the adenotome is opened and closed.

b. The soft palate is retracted in order to expose the orifice of the eustachian tube. Lymphoid tissue in this area is removed with various-shaped Ring punches.

appears in the pharynx and a silk suture (#0) is tied to this end. The catheter is removed from the nose and both ends of the string are tied externally. The string is cut and removed after a few hours if no bleeding has occurred.

Tonsillectomy. The upper medial aspect of the tonsil is grasped with an instrument such as an Allis forceps (Fig. 10.16a and b). It is pulled downward and forward, thus tenting out the mucous membrane superior to the tonsil between the anterior and posterior pillars. A small incision is made in this mucous membrane with the spade-shaped end of a tonsillectomy knife. The instrument is reversed and the right-angled end of the tonsil knife is inserted through the incision, under the mucous membrane just anterior to the posterior pillar (Fig. 10.16c). This mucous membrane is incised along the entire length of the posterior pillar. With the tonsil retracted slightly in a posterior direction, the right-angled knife is inserted beneath the mucous membrane immediately posterior to the anterior pillar by way of the same initial incision (Fig. 10.16d). This anterior incision is not performed first, for the resulting blood flow would obstruct a view of the posterior pillar.

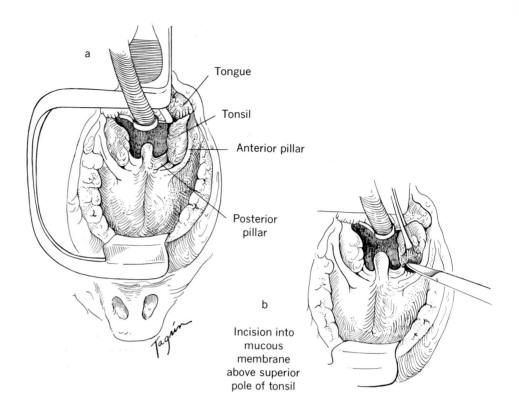

a

Tongue

Tonsil

Anterior pillar

Posterior pillar

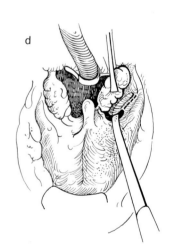

b

Incision into
mucous
membrane
above superior
pole of tonsil

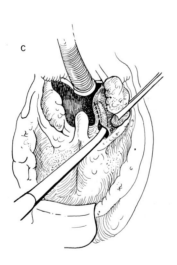

c

d

Incision
extended along
posterior and
anterior
pillars

FIGURE 10.16. Tonsillectomy.

a. An excellent view of the pharyngeal tonsils is obtained by placing the patient in the Rose position and exposing the pharynx with a Brown-Davis mouth gag. The surgeon sits at the head of the operating table.

b. The tonsil is grasped with Allis forceps and pulled downward medially. The mucous membrane superior to the tonsil, between the anterior and posterior pillar, is incised with the straight end of the tonsil knife.

c. The mucous membrane anterior to the posterior pillar is incised by inserting the right-angle end of the tonsil knife into the superior incision and dissecting inferiorly beneath the mucous membrane. This mucous membrane is incised along the entire length of the posterior pillar.

d. The mucous membrane posterior to the anterior pillar is incised by inserting the right-angle knife into the superior incision and dissecting inferiorly beneath the mucous membrane.

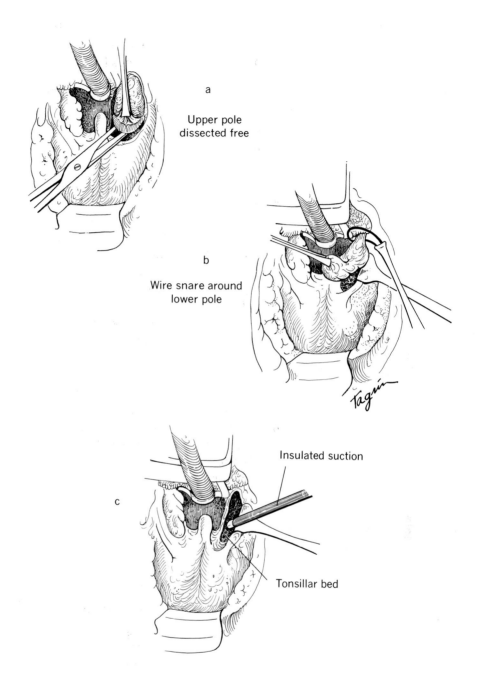

a

Upper pole
dissected free

b

Wire snare around
lower pole

Insulated suction

c

Tonsillar bed

FIGURE 10.17. *Tonsillectomy.*

a. The Allis clamp is re-applied so that it may be used to grasp the superior portion of the tonsil. The superior pole is carefully dissected in a plane between the fibrous capsule of the tonsil and the underlying muscles. Either a tonsil dissector or curved scissors can be used for this dissection. The superior pole of the tonsil is grasped with the Allis forceps and pulled downward. The remainder of the tonsil with the exception of the inferior pole is dissected by using the index finger, the tonsil dissector, or curved scissors.

b. A wire snare is placed over the tonsil. The snare is reflected inferiorly as it is being closed. Simultaneously, the tonsil is retracted superiorly. This completes the removal of the inferior pole.

c. Hemostasis is obtained by electrocoagulation with an insulated suction tip. A nonexplosive anesthetic must be used when electrocoagulation is employed. Many surgeons prefer to suture ligate all open blood vessels.

The Allis clamp is re-applied so that it may be used to grasp the superior aspect of the tonsil. The superior pole of the tonsil is then carefully dissected in the plane between the fibrous layer of the tonsil and the underlying muscles (Fig. 10.17a). A tonsil dissector or curved scissors is used for this dissection. As soon as the superior pole is in clear view it is grasped by the Allis forceps so that the tonsil can be more readily retracted inferiorly. The remainder of the tonsil, with the exception of the detachment of the inferior pole, is easily dissected, by using the index finger, tonsil dissector, and curved scissors.

A wire snare is placed around the tonsil. As the snare is tightened, it is pushed slightly inferiorly as the tonsil is being retracted superiorly (Fig. 10.17b). In so doing the inferior pole is completely excised.

Large vessels in the tonsillar fossae should be suture ligated with #2-0 or #3-0 catgut. If there is no significant bleeding, the tonsillar fossa is packed with a moist dental roll which remains untouched for at least 3 minutes. Providing a nonexplosive anesthetic agent is being used, the insulated suction tip with electro-cautery is an excellent way to obtain hemostasis in the tonsillar fossa (Fig. 10.17c).

With the exposure acquired by using a pillar retractor, the bleeding vessel is grasped with a hemostat. The needle is inserted in a postero-anterior direction, first below the hemostat and then above the hemostat. The hemostat is removed and the suture ligature tied. This type of suture ligature (Figure "8") is much more effective and secure than a slip tie placed around the vessel.

The patient is placed in a sitting position if the tonsillectomy is to be performed with local anesthesia. A metal tongue depressor is used in place of a mouth gag. The local anesthetic solution is injected into the tonsillar side of the pillars. The tonsil is grasped and pulled medially so that the anesthetic agent can be infiltrated posterior to the tonsil. The operative procedure is identical to that described above.

REFERENCES

Blocksma, R.: Silicone Implants for Velopharyngeal Incompetence: A Progress Report. Cleft Palate J. *1:*1:72–81 (Jan.) 1964.

Bloom, S. M.: Cancer of the Nasopharynx: with Special Reference to the Significance of Histopathology. Laryngoscope *71:*10:1207–1260 (Oct.) 1961.

Cherry, J., and Bordley, J. E.: Surgical Correction of Choanal Atresia. Ann. Otol. *75:*4:911–920 (Dec.) 1966.

Cocke, E. W., Jr.: Transpalatine Surgical Approach to the Nasopharynx and Posterior Nasal Cavity. Amer. J. Surg. *108:*517–525 (Oct.) 1964.

Ferguson, C. F.: Treatment of Airway Problems in the Newborn. Ann. Otol. *76:*4:762–774 (Oct.) 1967.

Fitz-Hugh, G. S., and Wallenborn, W. McK.: Tumors of the Nasopharynx, A review of Fifty-Two Cases. Laryngoscope *71:*5:457–479 (May) 1961.

Flake, C. G., and Ferguson, C. F.: Congenital Choanal Atresia in Infants and Children. Ann. Otol. *73:*458-473, 1964.

Fletcher, G. H., and Million, R. R.: Malignant Tumors of the Nasopharynx. Amer. J. Roentgen. *93:*1:44–55 (Jan.) 1965.

Lierle, D. M., Huffman, W. C., and Smith, J. L.: Palatal Insufficiency. Minnesota Med. (June) 1967, pp. 945–947.

Longacre, J. J., et al.: Combined Transoral, Transcervical and Transosseous Team Approach to Tumors of the Nasopharynx and Pharyngeal Region. Amer. J. Surg. *110:*4:644–648 (Oct.) 1965.

Matz, G. J., and Conner, G. H.: Nasopharyngeal Cancer. Laryngoscope *78:*10:1763–1767 (Aug.) 1967.

McGovern, F. H., and Fitz-Hugh, G. S.: Surgical Management of Congenital Choanal Atresia. Arch Otolaryng. *73:*627–634 (June) 1961.

Montgomery, W. W., Connelly, J. P., and Robinson, J. C.: Choanal Atresia, Part II; Surgical Management. Clin. Pediat. *4:*2:71–76 (Feb.) 1965.

Omerod, F. C.: Malignant Disease of the Nasopharynx. J. Laryngol. *65:*11:778–785 (Nov.) 1951.

Owens, H.: Observations in Treating Twenty-Five Cases of Choanal Atresia by the Transpalatine Approach. Laryngoscope 75:1:84–104 (Jan.) 1965.

Pang, L. Q.: Carcinoma of the Nasopharynx. Arch. Otolaryng. 82:622–628 (Dec.) 1965.

Smith, J. K., and McCabe, B. F.: Teflon Injection in the Nasopharynx to Improve Velopharyngeal Closure. Ann. Otol. 86:559–563 (July–Aug.) 1977.

Wang, C. C., and Schultz, M. D.: Cancer of the Nasopharynx: Its Clinical Course and Management. Geriatrics 20:864–870 (Oct.) 1965.

Wang, C. C., and Schultz, M. D.: Management of Locally Recurrent Carcinoma of the Nasopharynx. Radiology 86:5:900–903 (May) 1966.

Wilson, C. P.: Observations on the Surgery of the Nasopharynx. Ann. Otol. 66:1:5–36 (March) 1957.

11

Surgery of the Ear

SURGERY FOR ACOUSTIC NEURINOMA

The otolaryngologist has for the past decade and a half been involved with surgery for resection of the acoustic neurinoma. A more proper name for this tumor is vestibular schwannoma since it originates from the Schwann cells of either the superior or inferior vestibular nerve.

A small acoustic neurinoma (2 cm) is best removed by way of the translabyrinthine route. The operation is performed in a relatively short time and is attended with low morbidity and mortality rates. The one exception to this rule would be an acoustic neurinoma in a patient who is deaf in the other ear. In this instance, a suboccipital approach should be used in an attempt to preserve the hearing.

A total resection of a small acoustic neurinoma can be accomplished through the translabyrinthine route with a 75% chance for preservation of facial nerve function. This figure is in contrast to the below 20% usually reported when the tumor is approached from the posterior route. The intrameatal portion and petrous extensions of the tumor can be resected only through the translabyrinthine route. The importance of total removal cannot be overemphasized, for the mortality rate in patients with recurrent acoustic neurinomas rises sharply.

Total removal of a larger acoustic neurinoma (4 cm and larger) by way of the translabyrinthine route may not be practical, for the exposure of that portion of the tumor adherent to the brain stem and the exposure of vital arteries and cranial nerves may be difficult and hazardous. When the tumor is large, the translabyrinthine approach may be used for resection of the intrapetrous portion of the tumor, dissection of the intrapetrous and intracranial portions of the facial nerve, decompression of the tumor, and resection of the posterior surface of the petrous pyramid to the sigmoid portion of the lateral sinus in order to facilitate the suboccipital approach.

493

To complete the removal of the tumor, the suboccipital craniotomy is performed 1 to 2 weeks following the translabyrinthine procedure. This two-stage resection for large acoustic neurinomas is the safest and offers the patient the best chance for survival, preservation of the facial nerve, and complete removal of the tumor.

More recently, a one-stage suboccipital approach has been in vogue for resection of a large acoustic neurinoma (and in some institutions all acoustic neurinomas). This approach uses the combined efforts of the neurosurgeon and the otolaryngologist. We have used this approach for approximately 3 years. Recently, I compared the one-stage postoccipital approach to the two-stage translabyrinthine-suboccipital approach and found that the instance of total tumor removal is not as great with the one-stage approach. The instance of facial nerve injury is nearly doubled, and the incidence and severity of complications have increased along with the duration of hospitalization. It is thus my conclusion, at this time, that the two-stage procedure is the technique of choice.

The diagnosis and successful resection of an acoustic neurinoma is dependent upon a team effort. The team should include an audiologist, roentgenologist, otoneurologist, neurosurgeon, and otolaryngologist. Once the diagnostic procedures have been completed, the case should be reviewed at a meeting of all members of the team. It is my experience and that of my colleagues that all acoustic neurinomas should be approached first by the translabyrinthine route. The neurosurgeon should be present for the intracranial portion of this operation, or at least to inspect the field following the total resection of a small acoustic tumor. If the suboccipital approach is required as a second-stage procedure, the otolaryngologist should be present for that portion of the operation having to do with the facial nerve. Often he can be of valuable assistance with the identification and dissection of the lateral portion of this nerve.

Diagnosis

Advances in audiology have contributed considerably to the diagnosis of acoustic neurinomas. Since there is no specific pattern of audiologic findings, complete testing is necessary. For the most part this evaluation will either exclude the possibility of the presence of an acoustic tumor or present evidence which should initiate the stimulus to embark upon other diagnostic studies.

Audiologic Testing. For proper organization and simplicity it is best to divide the audiologic testing into six categories. Approximately 50% of patients with acoustic tumors will present positive findings in all of them. These categories are as follows:

1. *Testing with whispered and spoken voice.* With the patient's unaffected ear masked with a Bárány noise apparatus, phonetically balanced words are spoken at a distance of 1 foot from the patient. A moderate or marked loss of discrimination will be quite apparent. If the hearing loss is great, the use of a speaking tube is of value in detecting discrimination loss.
2. *Testing with a tuning fork.* If an acoustic neurinoma is present, it is obvious that the Weber test will show lateralization to the uninvolved ear. The reaction to the Rinne test should be positive, but should show a reduced bone and air conduction time. A marked increase of the bone

conduction time is indicative of tone decay. The Bing test, which is performed by placing the tuning fork over the mastoid process and intermittently occluding the external auditory canal, is of value. With a conductive hearing loss the patient notices very little or no difference in the hearing with the canal occluded, but with a sensorineural hearing loss he will usually state that bone conduction is louder when the ear canal is occluded. The tuning forks often give an excellent indication as to the presence of recruitment. This test is performed by lightly brushing 512, 1024, and 2048 tuning forks. With any significant hearing loss the patient will usually not hear one or all of these tuning forks. Unless the hearing loss is very severe, the patient will hear a tuning fork which has been moderately tapped with a rubber hammer. A positive reaction for recruitment is evident if the patient withdraws from the sound or states it is too loud or uncomfortable when the tuning fork, which has been struck by a sharp blow with the rubber hammer, is placed next to his ear.

3. *Audiogram.* Johnson and House, in their evaluation of pure-tone air-conduction threshold tests, in a series of 46 patients with acoustic neurinoma, found that there was no specific pattern associated with the tumor; 67.4% of the patients demonstrated a high-tone hearing loss, 24% a flat-tone loss, 4.3% a low-tone loss, and 4.3% a trough-shaped loss. Seventy-five percent of patients with acoustic neurinomas will have a type 3 or 4 Bekesy tracing. In a large series of these patients, at least 5% will have normal hearing. This is understandable, for the tumor does not involve or exert pressure on the cochlear nerve, nor does it interfere with the blood supply to the cochlea. Normal hearing or a slight hearing loss is not necessarily indicative of a small tumor.

4. *Recruitment.* Recruitment (determined by the alternate binaural loudness balanced test), which may or may not be present, is useful in differentiating cochlear from retrocochlear disease. Usually there is no recruitment when a neural lesion is present. Approximately 10% of patients with acoustic neurinomas, however, will have complete recruitment. Many others will demonstrate partial recruitment. This is quite understandable since an acoustic tumor may interfere with hearing, either by pressure on, or with involvement of, the cochlear nerve producing a neural-type loss. On the other hand, the tumor may interfere with the blood supply to the cochlea and thus produce an end-organ lesion.

5. *SISI (short increment sensitivity index) test.* This should be performed in all patients suspected of having an acoustic tumor. In the test a steady ring is administered at 20 decibels above the threshold and increased at 1 decibel increments. As a rule a cochlear lesion will respond to a 1-decibel increase in loudness. On the other hand, approximately 70% of patients with acoustic tumors will not respond and have a low (0 to 20%) Sisi score.

6. *Discrimination score.* A speech test should be conducted using the standard spondees and PB words. In approximately 70% of acoustic neurinoma patients the discrimination score will be at a 30% or lower level. Approximately 20% of the patients will show fairly good discrimination (60 to 100%). The remaining 10% will demonstrate a discrimination score between 30 and 60%.

Vestibular Testing. Approximately 95% of patients with acoustic neurinoma will show some evidence of vestibular dysfunction. Vertigo is usually not the presenting complaint associated with an acoustic neurinoma. Some symptoms suggestive of vestibular dysfunction can be elicited in approximately 80% of the patients; the remaining 20% will have no history of vertigo. A small percentage of patients will give a history of episodic vertigo. At least 6% of the patients with a positive history of vestibular dysfunction will admit only to a sensation of unsteadiness rather than that of true vertigo.

Caloric Test. The minimal caloric test is the first test used to determine vestibular function, for it is less apt to produce side effects than are the others. If the results of this testing show no abnormality on either side and equal response on both sides, additional testing is not indicated. The minimal caloric test is performed with the patient's head inclined backward at an angle of 60 degrees; 20 cc of water (at a temperature of 80° F) are instilled into the external auditory canal in 20 seconds. If there is no response to this test, then an icewater (Kobrak) test is performed. Icewater (5cc) is instilled into the external auditory canal with the patient's head inclined backward at a 60-degree angle. If there is no response, then 10 cc and finally 20 cc of icewater are instilled into the ear canal. No response to 20 cc of icewater is indicative of nonfunction.

Electronystagmography. Electronystagmography is of some value, but there are no consistent characteristic findings for localization of lesions. It will more readily demonstrate spontaneous nystagmus. Tracings are obtained after irrigating the ear canal with water both above and below the normal body temperature. The degree and type of response is recorded. The greatest value of electronystagmography is that it produces a permanent record which can be referred to, especially for comparison with future testing.

Trigeminal Nerve. The corneal reflexes are said to be absent in approximately 60% of patients with acoustic neurinoma. With careful testing, at least some slight degree of decreased facial sensation can be elicited in 30% of the patients. As a general rule there is normal fifth nerve function when the size of the tumor is less than 2 cm.

Facial Nerve. Less than 10% of patients with acoustic neurinomas will show either decreased function or irritability of the facial nerve. A loss of sensation in the posterior wall of the external auditory canal is rather difficult to evaluate. When pronounced, it should increase the index of suspicion that there is a lesion involving or compressing the facial nerve.

Hyperacusis is not a common finding. This may be confused with positive recruitment.

Pulec and House report that two thirds of patients with confirmed acoustic tumors had decreased taste function as determined by the electric taste-tester. Most of these patients were not aware of this loss, and only 8% showed a noticeable decreased taste.

The tear test (Schirmer) provides an evaluation of the parasympathetic fibers which accompany the facial nerve from the superior salivatory nucleus. The test is performed (Pulec) with two strips of filter paper 1 cm in width. Each is folded 5 mm from one end and placed over a lower lid. Normally 2 cm of filter paper will be saturated with tears in 1 minute. The unaffected side, of course, serves as a good control. Approximately 60% of the patients will show decreased tearing on the side of the lesion.

FIGURE 11.1. *X-ray diagnosis of acoustic neurinoma.*

a. Petrous apices viewed through the orbits in a patient with a one-year history of unilateral sensorineural hearing loss associated with poor discrimination and tone decay and absent caloric response. The left (arrow) appears to be very slightly enlarged as compared with the right.

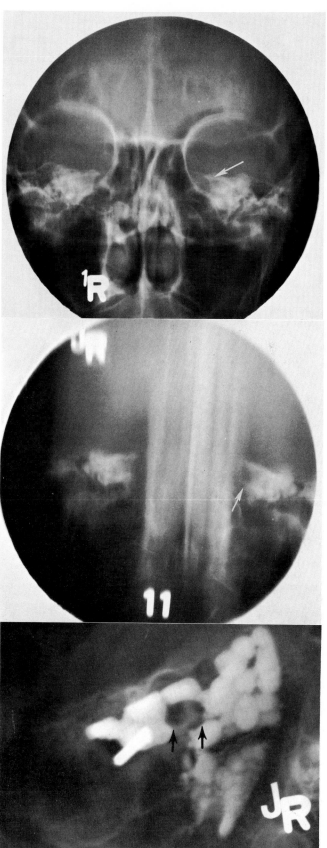

b. Laminogram demonstrating evidence of destruction (arrow). This also is not conclusive evidence of a tumor.

c. A contrast study clearly outlines a 1.5-cm tumor at the orifice of the internal auditory canal (arrows). Since the internal auditory canal did not appear to be enlarged, the tumor was resected by the translabyrinthine route with preservation of the function of the facial nerve.

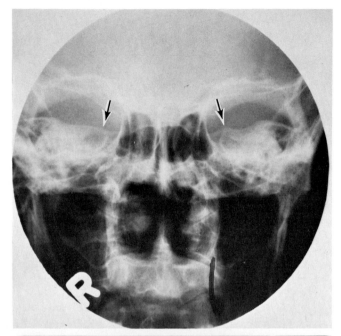

FIGURE 11.2.   *X-ray diagnosis of acoustic neurinoma (continued).*

a. An x ray of the petrous bone through the orbits does not show definite enlargement of the internal auditory canal (arrows) in a patient with clinical evidence of acoustic neurinoma. Laminograms also gave inconclusive evidence.

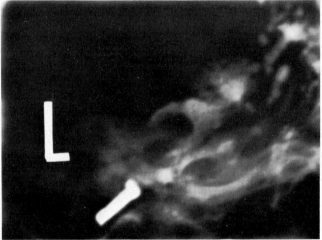

b. A contrast study, however, outlines a 2-cm tumor, which was resected by way of the translabyrinthine route with preservation of facial nerve function.

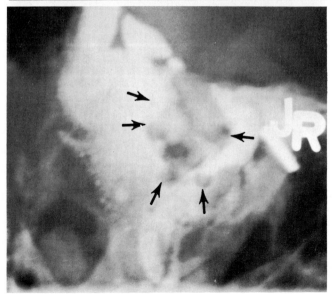

FIGURE 11.3.   *X-ray diagnosis of acoustic neurinoma (continued).*

a. Contrast study in a patient with a 10-year history of progressive sensorineural hearing loss and obvious clinical evidence of an acoustic neurinoma. The irregular outline is indicative of a multiloculated tumor or a tumor surrounded by cysts.

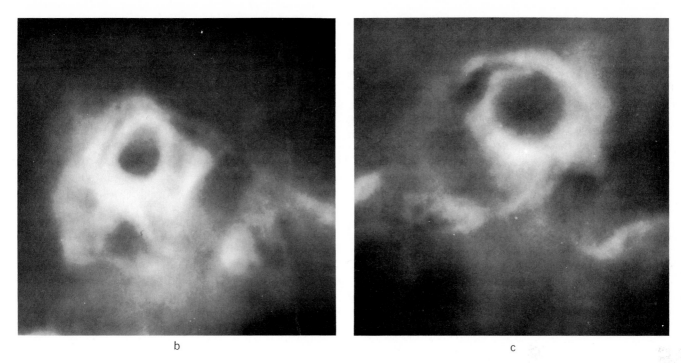

b

c

FIGURE 11.3 (Continued).

b and c. Lateral polytomography through the internal auditory canals of another patient. The normal left side (b) is compared with the enlarged right canal (c).

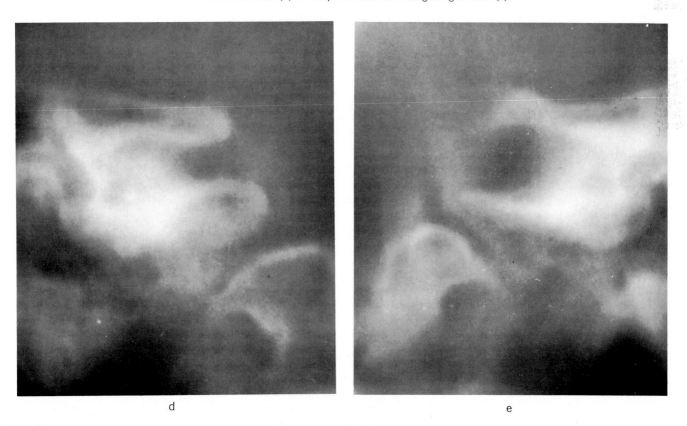

d

e

d and e. Anteroposterior polytomography of the internal auditory meatus. d is normal, and e is decidedly enlarged. A 2- x 3-cm right acoustic neurinoma was resected by the translabyrinthine route, with preservation of facial nerve function.

Other Cranial Nerves. Involvement of the ninth and tenth cranial nerves will be manifested by a decreased palatal or pharyngeal reflex and a vocal cord paralysis on the side of the lesion. Weakness or paralysis of the tongue musculature represents an involvement of the twelfth cranial nerve.

Involvement of the ninth, tenth, eleventh, and twelfth cranial nerves is evidence that the tumor has increased in size in an inferior and posterior direction and in the region of the jugular foramen. Cerebellar signs are rare; when manifest they signify the presence of a large tumor. The signs usually associated with cerebellar compression are past-pointing, a disturbance in the gait, or dysdiadochokinesia. As the size of the lesion increases, there may be signs of brain-stem compression, herniation of the cerebellar tonsils into the foramen magnum, increased cerebrospinal fluid pressure with resultant papilledema, and visual disturbance.

Spinal Fluid and Perilymph Protein Determination. An acoustic neurinoma does not necessarily cause a rise in the protein level of the spinal fluid. In 25% of the patients the spinal fluid protein value is less than 50 mg per 100 cc of fluid. Usually a normal protein level in a patient with an acoustic neurinoma denotes a relatively small tumor.

For perilymph protein determination, perilymph fluid is aspirated through a perforation made in the foot plate of the stapes. This test should not be performed if other evidence points to a positive diagnosis of an acoustic tumor or when the hearing is normal or slightly decreased. In a patient with an acoustic neurinoma the perilymph protein level is usually well in excess of 1000 mg per 100 cc.

X-ray Study. Of all the diagnostic procedures, radiographic evaluation is the most valuable. Routine x rays of the petrous bone should be taken if there is even a slight degree of suspicion that the patient has an acoustic tumor. These should include petrous views by way of the orbits, views at right angle to the long axis (Stenver views), and 30-degree angle fronto-occipital projections (Chamberlain-Towne views). Normally the diameter of the internal auditory canal is quite variable (2.5 to 11 mm) and there may be a 1- to 2-mm variation between the right and left sides. On the other hand, asymmetry between the two sides in a normal person is uncommon, and thus a 1-mm difference between the diameter of one internal auditory meatus and that of the other is significant, provided there is clinical evidence of the presence of an acoustic tumor. When a difference exists, laminograms or polytomography (Fig. 11.3) of the petrous bone are indicated. These will outline more clearly the differences in the diameters of the internal auditory canals and the areas of bone destruction.

If the index of suspicion of the presence of an acoustic tumor is high, contrast studies are indicated. This is especially true since the internal auditory canals are normal in 5% of persons with acoustic tumors. The myelography of the posterior fossa (Figs. 11.1–11.3) is by far the preferable contrast study. A pneumoencephalogram is indicated when the tumors are large.

Computed tomography has proven to be a very valuable technique to assist with the diagnosis of the acoustic neurinoma. The CT scan should follow polytomography in the diagnostic investigation of acoustic neurinomas for two reasons: The first is that CT scanning may demonstrate marked erosive changes in the bone whereas small changes are better appreciated by polytomography. Second, CT scanning should precede contrast study (Pantopaque cisternography), for residual Pantopaque droplets often interfere with CT scanning and in some cases cisternography may not be indicated for evaluation of the acoustic neurinoma. In cases

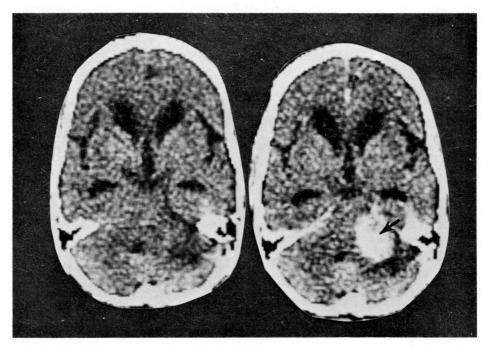

a

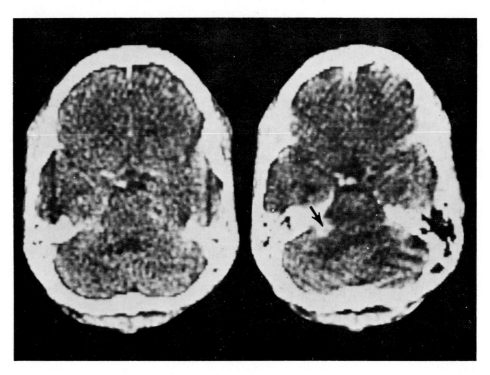

b

FIGURE 11.4.

   CT brain scan to confirm a strong suspicion of a right acoustic neurinoma.

   a. The large lesion is not shown in the plain study, but is quite clear with contrast enhancement (arrow).

   b. The plain CT scan (left) is normal. Contrast enhancement (right) clearly demonstrates a 1.5-cm mass medial to the left internal auditory canal (arrow).

where CT scanning is definitely positive and clinical features are suggestive of an angle tumor, operation may be planned without further study.

Parker and Davis report a 75% accuracy with the use of computed tomography for the diagnosis of an acoustic neurinoma. In this series, no intracanular lesions were visualized, and only 1 of 15 tumors less than 2 cm in the posterior fossa was diagnosed by CT scanning. The CT scanning is fairly accurate for the medium size tumors (2.0 to 3.0 cm). Only 4 of 16 tumors of this size had negative scans. CT scanning is quite accurate for large tumors. Only 2 of 45 large tumors were reported as negative. Both of these negative CT scans for large tumors were from patients who had undergone previous contrast studies.

Contrast enhanced scans have a much higher yield for demonstrating tumors as compared to plain scans. It is preferable, however, to perform a plain scan before one with contrast enhancement, for the former will sometimes permit differentiation of artifacts from tumor and meningioma from acoustic neurinoma (Figs. 11.4a and b).

Treatment

Middle Cranial Fossa Approach. This approach is similar to that used to approach the trigeminal ganglion. A window, approximately 4 cm square, is made in the squamous portion of the temporal bone. The temporal lobe dura is retracted superiorly after reducing the spinal fluid pressure. The greater superficial petrosal nerve is identified as it exits from the hiatus facialis on the anterior surface of the petrous pyramid. The bone over this nerve is removed by using a diamond bur and constant suction irrigation. The dissection is continued in a posterior direction, until the geniculate ganglion is identified. The bone superior to the facial nerve, medial to the geniculate ganglion, is removed in a similar fashion, until the internal auditory canal is identified. The roof of the internal auditory canal is removed, exposing the tumor.

This operation is technically difficult, for there is a fair chance of injury to the facial nerve as it is unroofed. The bony dissection is accomplished in an area between and very close to both the cochlea and the labyrinth. Injury to the internal auditory artery is another hazard and will result in loss of both auditory and vestibular function.

Translabyrinthine Approach to the Cerebellopontine Angle. *Anatomy.* The key to the translabyrinthine operation is a thorough knowledge of the anatomy of the petrous bone and its surrounding structures.

Figure 11.5a shows the anatomic relationships after the mastoid, middle ear, and labyrinth have been dissected. The important landmarks indicating the location of the horizontal portion of the facial nerve are the cochleariform process, incudal fossa, and the horizontal semicircular canal.

The ampullar ends of the horizontal and superior semicircular canals are close neighbors. The superior semicircular canal often extends above the level of the tegmen mastoideum. The common crus is deep and elusive. The posterior semicircular canal is found just posterior and at right angles to the horizontal semicircular canal.

The vertical portion of the facial nerve is found by a careful and thorough dissection of the superficial group of antero-inferior mastoid cells. The incudal fossa and digastric ridge are also useful landmarks.

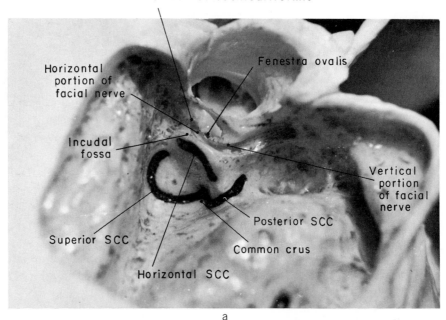

FIGURE 11.5. *Translabyrinthine approach to the internal auditory canal (right ear).*

a. Relationships of the semicircular canals and facial nerve. Note the close relationship between the ampullated ends of the superior and horizontal semicircular canals. The posterior canal is easily located behind, and at right angles to, the horizontal canal. The horizontal semicircular canal and incudal fossa provide landmarks in identifying the facial nerve.

b. The tegmen over the mastoid, as well as that over the antrum and posterior epitympanum, are in view.

Note the triangle formed by the labyrinth, tegmen mastoideum, and sigmoid sinus. The superior side of this triangle (between the labyrinth and sinodural angle) is known as Citelli's angle. This angle designates the position of the superior petrosal sinus at the junction of the dura of the middle and posterior cranial fossae.

The relationships of the cochleariform process, facial nerve, and horizontal semicircular canal are shown.

The digastric crest divides the superficial and deep groups of antero-inferior mastoid cells. Its anterior limit designates the inferior aspect of the vertical portion of the facial nerve.

The position of the sigmoid portion of the lateral sinus in relation to the labyrinth is variable. An anteriorly positioned sinus usually indicates underdevelopment of the mastoid cells and adds to the complexity of the operation.

The sinodural angle must be dissected (Fig. 11.5b). The tegmen over the dura of the posterior and middle fossae is identified. Citelli's angle, at the junction of the dural plates of the posterior and middle fossae is the landmark, in the mastoidectomy defect, for the superior petrosal sinus.

The superficial and deep groups of the antero-inferior mastoid cells are carefully dissected to determine the level of the jugular bulb and for location of the digastric crest.

A view of the posterior and middle cranial fossae is seen in Figure 11.6a. Of note are the branches of the middle meningeal artery, the sigmoid portion of the lateral sinus with the beginning of the jugular bulb, the superior and inferior petrosal sinuses, the anterior and posterior surfaces of the petrous pyramid, and the internal auditory meatus.

The translabyrinthine approach for small tumors is through the triangle bound by the superior petrosal sinus, the lateral sinus, and the jugular bulb.

The surgeon should have a clear mental picture of the components of the internal auditory meatus. A simple method of doing this is to visualize the internal auditory meatus as being divided into an upper and lower half by the horizontal crest (crista transversa).

The antero-inferior quadrant is occupied by the cochlear nerve. As would be expected from middle ear anatomy, the facial nerve enters the meatus (Fig. 11.6b) directly above in the anterosuperior quadrant.

Behind the facial nerve, in the posterosuperior quadrant, is the superior vestibular nerve with its branches to the utricle and horizontal and superior semicircular canals. There is a vertical crest between the superior vestibular nerve and the facial nerve.

The inferior vestibular nerve enters the meatus in the postero-inferior quadrant. It supplies the saccule. The nerve to the posterior semicircular canal usually enters behind the inferior vestibular nerve in a separate foramen.

Technique of Operation. The patient's auricle, postauricular region, and face are prepared and draped. The lower right quadrant of the abdomen is also prepared and draped so that an adipose autograft can be obtained in order to obliterate the mastoidectomy-labyrinthectomy defect following removal of the acoustic neurinoma (Fig. 11.7). The skin incision (Fig. 11.8) for the operation is made directly posterior to the entire length of the postauricular crease. It is extended superiorly over the temporal line and inferiorly over the mastoid process. The skin incision can be made with an electrosurgical knife, which, as a general rule, allows for excellent hemostasis (Fig. 11.9). The periosteum is elevated anteriorly, posteriorly, and superiorly so as to expose the entire superior and posterior rims of the bony external auditory canal, the temporal line, and the entire lateral surface of the mastoid process (Fig. 11.10).

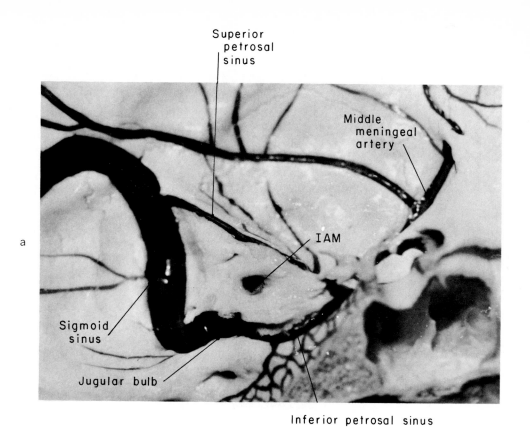

Superior
petrosal
sinus

Middle
meningeal
artery

a

IAM

Sigmoid
sinus

Jugular bulb

Inferior petrosal sinus

Crest dividing facial and
superior vestibular nerve

Nerve to utricle
(superior vestibular N.)

Facial nerve

Superior
semicircular canal

Horizontal
semicircular canal

b

Crista transversa

Nerve to saccule
(inferior vestibular N.)

Cochlea

Foramen singulare (posterior)

FIGURE 11.6

a. Intracranial view of the left internal auditory meatus (IAM). The exposure acquired using the translabyrinthine approach is that area bound by the sigmoid sinus posteriorly, the superior petrosal sinus superiorly, the internal auditory canal anteriorly, and the jugular bulb inferiorly.

b. The right internal auditory meatus. The crista transversa, crest between the facial and superior vestibular nerves, and the foramen singulare are important landmarks when identifying the components of the internal auditory meatus during the translabyrinthine approach to the acoustic neurinoma.

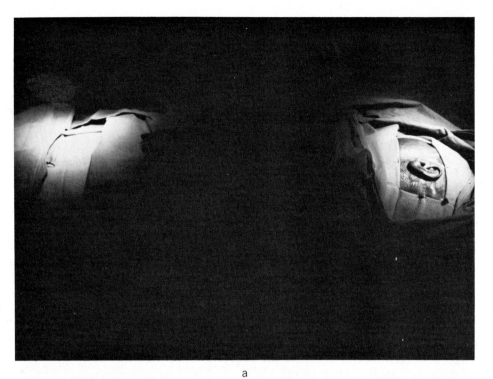

a

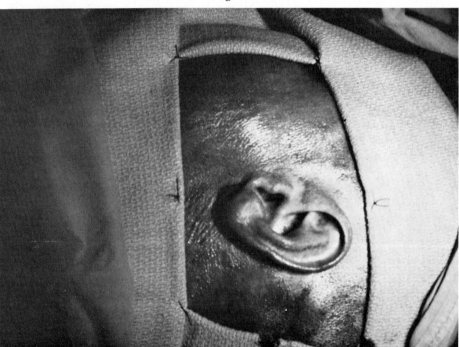

b

FIGURE 11.7.

a. The patient has been prepared for a translabyrinthine approach for resecting an acoustic neurinoma. It is important to leave exposed a portion of the face so that it will not be necessary for the surgeon to depend on others to monitor facial nerve function. The lower left abdomen is also prepared and draped so that an adipose tissue autograft can be obtained to obliterate the labyrinthectomy-mastoidectomy defect.

b. A close-up view of the technique for draping the auricle, postauricular region, and sufficient amount of the face so that the surgeon can monitor facial nerve function.

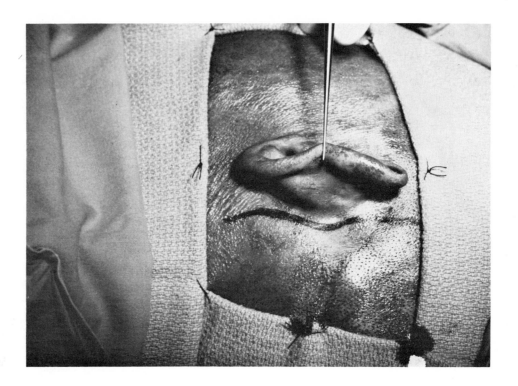

FIGURE 11.8.

The incision for the translabyrinthine approach extends slightly behind and along the full length of the postauricular crease. It then is extended up over the temporal line and down over the tip of the mastoid process.

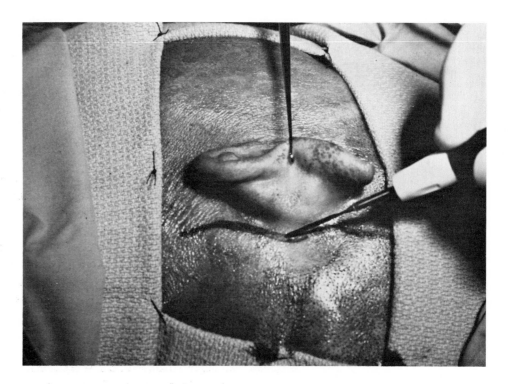

FIGURE 11.9.

The skin incision can be made with an electrosurgical knife in order to obtain better hemostasis.

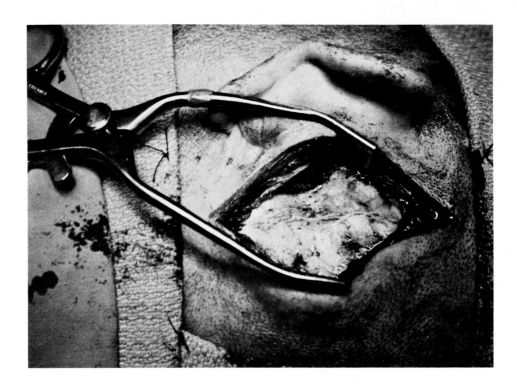

FIGURE 11.0.

   The periosteum is elevated anteriorly and posteriorly so as to have wide exposure and access to the posterior and superior bony external auditory canal walls and the root of the zygomatic portion of the temporal bone as well as the entire mastoid process and linea temporalis.

   The field for exposure can be accomplished using either one or two self-retaining retractors. It is imperative that all bleeding be controlled carefully by ligation of vessels and electrocautery in order to prevent blood flowing into the operative field as the cerebellopontine angle is approached and during resection of the acoustic neurinoma.

   A complete mastoidectomy is performed with dissection of all mastoid cell systems in an orderly fashion (Fig. 11.11). The anterior and posterior mastoid cells of the superior group are resected to expose the entire bony tegmen inferior and lateral to the middle cranial fossa, the sinodural angle, Citelli's angle (which identifies the position of the superior petrosal venous sinus), and the mastoid antrum.

   The superficial (behind the posterior bony wall of the external auditory canal) and deep (retrofacial) divisions of the anteroinferior group of mastoid cells are dissected so as to render the posterior external auditory canal wall as thin as possible, and to identify the vertical portion of the fallopian canal and the position of the digastric crest.

   The posteromedial mastoid cells (anterior, lateral, and posterior to the sigmoid portion of the lateral sinus) are removed in order to outline the entire bony plate over the sigmoid sinus and the bony plate anterior to the posterior cranial fossa dura. The latter bony plate (Trautmann's triangle) is triangular in shape and is outlined by Citelli's angle, the labyrinth and the sigmoid portion of the lateral sinus.

The mastoid antrum and the additus ad antrum are enlarged in order to expose the entire length of the horizontal semicircular canal and the short process of the incus. At this point a fenestration is made in the most prominent portion of the horizontal semicircular canal, using a diamond bur and constant suction irrigation (Fig. 11.12). Perilymph fluid is obtained for protein study if there is any doubt concerning the diagnosis of an acoustic neurinoma. The Silverstein micro-chemical kit for inner ear analysis can be used for this determination.

The horizontal semicircular canal is opened along its entire length with a cutting bur. By continuing the dissection directly posterior to the horizontal semi-circular canal, the posterior semicircular canal is easily identified, for its long axis is perpendicular to the direction of the dissection.

The ampullated end of the superior semicircular canal is found about 2 mm superior to the ampullated end of the horizontal semicircular canal (Fig. 11.13). The superior and posterior semicircular canals are opened exposing the common crus. As the bone becomes thin in this region, the endolymphatic duct can be identified, as it is passed medially to the common crus (Figs. 11.14 and 11.17).

The incus is removed in order to obtain a view of the horizontal portion of the fallopian canal in the middle ear space. The inferior portion of the horizontal semicircular canal is painstakingly removed to obtain maximum exposure and not injure the facial nerve. A large diamond bur with constant suction irrigation is best suited for this dissection. The facial nerve stimulator* (Fig. 11.15) is set at 2.0 V and tested for function by touching the temporalis muscle. The function of the nerve

*Richard's Manufacturing Co., Memphis, Tennessee

FIGURE 11.11.

A complete mastoidectomy has been performed. The superior group of mastoid cells have been resected, exposing the tegmen inferior and lateral to the middle cranial fossa dura from the sinodural angle to the antrum. The superficial group of the anterior inferior mastoid cells have been removed, exposing the bony posterior external auditory canal and the mastoid tip lateral to the digastric crest. The deep (retrofacial) mastoid cells have also been partially resected. The posteromedial cells are removed in order to expose the sigmoid sinus and bony plate anterior to the posterior cranial fossa dura. The angle at the junction of the middle and posterior cranial fossa dural plate (Citelli's angle) identifies the relative position of the superior petrosal venous sinus. The perilabyrinthine cells have not been disturbed. The horizontal semicircular canal and short process of the incus can be visualized.

a. Anterior superior cells
b. Perilabyrinthine cells
c. Tegmen middle fossa
d. Citelli's angle (superior petrosal sinus)
e. Bony plate anterior to posterior fossa dura
f. Posterior superior cells
g. Sigmoid sinus plate
h. Posteromedial cells
i. Digastric crest
j. Anterior inferior cells
k. Macewen's triangle (Henle's spine)
l. Horizontal semicircular canal
m. Short process of incus (Montgomery, 1973).

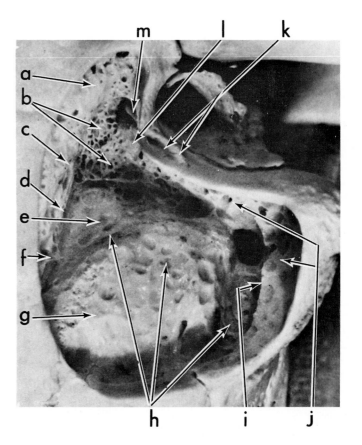

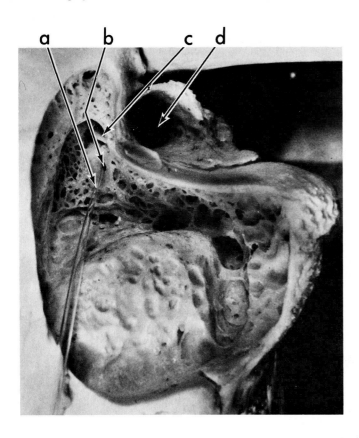

FIGURE 11.12.

A fenestration has been made in the horizontal semicircular canal in order to obtain perilymph fluid for protein study when necessary to verify the diagnosis of acoustic neurinoma. A capillary pipette is inserted into the fenestration.
   a. Capillary pipette in fenestration
   b. Horizontal semicircular canal (fenestration)
   c. Short process of incus
   d. External auditory canal (Montgomery, 1973).

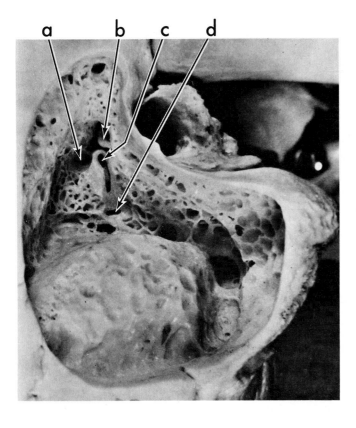

FIGURE 11.13.

The horizontal semicircular canal has been opened along its entire length. The posterior semicircular canal is identified by continuing the dissection directly posterior to the long axis of the horizontal semicircular canal. The ampullated end of the superior semicircular canal is found approximately 2 mm superior to the ampullated end of the horizontal semicircular canal. The heads of the malleus and incus can be visualized
   a. Ampullated end of superior semicircular canal
   b. Head of malleus and incus
   c. Ampullated end of horizontal semicircular canal
   d. Posterior semicircular canal (Montgomery, 1973).

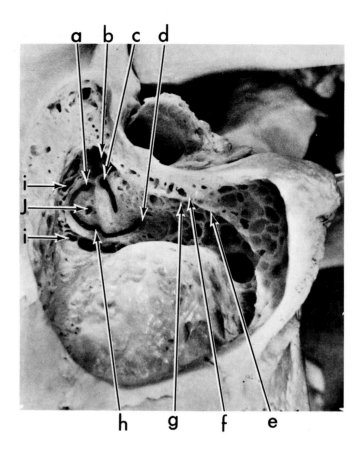

FIGURE 11.14.

The entire length of all three semicircular canals has been opened. The superior and posterior semicircular canals are joined posteriorly to form the common crus. The foramen for the subarcuate artery is identified. Before proceeding with further dissection it is best to remove the incus so the position of the horizontal portion of the facial nerve in the middle ear can be visualized. This view demonstrates the position of Korner's septum, which separates the superficial and deep groups of the anterior and inferior mastoid cells. The plane of Korner's septum is continuous with the digastric crest.

    a. Superior semicircular canal
    b. Head of malleus
    c. Horizontal semicircular canal
    d. Posterior semicircular canal
    e. Korner's septum
    f. Superficial group of anterior inferior cells
    g. Deep group of anterior inferior cells
    h. Common crus
    i. Perilabyrinthine cells
    j. Subarcuate artery foramen (Montgomery, 1973).

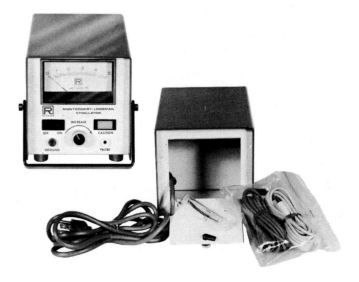

FIGURE 11.15.

Montgomery-Lingeman nerve stimulator.

stimulator can also be tested by touching the fallopian canal covering the horizontal portion of the facial nerve in the middle ear. The dissection for exposure of the fallopian canal inferior to the horizontal semicircular canal is continued with the nerve stimulator set at 1.0 V or less. As the facial nerve is approached, it can be readily stimulated by way of a branch of the stylomastoid artery which perforates the posterolateral aspect of the fallopian canal at its second genu. With this technique, the bony covering of the facial nerve can be thinned to a fraction of a millimeter (Fig. 11.16). The pinkish color of the nerve sheath is visualized through the thin layer of bone.

Having made certain of the exact location of the horizontal and vertical portions of the facial nerve, the medial aspect of the horizontal semicircular canal is removed in order to expose the vestibule of the labyrinth. This dissection includes bone medial to the horizontal portion of the fallopian canal. Exposure of the vestibule is increased as the superior and posterior semicircular canals are removed. Maximum exposure of the vestibule is essential before attempting to locate the internal auditory canal.

The bone anterior to the vestibule is gradually thinned, using a large diamond bur and constant suction irrigation until the dural reflection inside the posterior wall of the internal auditory meatus is identified (Fig. 11.17). The grayish color of the dura in this fenestration in contrast to the surrounding white bone reassures the surgeon of his position.

As a general rule, the tumor fills the internal auditory canal and can be identified anterior to the dural reflection. Even though the facial nerve is found superior and anterior to the fenestration in the posterior canal wall, it can be

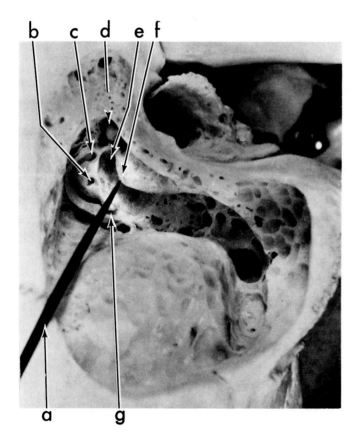

FIGURE 11.16.

The horizontal semicircular canal has been removed, exposing the horizontal portion and second genu of the fallopian canal. This dissection is monitored, using the nerve stimulator. The superior aspect of the vertical portion of the fallopian canal is also identified.

   a. Insulated tip from nerve stimulator
   b. Foramen for subarcuate artery
   c. Superior semicircular canal
   d. Head of malleus
   e. Vestibule of labyrinth
   f. Fallopian canal
   g. Posterior semicircular canal (Montgomery, 1973).

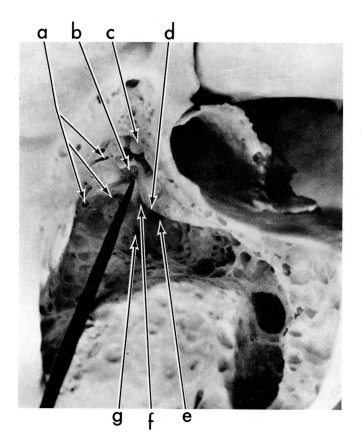

FIGURE 11.17.

The remaining semicircular canals have been removed and the wall of the vestibule thinned in all directions. A small fenestration has been made in the posterior wall of the internal auditory meatus, exposing the dural reflection in this region. As the bone of the vestibule is thinned posteroinferiorly, the jugular bulb may be exposed. The bony canal of the endolymphatic duct has been exposed, as this duct passes directly medial to the common crus.

    a. Perilabyrinthine cells
    b. Fenestration posterior wall of internal auditory meatus
    c. Head of malleus
    d. Fallopian canal
    e. Bony covering superior to dome of jugular bulb
    f. Vestibule of labyrinth
    g. Endolymphatic duct (Montgomery, 1973).

stimulated through the tumor with the nerve stimulator set at somewhere between 1.0 and 2.0 V. This check further assures the surgeon that his operation is properly directed.

The bone superior and inferior to the fenestration in the posterior wall of the internal auditory canal is carefully removed. In cases where there has been little or no erosion of the posterior wall of the internal auditory canal this dissection can be somewhat tedious. Encountering a pneumatized petrous tip and an enlarged internal auditory canal greatly facilitates this dissection. After the internal auditory canal has been exposed posterosuperiorly and posteroinferiorly, there remains a bridge of bone posteromedially which represents the posterior tip of the orifice of the internal auditory canal. This segment of bone can often be removed as one piece, especially in cases where the internal auditory canal has been markedly widened by the tumor.

The dural reflection covering the posterior aspect of the tumor and the vestibular nerves in the internal auditory canal is incised in a lateromedial direction, using a dural knife. A flap of this dura is reflected superiorly, in order to identify the facial nerve. Often it is possible to identify the facial nerve by reflecting the tumor inferiorly with a small, flat elevator (Fig. 11.18). If the tumor in the canal is quite large, it may not be possible to identify the facial nerve positively at this point. In such cases the nerve stimulator is gradually reduced until there is no stimulation of the facial nerve when the tumor or the vestibular nerves are touched. This setting is usually 0.1 or 0.2 V. The vestibular nerves are sectioned as they are identified. Often this is difficult if one or both are incorporated in the substance of the tumor.

a b c d e f g

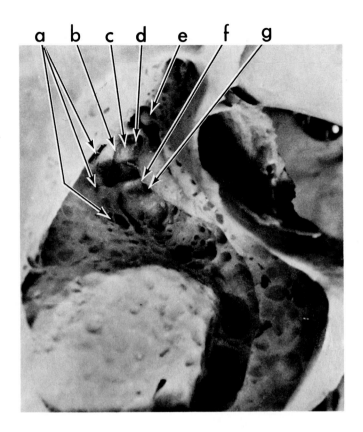

FIGURE 11.18.

The bony posterior wall of the internal auditory meatus has been removed, exposing the posterior aspect of the intracanalicular position of the tumor. At this point the facial nerve can be visualized by retracting the tumor inferiorly with a small, thin elevator, provided the nerve has not been flattened or displaced anteriorly. The position of the facial nerve can be verified by stimulating it with the nerve stimulator set at 0.1 V. A few perilabyrinthine cells which extend to the petrous tip remain to be dissected. The posterior aspect of the transverse crest can be visualized.

     a. Perilabyrinthine cells
     b. Posterosuperior rim of internal auditory canal
     c. Tumor (posterior surface)
     d. Transverse crest of internal auditory meatus
     e. Head of malleus
     f. Fallopian canal
     g. Region of jugular bulb dome (Montgomery, 1973).

Small portions of the tumor are resected superiorly until the facial nerve can be positively identified by a direct stimulus with the nerve stimulator set at 0.1 V or less, and by visualization. The facial nerve is thus identified by its relative antero-superior position in the internal auditory canal and by quantitatively stimulating it with the nerve stimulator during the dissection. The remainder of the tumor in the internal auditory canal is removed in its entirety to the internal auditory meatus. The vestibular (if not already sectioned) and cochlear nerves are sectioned as they exit from the porus acusticus. As a general rule, spinal fluid leakage is minimal or absent during the removal of the portion of the tumor in the internal auditory canal.

The medial aspect of the bony plate covering the posterior cranial fossa dura is partially removed using a diamond bur to expose the portion of the tumor medial to the internal auditory canal. Unless this portion of the tumor is small, it is best to resect the intracanalicular portion prior to opening the posterior fossa dura. By so doing, the course of the facial nerve can be directly visualized and its relation (which is quite variable) to the intracranial portion of the tumor can be more accurately speculated.

A profuse flow of cerebrospinal fluid occurs as the posterior fossa dura is incised unless the size of the tumor is very large. The spinal fluid is allowed to escape freely until the cerebrospinal fluid pressure has been reduced and the flow is minimal.

If the intracranial portion of the tumor is small (up to 2 cm), the remainder of the dissection is not difficult. The tumor capsule is easily separated from the facial nerve by reflecting the tumor in a posterior and inferior direction. Those instruments* designed for pterygomaxillary surgery are well suited for this dissection.

*Richard's Manufacturing Company, Memphis, Tennessee

The tumor is reflected superiorly in order to visualize the anteroinferior cerebellar artery. Before removing the tumor, the facial nerve must be dissected free so that it can be visualized at the point where it is attached to the brain stem. The eighth cranial nerve, which is attached to the medial aspect of the tumor, is sectioned at its exit from the brain stem using middle ear scissors, and the tumor is removed (Fig. 11.19).

With a large tumor, an intracapsular resection of the tumor must be accomplished to reduce its size. If the tumor is larger than 3 cm in diameter, or if at any point it is detected to be attached to the brain stem or lower cranial nerves, a subtotal intracapsular resection is accomplished and the field is prepared to facilitate the subsequent second stage suboccipital operation. The facial nerve is separated from the tumor to the brain stem, if possible. The posterior aspect of the facial nerve is covered with a small strip of either blue or green rayon material (Fig. 11.20). This "tag" will greatly facilitate identification of the facial nerve as it is approached by the suboccipital route. A complete removal of the bony plate anterior to the posterior fossa dura will also facilitate the second stage operation.

All bleeding points must be controlled after the tumor has been removed. This procedure often requires considerable patience. A few strands (and no more) of Surgicel, about 3 mm in length, are placed on a bleeding point, using alligator forceps. These strands are immediately covered with a small cottonoid pad, which has been saturated with thrombin solution. After 5 minutes the small pad is teased away. Other techniques for hemostasis include the use of small silver clips and cautery applied through an insulated #5 or #20 suction tip, or alligator forceps.

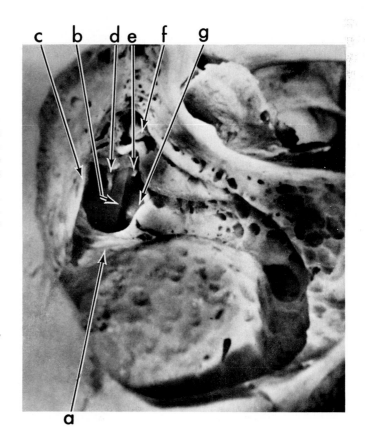

FIGURE 11.19.

The posterior lip of the internal auditory meatus and a portion of the bony plate anterior to the posterior fossa dura has been resected. The intracanalicular portion of the tumor has been resected with the vestibular and cochlear nerves. The facial nerve remains intact. The cells superior to the internal auditory meatus extend to the petrous tip. The transverse crest of the internal auditory meatus can be visualized. Sufficient exposure for resectioning the intracranial portion of the tumor has been accomplished. Additional posterior fossa dura plate can be removed if necessary.

    a. Posterior fossa dura plate
    b. Facial nerve
    c. Position of superior petrosal sinus
    d. Superior wall of internal auditory canal
    e. Transverse crest of internal auditory meatus
    f. Head of malleus
    g. Inferior wall of internal auditory canal (Montgomery, 1973).

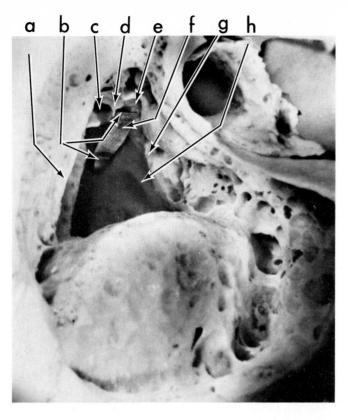

FIGURE 11.20.

    The field has been prepared for a second stage suboccipital approach for removal of a large acoustic neurinoma. The facial nerve has been tagged by placing a small strip of blue rayon cloth against its posterior surface. The bony plate anterior to the posterior fossa dura has been entirely removed. The position of the superior petrosal venous sinus is indicated as well as that of the dome of the jugular bulb.

    a. Superior petrosal venous sinus
    b. Facial nerve
    c. Mastoid cells extending to the petrous tip
    d. Anterior aspect—superior wall of internal auditory canal
    e. Transverse crest of internal auditory meatus
    f. Blue rayon cloth strip
    g. Region of jugular bulb
    h. Opposite internal auditory canal (Montgomery, 1973).

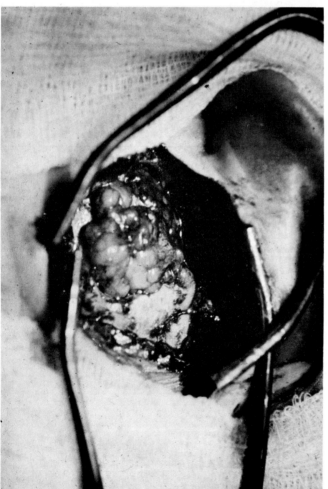

FIGURE 11.21.

    The acoustic neurinoma has been resected. Both the mastoidectomy and labyrinthectomy defects have been obliterated with adipose tissue immediately after it is obtained from the subcutaneous abdominal wall.

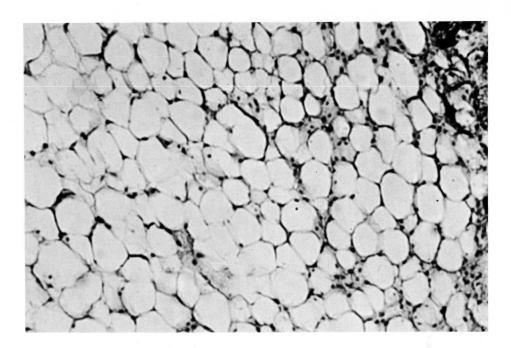

FIGURE 11.22

   A tissue section from an adipose autograft one month after being implanted into the mastoid cavity. There was no loss of adipose tissue and very little fibrous tissue.

   The entire field, including the mastoid, is packed while obtaining subcutaneous adipose tissue through a horizontal lower left abdomen incision. The packing is removed and the intracranial space observed for at least 15 minutes to make certain the cerebrospinal fluid is clear and that no bleeding occurs.

   A small piece of adipose tissue about 2 cm in diameter is placed in the labyrinthine defect. A second piece is inserted to completely fill the mastoidectomy defect. It is imperative, when obtaining this adipose tissue, that it not be injured by instrumentation. The adipose tissue serves to prevent postoperative contamination and leakage of spinal fluid (Figs. 11.21 and 11.22).

   The incision is closed in three layers and not drained (Fig. 11.23). A gauze wick is inserted into the internal auditory canal and a mastoidectomy-type dressing is applied.

   Postoperative Course. The postoperative course is similar to that for a mastoidectomy. The patient should be carefully observed for early signs of central nervous system complications. The usual duration of hospitalization is 1 week.

   Suboccipital Translabyrinthine Approach. Resection of large acoustic neurinomas, in excess of 4 cm in diameter, is rather difficult and hazardous by way of the translabyrinthine route. It is difficult to identify the antero-inferior cerebellar artery, and that portion of the tumor attached to the brain stem must be approached at right angles. Therefore, injury to the lower cranial nerves is likely. As a result, my colleagues and I have adopted a two-stage technique for resection of large tumors.

   The first-stage operation consists of a dissection and tagging of the facial nerve, decompression of the posterior fossa, and partial resection of the acoustic neurinoma. Of prime importance is the identification of the facial nerve. This is sometimes difficult when the tumor is large, for the nerve can be displaced and

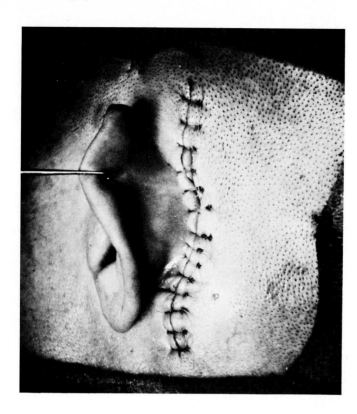

FIGURE 11.23.

The skin incision is closed in three layers without drainage.

may be broadened and thinned by pressure from the tumor. The tumor is carefully resected from the posterior aspect of the facial nerve, both in the internal auditory canal and intracranially. As much of the tumor is removed as is necessary for decompression of the posterior fossa. This is for the most part an intracapsular resection. It is important to remove as much bone as is possible on the posterior surface of the petrous pyramid in order to facilitate the dissection during the second-stage operation.

At the termination of the translabyrinthine operation, a narrow strip of blue rayon is placed on the posterior surface of the facial nerve. This is extremely useful as a "tag" for identification of the facial nerve during the second-stage procedure. The labyrinthectomy and mastoidectomy defects are obliterated with an adipose autograft, and the mastoid incision is closed without drainage.

The second-stage suboccipital operation should be performed as soon as the patient has recovered from the first-stage procedure. An interval of 1 to 2 weeks is usually required. During the second operation, the remainder of the tumor is dissected from its attachment to the lower cranial nerves, cerebellum, and brain stem. The rayon strip is identified and removed from the posterior surface of the facial nerve. The nerve stimulator, with a long insulated probe, is invaluable when outlining the course of the facial nerve from the brain stem to the internal auditory meatus. Once the course has been ascertained that portion of the tumor, which may extend forward and be attached to the fifth cranial nerve, can be readily resected.

A temporary facial paralysis may follow the resection of a large tumor. Anesthesia of the cornea is often present with large tumors. The cornea is thus in great danger of injury. The administration of antibiotic eye ointment is essential, beginning with the immediate postoperative period. If there is no evidence of return of facial nerve function in 3 to 5 days, a lateral tarsorrhaphy is indicated.

SURGERY OF THE AURICLE

Congenital Lop Ears

The term "congenital lop ears" covers a variety of anomalies of the external ear. Attempts to classify these various types of ear problems are confusing because one deformity may differ slightly from another and yet shade ever so slightly into still another category. There are, however, five basic defects, each with variations, which the surgeon will observe when analyzing congenital lop ear. These are:

1. Poor definition or absence of a component part of an ear, most often the anthelix
2. An excess of cartilage in the concha either uniformly, superiorly, or inferiorly
3. Abnormally small ears (microtia)
4. Excessive size of the ears (macrotia) or of a component part of the ears
5. Disparity in the size or shape of one ear as compared with the other

Many surgical techniques have been devised and advocated for the correction of these defects. That no one surgical procedure is a "cure-all" can be attested to by the number available. Each surgeon, therefore, should have a workable knowledge of a few basic procedures which he can vary to correct the unique defects of any particular ear.

The minimum age for surgical correction of lop ears should be around 4 to 5 years. Prior to this age, most children are not conscious of any deformity. At any earlier age the auricular cartilage may not be mature enough to make the procedure technically feasible.

(a)   **(b)**

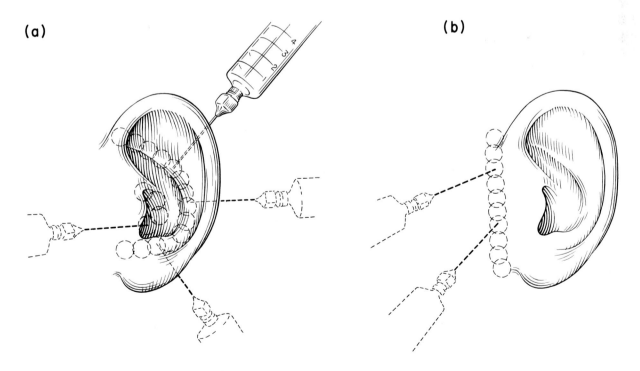

FIGURE 11.24

a and b. Technique of local anesthetic infiltration for surgery of the auricle.

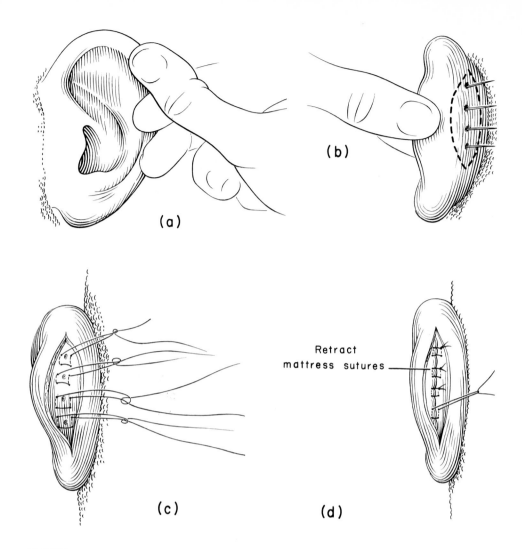

FIGURE 11.25. *Mattress-suture otoplasty for correction of lop ear (Mustarde technique).*

a and b. The ear is folded into the desired position, and the new anthelix is outlined with needles. An elliptical incision is made, and the surrounding skin is undermined.

c. Mattress sutures are placed to bridge a gap in the cartilage.

d. The sutures are tied as the ear is retracted into the desired contour.

Preoperative Preparation. Unless the patient is in his late teens, general anesthesia will prove invaluable. Local anesthesia can be used with older patients. Xylocaine with epinephrine is infiltrated circumferentially around the ear and around the external auditory meatus (Fig. 11.24). This works quite nicely with a well-premedicated patient.

After the patient is "prepped," he is draped so that contamination of an ear, either prior to the operation or following it, is avoided. This can be accomplished by placing a sterile stockinette, with holes cut for the ears, over the patient's head. A sterile sheet is placed under the head. After one ear has been operated upon, sterile batting is applied while working on the second. Many surgeons now prefer to use sterile adhesive drapes which are applied easily and provide a view of the patient's features.

Various Surgical Techniques. Space does not permit mention of the many procedures that have been devised for correction of the numerous auricular defects. Three widely used techniques will be described. A variation of one of these techniques will usually suffice to correct most cases of lop ears adequately. The surgeon's ability to use the right procedure for the right case and his own innovations will make the difference between mediocre and good results.

Mattress Suture Otoplasty (Mustarde Technique) (Fig. 11.25). This is a simple method which has recently become quite popular.

The ear is folded into the desired position (Fig. 11.25a) and straight needles are passed through the apex of the "new" anthelix (Fig. 11.25b). The needles are tipped with methylene blue and withdrawn, leaving a series of dots along the posterior surface of the apex of the new anthelix. An elliptical excision of skin is made on the posterior aspect of the ear down to perichondrium. The skin is undermined 5 to 10 mm in all directions.

Using #4-0 white silk or braided dacron, with an atraumatic needle, at least four mattress sutures are placed in position to bridge a gap in the cartilage. These are tied when all the sutures are in place (Fig. 11.25c). The degree of tightening of the sutures determines the contour of the anthelix. The skin is closed with interrupted sutures of #5-0 nylon.

This is a simple procedure which will correct a poorly developed anthelix, but other techniques or variations of this technique may be necessary in patients with abnormalities of the conchal cartilage, grossly enlarged ears, or disparity of ear size.

Cutting, Thinning, and Tubing the Cartilage. This technique was described by Converse and associates in 1955 (Fig. 11.26). An elliptical piece of postauricular skin is excised to expose the auricular cartilage posteriorly. The anthelix is outlined with straight needles introduced anteriorly when the ear is positioned into proper alignment (Fig. 11.26a). The needles are tipped with ink and withdrawn. The cartilage is incised along the inked lines provided by this maneuver. It should be noted that the superior incision does not join the lateral incision. Another incision is also made along the lateral border of the conchal cartilage. The auricular cartilage between these incisions is thinned with a wire brush (Fig. 11.26b), then folded back and sutured to the proper width (Fig. 11.26c). This technique can be combined with the excision of conchal cartilage when necessary.

Linear Incisions and Fish-Scaling. Luckett, in 1910, advocated "breaking the spring" of the cartilage with a single linear incision to help form a new anthelix. This procedure is seldom used today for occasionally it produces a sharp crease in the ear rather than the natural-appearing, rounded anthelix desired. This method was modified later by others who preferred multiple partial-thickness incisions parallel to the new anthelix (Fig. 11.27). Those experienced with this technique can produce a normal-appearing anthelix.

Another method for "breaking the spring" of the auricular cartilage, involving multiple gouges in the posterior aspect of the cartilage, was introduced by Holmes in 1966 (Fig. 11.28). This operation is performed by making rows of interdigitating pieces of cartilage with only partial thickness (Fig. 11.28a and b). According to Holmes, this adequately breaks the spring and forms a surface area for fibrosis to occur so that the ear will remain in this position, once the stay sutures are removed.

Surgery of the Lobule. Excessive lobule size may be decreased by a simple wedge incision (Fig. 11.29a). The protruding lobule may be corrected at the time of an otoplasty by a "W" excision of postauricular skin as is shown in Figure 11.29b and c.

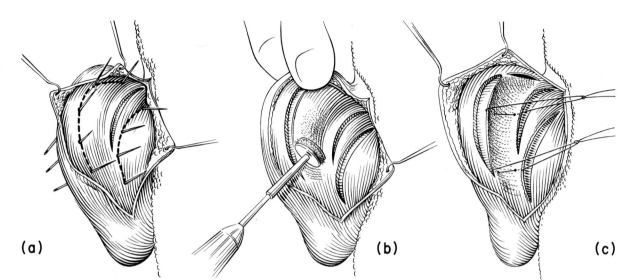

FIGURE 11.26. *Cutting, thinning, and tubing the cartilage (Converse technique).*

a. Straight needles are passed along the borders of the anthelix to mark the cartilaginous incisions. An incision is made through the cartilage between the needles to correspond to the new anthelix.

b. An electrical brush is used to thin the cartilage in the area of the anthelix to "break the spring." If excessive conchal cartilage is present it can be excised at this time.

c. It should be noted that the lateral incision of the anthelix does not continue superiorly. Sutures are in place and are used to form the anthelix into the desired position by the proper amount of tension. The skin is then closed with interrupted nylon sutures.

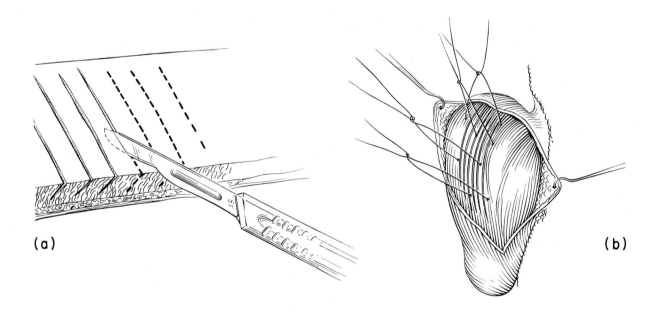

FIGURE 11.27. *Cutting, thinning, and tubing the cartilage (Kazanjian technique).*

a. The partial-thickness incisions are made in the posterior conchal cartilage which remains adherent to the auricular skin anteriorly.

b. Multiple partial-thickness linear incisions are made posteriorly along the anthelix, and sutures are placed. The sutures are tied to determine the auriculocephalic angle.

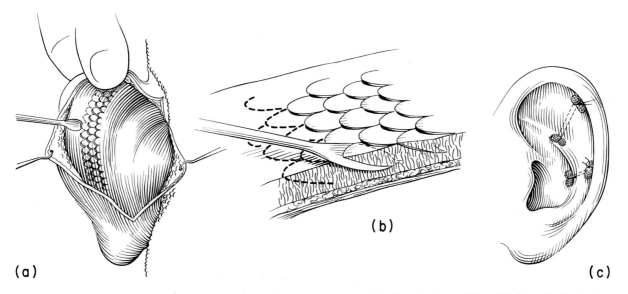

FIGURE 11.28. *"Breaking the spring" of auricular cartilage (Holmes technique).*

 a. A row of interdigitating gouges is fashioned along the posterior aspect of the anthelix after the elliptical excision of posterior auricular skin has been made.

 b. A closer view of the partial-thickness posterior gouges which have a "fish-scale" appearance. The purpose of the gouges is to "break the spring" of the auricular cartilage.

 c. Stay sutures are placed prior to dressing the ear. Mattress sutures are used in the cartilage posteriorly.

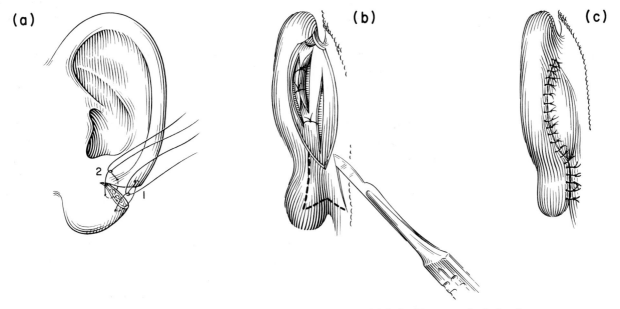

FIGURE 11.29. *Corrective surgery of lobule (Converse technique).*

 a. A wedge incision with sutures in place. In many instances this simple procedure suffices for correction of excessive size of lobule. The initial suture, or "key suture," should be placed at the rim of the ear to obtain exact approximation.

 b and c. Another method for decreasing lobule size is that of making a W-shaped incision, as shown, at the time of otoplasty. The intervening skin is removed and the edges approximated in continuity with the otoplasty incision.

Dressing and Postoperative Care. Dressing and packing of the ear is most important to prevent the formation of hematomas and to hold the ears relatively immobile during the initial healing phase. Cotton, impregnated with either an antibiotic ointment or tincture of benzoin, is packed into the convolutions of the ear and covered carefully with cotton fluff. The postauricular incision is covered with petrolatum gauze and the proper amount of cotton fluff. Cotton pads are then placed over the ears and a mild compression dressing is taped into place to remain for 5 to 7 days. The ear should be examined for hematomas the day following the operation.

Excision of Auricular Lesions

A natural-appearing or cosmetically acceptable external ear following trauma or surgical removal of a tumor is the result of a gentle surgical technique plus a basic knowledge of flaps, grafts, and pedicles.

The most commonly excised tumors of the external ear and auricle are squamous cell and basal cell carcinomas. Excision of these lesions is usually performed with the area locally anesthetized. A small tumor presents no difficulty since it may be excised by a simple V incision which is closed primarily (Fig. 11.30a and b). As the size of the lesion increases it becomes more difficult to approximate the edges of the helix; when closure is difficult two additional small V incisions are most helpful. A 1-cm margin should be obtained around the lesion. The results of a frozen section should be checked before the wound is closed.

In some instances up to one third of the auricle may be excised in this manner without disturbing the contour of the ear.

For larger defects, the surgeon must resort to local flaps and pedicles. For complete or nearly complete loss of the auricle there is no good method of total reconstruction. Numerous procedures have been employed, but none have given consistently good, cosmetically acceptable results in even the most skilled hands. This is a problem that remains sorely in need of a solution.

The surgeon may use one of a variety of flaps, pedicles, or grafts for reconstruction when partial loss of the auricle does not permit primary closure.

Postauricular Flap (Fig. 11.31). This flap, also known as an auriculomastoid flap, can be used in a number of ways. Figure 11.31 depicts a typical application. In this instance the flap is based posteriorly and outlined to fit the defect of the auricle. It is sutured in place with a strip of cartilage graft from the opposite ear, or nasal septum, embedded to conform to the helix. After 3 weeks, the base of the flap is severed and the flap is raised and sutured in place to form the posterior surface of the auricle.

Chondrocutaneous Flap (Fig. 11.32). For a similar lesion, Millard has described an ingenious method which employs a composite flap using cartilage from the ear being operated upon to re-form the rim of the helix. The flap is based on the anterior auricular skin (Fig. 11.32a) and has intervening scar tissue which makes a delay imperative. After a 2-week delay, the flap is raised again, and a piece of cartilage, 0.33 cm in width, is excised and left attached to the skin (Fig. 11.32b). This is fashioned to form a cartilaginous support for the length of the reconstructed helix. The distal skin is sutured into place to form the posterior surface of the auricle (Fig. 11.32c). A split-thickness graft is needed to complete the posterior surface of the auricle and to resurface the donor site.

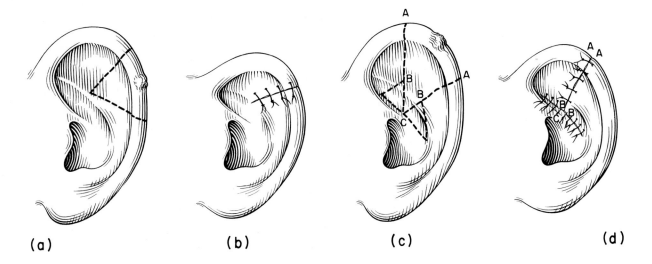

FIGURE 11.30. *Excision of auricular lesion.*

    a. A simple wedge excision of a small lesion.

    b. Direct approximation of the edges is made with interrupted sutures.

    c and d. When the triangular defect caused by the initial wedge incision is too large to permit closure without producing a striking deformity of the auricle, two smaller triangular areas are excised at the apex of the first triangle as indicated in (c). Primary closure is accomplished with interrupted sutures.

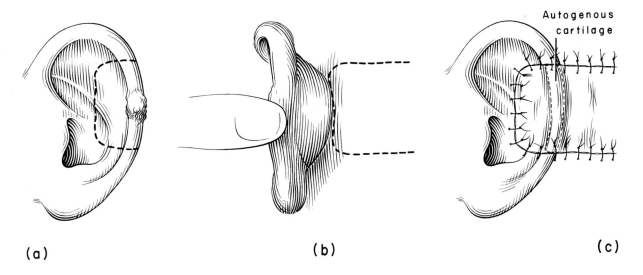

FIGURE 11.31. *Postauricular flap.*

    a. The lesion and surrounding tissue to be excised.

    b. The ear is held forward and a postauricular flap is outlined.

    c. The postauricular flap has been elevated and sutured into the defect. A piece of autogenous cartilage may be embedded to give additional form to the new helix. After 3 weeks the flap is detached from the base and sutured into place to fill the postauricular defect. Split-thickness skin grafts are used to complete the coverage in the postauricular area and donor site.

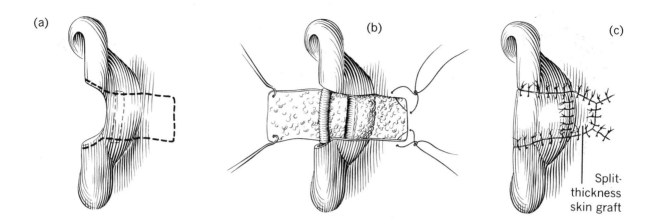

(a)   (b)   (c)

Split-
thickness
skin graft

FIGURE 11.32. *Chondrocutaneous flap (Millard technique).*

a. An anteriorly based ear flap is outlined. The flap is delayed by elevating the postauricular portion and then continuing the incisions along the lateral border to the base of the flap.

b. After 2 weeks, the flap is elevated with a piece of conchal cartilage attached. This cartilage will form the new helix.

c. The flap is sutured into place and a split-thickness skin graft is used to complete the postauricular coverage and to cover the donor site.

Advancement of a Helical Flap for Superior Auricular Defects (Fig. 11.33). This procedure is advantageous for relatively small- to medium-sized superior marginal defects. It has a cosmetic advantage in that duplication of the helix is not attempted. Instead, the remaining helix is advanced superiorly. A composite advancement is fashioned with the incision carried just anterior to the remaining helix and through the sides of the defect (Fig. 11.33a). The flap is based on the postauricular skin which must be freed from the posterior surface of the aural cartilage. It is then advanced and sutured (Fig. 11.33b, c, and d). If the decrease in vertical height is noticeable, the height of the opposite ear may be reduced by the wedge-incision technique.

Scalp Flap for Superior Auricular Defects (Fig. 11.34). If the hairline permits, this procedure is useful for the repair of the superior auricular defects. A local scalp flap is raised superiorly, and autogenous cartilage is embedded (Fig. 11.34a and b). The freshened edges of the auricle are sutured to the flap. After an appropriate delay (usually 3 weeks), the scalp flap is excised and sutured in place to re-form the contour of the ear (Fig. 11.34c). The scalp is closed primarily and a split-thickness skin graft is needed for the posterior surface of the auricle.

Tubed Pedicle Flap (Fig. 11.35). The tubed pedicle flap can be used for subtotal or total loss of the helix. Based posteriorly near the auricle, the flap can be delayed and attached to the remaining auricle to form a helix. This procedure requires multiple steps and often the results are not entirely satisfactory.

Preauricular Flaps (Fig. 11.36). These are superiorly based flaps which are rotated 90 degrees without delay. The donor site is closed primarily. They have proven satisfactory for correction of defects of the anterosuperior area of the auricle.

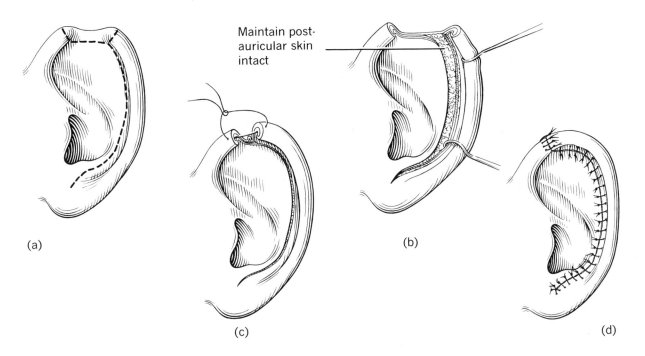

FIGURE 11.33. *Advancement of helical flap.*

a. A defect of the superior portion of the helix is outlined. The incision is carried just anterior to the remaining helix on both sides of the defect.

b. Incisions are made to freshen the edges of the defect and to form an advancement composite flap based inferiorly and posteriorly on the postauricular skin.

c. The chondrocutaneous flap is advanced and a "key suture" is placed.

d. The advancement flap is sewn into place with interrupted sutures.

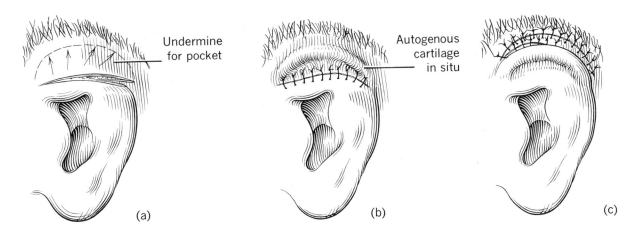

FIGURE 11.34. *Scalp flap.*

a. The incision for the scalp flap and the extent of undermining is shown. Autogenous cartilage is embedded to form the superior helix.

b. The superior margin of the auricle is sutured to the scalp.

c. After a 3-week delay the scalp flap is excised from its base. The scalp is closed primarily or with a split-thickness skin graft, depending on the size of the defect.

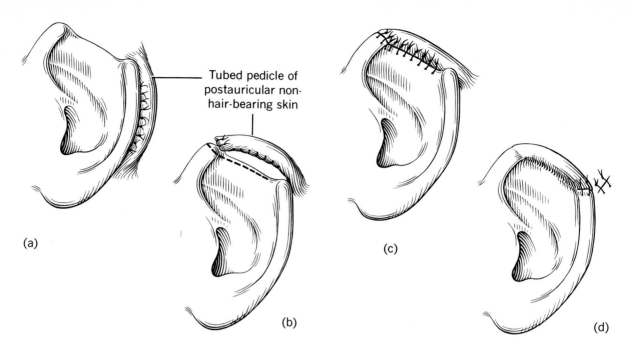

Tubed pedicle of postauricular non-hair-bearing skin

(a)

(b)

(c)

(d)

FIGURE 11.35.   *Tubed pedicle flap.*

a. The helical defect. A bipedicled tube has been raised from the postauricular skin.

b. After 3 weeks the inferior base of the tubed pedicle is cut and is sutured to the superior aspect of the auricle. The posterior base of the pedicle is left intact.

c. Three weeks later the pedicle base is cut and sutured to the auricle to complete the new helix.

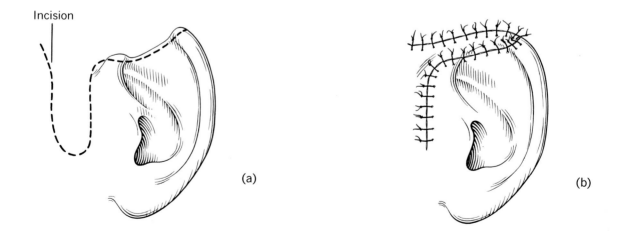

Incision

(a)

(b)

FIGURE 11.36.   *Preauricular flap.*

a. A defect of the anterosuperior portion of the auricle. The flap, which in this instance is based superiorly, is outlined.

b. After freshening the edges of the auricle the flap is sutured into place. The donor site is closed primarily.

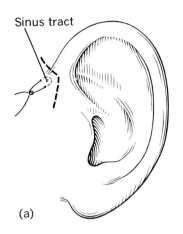 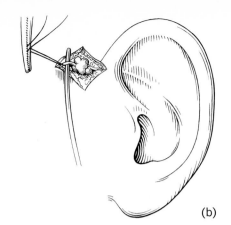 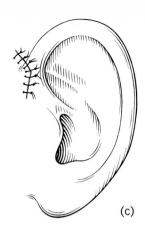

Sinus tract

(a)   (b)   (c)

FIGURE 11.37. *Excision of preauricular cyst.*

　　a. A suture is placed around the sinus tract and a wedge incision is made into subcutaneous tissue.

　　b. The duct, cyst, and ligament are exposed and excised.

　　c. Closure is completed with interrupted sutures.

Special Problems

Excision of Preauricular Cysts (Fig. 11.37). Preauricular cysts are common congenital cystic structures located anterior to the base of the helix. The small, intermittently draining sinus tract can usually be probed without difficulty. These cysts produce very few symptoms until they become infected. Prophylactic excision is indicated.

The external tract is ligated with a silk suture (Fig. 11.37a). A triangular flap is then raised exposing the cystic system (Fig. 11.37b). This conglomerate of cyst, fibrosis, and subcutaneous tissue is removed along with the duct. The triangular flap is then sutured into place (Fig. 11.37c).

Chondritis Following a Burn. The progress of a burned ear should be followed very closely. The usual time for onset of chondritis is 3 to 5 weeks following the accident. Dull pain heralds the onset; usually the pain increases in severity. The ear develops inflammation and edema causing its protrusion from the head. Fluctuance develops and drainage may occur spontaneously.

Dowling attributed a decrease of from 19 to 29% of chondritis of the auricle, occurring in association with all burns of the face, to open-air treatment and the use of Sulfamylon.

The cartilage involved with chondritis should be excised along with the overlying skin. If possible, the underlying skin, upon which a graft may be placed, should be preserved. The incidence of recurrence is high and, when this takes place, additional auricle must be excised. Chondritis of the ear usually is attended with at least some degree of auricular deformity.

The Cauliflower Ear. This is the "boxer's ear" in which scar contraction has occurred following trauma and hematoma formation.

Prevention is, of course, the best treatment. The blood and serum in an acute hematoma of the auricle should be evacuated as soon as feasible. A problem arises in that the hematoma may continue to re-form. To avoid this, a pressure dressing should be applied. One method is to tie through-and-through sutures over moist cotton; this will provide firm pressure and prevent the reaccumulation of serum and blood. Cotton, impregnated with tincture of benzoin, is then tucked into all the spaces of the auricle, and a pressure dressing is applied.

TEMPORAL BONE RESECTION

Block resection of the temporal bone, with or without a radical neck dissection, as pioneered by John S. Lewis, has increased the 5-year survival rate for carcinoma involving the temporal bone. Prior to instigation of this method of therapy the treatment consisted of a radical mastoidectomy followed by radiation therapy, with a resultant 5-year cure rate of less than 10%. The osteonecrosis and injury to the intracranial structures (pons and medulla), following a full course of radiation therapy to the temporal bone, were often devastating.

Temporal bone resection, with or without preoperative radiation therapy, has increased the 5-year survival rate to approximately 30% (Lewis, 1966). The preoperative radiation therapy, however, should *not* exceed 4000r.

Pathology of Carcinoma Involving the Ear

Carcinoma of the external ear and outer ear canal is most frequently of the basal cell variety (in two thirds of cases) and most often is found in the elderly white male. Basal cell carcinoma of the auricle, which is located well away from the external auditory canal, is not a serious disease and can be treated by radiation therapy or local excision as is prescribed for similar lesions in other areas of the head and neck. A lesion within 1 cm of the external auditory canal is a much more serious disease and must be treated by radical surgery. The extensive lymphatics in this region account for the seriousness of this disease (Miller).

Squamous cell carcinoma is the most common type of tumor found in the deep external auditory canal, middle ear, and mastoid. It is more prevalent among females than among males and occasionally is associated with chronic otitis media.

Adenocarcinoma of the temporal bone arising from the parotid, ceruminous glands, or middle ear mucosa, is rather rare. Numerous other malignant tumors have been reported in this area. The most common are rhabdomyosarcoma, malignant melanoma, and spindle-cell sarcoma.

Signs and Symptoms of Carcinoma Involving the Temporal Bone

1. *Pain* can result from secondary external otitis or otitis media, but may be due to invasion of bone by tumor.
2. *Hearing loss* is a common symptom and is due to either obstruction of the external auditory canal by the tumor, the presence of tumor or secondary infection involving the tympanic membrane or middle ear, or the extension of disease into the inner ear. It is thus important to differentiate between a conductive and perceptive hearing loss.
3. *Bleeding* from the external auditory canal can be the first and only symptom of disease. Severe hemorrhage from the external auditory canal is encountered with the rhabdomyosarcoma.
4. *Otorrhea* associated with a long history of chronic otitis media occasionally precedes the onset of carcinoma. Usually, however, the otorrhea is caused by secondary otitis externa or otitis media. A biopsy of the external auditory canal should be performed in those cases of chronic otitis externa which do not respond to the usual conservative measures, especially when granulation tissue is present.

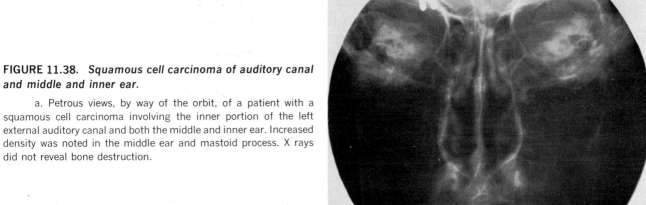

FIGURE 11.38. *Squamous cell carcinoma of auditory canal and middle and inner ear.*

a. Petrous views, by way of the orbit, of a patient with a squamous cell carcinoma involving the inner portion of the left external auditory canal and both the middle and inner ear. Increased density was noted in the middle ear and mastoid process. X rays did not reveal bone destruction.

b. During surgery the petrous bone was found to be extensively involved with the carcinoma, and thus a complete resection of the temporal bone was necessary. The resulting defect was not obliterated with adipose tissue, and the postoperative course was complicated by cerebrospinal fluid leakage and meningitis.

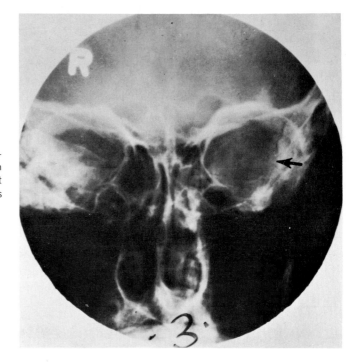

5. *A facial nerve paralysis* may occur when the disease extends to the middle ear and beyond. Rather extensive disease can be expected when facial nerve paralysis complicates a malignant lesion in this region.
6. *Vertigo* is usually indicative of extension of disease to the inner ear, but may be the result of secondary infection.
7. *External swelling* can be present and is due to extension of disease into the parotid gland or the sternocleidomastoid muscle.

Diagnosis of Carcinoma Involving the Temporal Bone

Routine x rays (Fig. 11.38) of the mastoid bone will show evidence of bone destruction in approximately 40% of the cases. Polytomography of the temporal bone has somewhat increased this percentage. It must be kept in mind that the exact extent of disease cannot be determined until the time of operation.

The functions of the facial, auditory, and vestibular nerves should be carefully studied. Any evidence of extension of disease beyond the confines of the temporal bone must be evaluated. The surgeon should search carefully for enlarged cervical lymph nodes.

The diagnostician must be careful not to be fooled by a pathologic report indicating no malignant disease as ascertained from a study of granulation tissue or of a polyp overlying the lesion itself. A repeat biopsy is indicated if there is any suspicion of malignant tumor.

It can be assumed that there is disease in the middle ear if the lesion in the external auditory canal has extended to the region of the tympanic membrane. The tympanic membrane may remain entirely normal when the tumor extends around the annular ligament to the middle ear.

Radiation Therapy of Carcinoma Involving the Temporal Bone

It is the considered opinion of most radiotherapists that any form of radiation therapy to a carcinoma which has invaded the bone is of little value. Most reports in the literature indicate a 5-year survival rate of less than 10% for patients with carcinoma of the temporal bone treated by radiation therapy. The complications of a full course of radiation therapy for temporal bone carcinoma have been mentioned.

Postoperative radiation therapy is indicated for those patients who had had one or more surgical procedures prior to the temporal bone resection. The amount of postoperative supra-voltage radiation should not exceed 4500r.

Preoperative radiation therapy is indicated for patients with more advanced disease in whom the cancer extends to the dura. These patients have severe pain that is difficult to control, even with narcotics. The amount of preoperative supra-voltage radiation should not exceed 4000r.

Indications for Temporal Bone Resection

Positive indications for temporal bone resections are:
1. Disease of recent onset
2. Evidence of slight bone destruction
3. More advanced disease in a patient who has received preoperative radiation therapy

Preoperative Care

At least six units of whole blood should be in readiness prior to this extensive operation. The patient's scalp is shaved completely if the entire auricle is to be removed, otherwise the shaved area can be limited to the preauricular region, the scalp over the squamous portion of the temporal bone, and the region behind the mastoid bone.

Anatomic Considerations

The surgeon must have a thorough knowledge of the vascularity surrounding the temporal bone (Fig. 11.6a). The sigmoid portion of the lateral sinus lies posteromedial to the mastoid bone and extends inferiorly to the jugular bulb at the base of the skull. The superior and inferior petrosal venous sinuses are also important landmarks during this dissection. Medial to the petrosal bone is the cavernous sinus. The carotid artery is located inferior, anterior, and medial in the petrous pyramid and fortunately is less vulnerable to injury during a temporal bone resection than are the other vascular structures.

It is usually necessary to sacrifice the facial nerve when the temporal bone is resected. The condylar process of the mandible and parotid gland are also included in the resection. The cochlea and semicircular canals are transected or resected during the procedure. A radical neck dissection is performed if there is evidence of cervical metastasis or if evidence of carcinoma in the inframastoid lymph nodes is found on frozen section at the time of the operation.

The location of the hypoglossal and vagus nerves at the base of the skull should be kept in mind during the operation in order to avoid their injury.

Surgical Technique

In general there are two variations of the primary incisions, depending upon whether or not there is to be partial preservation of the auricle. The peripheral auricle can be preserved when the tumor lies deep in the external auditory canal. The incisions for this resection are illustrated in Figure 11.39.

The entire auricle must be sacrificed when the tumor is present in the region of the concha. The incisions to be used when the entire auricle is removed along with the temporal bone resection are illustrated in Figure 11.40.

After elevating the flap over the tip of the mastoid bone and the sternocleido-mastoid muscle, a careful search for lymph nodes is conducted. The nodes are removed and sent to the pathology department for frozen-section diagnosis. A radical neck dissection is included with the operation if the lymph nodes show evidence of tumor involvement. Skin flaps are elevated anteriorly over the parotid gland, superiorly over the squamous portion of the temporal bone, posteriorly over and behind the mastoid bone, and inferiorly to expose the sternocleidomastoid and digastric muscles. The incisions for rotation and advancement of the flaps, to be used for repair of the defect when the entire auricle is removed (Fig. 11.40), are not made until the temporal bone resection has been completed. The medial and lateral outline of the bone incisions for temporal bone resection are shown in Figures 11.41 and 11.42.

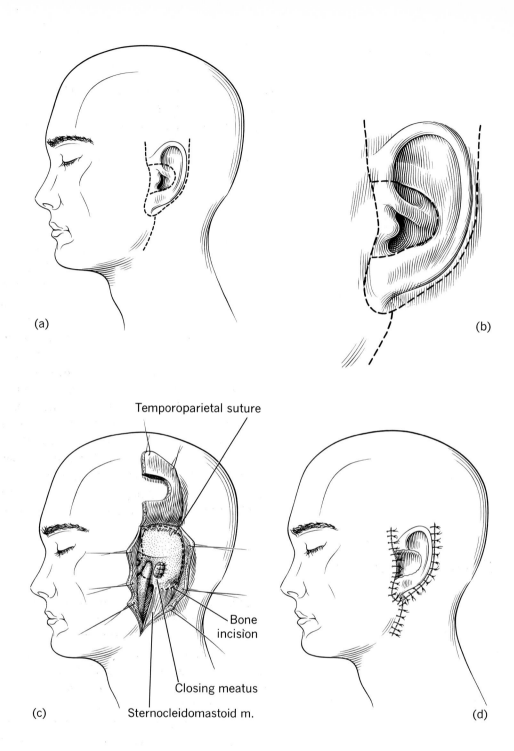

Temporoparietal suture

(a)

(b)

Bone incision

Closing meatus

Sternocleidomastoid m.

(c)

(d)

FIGURE 11.39. *Incisions for temporal bone resection with partial preservation of the auricle.*

a. An incision begins anterior and superior to the root of the helix and extends downward in the preauricular crease to join a second incision which extends downward over the posterior aspect of the mastoid bone. A third incision begins at the junction of the above incisions and follows the anterior border of the sternocleidomastoid muscle.

b. The incision around the external

auditory canal is extended across the root of the helix to the inferior root of the anthelix. It progresses along the anthelix to its inferior extent and is finally directed anteriorly below the tragus, to rejoin the preauricular incision.

c. The portion of the auricle to be preserved is dissected in a plane above the periosteum of the underlying temporal bone and reflected superiorly. The core of the

external auditory meatus is closed with a few interrupted sutures.

d. The skin incisions are approximated following the temporal bone resection. A split-thickness skin graft is sutured anteriorly. The center of the graft is reflected into the cavity and packed in place with antibiotic ointment-impregnated iodoform gauze. It is usually not necessary to suture the skin graft to the remaining skin margin.

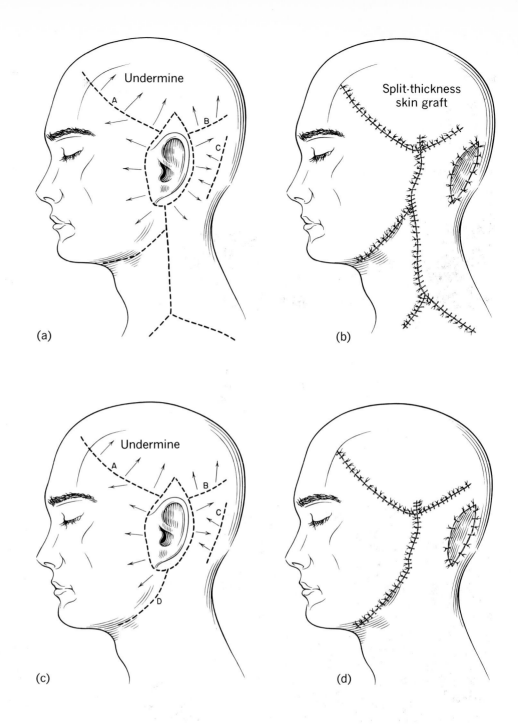

(a)

(b)

(c)

(d)

FIGURE 11.40. *Incisions for temporal bone resection that includes the entire auricle.*

a. The first incision begins directly above the auricle over the squamous portion of the temporal bone. It is extended inferiorly in the preauricular crease. A second incision begins at the same point above the auricle and is extended down over the posterior aspect of the mastoid bone to join the preauricular incision. A third incision begins at the junction of the first two inferiorly and is extended downward over the sternoclei-domastoid muscle. The anterior and inferior skin incisions for radical neck dissection are made according to the surgeon's preference. The incisions for rotation of scalp

flaps are made as shown (A and B). Extensive undermining of flaps is necessary to provide for a primary closure of the defect over the resected temporal bone. It may be necessary to make a relaxing incision (C) in the occipital region in order to close the defect.

b. A primary closure of the defect over the temporal bone has been made. The defect in the occipital region is repaired with a split-thickness skin graft. It is imperative to close the skin over the site of temporal bone resection and to use an adipose autograft to fill the underlying cavity in order to

prevent leakage of spinal fluid.

c. The cervical incision is modified, as is shown, when a radical neck dissection is not included in the procedure. This incision (D) is directed anteriorly over the digastric muscle.

d. The final result of the repair following a temporal bone resection that does not include a radical neck dissection is illustrated. The incision and resultant defect in the occipital region may be necessary in order to prevent tension on the suture line over the site of resection of the temporal bone.

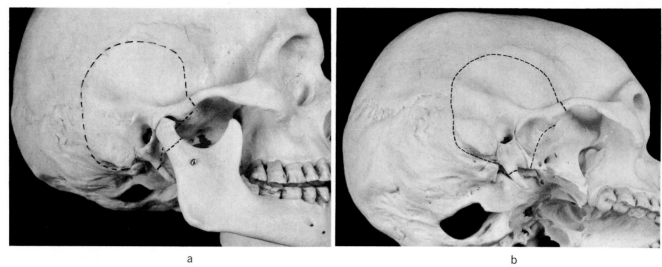

a   b

FIGURE 11.41.   *Temporal bone resection.*

a. A lateral view of the outline of the temporal bone resection, beginning at the temporal line. The dissection continues superiorly, anteriorly, and inferiorly to include a large segment of the squamous portion of the temporal bone. The dissection continues across the root of the zygomatic portion of the temporal bone, the glenoid fossa, and the neck of the condylar process of the mandible.

b. The mandible has been removed to demonstrate the line of dissection, across the styloid process of the glenoid fossa, the base of the temporal bone, and posterior to the mastoid process where the sigmoid portion of the lateral sinus is identified and reflected posteriorly.

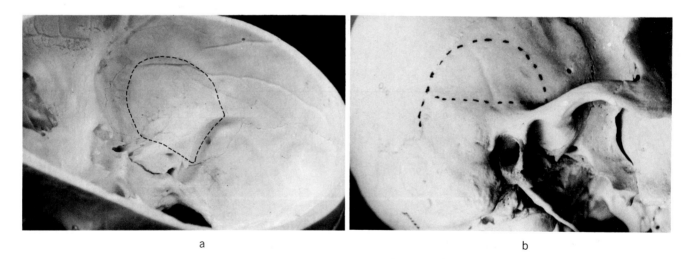

a   b

FIGURE 11.42.   *Temporal bone resection.*

a. An intracranial view of the area of temporal bone to be resected. Beginning superiorly in the squamous portion of the temporal bone and progressing in a clockwise fashion, the incision is continued to the inferior aspect of the squamous portion of the bone to the posterior margin of the mastoid bone. Here the junction of the lateral sinus and sigmoid portion of the lateral sinus are identified. The sigmoid portion of the lateral sinus is dissected free to the jugular foramen. The petrous portion of the temporal bone is transected immediately lateral to the internal auditory meatus. Anteriorly the dissection involves the root of the zygomatic portion of the temporal bone and the glenoid fossa.

b. The interrupted lines indicate the amount of squamous portion of the temporal bone to be resected. The posterior limit is the suture line between the temporal bone and the occipital bone. The anterior limit is the root of the zygomatic portion of the temporal bone. The inferior line follows the temporal line.

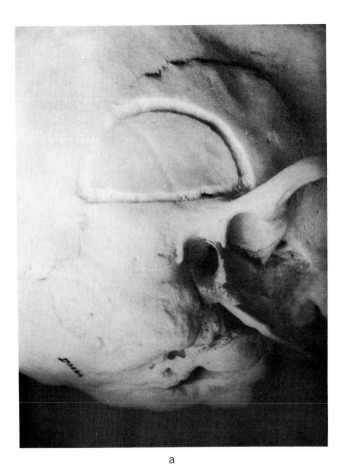
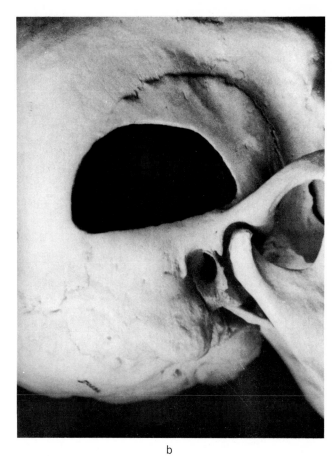

a

b

FIGURE 11.43. *Temporal bone resection.*

a. The squamous portion of the temporal bone, as outlined, can be removed with a rotating cutting bur. A second method is that of removing a small portion of bone superiorly with a bur or a trephine; following this the desired amount of bone is removed with Kerrison forceps.

b. A goodly amount of the squamous portion of the temporal bone has been resected, exposing the temporal lobe dura. A curved, blunt, round-ended elevator is used to separate the dura from the inner table of the bone in order to avoid injury to the dura and the numerous blood vessels on its surface. If destruction in the inferior aspect of the bone has been demonstrated by preoperative x rays, or involvement of either bone or dura with the tumor is encountered during this portion of the operation, the resection is discontinued in this area. Following resection of the temporal bone the involved dura is resected and repaired with temporal muscle fascia.

The squamous portion of the temporal bone is carefully inspected for evidence of bone destruction. The bone incision in this area is made with a rotating cutting bur (Figs. 11.42b and 11.43). This incision begins anteriorly over the root of the zygomatic portion of the temporal bone, and extends superiorly to a point at least 4 cm above the level of the temporal line. The posterior limit of the bone incision, which extends across the squamous bone superiorly, is continued to a vertical line drawn from behind the mastoid bone. The posterior bone incision is made along this vertical line. The squamous bone can be removed, either piecemeal with a rongeur or in one piece by making a bone incision above the temporal line.

It is not uncommon for carcinoma to involve a portion of the dura in the region over the roof of the epitympanum. The area of involvement is excised with a wide margin and repaired with temporal fascia.

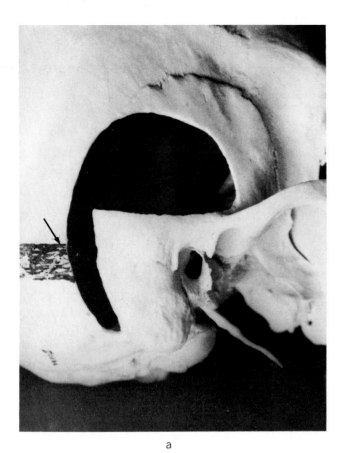

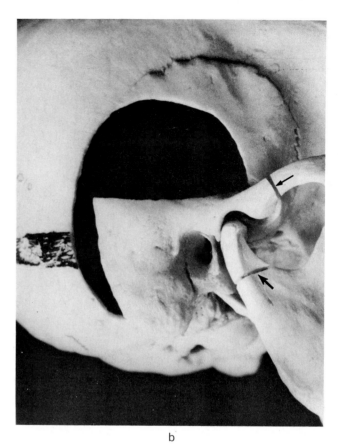

a   b

FIGURE 11.44. *Temporal bone resection.*

a. By elevating the dura in the region of the posterior and inferior aspect of the squamous defect, the beginning of the sigmoid portion of the lateral sinus is identified (arrow). The bone in the posterior aspect of the mastoid process is removed with a bur. As this is accomplished the sigmoid sinus is carefully separated from the bone and reflected posteriorly. This dissection is continued until the jugular bulb is identified.

b. The root of the zygomatic portion of the temporal bone (small arrow) and the neck of the condylar process of the mandible (large arrow) are exposed and transected either with a Gigli or Stryker saw. It is important to elevate the periosteum from the neck of the condylar process carefully and to use extreme care when cutting through this structure in order to avoid the venous plexus anterior and medial to this area.

The attachments of the sternocleidomastoid and digastric muscles to the mastoid bone are severed. The jugular vein, carotid artery, and vagus, hypoglossal, glossopharyngeal, and facial nerves are exposed. A ligature is placed around both the internal carotid artery and the internal jugular vein to be tightened if either vessel is inadvertently opened during the temporal bone resection.

The beginning of the sigmoid portion of the lateral sinus is identified by additional bone removal in the postero-inferior aspect of the defect made by resection of the squamous portion of the temporal bone (Fig. 11.44a). The entire sigmoid portion of the lateral sinus is exposed and dissected posteriorly, away from the temporal bone, so that it will not be injured as the temporal bone is removed.

The head and neck of the condylar process of the mandible are exposed and an incision is made through the neck of the mandible with a Stryker or Gigli

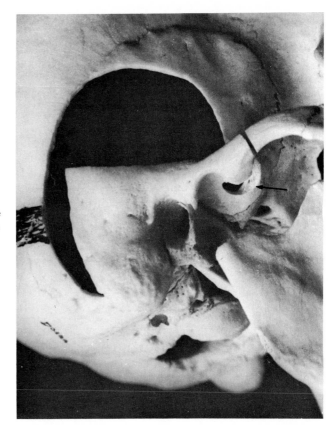

FIGURE 11.45. *Temporal bone resection.*

a. The head and neck of the mandible have been removed. The rather thick bone between the squamosal defect and the glenoid fossa is resected with a bur (arrow), exposing the underlying dura.

b. The bone dissection is continued inferiorly across the glenoid fossa, exposing the eustachian tube (black arrow). There then remains a thin segment of bone between the line of dissection and the carotid canal. The muscles are separated from the base of the styloid process and this base is transected (white arrow).

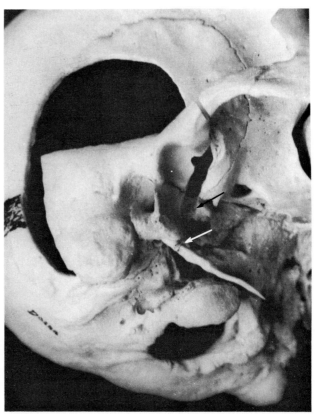

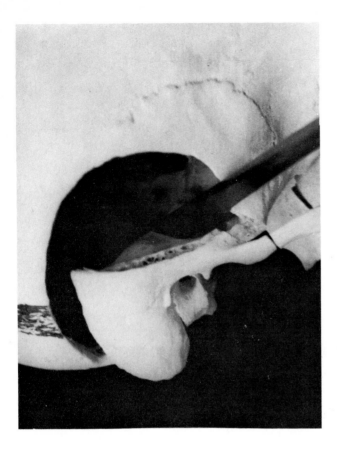

FIGURE 11.46. *Temporal bone resection.*

a. The spinal fluid pressure is reduced by making a small linear incision through the dura in an area which is surrounded by a purse-string suture. A catheter is inserted and approximately 40 cc of spinal fluid are withdrawn. The spinal fluid pressure can also be reduced by the intravenous administration of mannitol solution. It is important that a urinary catheter be in place if this drug is used. A third method for reducing the spinal fluid pressure is by way of an indwelling spinal catheter which is inserted prior to the operation.

The dura is elevated from the anterior and posterior surfaces of the petrous bone. Careful dissection is necessary in the region of the petrosal sinuses. An osteotome is placed on the anterior surface of the petrous pyramid, posterior to the arcuate eminence and anterior to the internal auditory meatus. The petrous pyramid is carefully transected with this osteotome.

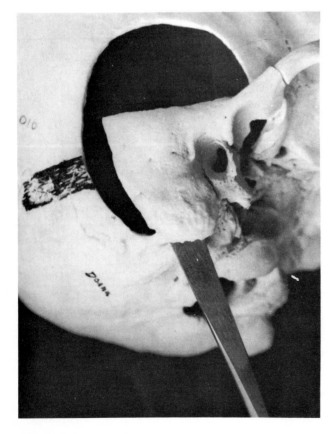

b. The sternocleidomastoid and digastric muscles have been resected from the mastoid bone. The internal jugular vein and carotid artery are carefully identified. A chisel is placed posterior to the digastric crest, and the base of the petrous bone is transected with an osteotome.

saw (Fig. 11.44b). The condylar process above this incision is resected, exposing the glenoid fossa (Fig. 11.45a). Beginning in the antero-inferior aspect of the defect made by resecting the squamous portion of the temporal bone, an incision is made through the root of the zygomatic portion of the temporal bone with a rotating cutting bur, Kerrison forceps, or Stryker saw. The middle meningeal artery, or one of its branches, is usually present in this location and must be carefully avoided. The bone dissection is continued inferiorly across the glenoid fossa exposing the eustachian tube (black arrow). There then remains a thin segment of bone between the line of dissection and the carotid canal.

The parotid gland, along with the facial nerve, is resected at this point. On occasion, when the tumor involves only the outer half of the external auditory canal and the surgeon is certain that there is no extension of disease around the annular ligament into the middle ear, it may be possible to preserve the continuity of the facial nerve. In such a case the facial nerve is clearly exposed at the stylomastoid foramen and a superficial and deep lobe parotidectomy is performed.

The styloid process is identified and transected near its base (Fig. 11.45b). The muscles attached to the base of the styloid process and the inferior surface of the temporal bone are transected at this time. A vertical bone incision is made in the glenoid fossa, exposing the eustachian tube.

The spinal fluid pressure must be reduced prior to dissecting the dura from the anterior and posterior surfaces of the petrous bone. This is accomplished by using either an intravenous sodium mannitol solution or an indwelling spinal catheter, or by making a small linear incision through the dura over the temporal lobe. A purse-string suture is then placed around this incision and the catheter is inserted for drainage of spinal fluid. Approximately 40 cc of spinal fluid are removed. Dissection of the dura in the region of the superior petrosal sinus is rather difficult. A tear in the superior petrosal vein is repaired with silver clips or silk sutures.

The dura of the temporal lobe is retracted medially and superiorly, exposing the petrous bone to the level of the internal auditory meatus. A curved osteotome is placed medial to the arcuate eminence and immediately lateral to the internal auditory meatus on the anterior surface of the petrous pyramid (Fig. 11.46a). An incision is made in a posterior and inferior direction, with extreme care, and only through bone, in order to avoid injury to the internal carotid artery.

The inferior surface of the temporal bone is exposed. A chisel is placed medial to the digastric groove and a bone incision is made in a superior direction (Fig. 11.46b). At this point the temporal bone should be free with the exception of a small area of bony attachment in the region of the glenoid fossa. The attachments are easily severed with a straight osteotome.

As the remaining soft tissue attachments of the temporal bone are incised and the temporal bone is removed (Fig. 11.47), one or more tears may be made in the dura, resulting in spinal fluid leakage. Subcutaneous adipose tissue is obtained from the abdominal wall and used to repair the defects in the dura and also to obliterate the cavity resulting from the temporal bone resection. The catheter is removed from the dura of the temporal bone and a purse-string suture is tied.

At this point a radical neck dissection is carried out if indicated. If available a second team of surgeons should be called in to perform this operation. A radical neck dissection is usually unnecessary with resection of a temporal bone carcinoma for metastasis to the neck occurs in only 16% of uncontrolled cases. Almost all patients die of local disease with possible extension into the brain.

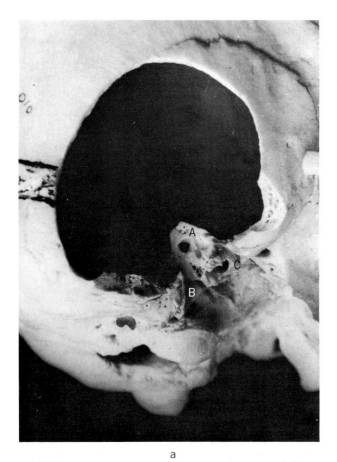

a

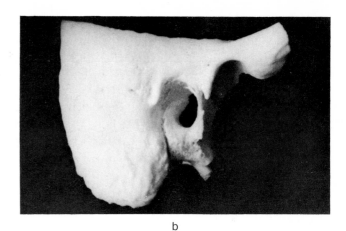

b

FIGURE 11.47.   *Temporal bone resection.*

a. The remaining bony attachments of the temporal bone are easily severed, and the temporal bone is removed following section of the remaining soft tissue attachments. The tip of the petrous bone remains in place. The internal auditory meatus (A), jugular foramen (B), and carotid canal (C) are in view.

b. A photograph of the resected temporal bone. Note the root of the zygomatic portion of the temporal bone, the glenoid fossa, the base of the squamous portion of the temporal bone, the mastoid bone, and the base of the styloid process.

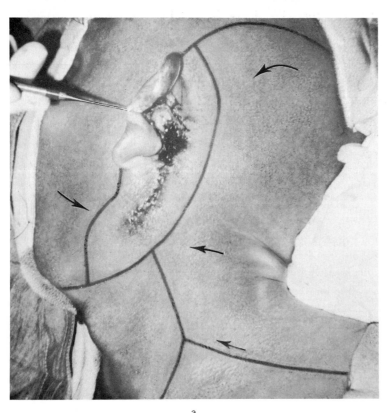

a

FIGURE 11.48.   *Temporal bone resection.*

a. A 36-year-old male with a history of a "black mole" with satellite lesions behind the left auricle of 2 months' duration. Ten days before this photograph was taken an attempt was made to excise the lesion. The operation was discontinued when a large metastatic node was encountered on, and invading, the mastoid bone (note the incision with sutures in place). The incisions to accomplish resection of the mastoid bone, radical neck dissection, and repair are shown. The arrows indicate the direction for rotation and advancement of the skin flaps. A temporal flap was not necessary in this case.

b. A photograph showing the repair following resection of the auricle, skin surrounding the recent operation, parotid gland, and mastoid bone, and a radical neck dissection. The facial nerve was grafted using the spinal accessory nerve and its branches to the trapezius muscle. The external auditory canal was reconstituted by packing the flap margins (arrow) into the remaining portion of the bony ear canal.

c. A photograph of the patient 2 months following the operation. The face lift accomplished as the surgical defect was repaired minimizes the left facial paralysis.

d. Facial nerve function returned after 10 months. The patient remains without recurrent disease 6 years following the operation.

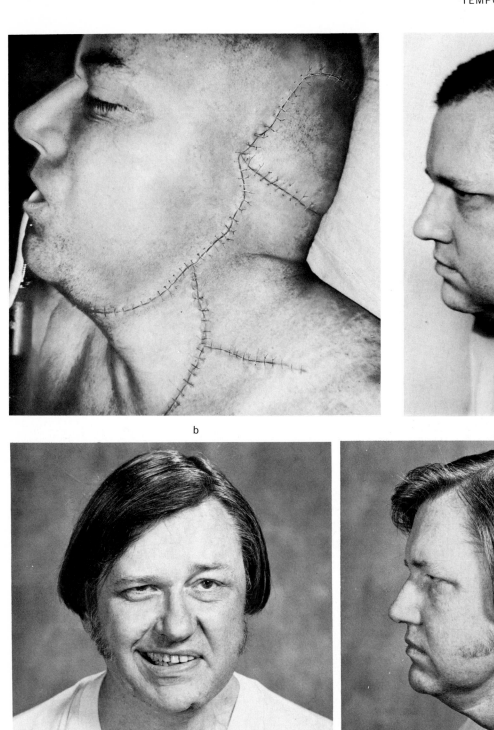

b

c

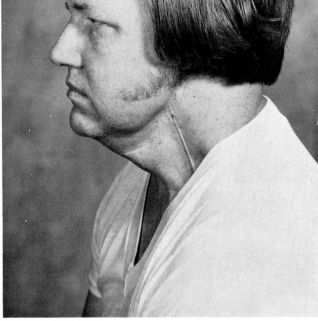

d

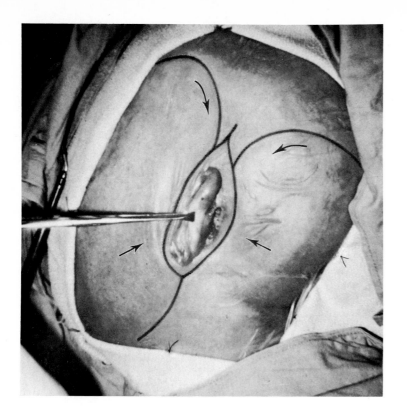

FIGURE 11.49. *Temporal bone resection.*

a. Photograph showing irreversible necrosis of the auricular cartilages involving the temporal bone in a 67-year-old woman who, 4 years previously, had x-ray therapy (6000r) for carcinoma of the external auditory canal and middle ear. At the time this picture was taken, no evidence of carcinoma could be found, but the patient had constant discharge and severe pain due to secondary infection. The auricle, surrounding necrotic skin, and temporal bone were resected. The defect was obliterated with subcutaneous abdominal adipose tissue.

Flaps were elevated and advanced as indicated by the arrows to accomplish a primary closure. All incisions healed without complication.

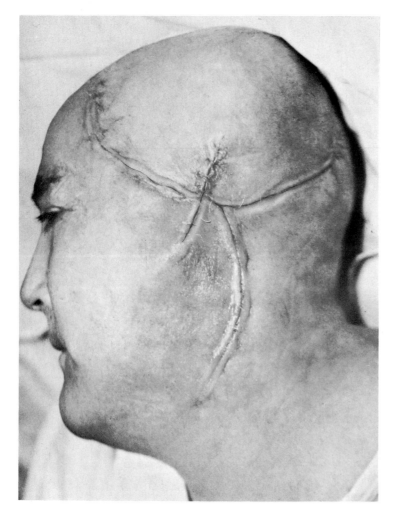

b. The appearance of the repair 10 days following the operation. The incisions were well healed. The patient was discharged from the hospital at this time, wearing a wig to cover the defect and missing auricle.

The hypoglossal nerve is identified, dissected free, and transected peripherally, so that it can be re-directed and sutured to the peripheral end of the transected facial nerve. The results of hypoglossal facial anastomosis are quite gratifying, for a good facial tone is obtained and there is motion of the face when the patient attempts to move the tongue or swallow.

Postoperative Management

In the past, cerebral fluid leakage has been a serious complication with the additional hazards of meningitis and brain abscess. The incidence of these complications has been markedly reduced with the use of adipose autografts.

If postoperative hemorrhage occurs, the site of bleeding may be a lateral sinus or the superior petrosal sinus. Bleeding is easily detected for it will either saturate the dressing or cause swelling, as the blood infiltrates the subcutaneous spaces.

Infection is a likely complication because of the length of time required for the operation and the existing secondary infection superimposed on the carcinoma. It is wise to place the patient on intravenous antibiotic therapy to cover both gram-positive and gram-negative organisms for a period of at least 5 days following the operation.

A facial nerve paralysis is managed as has been mentioned (p. 518).

Varying degrees of vertigo will persist for 3 to 6 weeks postoperatively unless the labyrinth was functionless prior to surgery. A careful explanation of the cause of this vertigo, along with antivertiginous medication, will be beneficial.

For a patient in whom the tumor was not completely resected, postoperative radiation therapy is instituted as soon as wound healing is complete. The use of cryosurgery for treatment of residual or recurrent disease may be of value.

REFERENCES

Busis, S. N.: Neuro-otologic Tests and Examination. Arch. Otolaryng. 89:1–10 (Jan.) 1969.

Coleman, C. C., Jr.: Removal of the Temporal Bone for Cancer. Amer. J. Surg. 112:4:583–590 (Oct.) 1966.

Conley, J. J.: Tumors of the Infratemporal Fossa. Arch. Otolaryng. 79:498–504 (May) 1964.

Conley, J. J., Pack, G. T., and Trinidad, S. S.: Surgical Technique of Removal of Infratemporal Meningioma. Laryngoscope 66:5:540–549 (May) 1956.

Converse, J. M., Nigro, A., Wilson, F., and Johnson, N.: A Technique for Surgical Correction of Lop Ears. Plast. Reconstr. Surg. 15:411–418 (May) 1955.

Dowling, J. A., Boley, F. D., and Moncrief, J. H.: Chondritis of the Burned Ear. Plast. Reconstr. Surg. 42:2:115, 1968.

Hitselberger, W. E., and House, W. F.: Acoustic Tumor Surgery. Arch. Otolaryng. 84:255–265 (Sept.) 1966.

Hitselberger, W. E., and House, W. F.: Surgical Approaches to Acoustic Tumors. Arch. Otolaryng. 84:286–291 (Sept.) 1966.

Holmes, E. M.: Otoplasty. Arch. Otolaryng. 83:156–159 (Feb.) 1966.

House, W. F.: Surgical Exposure of the Internal Auditory Canal and Its Contents through the Middle Cranial Fossa. Laryngoscope 11:1363–85 (Nov.) 1961.

House, W. F.: Surgery of the Petrous Portion of the VIIth Nerve. Ann. Otol. 3:802 (Sept.) 1963.

House, W. F.: Middle Cranial Fossa Approach to the Petrous Pyramid. Arch. Otolaryng. 78:460–469 (Oct.) 1963.

House, W. F. (Ed.): Transtemporal Bone Microsurgical Removal of Acoustic Neuromas. A monograph in Arch. Otolaryng. 80:6:601–757 (Dec.) 1964.

House, H. P., and House, W. F.: Historical Review and Problem of Acoustic Neuroma. Arch. Otolaryng. 80:6:601–604 (Dec.) 1964.

Johnson, E. W., and House, W. F.: Auditory Findings in 53 Cases of Acoustic Neuromas. Arch. Otolaryng. 80:6:667–677 (Dec.) 1964.

Lewis, J. S., and Page, R.: Radical Surgery for Malignant Tumors of the Ear. Arch. Otolaryng. 83:114–119 (Feb.) 1966.

Lewis, J. S., and Parsons, H.: Surgery for Advanced Ear Cancer. Ann. Otol. 67:2:364–372 (June) 1958.

Luckett, W. H.: A New Operation for Prominent Ears Based on the Anatomy of the Deformity. Surg. Gynec. Obstet. 10:635, 1910.

Millard, D. R.: The Chondrocutaneous Flap in Partial Auricular Repair. Plast. Reconstr. Surg. 37:6:523, 1966.

Miller, D.: Cancer of the External Auditory Meatus. Laryngoscope 65:6:448–461 (June) 1955.

Montgomery, W. W.: The Fate of Adipose Implants in a Bony Cavity. Laryngoscope 74:6:816–827 (June) 1964.

Montgomery, W. W.: Translabyrinthine Resection of the Small Acoustic Neuroma. Arch. Otolaryng. 89:319–326 (Feb.) 1969.

Montgomery, W. W., Weis, A. D., and Ojemann, R. G.: Suboccipital Translabyrinthine Approach to Acoustic Neuroma. Arch. Otolaryng. 83:566–569 (June) 1966.

Montgomery, W. W.: Surgery for Acoustic Neurinoma. Ann. Otol. Rhinol. Laryngol. 82:428–441, (July–Aug.) 1973.

Mullan, J. F.: Intracranial Removal of Acoustic Tumors. Arch. Otolaryng. 83:591 (June) 1966.

Mustarde, J. C.: The Correction of Prominent Ears Using Simple Mattress Sutures. Brit. J. Plast. Surg. 16:170, 1963.

Owens, E.: The Sisi Test and VIIIth Nerve Versus Cochlear Involvement. J. Speech Hearing Dis. 30:252–262 (Aug.) 1965.

Parker, S. W., and Davis, K. R.: Limitations of Computed Tomography in the Investigation of Acoustic Neurinomas. Ann. Otol. Rhinol. Laryngol. 86(4):436 (July–Aug.) 1977.

Parsons, H., and Lewis, J. S.: Subtotal Resection of the Temporal Bone for Cancer of the Ear. Cancer 7:5:995–1001 (Sept.) 1954.

Pulec, J. L.: Comments on Translabyrinthine Approach to Acoustic Neuromas. Arch. Otolaryng. 83:592–94 (June) 1966.

Pulec, J. L., and House, W. F.: Trigeminal Nerve Testing in Acoustic Tumors. Arch. Otolaryng. 80:6:681–684 (Dec.) 1964.

Pulec, J. L., and House W. F.: Facial Nerve Involvement and Testing in Acoustic Neuromas. Arch. Otolaryng. 80:6:685–692 (Dec.) 1964.

Pulec, J. L., House, W. F., and Hughes, R. L.: Vestibular Involvement and Testing in Acoustic Neuromas. Arch. Otolaryng. 80:6:677–681 (Dec.) 1964.

Sachs, E., Jr.: Translabyrinthine Microsurgery for Acoustic Neuromas. J. Neurosurg. 22:399–401 (Apr.) 1965.

Shambaugh, G. E., Jr.: Team Approach to Early Diagnosis and Removal of Acoustic Neuromas. Arch. Otolaryng. 83:570–573 (June) 1966.

Silverstein, H., and Schuknecht, H. F.: Biochemical Studies of Inner Ear Fluid in Man. Arch. Otolaryng. 84:395–402 (Oct.) 1966.

Temporal Bone Bank: The Technique for Acquiring and Preparing the Human Temporal Bone for the Study of Middle Ear Pathology. Trans. Amer. Acad Ophthal. Otolaryng. 65:784–788 (Sept.-Oct.) 1961.

Walsh, L.: The Surgery of Acoustic Neuromas. Proc. Roy. Soc. Med. 58:1073–76, 1965.

Index

Numerals in *italic* refer to illustration